VOLUME II

THIRD EDITION

CLINICAL UROGRAPHY

An Atlas and Textbook of Roentgenologic Diagnosis

JOHN L. EMMETT, M.D., M.S. (Urology)

Emeritus Consultant, Section of Urology, Mayo Clinic;
Emeritus Professor of Urology, Mayo Graduate School of
Medicine (University of Minnesota); Rochester, Minnesota.

DAVID M. WITTEN, M.D., M.S. (Radiology)

Professor and Chairman, Department of Diagnostic Radiology,
University of Alabama Medical School, Birmingham, Alabama;
Formerly Consultant, Section of Diagnostic Roentgenology,
Mayo Clinic; Assistant Professor of Radiology, Mayo Graduate
School of Medicine (University of Minnesota); Rochester, Minnesota.

W. B. SAUNDERS COMPANY

Philadelphia • London • Toronto

W. B. Saunders Company: West Washington Square
                          Philadelphia, Pa.

                          12 Dyott Street
                          London, WC1A   1DB

                          833 Oxford Street
                          Toronto 18, Ontario

Vol. II   SBN 0-7216-3378-1

CLINICAL UROGRAPHY

Print No.   9   8   7   6   5   4

CONTENTS

CHAPTER 6

Calculous Disease of the Genitourinary Tract

The urographic diagnostic problems associated with urinary calculi can be classified in four categories: (1) the identification of calcific shadows which appear in the plain film; (2) localization of those calcific shadows which prove to be stones in the urinary tract; (3) the demonstration of nonopaque urinary calculi which are not apparent in the plain film; and (4) appraisal of pathologic and physiologic changes in the urinary tract produced by calculi.

IMPORTANCE OF PRELIMINARY PLAIN FILM (KUB)

In Chapter 1 (see Figs. 1-1 and 1-2) and Chapter 3 (see Figs. 3-5 through 3-8) the importance of a preliminary plain film before urograms are made was discussed at length. As was stated in those chapters, nowhere is a plain film more important than in the diagnosis of urinary calculi. The reason for this is apparent. Urographic medium may completely obscure calculi so that they would not be suspected if no preliminary plain film were available. Likewise, localized collections of urographic medium in a ureter bent back on itself or in a calyx projected in the anteroposterior plane might suggest a calculus when none was present. *It is axiomatic that one should never attempt the interpretation of urograms if no preliminary plain film is available.*

Radiographic Characteristics of Urinary Calculi

Most urinary calculi are sufficiently opaque to roentgen rays to cast a shadow in the plain film. Stones vary greatly in density (or opacity). All stones have some degree of opacity to roentgen rays, but when the density of the stones is no greater than the surrounding soft tissues, they will not cast shadows on the film.

The roentgenographic density of a stone varies according to the atomic weight of the salt of which it is composed (Arcelin). The greater the atomic weight, the greater the density of the stone. *Stones which are regarded as opaque to roentgen rays* are (in decreasing order of density) calcium oxalate, calcium carbonate, and the phosphates (Lagergren and Öhrling; Winsbury-

White). Cystine stones vary considerably in density. *Stones which are considered to be of poor density* (or nonopaque) are composed of uric acid and the urates (ammonium, sodium, magnesium, and potassium), xanthine (Prien and Frondel), and "matrix" concretions. "Pure" stones, those containing only one chemical substance, are rare. Most stones are mixtures of the various chemical substances so that all degrees of density and opacity are encountered.

Boyce and co-workers have stated that urinary concretions consist of an aggregation of crystalline components within an organic matrix. Eleven distinct crystalline components have been identified by x-ray diffraction patterns (Lagergren). Approximately 95% of all renal and ureteral calculi are composed of (in decreasing order of radiopacity) calcium phosphate (hydroxyapatite), calcium oxalate, and magnesium ammonium phosphate hexahydrate. Uric acid and urates account for about 4% and cystine for about 1%.

The roentgen appearance of calculi may suggest their composition. For instance, **calcium phosphate calculi** usually have smooth contours and are of uniform maximum density (Fig. 6–1). **Calcium oxalate calculi** are also very radiopaque and are difficult to distinguish from calcium phosphate (see Figs 6–100 through 6–104). On the other hand, **magnesium ammonium phosphate hexahydrate calculi** are of considerably less density (Fig. 6–2); they are the type of calculi often seen in patients with persistent urinary infection. **Laminated calculi** result from the deposition of alternate layers of dense radiopaque material (such as calcium phosphate or calcium oxalate) and material of relatively low radiopacity such as magnesium ammonium phosphate hexahydrate or urates (Fig. 6–3). Calcium oxalate is present in more than half of all urinary calculi. A "pure" calcium oxalate calculus is rarely encountered.

Cystine calculi have been thought of as essentially nonopaque but in reality they are moderately opaque and present a "frosted" or "ground-glass" appearance (Fig. 6–4). These calculi are thought to result from a hereditary defect in renal tubular transport and have responded to d-penicillamine therapy (Crawhall, Scowen, and Watts).

The only **completely radiolucent calculi are pure uric acid or urates** (ammonium, sodium, magnesium, or potassium) and matrix concretions. Such calculi can be diagnosed radiologically only as negative filling defects in the urograms. In this case, differential diagnosis must include blood clots, papillomas, and malignant tumors. Uric acid and pure urate stones may be seen in patients with gout and also in patients with leukemia. It should not be forgotten, however, that radiopaque calcigerous calculi are encountered in approximately 20% of gouty patients who form calculi. Large uric acid or pure urate calculi are commonly found in the bladder of males with urinary obstruction from an enlarged prostate gland.

Matrix concretions are composed largely of a mucoprotein matrix laminated with sparsely distributed crystals of magnesium ammonium phosphate and basic calcium phosphate as dioxyapatite (Boyce). The calcific material is in such low concentration, however, that it casts no shadow in the plain film (Fig. 6–5A). Grossly the specimen has a "waxy" surface and is yellow (Fig. 6–5B).

A peculiar, poorly understood type of small calculi presents in such conditions as nephrocalcinosis, sponge kidney, and calyceal diverticula or cysts filled with "milk of calcium stone." Boyce has grouped these under the heading **seed calculi**. He has described them as perfect spherules usually composed of calcium phosphate as hydroxyapatite in an organic matrix which vary in size from microscopic to 1 mm in diameter. They may be formed in the renal tubular cells, peritubular interstitium, or even the glomerulus. If they enter larger drainage ducts, they frequently acquire additional layers of calcium oxalate and become larger as may be the case in nephrocalcinosis (both with and without associated sponge kidney).* If excreted into a relatively closed calyceal "diverticulum" or calyceal "cyst," they may remain small and discrete and are spoken of as "milk of calcium" stone (see discussion below).

The etiology of urinary calculi is poorly understood and a discussion of it is not indicated in a book of this kind. It should be mentioned in passing, however, that some "associated" diseases appear to predispose to the formation of renal calculi. Among these may be mentioned multiple myeloma, sarcoidosis (see discussion later in this chapter), Paget's disease, postmenopausal and senile osteoporosis, osteolytic metastasis (especially from breast carcinoma), leukemia, and squamous cell epithelioma of the renal pelvis (see discussion in Chapter 10, pages 1131–1132 and 1154).

CONFUSING EXTRAURINARY CALCIFIC SHADOWS

The problem of extraurinary shadows was discussed in detail in Chapter 3 (see Figs. 3–14 through 3–114). For emphasis, a few of the commonly confusing extraurinary shadows will be mentioned again. *Calcified costal cartilages* are a common source of confusion, since they may appear in such fragmentary outline as to suggest renal stone (Fig. 6–6A and B; see also Fig. 3–14). *Calcified mesenteric lymph nodes* must always be kept in mind. Their more or less characteristic appearance, plus the fact that they change position in relation to each other, as well as to the bony pelvis, makes their recognition quite easy (Fig. 6–7A and B;

*See also discussion of primary renal oxaluria later in this chapter (page 675).

see also Figs. 3–57 through 3–60). Increased density of the tips of the transverse processes of the lumbar vertebrae may suggest ureteral stone if not closely scrutinized (Fig. 6–8). *Fragmentary calcification of the iliac vessels* just below the sacro-iliac joints is commonly mistaken for ureteral calculi. Although the physician experienced in urographic interpretation often is able to identify these shadows in the plain film, urographic methods frequently must be used for their identification (Fig. 6–9; see also Fig. 3–24). *Phleboliths* are not difficult to recognize in most cases because of their smooth outline, dense periphery, and less dense centers. However, the fact that they are nearly always located in the areas of the lower portions of the ureters may make identification with a lead catheter or a urogram necessary (Fig. 6–10A and B; see also Fig. 3–21). Laminated and faceted shadows over the right renal area should always make one suspect gallstones (Fig. 6–11A and B; see also Figs. 3–39 through 3–42). Laminated renal stones, however, do occur (see Fig. 3–45).

Because they tend to produce urinary stasis of some degree, urinary calculi furnish an ideal situation for the use of excretory urography. The stasis prevents too rapid excretion of medium so that delineation of the urinary tract may be better than in normal patients who have no obstruction. In some cases, however, it is necessary to resort to retrograde pyelography for adequate diagnosis.

Small calculi may be exceedingly difficult to visualize, either in the kidneys or in the ureters. It has been the not uncommon experience of every urologist to have a patient spontaneously pass a small stone after a most exhaustive urologic examination had failed to disclose its presence. The reason for this diagnostic difficulty is not only the small size of the stone but other factors such as the degree of density, overlying fluid or gas in the intestine, or adjacent bony structures.

(Text continued on page 615.)

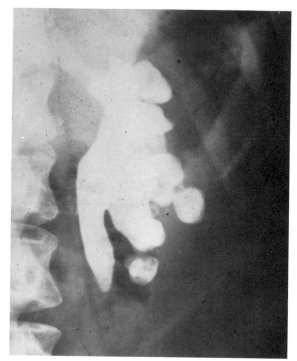

Figure 6–1. *Plain film.* Branched calculus composed of calcium phosphate. Note uniform dense radiopacity. (From Boyce, W. H.)

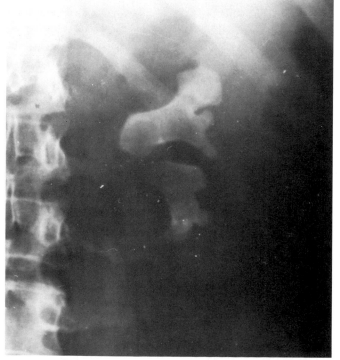

Figure 6–2. *Plain film.* Branched calculus composed of magnesium ammonium phosphate hexahydrate. Note relative radiolucency as compared with calcium phosphate stone (Fig. 6–1). Fine laminations are composed of calcium phosphate as hydroxyapatite. (From Boyce, W. H.)

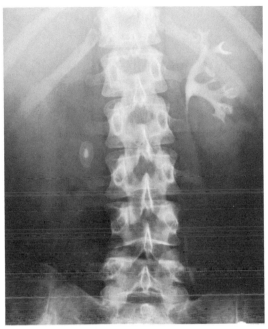

Figure 6–3. *Excretory urogram, 15-minute film.* Laminated stone with very dense center (probably calcium oxalate). Stone situated at right ureteropelvic junction. No function seen. Left kidney normal.

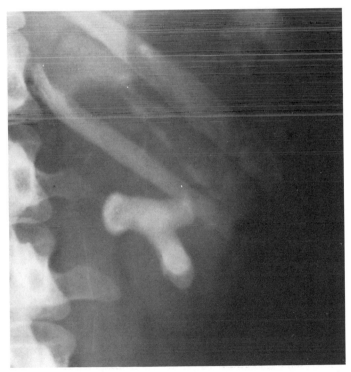

Figure 6–4. *Plain film.* Cystine calculus. Typical "ground-glass" appearance with uniform radiopacity and absence of laminations. (From Boyce, W. H.)

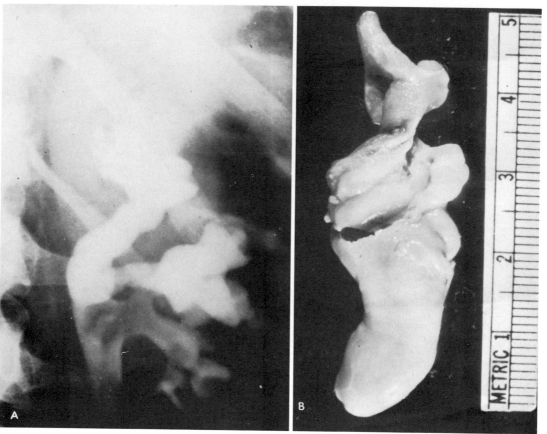

Figure 6–5. A, *Retrograde pyelogram.* Filling defect in pelvis and lower calyx from radiolucent matrix-type "stone" composed largely of mucoprotein. B, Surgical specimen. Has a "waxy" surface and yellow color. (From Boyce, W. H.)

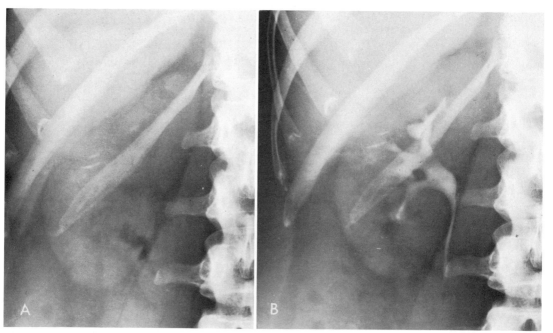

Figure 6–6. A, *Plain film.* Shadows over renal area caused by calcified costal cartilages. Could be mistaken for renal calculi. B, *Excretory urogram.* Calcific shadows excluded.

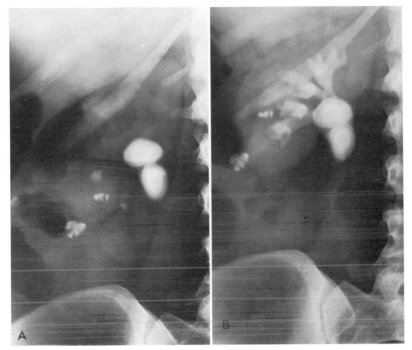

Figure 6–7.   Calcified mesenteric lymph nodes and renal calculi. **A,** *Plain film.* Multiple shadows over right renal area suggest calcified mesenteric lymph nodes and renal calculi. Identification with urogram will be necessary. **B,** *Excretory urogram.* Large shadows are two stones in right renal pelvis. Remainder of shadows are calcified mesenteric lymph nodes. Note how shadows of calcified lymph nodes change position in relation to each other, as well as to renal calculi.

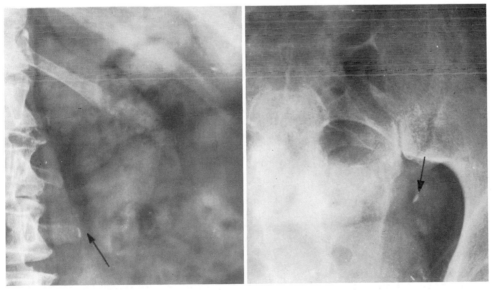

Fig. 6–8   Fig. 6–9

Figure 6–8.   *Plain film.* Increased density of left transverse process of third lumbar vertebra, which could be mistaken for ureteral calculus.

Figure 6–9.   *Plain film.* Fragmentary calcification of iliac vessel below left sacro-iliac joint, which is commonly confused with ureteral calculus.

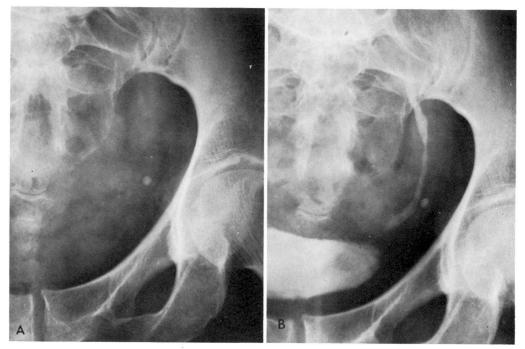

Figure 6–10.   A, *Plain film.* **Phlebolith could be confused with ureteral stone.** Shadow opposite left ischial spine, circular in outline, with dense periphery and less dense center, suggests phlebolith. **B,** *Excretory urogram.* Left ureter is outlined and shadow is excluded and demonstrated to be phlebolith.

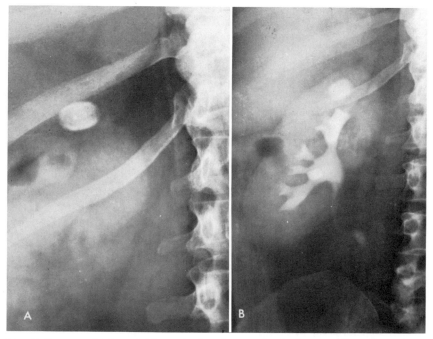

Figure 6–11.   **Gallstone which could be mistaken for renal calculus.** **A,** *Plain film.* Laminated shadow overlying upper border of right kidney. **B,** *Excretory urogram.* Shadow excluded; it is definitely produced by gallstone.

RENAL CALCULI

Opaque Calcific Shadows

METHODS OF IDENTIFICATION AND LOCALIZATION

One suspects a urinary calculus in the plain film when a calcific shadow overlies the areas where the kidneys, ureters, bladder, and prostate gland are normally situated. Shadows in other areas, however, cannot be entirely identified in this manner because of possible mobility of the kidneys and ureters, not to mention other factors such as the possibility of anomalous renal position, large hydronephrosis, and distended urinary bladder or diverticula. Factors other than position, therefore, should be relied on for identification of urinary calculi. Data obtained by use of the lead catheter and by means of urography also may be necessary.

Shape or Contour of Shadow

The shape or contour of a shadow is of great diagnostic importance. Often a calculus assumes the *shape of a calyx* or may even form a *cast of the pelvis and calyces*. In the latter case it is spoken of as a *branched* or *staghorn calculus* (Figs. 6–12, 6–13, and 6–14).

Use of Opaque Ureteral Catheter and Additional Plain Films

Although identification of shadows in the plain film when an opaque catheter is in place may be feasible, it is not so accurate a procedure as urography. However, if one can introduce an opaque catheter so that in the plain film the catheter or its tip is adjacent to the shadow and maintains its position in oblique and lateral views, one can assume with reasonable assurance that the shadow in question is a urinary calculus. Parenthetically, it should be stated that opaque catheters are of more value in the identification of ureteral than renal calculi (Figs. 6–15A and B and 6–16).

Urograms

Urography is by far the most useful method for identification and localization of urinary calculi. Both the excretory and retrograde methods are useful, one complementing the other. The problem of which to use has been discussed in detail in Chapter 1. An excretory urogram is the procedure to employ first in nearly all cases. If visualization is sufficient for identification, then one obviates the danger of introducing contrast medium above an obstructing stone by retrograde means, which always carries some risk of febrile reaction and pain.

The object of the urogram, of course, is to show that the shadow in question is within some portion of the pelviocalyceal system. Often this is possible by simply making an anteroposterior urogram. If the shadow and the opaque medium coincide and the stone produces an increase or decrease in density of the contrast medium or a "negative" shadow, or its shape coincides with the contour of some part of the pelviocalyceal system, one may be reasonably sure of its identification. If, however, the positions of the contrast medium and of the stone coincide, but the medium is so dense that it obscures the shadow completely or the shape of the stone is not of diagnostic value, or both, one could assume that the shadow in question could be outside the kidney but lying in such a position that it coincides with the pelviocalyceal system in the anteroposterior view. In such a case *oblique* or *lateral* views or both are necessary for diagnosis. Films made with patient erect may help "throw out" shadows which lie over the kidney or ureter in the routine film made with patient supine. If the shadow cannot be "thrown out" in these urograms, it is usually reasonably safe to assume that the shadow is a renal calculus (Figs. 6–17 through 6–27). If still in doubt one may resort either to pyelograms made with medium of less density or to air pyelograms (Figs. 6–28, 6–29, and 6–30).

(Text continued on page 627.)

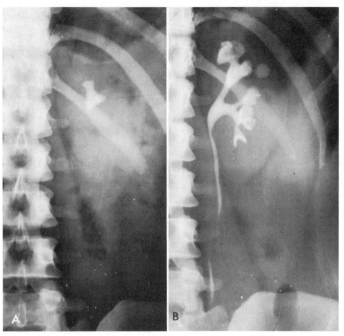

Figure 6–12.   A, *Plain film.* **Stone forming cast of upper calyx.** Calcific shadow overlying upper pole of left kidney, assuming contour of renal calyx. **B,** *Excretory urogram.* Stone is seen forming cast of portion of upper calyx, with resulting calycectasis. Small calyceal diverticulum adjacent to lateral branch of upper calyx.

Fig. 6–13

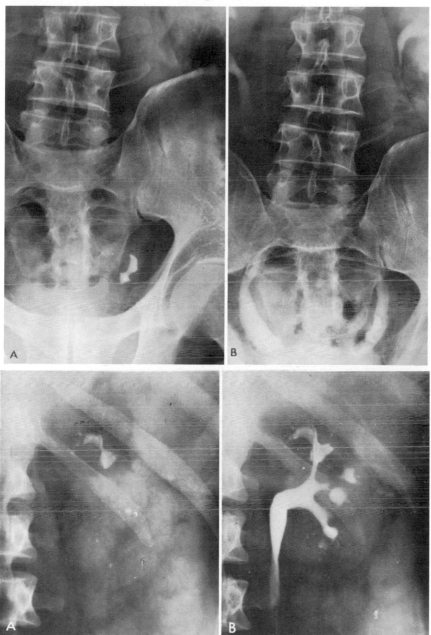

Fig. 6–14

Figure 6–13.   A, *Plain film.* Shadow of stone forming cast of composite calyx of left kidney, which has dropped into lower segment of ureter. B, *Excretory urogram.* Both ureters dilated. Shadow is demonstrated to be included in lower portion of left ureter.

Figure 6–14.   A, *Plain film.* Multiple calcific shadows overlying left renal area. Largest shadow appears to be cast of composite calyx. B, *Left retrograde pyelogram.* Largest shadow is seen to be stone forming cast of composite upper calyx. Other shadows are smaller stones in various calyces.

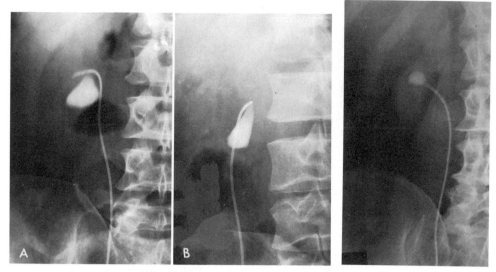

Fig. 6–15   **Fig. 6–16**

Figure 6–15. A, *Plain film*. Identification of renal calculus with opaque catheter. In anteroposterior view, catheter surrounds and is adjacent to shadow. **B,** *In oblique view*, catheter is still adjacent to shadow, a fact which would seem to indicate that it is definitely renal stone.

    Figure 6–16. *Plain film.* Identification of renal calculus with opaque catheter. Lead catheter in right ureter. Shadow overlying middle portion of right kidney. Tip of catheter adjacent to shadow, suggesting that it is definitely renal calculus. Oblique view would be necessary to be certain of this diagnosis, as it is possible that shadow in question could be in plane anterior or posterior to that of kidney.

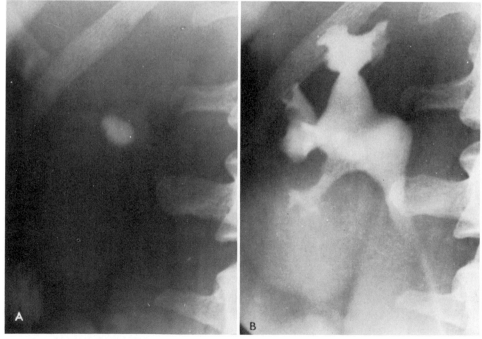

    Figure 6–17. Identification of renal calculus by means of urogram. **A,** *Plain film.* Calcific shadow overlying right midrenal area. **B,** *Right retrograde pyelogram.* Shadow is seen to be stone in renal pelvis; it is of greater density than pyelographic medium and can be seen through it.

Fig. 6-18

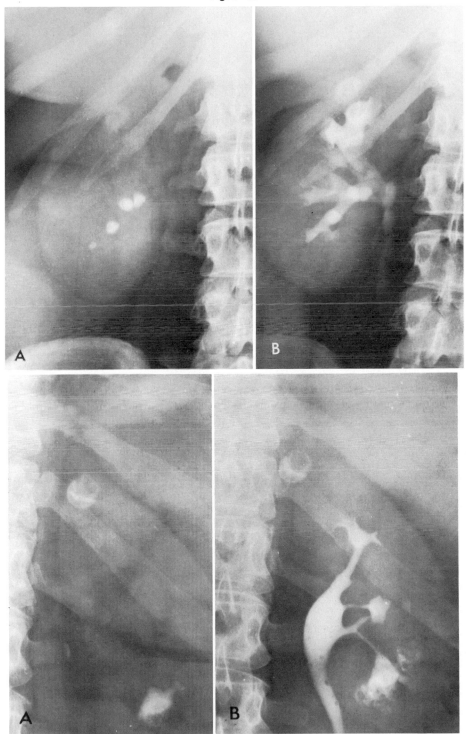

Fig. 6-19

Figure 6-18. Multiple renal calculi of greater density than contrast medium. **A,** *Plain film.* Multiple calcific shadows over lower pole of right kidney. **B,** *Excretory urogram.* Shadows are seen to be stones in renal pelvis and in lower calyces of right kidney.

Figure 6-19. **A,** *Plain film.* **Stone in lower calyx of left kidney; calcified splenic vessel.** Irregular calcific shadow overlying lower pole of left kidney. Shadow suggesting calcified splenic vessel overlying upper pole. **B,** *Left retrograde pyelogram.* Lower shadow definitely included in calyx, which can be demonstrated by contour of lower calyx, which matches that of stone. Oblique view would be unnecessary for accurate identification.

Fig. 6–20

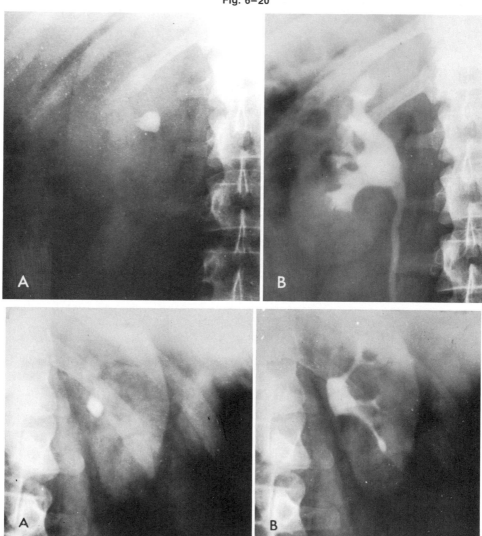

Fig. 6–21

Figure 6–20.   Stone in renal pelvis of almost same density as contrast medium. **A,** *Plain film.* Calcific shadow overlying right renal area. **B,** *Excretory urogram.* Shadow obscured by pelviocalyceal system. One would need oblique view to be absolutely sure that shadow is renal stone.

Figure 6–21.   Stone in left renal pelvis. Essentially same diagnostic situation as in Figure 6–20. **A,** *Plain film.* Calcific shadow overlying left renal area. **B,** *Left retrograde pyelogram.*

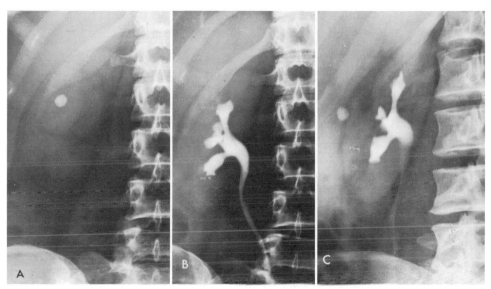

Figure 6–22. Extraurinary shadow suggests renal stone. Was excluded only with oblique urogram. **A,** *Plain film.* Calcific shadow overlying right renal area. **B,** *Right retrograde pyelogram. Anteroposterior view* shows shadow obscured by pelviocalyceal system. Suggests that shadow is renal stone. **C,** *Oblique view.* Shadow definitely excluded from kidney. This case illustrates ease of error in diagnosis if oblique views are not made when indicated.

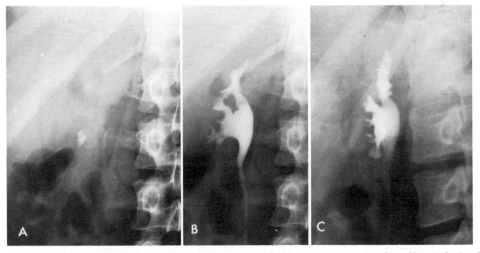

Figure 6–23. Right renal calculus. Identification required oblique urogram. **A,** *Plain film.* Calcific shadow overlying lower pole of right kidney. **B,** *Right retrograde pyelogram, anteroposterior view.* Shadow obscured by pelviocalyceal system, suggesting that it is included in pelvis or lower calyces. **C,** *Oblique view.* Shadow is not excluded, corroborating diagnosis of right renal stone.

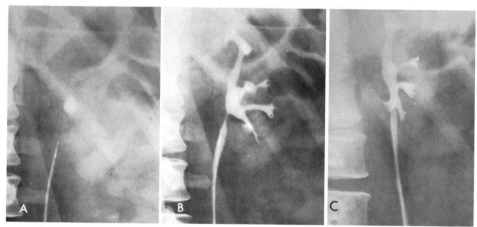

Figure 6–24.   Stone in left renal pelvis. Identification required lateral pyelogram. **A,** *Plain film.* Calcific shadow overlying left kidney. **B,** *Left retrograde pyelogram, anteroposterior view.* Shadow obscured by renal pelvis, suggesting that shadow is included in pelvis. **C,** *Lateral view.* Shadow is not excluded, corroborating diagnosis of left renal stone.

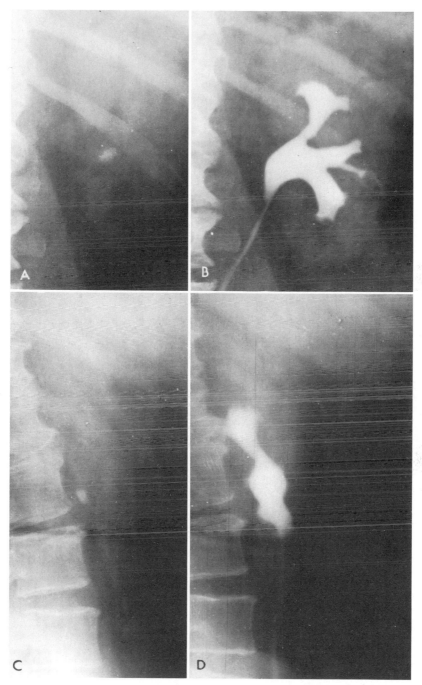

Figure 6–25.   Stone in left renal pelvis. Identification required lateral pyelogram. A, *Plain film.* Calcific shadow overlying left midrenal area. **B,** *Left retrograde pyelogram, anteroposterior view.* Shadow of stone is obscured by contrast medium filling pelvis, but is not accurately identified. **C,** *Lateral plain film.* Shadow lying just anterior to bony structure of third lumbar vertebra. **D,** *Left lateral retrograde pyelogram.* Stone definitely included in pelvis.

Fig. 6–26

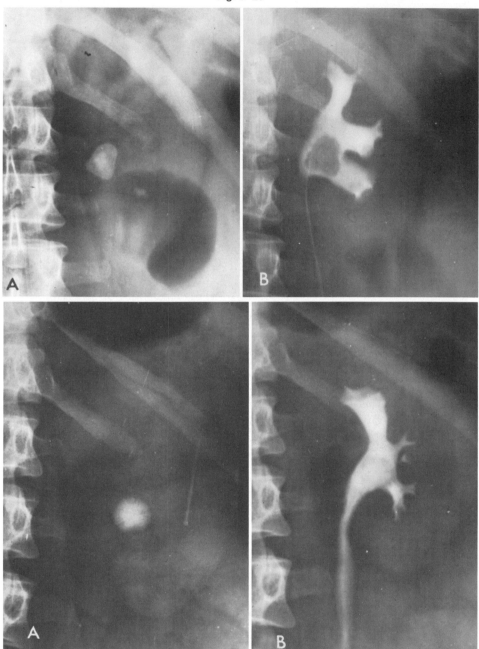

Fig. 6–27

Figure 6–26.   Laminated stones in left renal pelvis and lower calyx, producing "negative" filling defects in pyelogram. **A,** *Plain film.* Two calcific shadows of good density. **B,** *Left retrograde pyelogram.* Stones displace contrast medium and cast "negative" shadow in renal pelvis and tip of lower calyx. Oblique views would not be necessary for accurate diagnosis.

Figure 6–27.   Laminated stone in left renal pelvis producing partial "negative" filling defect in pyelogram. **A,** *Plain film.* Calcific shadow of good density overlying midrenal area. **B,** *Left retrograde pyelogram.* Stone displaces contrast medium and produces partial negative shadow in pelvis, making accurate diagnosis possible without use of oblique views.

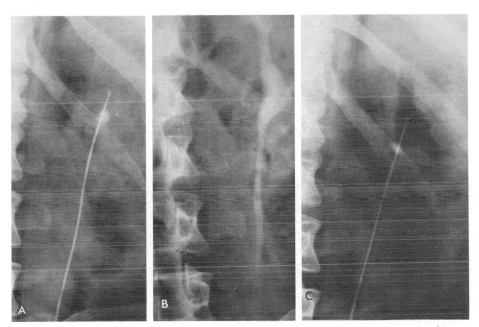

Figure 6–28. Stone at left ureteropelvic junction identified with an air pyelogram. **A,** *Plain film.* Lead catheter in left ureter. Calcific shadow over left midrenal area suggests stone in renal pelvis. **B,** *Left retrograde pyelogram using contrast medium.* Shadow obscured by pelviocalyceal system, but identity of shadow cannot be accurately determined from this pyelogram, because shadow and contrast medium are apparently of equal density. **C,** *Left retrograde air pyelogram.* Shadow is seen to be stone localized at ureteropelvic junction.

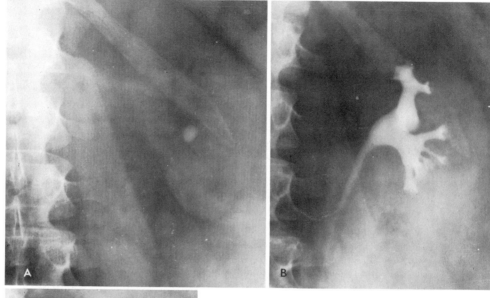

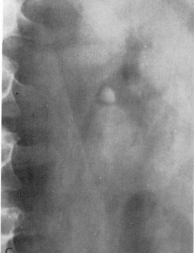

Figure 6–29. Stone in left renal pelvis identified with an air pyelogram. **A,** *Plain film.* Calcific shadow over left midrenal area suggests renal stone. **B,** *Left retrograde pyelogram, using contrast medium.* Shadow obscured by pelviocalyceal system, but shadow cannot be accurately identified because shadow and contrast medium are apparently of equal density. **C,** *Left retrograde air pyelogram.* Shadow is seen to be stone in renal pelvis.

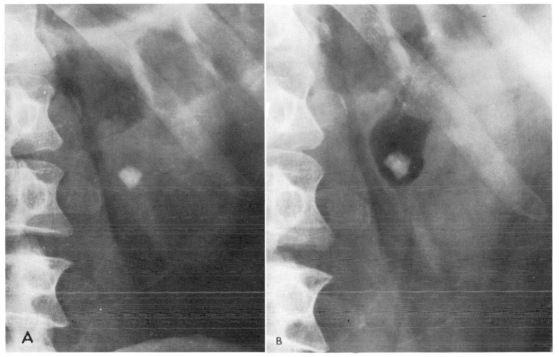

Figure 6–30. Stone in left renal pelvis identified with an air pyelogram. A, *Plain film.* Calcific shadow over left midrenal area. B, *Left retrograde air pyelogram.* Shadow demonstrated to be stone in pelvis of left kidney.

Nonopaque Calculi and Calculi of Poor Density

Stones of poor density and completely *nonopaque stones* are easily overlooked in both plain films and urograms. Stones of poor density may cast shadows so dim that they are easily obscured by gas in the intestine. They can be seen only if carefully looked for. *Soft* stones composed of putty-like material and organic substance, so-called matrix calculi, may fall into this category. Urographic medium may help interpretation by casting a negative shadow of the stone. Just as often, however, it will obscure the stone, which would not be recognized unless the plain film were closely scrutinized. Various combinations, such as dense center and less dense periphery, or vice versa, yield roentgenograms of unusual appearance (Figs. 6–31 through 6–39). *Completely nonopaque stones* are the bugaboo of the urologist. If small, they may be almost impossible to demonstrate. When of sufficient size and volume, they cast a *negative shadow or filling defect* which furnishes excellent visualization (Figs. 6–40 through 6–44). Negative shadows and filling defects, however, are also found with tumors of the renal pelvis and blood clots and may be simulated by air bubbles. When the diagnosis is in doubt, subsequent roentgenograms made several days or weeks later will show a change in contour or absence of the negative shadow (Fig. 6–45; see also Fig. 10–153).

(*Text continued on page 636.*)

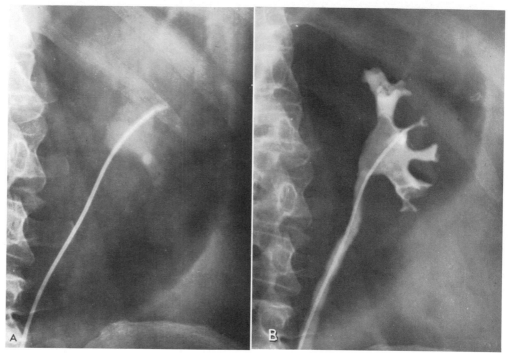

Figure 6–31. Branched stone of poor density yields "negative" shadow in pyelogram. **A,** *Plain film.* Shadow of soft stone of poor density outlining pelvis and lower calyces of left kidney. **B,** *Left retrograde pyelogram.* Contrast medium is displaced by stone, forming partially negative shadow. Stone forms cast of pelvis and lower calyx.

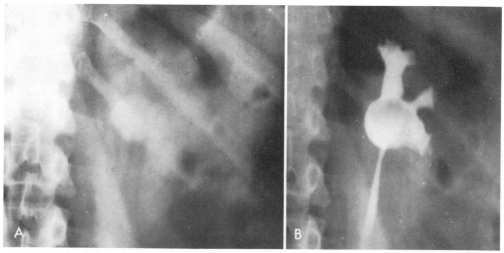

Figure 6–32. Renal calculus of poor density identified as "negative" shadow in pyelogram. **A,** *Plain film.* Indefinite shadow suggesting soft stone of poor density overlying left midrenal area. **B,** *Left retrograde pyelogram.* Medium displaced by stone. Partial filling defect of left renal pelvis, indicating that stone is in pelvis and portion of lower calyx.

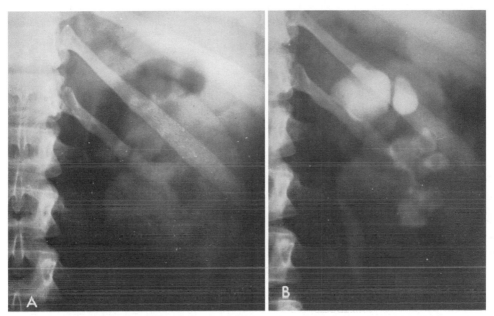

Figure 6–33. Branched stone of poor density. **A,** *Plain film.* Branched stone of poor density filling pelvis and calyces of left kidney. **B,** *Excretory urogram.* Moderate calycectasis beyond projections of stone. Pelvis does not fill with medium because of being completely filled with stone.

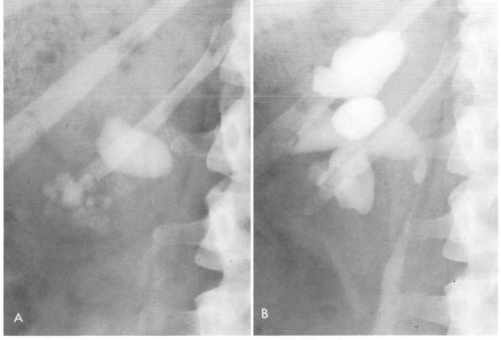

Figure 6–34. Cystine stones. Note "ground-glass" appearance in plain film. **A,** *Plain film.* **B,** *Excretory urogram.* Cystine stones in pelvis and lower calyx of right kidney. Density of stone is less than that of contrast medium.

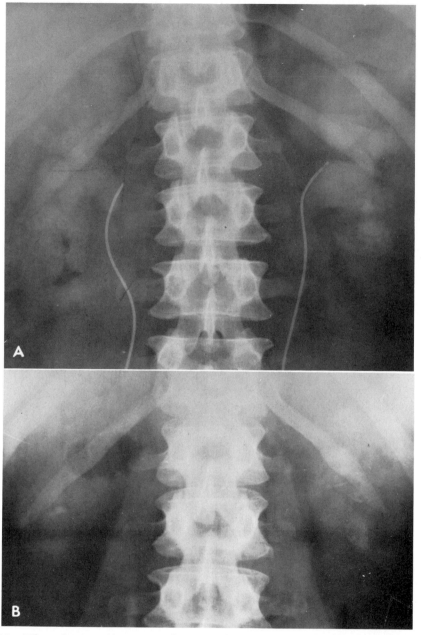

Figure 6–35. Bilateral uric acid stones with some calcium content. Poor density. Partial disintegration as result of dietary control and alkalinization of urine. **A,** *Plain film* with opaque ureteral catheters in place. Branched calculi of poor density filling pelvis and calyces of both kidneys. **B,** *Plain film,* 6 months later. Most of stones are gone on right. Much improved on left.

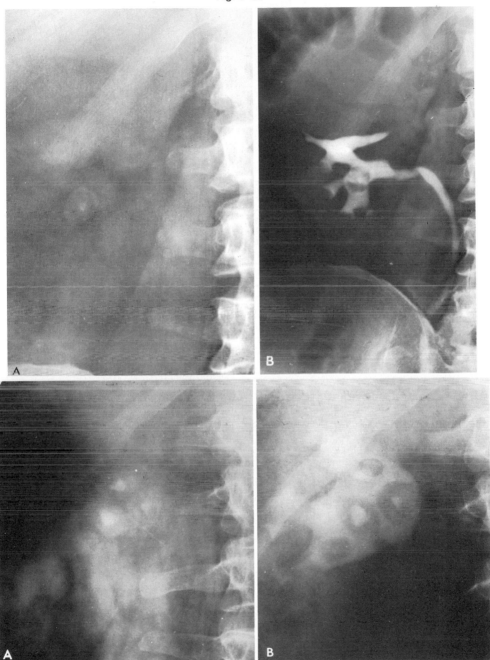

Fig. 6–37

Figure 6–36.   Laminated renal stone with dense center and less dense periphery. **A,** *Plain film.* Shadow over right renal area, with dense center, but remainder of poor density. **B,** *Right retrograde pyelogram.* Shadow is seen to be stone with dense center and periphery, situated in pelvis. Because of its poor density, stone casts negative shadow. Simple cyst in upper pole of kidney.

Figure 6–37.   Laminated calculi with dense centers but peripheries of poor density which could be easily overlooked in plain film. Well-demonstrated as "negative" shadows in pyelogram. **A,** *Plain film.* Three triangular calcific shadows over right renal area. **B,** *Right retrograde pyelogram.* Four filling defects in dilated renal pelvis. Filling defects are larger than shadows seen in plain film. They are caused by four stones, one of which is completely nonopaque and three of which have nonopaque peripheries.

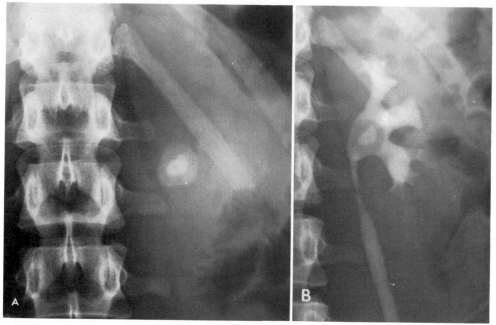

Figure 6–38. **A,** *Plain film.* **Stone** with dense center and less dense periphery. **B,** *Left retrograde pyelogram.* Negative shadow cast by **laminated stone** as it displaces contrast medium. Note that dense center of stone is easily visualized.

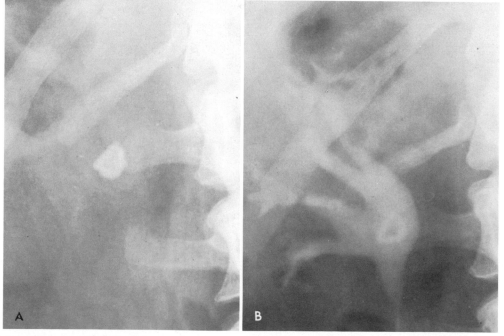

Figure 6–39.   Laminated stone; periphery is more dense than center. **A,** *Plain film.* **B,** *Excretory urogram.* Stone is in renal pelvis; "negative" shadow of center of stone is most prominent.

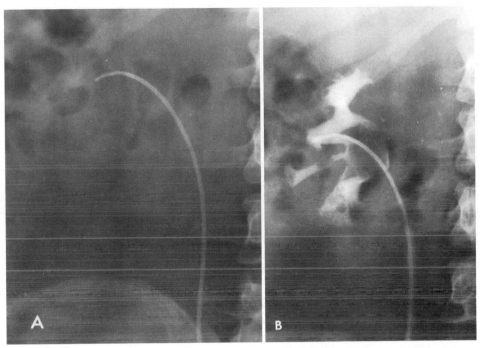

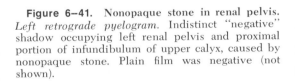

Figure 6–40. Nonopaque stone in renal pelvis. A, *Plain film.* Catheter in right ureter. Otherwise negative. B, *Right retrograde pyelogram.* Nonopaque stone. Negative shadow occupying most of renal pelvis, due to nonopaque stone.

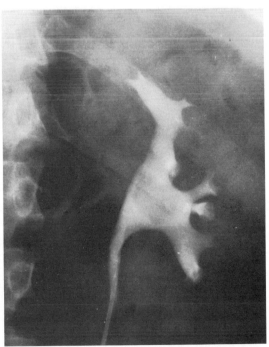

Figure 6–41. Nonopaque stone in renal pelvis. *Left retrograde pyelogram.* Indistinct "negative" shadow occupying left renal pelvis and proximal portion of infundibulum of upper calyx, caused by nonopaque stone. Plain film was negative (not shown).

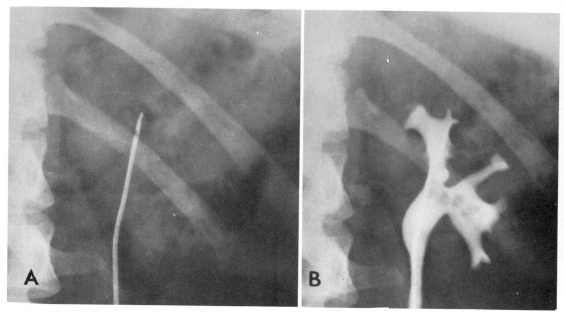

Figure 6–42.   Nonopaque calculi in pelvis and lower calyces. **A,** *Plain film.* Negative. **B,** *Left retrograde pyelogram.* Multiple negative shadows caused by nonopaque stones in pelvis and lower calyx of left kidney.

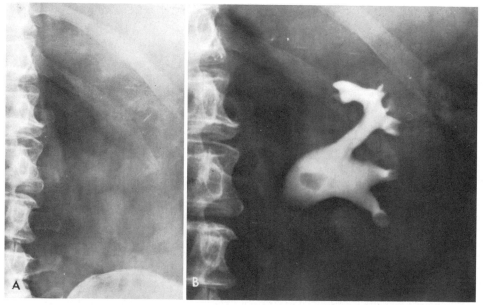

Figure 6–43.   Nonopaque renal calculi. **A,** *Plain film.* Negative. **B,** *Left retrograde pyelogram.* Two discrete negative shadows in pelvis of left kidney, indicating nonopaque stones.

Fig. 6–44

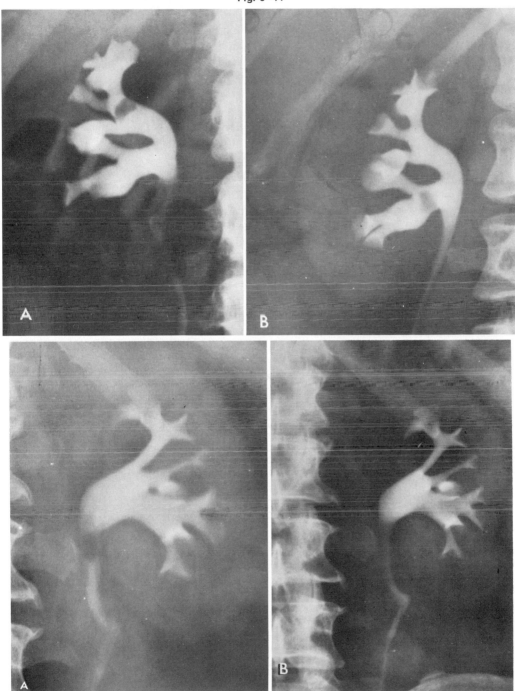

Fig. 6–45

Figure 6–44. "Migratory" nonopaque stone. **A,** *Right retrograde pyelogram.* Filling defect in upper major calyx, caused by nonopaque stone. Plain film was negative (not shown). **B,** *Right retrograde pyelogram,* made 2 days later. Stone is now in lower major calyx, indicating migratory stone.

Figure 6–45. Air bubble simulating nonopaque stone. **A,** *Left retrograde pyelogram.* Oval negative shadow at or just below ureteropelvic juncture suggests nonopaque stone. **B,** *Left retrograde pyelogram* made 2 days later. Filling defect has disappeared. It was apparently result of air bubble.

Pathologic Changes in Kidneys, Resulting From Calculi

As might be expected, the most common pathologic condition produced by stone is *obstruction with dilatation of the pelvis or calyces or both.* The location and degree of dilatation depend on the position and degree of obstruction of the stone. A stone lodged in the infundibulum of a calyx may produce *localized calycectasis* or *hydrocalyx.** Stones in calyces may produce dilatation simply because of their presence and associated infection. Stones in dilated calyces usually are recognized quite easily, especially if the stone assumes somewhat the shape of the calyx (Figs. 6–46, 6–47, and 6–48). A stone in the renal pelvis may produce pyelectasis or calycectasis or both (Figs. 6–49, 6–50, and 6–51).

The presence of a stone in the renal pelvis may cause spasm and contraction of the pelvis rather than dilatation. In such cases the pelvis is seen tightly contracted around the stone, with an associated spasticity and contracture of the ureteropelvic juncture, apparently a result of irritation (Figs. 6–52, 6–53, and 6–54).

SECONDARY CALCULI

Calculi may be the result of, rather than the cause of, urinary stasis. One ex-

*See discussion of hydrocalyx and calyceal diverticulum in Chapter 5, page 394.

ample of this is the *calculi of recumbency,* which occur in patients who are bedridden for a long time, usually after accidents which have caused multiple fractures (Fig. 6–55). Another example is the patient with obstruction of the ureteropelvic juncture and associated pyelectasis (Figs. 6–56 through 6–61).

At times it may be difficult to know whether there is sufficient functioning renal tissue to permit a conservative operation (removal of calculi) or whether a nephrectomy will be required. The absence or diminution of function indicated by the excretory urogram is not always accurate. When the functioning ability of the kidney with secondary calculi is in question, the demonstration of good blood supply by means of an aortogram may be distinctly helpful (Figs. 6–62 and 6–63).

CALYCECTASIS WITH CALCULI SIMULATING TUBERCULOSIS WITH CALCIFICATION

At times stones may be of such contour and density and may produce such calycectasis that they *suggest renal tuberculosis with calcification.* This type of stone usually is irregular, with many fragments lying closely together in an irregularly dilated calyx that simulates the cortical destruction characteristic of tuberculosis (Figs. 6–64 and 6–65). (See also Chapter 8, Renal Tuberculosis.)

(Text continued on page 647.)

Fig. 6–46

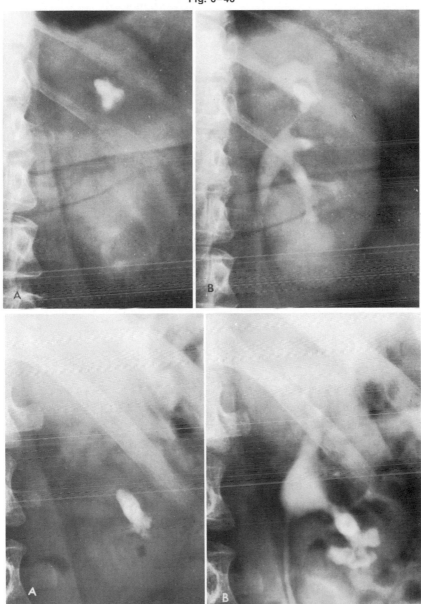

Fig. 6–47

Figure 6–46. **Stone obstructing upper calyx. A,** *Plain film.* Calcific shadow overlying upper pole of left kidney, suggesting stone forming cast of portion of upper calyx. **B,** *Excretory urogram.* Dilatation of upper calyx caused by stone which obstructs minor calyx and infundibulum. Remainder of kidney normal.

Figure 6–47. **Stone obstructing lower calyx. A,** *Plain film.* Irregular calcific shadow overlying lower pole of left kidney. **B,** *Excretory urogram.* Shadow is stone impacted in infundibulum of lower calyx, producing localized dilatation of lower minor calyx.

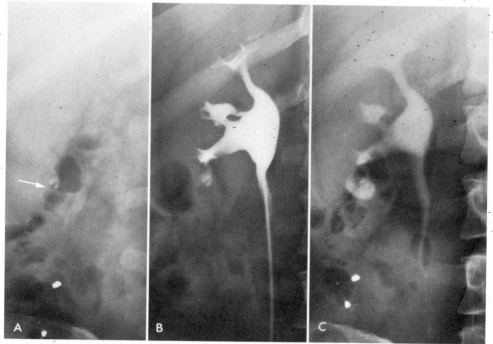

Figure 6–48. Stone obstructing lower calyx. Calycectasis cephalad to stone demonstrated by excretory urogram. **A,** *Plain film.* Irregular calcific shadow overlying lower pole of right kidney (*arrow*). **B,** *Right retrograde pyelogram.* Shadow is included in branch of lower calyx, which does not appear to be greatly dilated. **C,** *Excretory urogram.* Marked dilatation of lower calyx proximal to stone. This would have been missed if excretory urogram had not been made.

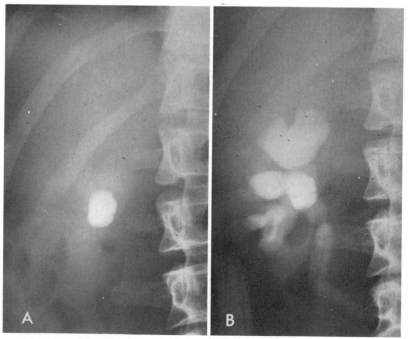

Figure 6–49. Stone in renal pelvis obstructing calyces. **A,** *Plain film.* Large calcific shadow overlying right renal pelvis. **B,** *Excretory urogram.* Shadow is stone in pelvis of kidney, causing moderate calycectasis and adjacent ureterectasis.

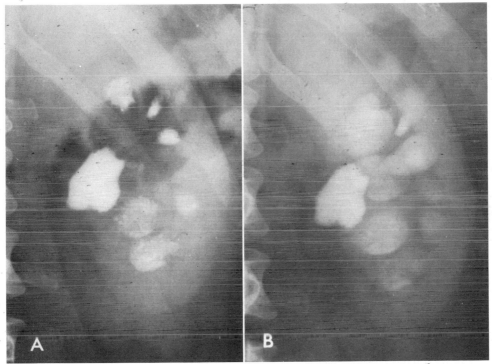

Figure 6–50.   Stone in renal pelvis with secondary (?) calculi in dilated (obstructed) calyces. **A,** *Plain film.* Calcific shadows outlining pelvis and calyces of left kidney. **B,** *Excretory urogram.* Larger shadow is stone filling pelvis and producing marked calycectasis. There are secondary calculi in all of calyces, resulting from obstructive dilatation.

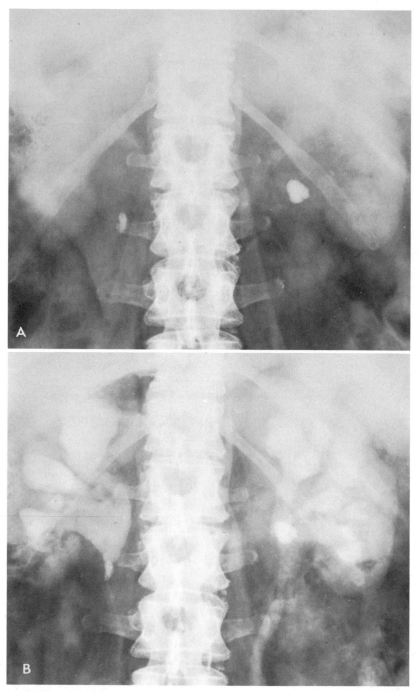

Figure 6–51. A, *Plain film.* B, *Excretory urogram.* Stone is blocking each ureteropelvic juncture and producing calycectasis, especially marked on right.

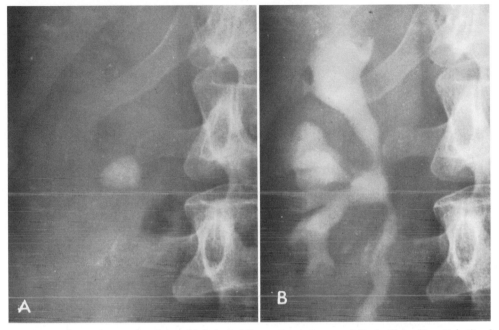

Figure 6–52. Stone in renal pelvis which is tightly contracted around it. A, *Plain film.* Calcific shadow overlying right renal area. B, *Right retrograde pyelogram.* Some evidence of calycectasis.

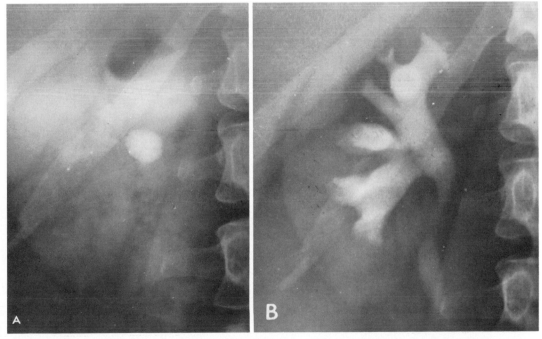

Figure 6–53. A, *Plain film.* Irregular calcific shadow overlying right renal area. B, *Excretory urogram.* Right renal pelvis and adjacent portion of ureter spastic and contracted around pelvic stone, with some evidence of calycectasis. Very little obstruction is present.

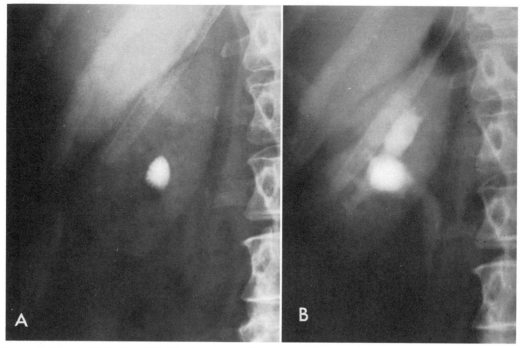

Figure 6–54. A, *Plain film.* Calcific shadow overlying right renal area. **B,** *Excretory urogram.* **Right renal pelvis contracted around stone, causing moderate calycectasis.**

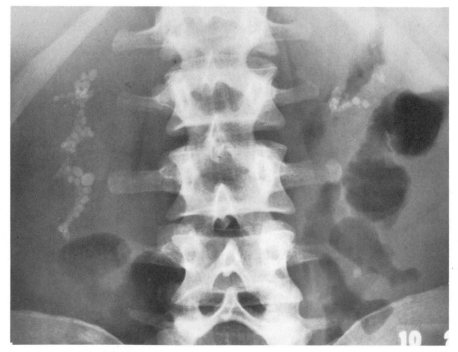

Figure 6–55. *Plain film.* **Calculi of recumbency.** Multiple small calculi in calyces. (Patient immobilized with fracture of pelvis.) Might be confused with nephrocalcinosis.

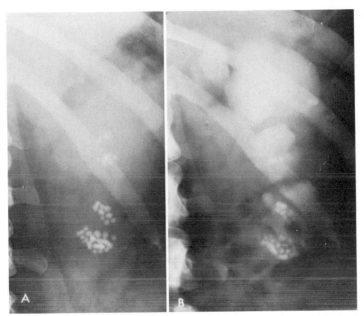

Figure 6–56.   Secondary calculi in hydronephrosis. **A,** *Plain film.* Multiple small calculi scattered throughout left renal area. **B,** *Excretory urogram.* Incomplete filling of left renal pelvis. Marked calycectasis. Stones are grouped in large dilated calyces.

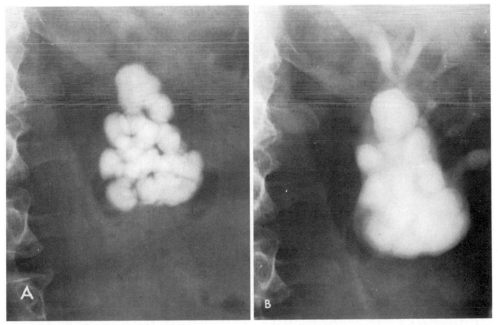

Figure 6–57.   Secondary calculi in hydronephrosis. **A,** *Plain film.* Large number of calculi overlying left renal area. **B,** *Excretory urogram.* Marked pyelectasis with minimal calycectasis. Large pelvis is filled with calculi. Obstruction at ureteropelvic junction. Left nephrectomy.

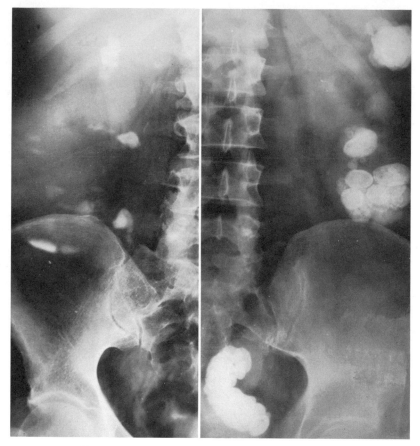

Fig. 6–58   Fig. 6–59

Figure 6–58.   Secondary calculi in hydronephrosis. *Plain film.* Multiple calcific shadows overlying entire right side of abdomen. Excretory urogram (not shown here) showed no function on right. Left kidney normal. Exploration showed huge hydronephrosis with secondary calculi. Right nephrectomy. Hydronephrosis and stones.

Figure 6–59.   Secondary calculi in hydronephrosis and hydroureter. *Excretory urogram.* Nonfunctioning left kidney, which is site of extreme hydronephrosis and ureterectasis. Large secondary calculi situated in kidney and lower portion of ureter. Right kidney was normal.

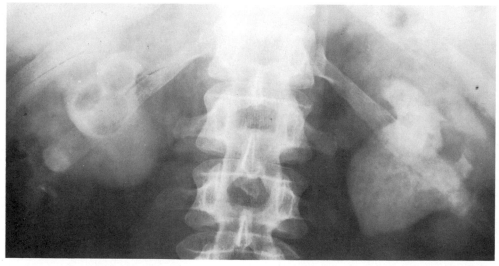

Figure 6–60.   *Excretory urogram.* Bilateral obstruction of ureteropelvic junctures, with secondary non-opaque calculi. On right, three large oval calculi produce negative shadows. On left, pelvis and calyces are filled with numerous small nonopaque calculi which give a mottled appearance. Both kidneys explored; calculi removed and plastic operation on ureteropelvic juncture.

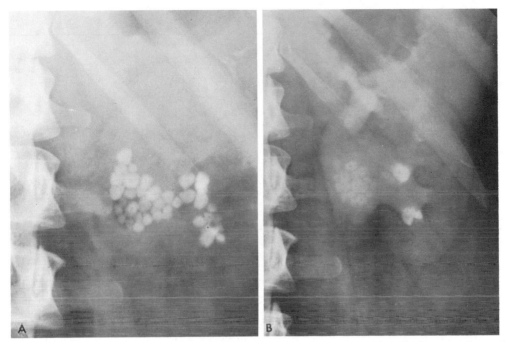

Figure 6–61. Obstruction of ureteropelvic juncture, with pyelectasis and multiple secondary calculi. A, *Plain film.* B, *Excretory urogram.*

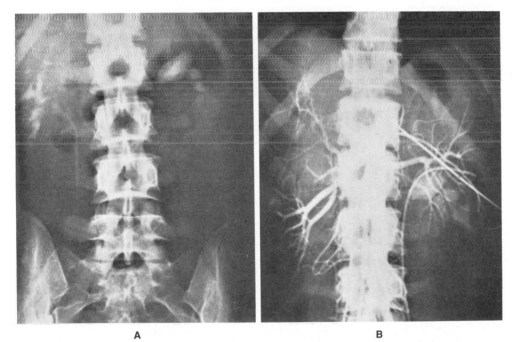

A   B

Figure 6–62. Evaluation of "recovery potential" of damaged kidney by arteriography. A, *Excretory urogram.* Multiple stones in nonfunctioning left kidney. Normal right kidney. B, *Aortogram* shows excellent arterial supply to both right and left kidneys. *Comment:* In this case excretory urogram suggested presence of partially destroyed, nonfunctioning left kidney. Aortogram, by virtue of demonstrating equally good arterial supply bilaterally, suggested that conservative operation, with preservation of kidney, was indicated. Excretory urogram made 5 months after removal of stone showed excellent function of left kidney. (Courtesy of Dr. A. K. Doss.)

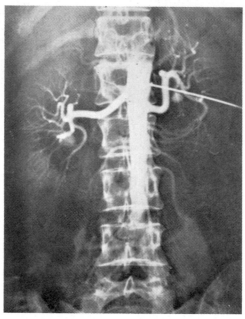

Figure 6–63.   *Aortogram* in patient with stones in both renal pelves. (Previous excretory urogram showed stones in each pelvis.) **Aortogram shows excellent blood supply to both right and left kidneys,** with visualization of larger and smaller intrarenal vessels. Corticomedullogram is also present bilaterally. This is good example of normal arteriogram. (Courtesy of Dr. A. K. Doss.)

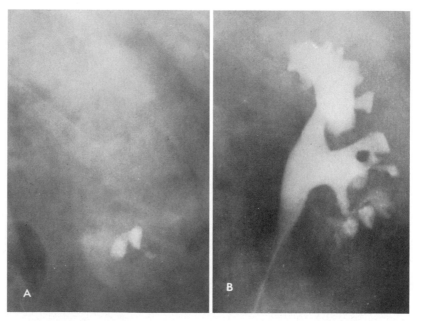

Figure 6–64.   **Renal calculi simulating tuberculosis with calcification. A,** *Plain film.* Irregular areas of calcification over lower pole of left kidney. **B,** *Left retrograde pyelogram.* Marked irregularity of lower calyx, which could suggest cortical destruction with calcification from tuberculosis. This, however, was stone in dilated, infected lower calyx. Inoculated guinea pigs were negative for tuberculosis.

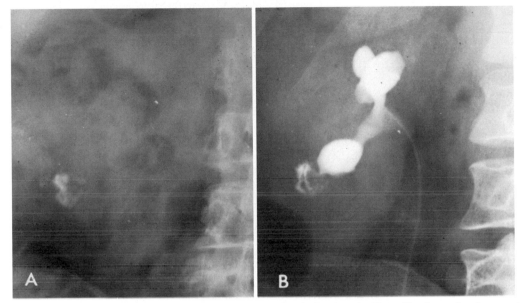

Figure 6–65. Renal stone simulating tuberculosis with calcification. A, *Plain film.* Irregular, fragmentary type of calcification in lower pole of right kidney. B, *Right retrograde pyelogram.* Unusual calycectasis, with apparent absence of middle calyx. Calcification seems to communicate with, is adjacent to, and below dilated lower calyx. Could easily be mistaken for tuberculous calcification.

Miscellaneous Types and Locations of Calculi

Laminated calculi are occasionally seen (see Fig. 6–3). "Burr-like" stones, more common in the bladder, are also seen in the renal pelvis (Figs. 6–66 through 6–69).

BRANCHED (STAGHORN) CALCULI

Branched calculi produce the most dramatic-appearing roentgenograms in urography. Forming a cast of part or all of the pelviocalyceal system, they may reach enormous proportions, especially in cases in which pyelectasis becomes marked. There is usually no problem in identification or localization of such calculi, but it may be extremely difficult to estimate renal function by means of excretory urography. The reason for this is that often the stone completely fills the pelvis and calyces so that no medium can collect around its periphery. If contrast medium cannot be demonstrated in the ureter, some other test of renal function must be used. In some cases the calyces are dilated beyond the tips of the branched calculi so that varying degrees of calycectasis may be demonstrated (Figs. 6–70 through 6–73).

RECURRING CALCULI

Calculi that recur following surgical removal may assume bizarre shapes because of postoperative deformity of the pelvis and calyces including calyceal deformity caused by nephrostomy tubes (Figs. 6–74A and B and 6–75A and B). Calculi that have been spilled in the wound during operation may present some problem in identification (Fig. 6–76).

CALCULI IN ANOMALIES

Calculi in anomalous conditions of the kidneys and ureters will be discussed in Chapter 12.

CORTICAL STONES; STONES IN CALYCEAL DIVERTICULA OR PYELOGENIC CYSTS

"Cortical" stones may present difficult problems in diagnosis. In most cases they are situated near the calyces, so that the problem nearly always is one of determining whether the stone is in the tip of a calyx, in a walled-off portion of the calyx, in a pyelogenic cyst, diverticulum* or hydrocalyx, or in the adjacent cortex, not communicating with the pelvi-ocalyceal system. Differential diagnosis here requires use of an excretory urogram to determine whether medium surrounds the stone, showing that it communicates with the calyx, or whether there is no communication. Urograms must be made in various oblique positions as well as in the lateral position. In many cases it is not possible to make the distinction accurately until the involved kidney has been explored surgically (Fig. 6–77 through 6–81).

"MILK OF CALCIUM" RENAL STONE

Approximately seven cases of "milk of calcium" renal stone have been reported in the literature (Benendo and Litwak; Henken; Howell; Maurer and Wildin; Pullman and King; Rosenberg; Walker, Pearson, and Johnson). The term "milk of calcium" has been borrowed from a somewhat similar condition encountered in the gallbladder. The "milky" fluid is a

---

*See discussion of calyceal diverticulum and pyelo-genic cyst, Chapter 5, page 394.

suspension of a fine calcific sediment which has been alleged to be calcium carbonate.

In all seven reported cases the "milk of calcium" fluid has been contained either in a calyceal diverticulum with restricted drainage into the calyx or in a pyelogenic cyst (calyceal cyst*) in which no communication with the calyx could be found.

In most cases the condition was asymptomatic and found only accidentally. In the plain film taken with the patient supine, the appearance suggests an ordinary round or oval solid calculus. However, with the patient upright or sitting, the calcific material gravitates to the bottom of the cyst resulting in the characteristic "half-moon" contour (Figs. 6–82 and 6–83).

In all of the case reports it has been stated that the material consists of calcium carbonate as is the case in the gallbladder. However, in only one of the seven cases (autopsy case of Walker, Pearson, and Johnson) was the material analyzed, the authors stating that it was calcium carbonate. Boyce reports that the material is small spherules of calcium phosphate (see discussion of "seed calculi" above). Three of the seven patients have been operated on. In Howell's case (the first reported) the true diagnosis was not suspected before operation as no film had been made with the patient upright. The condition was considered to be a solid stone and it could not be found at operation. Postoperative films in the upright and lateral positions disclosed the true nature of the lesion.

---

*See discussion in Chapter 5, page 394.

(Text continued on page 661.)

Fig. 6–66   Fig. 6–67

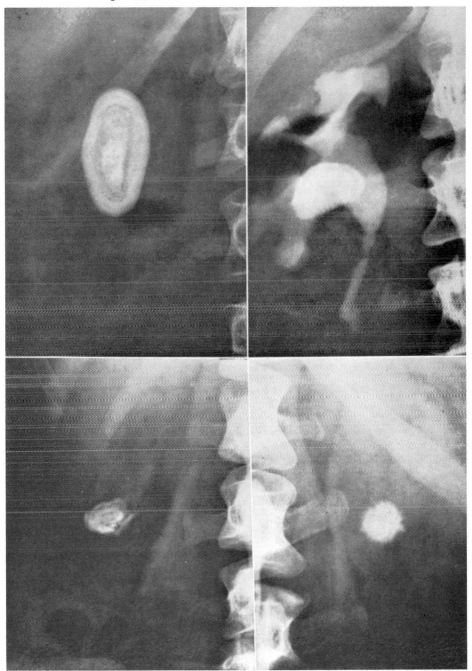

Fig. 6–68   Fig. 6–69

Figure 6–66.   *Plain film.* Large laminated stone in right kidney, associated with marked pyelectasis.
Figure 6–67.   Laminated stone in renal area. *Right retrograde pyelogram.* Stone free in renal pelvis.
Figure 6–68.   *Plain film.* Unusual type of laminated stone in lower calyx of right kidney.
Figure 6–69.   *Plain film.* Burr-like type of renal stone situated in left renal pelvis.

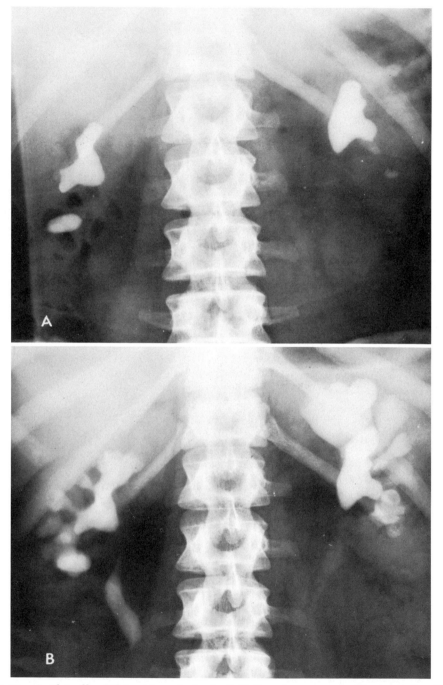

Figure 6–70.   A, *Plain film.* **Bilateral branched calculi.** B, *Excretory urogram, 20-minute film.* Moderately good function bilaterally. Considerable calycectasis on left due to obstruction from stone.

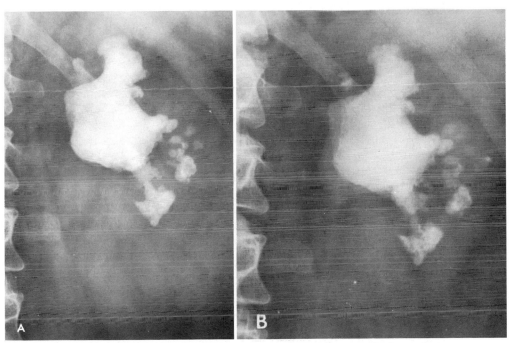

Figure 6–71. A, *Plain film.* Large branched stone forming cast of pelvis and calyces. B, *Excretory urogram, 20-minute film.* Moderately good function, as seen by areas of medium in pelvis and upper ureter just medial to margin of stone.

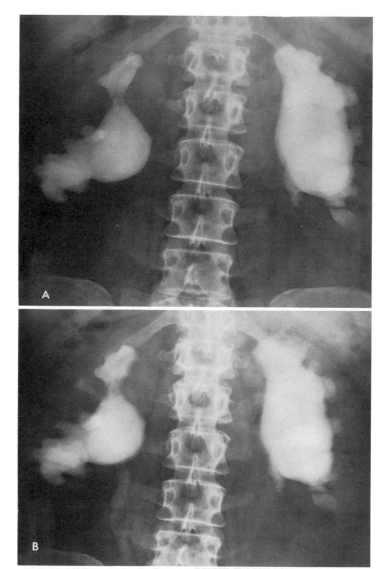

Figure 6–72.   A, *Plain film.* Huge bilateral branched calculi filling pelvis and calyces of both kidneys. B, *Excretory urogram, 20-minute film.* Evidence of function on right, as shown by contrast medium in lateral branch of upper calyx and ureter. Function also retained in left kidney, as shown by collection of contrast medium around periphery of stone.

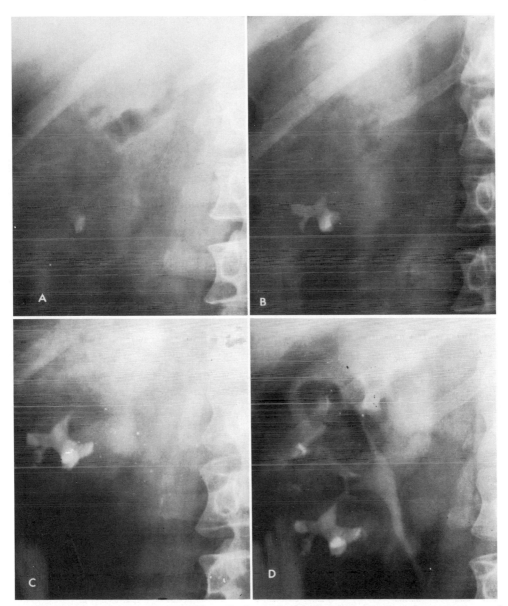

Figure 6–73.   Progression in growth of branched calculus from single calculus in tip of minor calyx to one filling entire lower group of calyces, including infundibulum of major calyx. **A**, *Plain film*. Small stone in tip of lower calyx of right kidney. **B**, *Plain film*, 6 months later than **A**. Stone has grown and now fills two branches of lower calyces. **C**, *Plain film*, 19 months later than **B**. Stone has increased in size and now fills larger group of calyces, part of major calyx, and infundibulum. **D**, *Excretory urogram*, same date as **C**. Pelvis and middle and upper calyces normal. Lower group of calyces completely filled by branched calculus.

Fig. 6–74

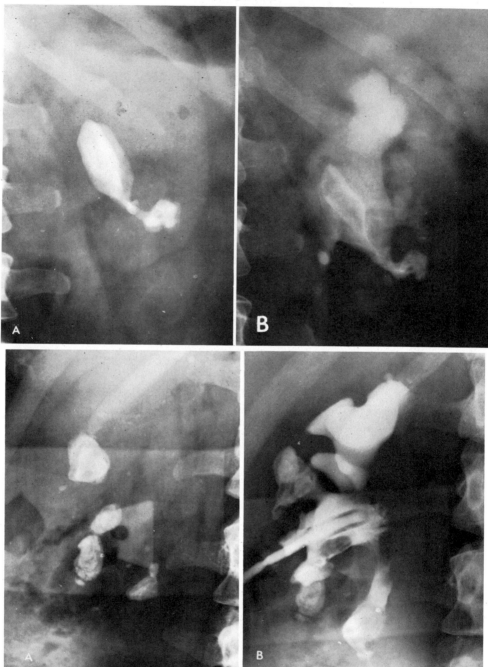

Fig. 6–75

Figure 6–74. **Recurring calculi in postoperative deformed kidney. A,** *Plain film.* **Laminated calculus of unusual shape** in left renal area. **B,** *Excretory urogram.* Stone is seen lying in pelvis and postoperatively deformed lower calyx. Moderate pyelectasis.

Figure 6–75. **Recurring calculi in postoperatively deformed right kidney and upper part of ureter. A,** *Plain film.* Multiple calculi of varying sizes, some of which are laminated, overlying right kidney. Adhesive tape, which is securing nephrostomy tube, is also visible. The tube is nonopaque, so it can be seen only with difficulty. **B,** *Right retrograde pyelogram.* Medium injected through nephrostomy tube, which is now visible. Marked deformity, cicatrization, and dilatation of calyces. Stones located in upper and lower calyces and in pelvis. Lowermost large stone is included in deformed, dilated upper part of ureter, just below ureteropelvic junction.

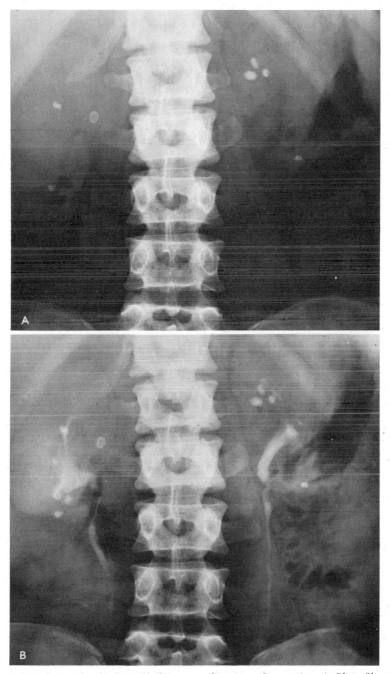

Figure 6–76.   Multiple renal calculi, spilled in wound at time of operation. **A,** *Plain film.* Multiple calculi overlying and in vicinity of both kidneys. **B,** *Excretory urogram.* Postoperative deformity of pelves and calyces. Stones are seen to lie outside pelviocalyceal system.

Fig. 6–77

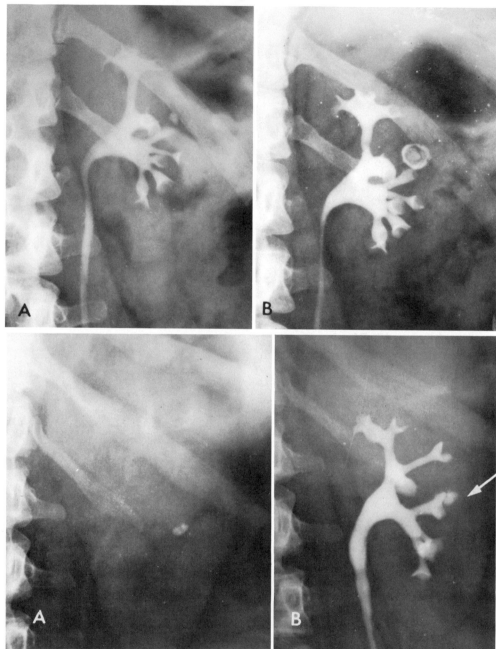

Fig. 6–78

Figure 6–77. Renal cortical or encysted stone. **A,** *Left retrograde pyelogram.* Stone adjacent to, but well removed from, tips of middle and upper calyces. **B,** *Left retrograde pyelogram* made 4 years later. Marked increase in size of cortical stone, which still occupies same position and apparently does not communicate with pelviocalyceal system.

Figure 6–78. Renal cortical or encysted stone. **A,** *Plain film* (made following retrograde pyelography—a little contrast medium remains in upper calyx and ureter). Calcific shadow overlying left renal area. **B,** *Left retrograde pyelogram.* Shadow adjacent to and beyond middle calyx (*arrow*); impossible to tell from these films whether contrast medium surrounds stone.

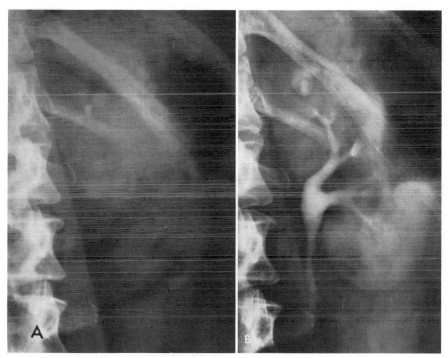

Figure 6–79.   A, *Plain film.* **Stone in calyceal diverticulum.** Renal cortical or encysted stone over upper pole of left kidney? **B,** *Excretory urogram.* Shadow seems to be at least 1 cm beyond tip of upper calyx. However, contrast medium surrounds stone, suggesting stone in calyceal diverticulum.

Fig. 6–80

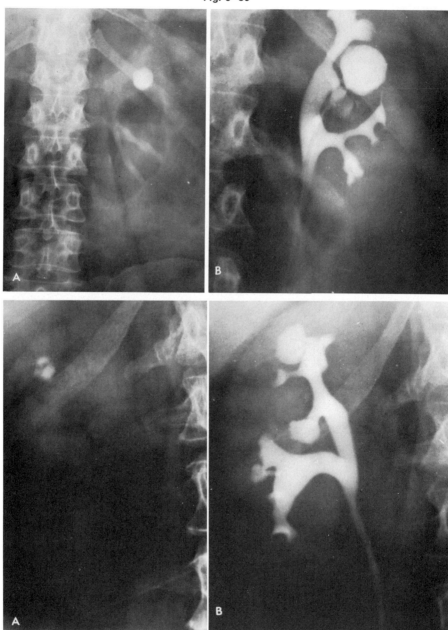

Fig. 6–81

Figure 6–80. **Stone in calyceal diverticulum. A,** *Plain film.* Calcific shadow over upper pole of left kidney. **B,** *Left retrograde pyelogram.* Medium fills diverticulum and surrounds stone; there apparently is communication with branch of upper calyx.

Figure 6–81. **Stone in calyceal diverticulum. A,** *Plain film.* Irregular calcific shadow over upper pole of right kidney. **B,** *Right retrograde pyelogram.* Contrast medium fills circular pocket which surrounds stone and apparently communicates with upper calyx.

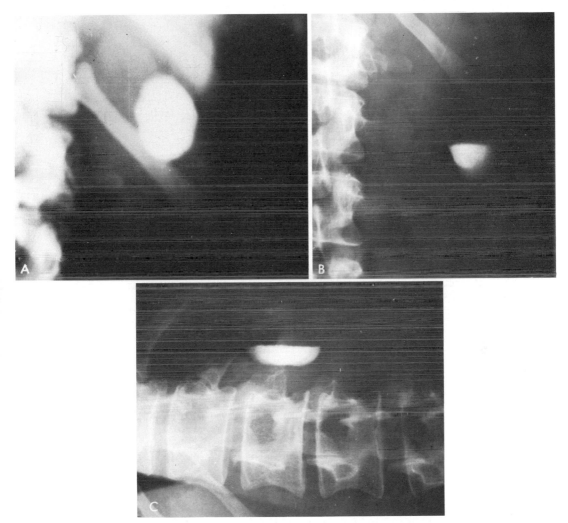

Figure 6–82. "Milk of calcium" stone. **A,** *Plain film,* supine position. Shadow appears to be oval-shaped solid calculus over upper pole of kidney. **B,** *Upright film.* Calcium material has "layered out," resulting in typical "half-moon" shape. **C,** *Horizontal right lateral position.* "Half-moon" appearance with convex border projected against spine. (From Boyce, W. H.)

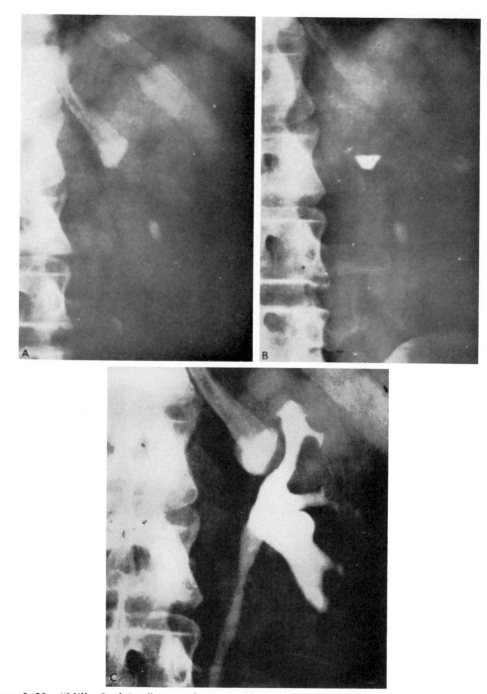

Figure 6–83. "Milk of calcium" in renal cyst. **A,** *Plain film,* supine position. Large oval-shaped calculus in upper pole of left kidney. Smaller stone of less density over lower pole. **B,** *Plain film* in erect position. Upper shadow has "layered out," causing shadow to assume typical "half-moon" contour. Lower shadow unchanged. **C,** *Retrograde pyelogram,* supine position. Upper shadow now assumes original shape and is "milk of calcium" material in cyst adjacent to upper calyx. No apparent communication with calyx or pelvis. Lower stone is in lower calyx and is obscured by contrast medium. (From Benendo, B., and Litwak, A.)

NEPHROCALCINOSIS

by

Denis C. O'Sullivan

"Nephrocalcinosis" is a term used to describe calcium deposits in the parenchyma of the kidney (Albright, Aub, and Bauer; Albright and associates). The deposits are commonly located in the renal pyramids, but may be scattered diffusely throughout the cortex and medulla of the kidney (Mortensen; Mortensen and Emmett). They may or may not be demonstrable roentgenographically. Nephrocalcinosis is usually a bilateral disease, but occasionally is confined to only one kidney (Fig. 6–84). Two types are recognized: medullary and cortical.

MEDULLARY TYPE

The medullary type is by far the most common, accounting for more than 95% of cases (Huth). The distal tubules and the loop of Henle are involved, which confines the calcification to the renal pyramids. The calcium deposits may be located (1) in the basement membrane of the collecting tubules, (2) in the cytoplasm of the tubular epithelial cells, (3) in the interstitial tissue, and (4) as small tubular calculi (Mortensen). The formation of the tubular calculi may be the result of erosion of calcium deposits from the lining epithelium into the tubular lumen or may result from the precipitation of calcium salts in dilated tubules. Tubular dilatation, sometimes referred to as intrarenal hydronephrosis (Shanks and MacDonald), may be congenital or the end result of infection or toxemia (see "Sponge Kidney," Chapter 9, pages 1013–1014). Tubular degeneration may follow an episode of inflammation or toxemia; fibrotic changes may occur in the healing phase and cause constriction of the tubules and proximal dilatation. Tubular dilatation, especially in the presence of increased calcium concentration, would predispose to the precipitation of tubular calculi. Tubular calculi apparently may be the nidus for the formation of renal calculi, as some patients with nephrocalcinosis repeatedly form calculi also (Fig. 6–85).

Etiology

Nephrocalcinosis may be the end result of a number of unrelated pathologic conditions. These include hyperparathyroidism (Albright and associates; Keating), chronic pyelonephritis (Albright, Dienes, and Sulkowitch; Beeson, Rocha, and Guez), chronic glomerulonephritis (Arons, Christensen, and Sosman; Geraci, Harris, and Keith; Randall, Strauss, and McNeely), hypervitaminosis D, milk alkali syndrome (Burnett and associates; Scholz and Keating), sarcoidosis (Richtsmeier; Wilson and Brown), renal tubular acidosis (Bauld, MacDonald, and Hill; Faconi; Schreiner, Smith, and Kyle), idiopathic hypercalcemia in children (Lightwood and Payne; Snyder), sulfonamide intoxication (Engel), medullary sponge kidney (Vermooten), thyrotoxicosis (Epstein, Freedman, and Levitin; Sallin), neoplastic disease with or without demonstrable metastatic deposits in bone (Plimpton and Gellhorn; Thomas, Connor, and Morgan), primary oxaluria (Pyrah and associates), and skeletal atrophy due to misuse (Thomas, Connor, and Morgan). In some cases the cause is unknown.

Roentgenographic Appearance

Calcium deposits confined to the region of the renal pyramids are the commonest x-ray finding. The calcium deposits may be fine and feathery (Figs. 6–86 and 6–87) or may be in the form of coarser granules (Figs. 6–88 through 6–92).

CORTICAL TYPE

The cortical type of nephrocalcinosis differs considerably in appearance from the medullary type. It appears as a generalized cortical involvement consisting of diffuse stippled calcification that provides a faint "calcium shadow" of minimal density which outlines the entire kidney (Figs. 6–93 through 6–97). This type of nephrocalcinosis is thought to be the result of *chronic glomerulonephritis* (Esposito; Geraci, Harris, and Keith; Pyrah and Hodgkinson); it may be aggravated by excessive milk intake.

Acute renal cortical necrosis may also result in calcification which is somewhat of this type (see discussion, Chapter 17, pages 1908–1910). In the past this type of nephrocalcinosis was rarely encountered because few patients survived the condition. With modern artificial dialysis, which carries patients over the acute phase of the disease, more are now living long enough to develop this calcification (Riesz and Wagner; Walls, Schorr, and Kerr).

Renal Manifestations of Sarcoidosis

by

Harold W. Calhoun

Sarcoidosis (Boeck's sarcoid) is a systemic disease with protean clinical manifestations. The characteristic noncaseating granulomatous lesions may be found in most organ systems. Despite intensive research, the etiology of this disease remains obscure (Utz and associates). Most authors state that tuberculosis must be excluded by culture and allergy tests before diagnosing sarcoidosis (Kirklin and Morton); however, both disease processes have been reported in the same patient (Davidson and associates).

Pulmonary involvement with bilateral linear diffuse infiltrations extending peripherally from the hilum is the commonest objective evidence of this disease (Fig. 6–98). Usually only the lower two thirds of the lung fields are involved (Kirklin and Morton). Hilar lymphadenopathy is commonly present, and reports of "middle-lobe syndrome" as a result of bronchial compression can be found in the literature (Goldenberg and Greenspan). Superficial lymphadenopathy and splenomegaly are present in roughly 20% of cases reported. Anterior uveitis has been seen in 25% of some series, and, unless actively treated, will usually progress to glaucoma or cataract formation or both (Utz and associates). Skin lesions are an initial complaint in only 10% of the patients (Lorincz, Malkinson, and Rothman). *Bone lesions* vary from a coarse reticular pattern in the shaft to punched-out cyst-like lesions in the middle and distal phalanges of the hands and feet (Goetz; Mather; Solomon and Channick). The incidence (Kirklin and Morton) of bone lesions varies considerably depending on the reports read. Granulomatous lesions have been found in the synovial membrane, and 10 to 15% of the patients have symptoms of arthritis (Utz and associates).

Females having sarcoidosis outnumber men by three to two. However, life-threatening complications of this disease are more likely to develop in males. The prognosis usually appears good unless pulmonary decompensation or renal insufficiency occurs.

Prior to 1948, *renal insufficiency* was generally attributed to massive renal involvement with sarcoidosis. In fact, some degree of renal involvement is found in 20% of cases studied at necropsy, but massive invasion is not found frequently enough to account for the large group of cases of associated renal insufficiency (Jackson and Dancaster; Klatskin and Gordon). *Hypercalcemia* was first associated with sarcoidosis in 1939 (Harrell and Fisher). Since that time, the incidence of hypercalcemia in association with sarcoidosis has been estimated as from 5 to 30% of cases (Jackson and Dancaster; Scholz and Keating). Despite numerous interesting theories, the exact cause of hypercalcemia has not been found. It has been proved that vitamin D adversely affects the calcium levels in some, but not all, cases of hypercalcemia (Anderson and associates; Burr, Farrell, and Hills; Goetz).

Hypercalciuria, whether secondary to hypercalcemia or the reverse, as suggested by some authors, is a common denominator to many disease processes. Renal calculi or nephrocalcinosis or both are the inevitable sequelae to hypercal-

ciuria. Since 1948, sarcoidosis with hypercalcemia, hypercalciuria, and *subsequent renal calculi or nephrocalcinosis or both* have been more fully appreciated (Jackson and Dancaster; Klatskin and Gordon; Snapper and Gechman) (Fig. 6–99). Pyelonephritis and renal insufficiency commonly accompany this complication. To the unwary, the renal complications of this disease may so dominate the clinical picture that the primary disease may be obscured and the condition may masquerade as hyperparathyroidism or primary renal disease (Klatskin and Gordon).

(Text continued on page 675.)

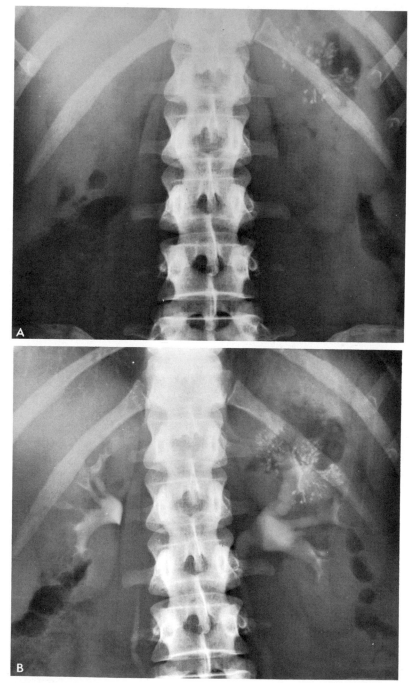

Figure 6–84.   Unilateral nephrocalcinosis (medullary type) confined to upper pole of left kidney in woman, 26 years of age. **A,** *Plain film.* **B,** *Excretory urogram.* Heminephrectomy done by Dr. Edward H. Ray, Jr., with good result.

Fig. 6–85

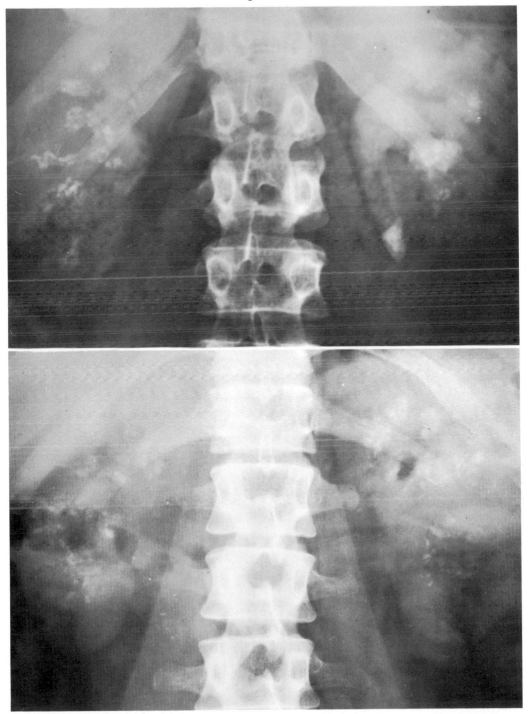

Fig. 6–86

Figure 6–85.   Medullary type of nephrocalcinosis and nephrolithiasis. *Excretory urogram.* Stone impacted just below left ureteropelvic juncture. Pelviolithotomy.

Figure 6–86.   *Plain film.* Nephrocalcinosis. Feathery type of calcification.

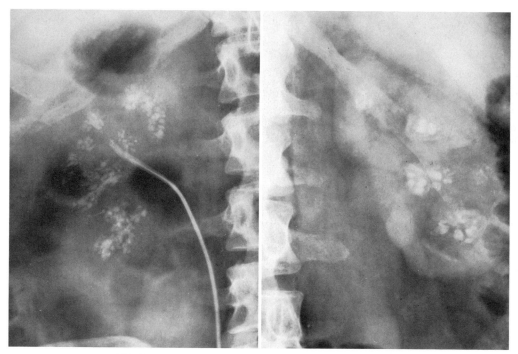

Fig. 6–87   **Fig. 6–88**

Figure 6–87.   *Plain film.* With opaque catheter in right ureter. Nephrocalcinosis (medullary type). Feathery type of calcification.

Figure 6–88.   *Plain film.* Nephrocalcinosis. Coarse granular type involving renal pyramids.

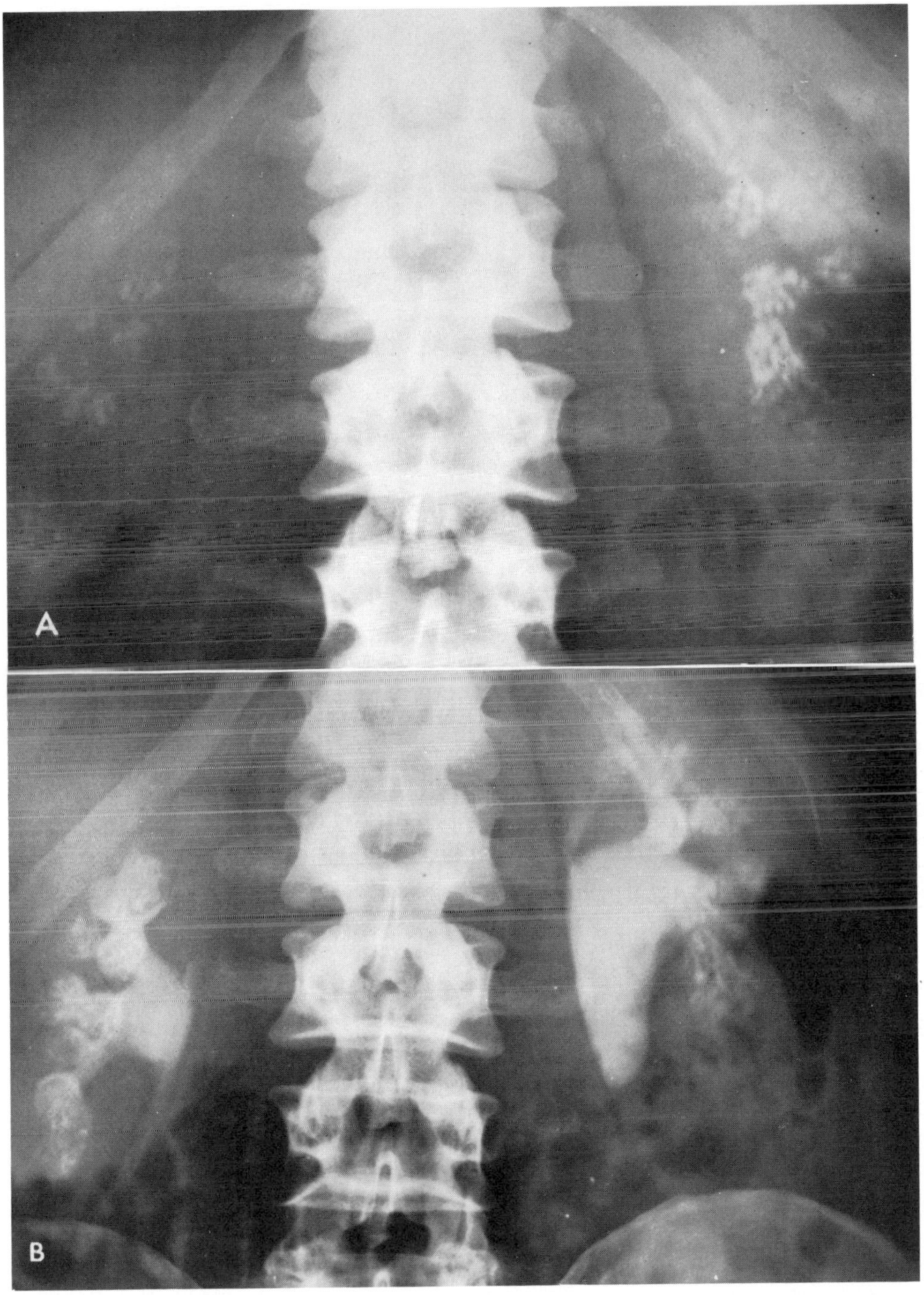

Figure 6–89. A, *Plain film.* **Medullary type of nephrocalcinosis. Granular type of calcification. B,** *Excretory urogram.* Typical relationship of calcific shadows to wide, cup-shaped calyces, showing calcification in tips of pyramids as they project into calyces.

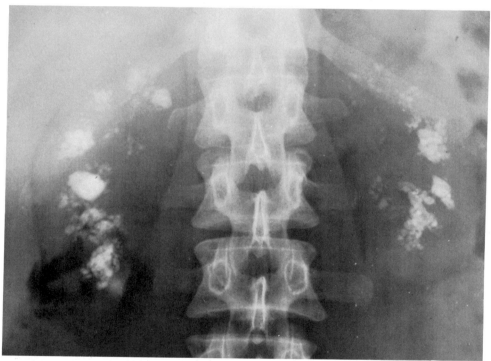

Figure 6–90. *Plain film.* Nephrocalcinosis (medullary type). Coarse granular type of calcification.

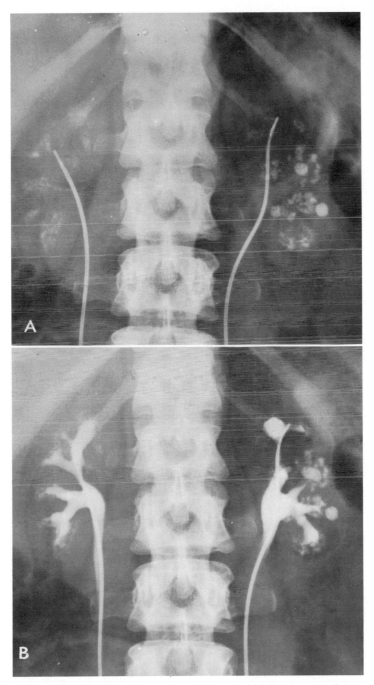

Figure 6–91. A, *Plain film.* Nephrocalcinosis (medullary type). Coarse granular type of calcification. B, *Bilateral retrograde pyelogram.* Typical involvement of renal pyramids.

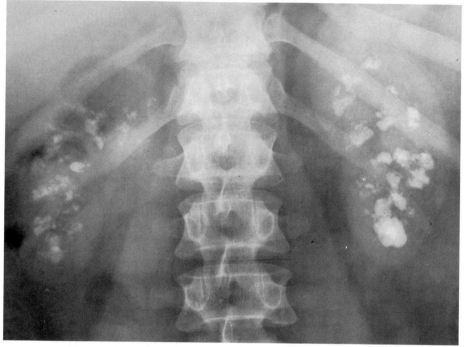

Figure 6–92. *Plain film.* Advanced nephrocalcinosis (medullary type). Coarse granular type of calcification.

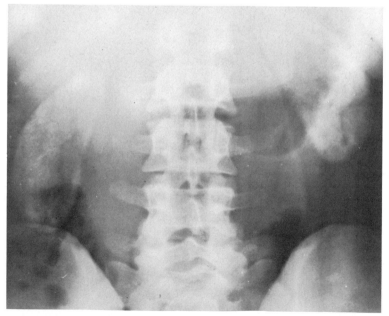

Figure 6–93. *Plain film.* Specific nephrocalcinosis of chronic glomerulonephritis. Increase in renal density caused by diffuse granular calcifications in parenchyma. Note small regular renal outlines. (From Esposito, W. J.)

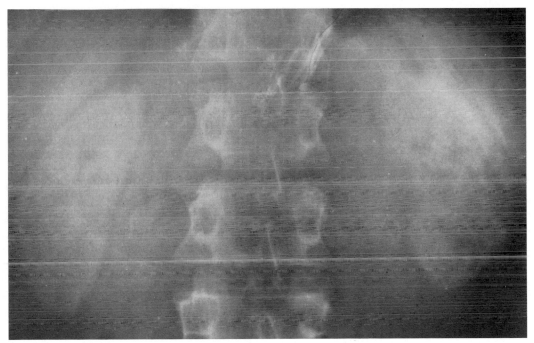

Figure 6–94.   *Plain film.* **Specific nephrocalcinosis of glomerulonephritis.** Note innumerable fine granular calcifications that are primarily cortical in location. (From Esposito, W. J.)

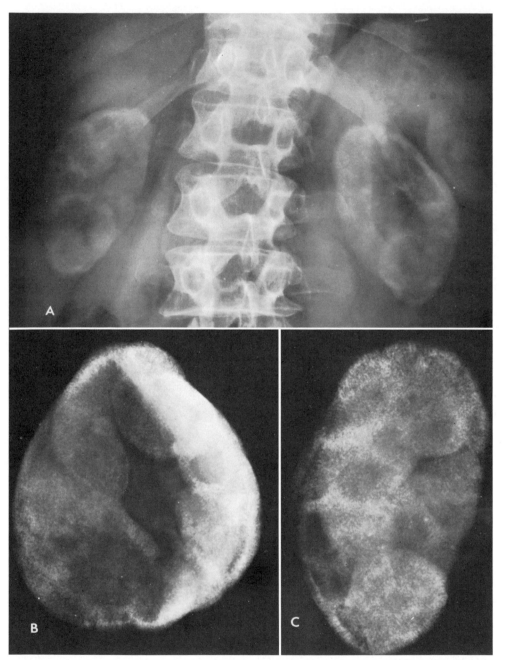

Figure 6–95. A, *Plain film.* Cortical type of nephrocalcinosis. Diffuse involvement of entire kidneys. B and C, *Roentgenograms made of kidneys removed at necropsy.* (Courtesy of Dr. Richard Lyons.)

Fig. 6–96

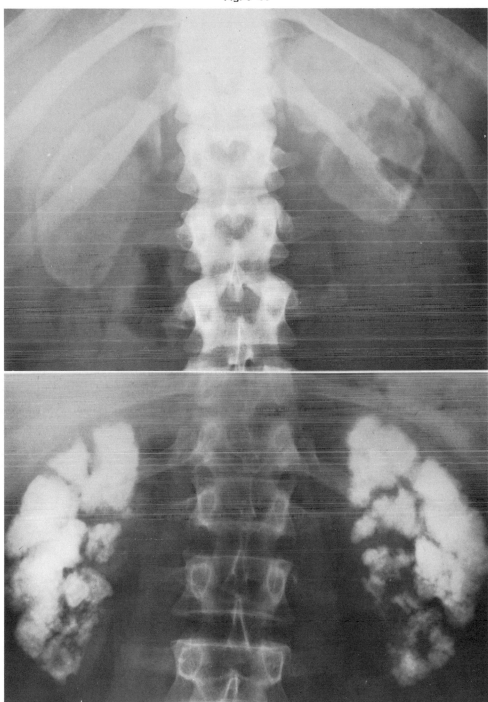

Fig. 6–97

Figure 6–96. *Plain film.* Nephrocalcinosis from chronic glomerulonephritis. Fine granular stippling diffusely distributed throughout entire kidney of man, 23 years of age, with renal insufficiency. Apparently end result of glomerulonephritis.

Figure 6–97. *Plain film.* Advanced nephrocalcinosis.

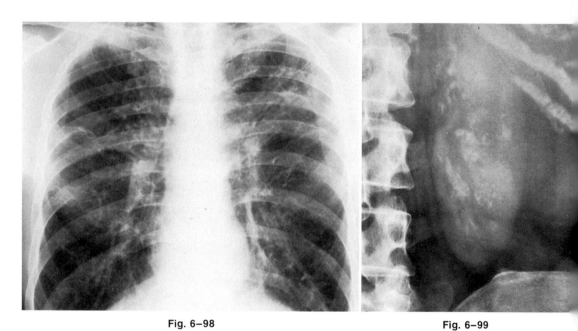

Fig. 6–98   **Fig. 6–99**

Figure 6–98.   Sarcoidosis. Pulmonary involvement.
Figure 6–99.   *Excretory urogram.* Nephrocalcinosis in woman, 64 years of age, with sarcoidosis of many years' standing.

Primary Hyperoxaluria

by
Lynwood H. Smith

Primary hyperoxaluria is a rare genetic disorder of glyoxylic acid metabolism characterized by increased excretion of oxalic acid, glycolic acid, and glyoxylic acid in the urine (Wyngaarden and Elder). The condition results in deposition of poorly soluble calcium oxalate in the urinary tract as nephrolithiasis and nephrocalcinosis; subsequent renal failure and death may occur in as many as half the patients with this condition. In some patients after the onset of renal insufficiency, extrarenal deposition of calcium oxalate occurs and is termed "oxalosis." The inheritance of primary hyperoxaluria is consistent with transmission as an autosomal recessive trait in most families.

Hockaday and colleagues summarized the clinical course of 63 patients with typical primary hyperoxaluria. Symptoms began before the age of 30 in all the patients, and only one of the group had lived beyond the age of 40. Twenty-eight of the patients died before age 20. Recently a more benign form of the disease has been reported with onset in adult life, only moderate increase in oxalate excretion in the urine, and less difficulty with renal complications (Cochran and associates; Smith, Jones, and Keating). For a complete review of primary hyperoxaluria, the reader is referred to excellent summaries (Hockaday and associates; Williams and Smith; Wyngaarden and Elder).

The roentgenographic findings in the kidney in primary hyperoxaluria can be quite suggestive of the disease and will be discussed from the standpoint of two conditions, namely nephrolithiasis and nephrocalcinosis. This is being done only for convenience, as both conditions can be seen in the same patient.

NEPHROLITHIASIS IN PRIMARY OXALURIA

When the crystalline structure of kidney stones is predominantly calcium oxalate, the stones appear as very dense, homogeneous, radiopaque shadows. The larger the stone the more dense it is, yet it retains its homogeneous pattern without evidence of lamination. Though there can be some degree of branching, this appears to be unusual. Instead, the stones tend to remain as individual ones of large size. Figures 6–100 through 6–104 illustrate the types of stones seen in five patients with primary hyperoxaluria. In Figure 6–104A the patient originally presented with very dense, homogeneous stones which proved to be calcium oxalate. They were removed surgically. The patient later developed an infection of the urinary tract with *Proteus* species and formed several laminated stones in the same kidney (Fig. 6-104B). These stones contained small amounts of calcium oxalate when removed but the major crystal component was struvite, $Mg(NH_4)(PO_4) \cdot 6H_2O$. The difference in appearance was striking.

Kidney stones composed mainly of calcium oxalate are commonly formed in patients with idiopathic renal lithiasis, hyperparathyroidism, and renal tubular acidosis, yet these stones often remain quite small as compared to the stones formed in patients with primary hyperoxaluria. The differentiation may only be suggested by the roentgenograms and is based on adequate metabolic studies.

NEPHROCALCINOSIS IN HYPEROXALURIA

Extensive nephrocalcinosis may occur in patients with primary hyperoxaluria though it is often associated with stone formation. There are no characteristic roentgenographic features of this nephrocalcinosis, and one must differentiate it from that due to other causes such as renal tubular acidosis, hyperparathyroidism, hypervitaminosis D, sarcoidosis, and cortical infarction. (See discussion above, pages 661–662). When severe it may be more widespread, extending to the renal capsule as is shown in Figure 6–105, which represents a patient who had only one kidney, with diffuse nephrocalcinosis involving most of the renal parenchyma.

In summary, the diagnosis of primary hyperoxaluria may be suggested on roentgenograms of the kidney areas by the presence of large, dense, homogeneous, radiopaque stones or the presence of nephrocalcinosis. These findings have especial significance in children and young adults, in whom renal lithiasis or nephrocalcinosis is relatively rare. The diagnosis is made through adequate metabolic studies, which demonstrate an increased urinary excretion of oxalate in the absence of other causes of stone formation or nephrocalcinosis.

(Text continued on page 679.)

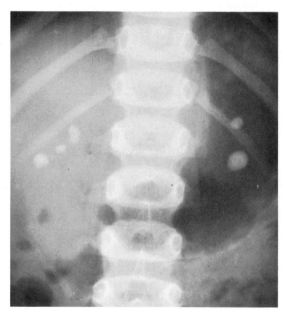

Figure 6–100. *Plain film.* **Primary hyperoxaluria** in 3-year-old girl with bilateral stones, which are large, dense, and homogeneous.

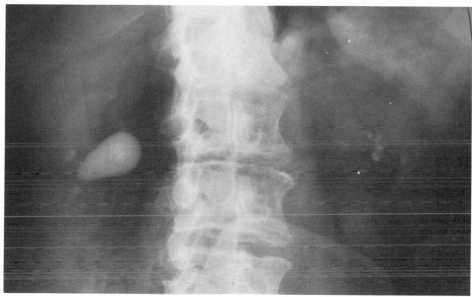

Figure 6–101. *Plain film.* Primary hyperoxaluria in 62-year-old woman with both large and small radio-opaque stones yet without staghorn formation.

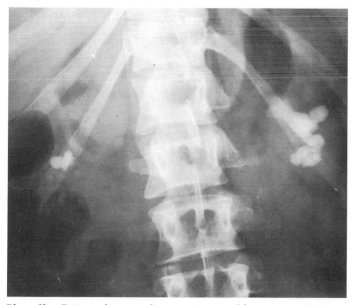

Figure 6–102. *Plain film.* Primary hyperoxaluria in 35-year-old woman with dense, bilateral stones.

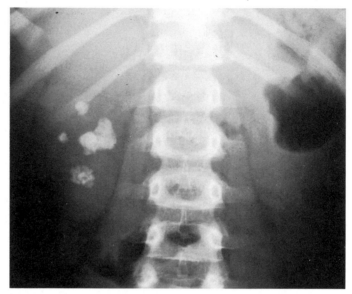

Figure 6–103.   *Plain film.* **Primary hyperoxaluria, bilateral ureterovesical reflux, and urinary tract infection** in 5-year-old girl with dense stones in right kidney which proved to be calcium oxalate-hydroxyapatite on analysis when removed.

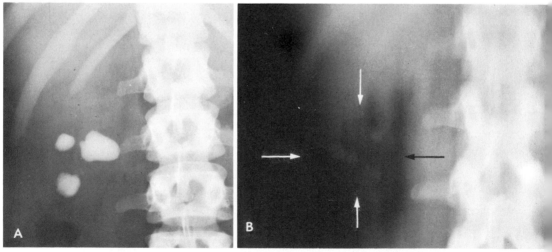

Figure 6–104.   **Primary hyperoxaluria. A,** *Plain film.* Original stones present in right kidney in 1959 were dense and homogeneous. **B,** *Plain film.* Patient developed *Proteus* bacteruria postoperatively and formed five stones which contained small amounts of calcium oxalate but the major crystal component was struvite (magnesium ammonium phosphate). The stones were much less dense on roentgenograms.

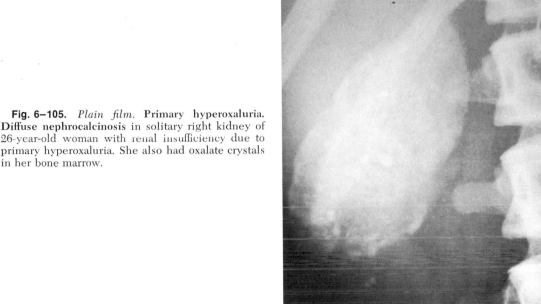

Fig. 6–105. *Plain film.* **Primary hyperoxaluria. Diffuse nephrocalcinosis** in solitary right kidney of 26-year-old woman with renal insufficiency due to primary hyperoxaluria. She also had oxalate crystals in her bone marrow.

Hyperparathyroidism

by
Denis C. O'Sullivan

PRIMARY HYPERPARATHYROIDISM

Primary hyperparathyroidism is characterized by excessive production of parathyroid hormone and failure of the homeostatic mechanism, which inhibits production of parathyroid hormone when serum calcium becomes increased. This mechanism maintains the calcium in the extracellular fluid within narrow limits. The incidence of this condition is difficult to determine but the diagnosis is being made with increasing frequency (McGeown). The accuracy of calcium determination by the laboratory plays a large part in confirming the diagnosis. The ratio of females to males in most series is 2 to 1 (Irvine).

Pathology

Keating's series from the Mayo Clinic is representative of most series. He found a single adenoma in 335 (88%), two or more adenomas in 23 (6%), primary hyperplasia in 19 (5%), and carcinoma in 3 (1%). Multiple parathyroid adenomas may be asssociated with adenomas of other endocrine glands (Moldawer, Nardi, and Raker; Underdahl, Woolner, and Black). Parathyroid hormone acts on the kidneys, bone, and bowel. It causes increased reabsorption of calcium from the distal tubules (Widrow and Levinsky), mobilization of calcium from the bones, and increased absorption of calcium from the small bowel, thus increasing the calcium level in the extracellular fluid. As the serum calcium level rises the ability of the renal tubules to reabsorb calcium is exceeded and hypercalciuria develops (Talmage and Kraintz). This in turn is the basis for stone formation and nephrocalcinosis in this disease. Thyrocalcitonin is a thyroid hormone (Foster and associates; Hirsch, Gauthier, and Munson) which lowers the serum calcium level but its role in calcium homeostasis is uncertain at present.

Symptoms

Stone formation in the urinary tract and the symptoms associated with it are present in more than two thirds of patients with hyperparathyroidism. Any patient with calculi in the kidney, ureter, or bladder should be checked for hyperparathyroidism. Bone involvement with bone pain, skeletal deformities, cyst formation, or pathologic fracture is the second commonest mode of presentation. Gastrointestinal symptoms associated with hypercalcemia are anorexia, nausea, vomiting, and constipation. An association between hyperparathyroidism and pancreatitis has also been described (Herskovic, Keating, and Gross). Approximately 10% of patients with hyperparathyroidism have peptic ulcer. In a few of these the ulcer has been proven to be part of the Zollinger-Ellison syndrome. Occasional instances of peptic ulcer have been observed (Condon and associates) which did not respond to treatment until the parathyroid adenoma had been removed. In the majority of cases, however, it is reasonably certain that the coexistence of peptic ulcer and hyperparathyroidism is fortuitous. The symptoms of hypercalcemia are sometimes so vague as to suggest a psychoneurotic origin. The polyuria and polydipsia associated with this condition may suggest the diagnosis of diabetes mellitus or diabetes insipidus. Unusual modes of presentation are occasionally reported; for example, tetany in a newborn infant can occur when the mother has unrecognized hyperparathyroidism, and giant cell tumor of a vertebra has presented as paraplegia (Shaw and Davies).

Laboratory Findings

Increase of serum calcium is the *sole* reliable diagnostic criterion of this disease. The concentration of serum inorganic phosphorus is sometimes decreased as is the tubular reabsorption of phosphorus, but these are unreliable diagnostic criteria since they are frequently normal in hyperparathyroidism and frequently altered in other conditions. Although the concentration of serum inorganic phosphorus may be within normal limits in many cases of hyperparathyroidism it is generally at the lower end of the normal range so that some additional insight is often provided by measuring it. Other tests such as the response to calcium infusion or the excretion of phosphate in the urine have not proved consistently reliable. The estimation of human parathyroid hormone by radioimmunoassay is the most sensitive test available (Williams) and holds promise as a diagnostic aid, but the difficulty in procuring a satisfactory human antigen has not been overcome. The hypercalcemia of hyperparathyroidism persists when cortisone is administered; this helps distinguish it from the hypercalcemia of other conditions.

Roentgenographic Findings

Calculi in the kidneys, ureters, or bladder are present in more than two thirds of the cases of hyperparathyroidism (Black and Zimmer; Welbourn and Selwood) (Figs. 6–106 and 6–107). Nephrocalcinosis is a much rarer manifestation of this condition. The presence of bladder calculi, even when not associated with renal or ureteral calculi, should remind one to search for hyperparathyroidism (Potter, Greene, and Keating).

Skeletal changes indicate a more severe and rapidly progressive form of parathyroid overactivity. It has been postulated that there may be two types of hyperparathyroidism: one involving the kidneys and the other involving bone (Dent). It would appear, however, that the severity of the hyperparathyroidism is the deciding factor. Thus, Black and Zimmer found no case of skeletal involvement when the serum calcium value was less than 11 mg per 100 ml. Levinson and Cooper found that the average calcium level in hyperparathyroidism with calculi was 12.3 mg per 100 ml, whereas with skeletal involvement it was 15.1 mg per 100 ml. Lloyd's findings were similar to these; he pointed out that bone disease is associated with larger tumors, very high levels of serum calcium, and a history of short-term disease, while calculi are associated with smaller tumors, a longer history, and lower levels of serum calcium than in bone involvement. An early radiographic finding is subperiosteal resorption of bone (Fig. 6-108), seen typically in the middle phalanges. Other early changes are resorption of the lamina dura and decalcification of the spongy bone around the teeth. Generalized skeletal decalcification, cyst formation, bone deformities due to demineralization, and pathologic fractures are the more severe bone complications of the disease.

Treatment

The only treatment is removal of the overactive gland or glands. Good exposure in an avascular field is essential for successful parathyroid surgery (see Figs. 6-106 and 6-107). Failure of the serum calcium level to return to normal after removal of a parathyroid adenoma indicates that one or more adenomas are most likely still present. When hyperplasia is the cause, three glands should be removed and only a portion of the remaining gland with an intact blood supply should be left. Hyperparathyroidism does not recur when all adenomas are removed or after resection in cases of primary hyperplasia except when these lesions occur in patients with familial hyperparathyroidism or multiple endocrine adenomatosis. Recurrence is the rule in parathyroid carcinoma.

SECONDARY HYPERPARATHYROIDISM

Hyperparathyroidism, secondary to renal failure, has assumed increasing importance with the expansion of maintenance dialysis and renal transplantation facilities. Hyperparathyroidism in renal failure is thought to be secondary to the hypocalcemia present in a large number of these cases with resulting hyperplasia of the parathyroid glands. Berson and Yalow have demonstrated by radioimmunoassay techniques very high levels of parathyroid hormone in chronic renal failure.

Parathyroid autonomy may occur during chronic dialysis (Wing and colleagues) or after renal transplantation (McIntosh, Peterson, and McPhaul), necessitating parathyroidectomy to prevent damage to the transplanted kidney and promote healing of osteitis fibrosa. Stanbury pointed out that when normal renal function is restored by transplantation the patient still possesses a much greater mass of hyperplastic parathyroid tissue than is now needed. This may cause persistent hypercalcemia and hypophosphatemia and necessitate removal of the hyperplastic tissue.

(Text continued on page 684.)

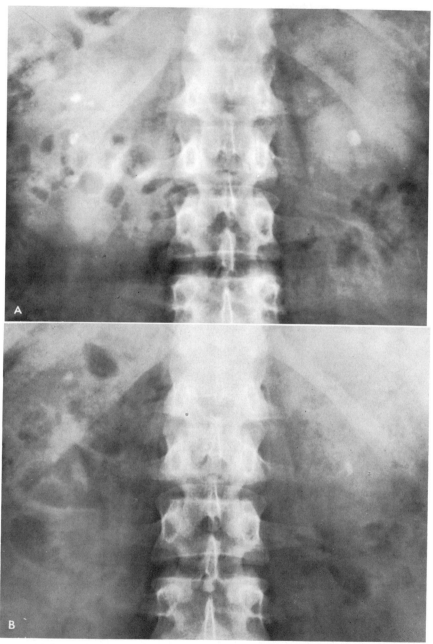

Figure 6–106.   Partial dissolution of calculi following removal of parathyroid adenoma. Bilateral renal calculi in woman, 27 years of age, with hyperparathyroidism (serum calcium, 15.0 mg; serum phosphate, 1.9 mg per 100 ml). **A,** *Plain film* before excision of right superior parathyroid gland because of parathyroid adenoma, chief cell type. **B,** *Plain film* 6 months after operation. Note substantial reduction in size of all calculi.

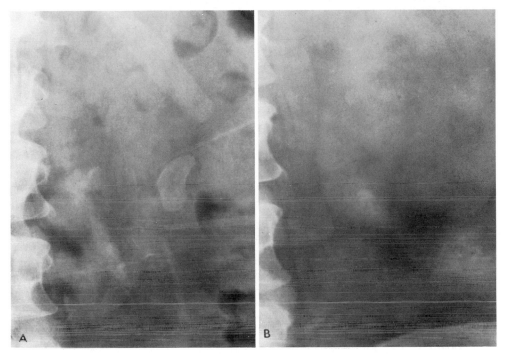

Figure 6–107.   Partial dissolution of calculi following removal of parathyroid adenoma. Left renal calculus and hyperparathyroidism in man, 48 years of age. **A,** *Plain film* shows large calculus in lower pole of left kidney. **B,** *Plain film* made 4 months after surgical removal of parathyroid adenoma. Great reduction in size of stone.

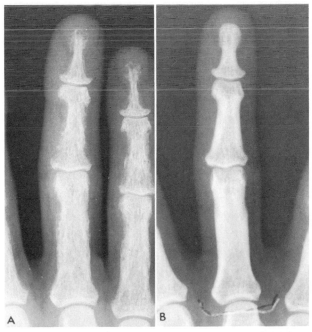

Figure 6–108.   Primary hyperparathyroidism. **A,** Before operation, showing extensive subperiosteal resorption of bone. **B,** Three years after removal of **parathyroid adenoma.** Subperiosteal bone has been restored completely. (From Pugh, D. G.)

URETERAL CALCULI

Reasons for Difficulties in Demonstrating Calculi in Plain Films

Difficulties in diagnosis of ureteral stones arise when they are of *small size* or *poor density*, or are *obscured by gas* in the intestine or *by bony structures* which they overlie. The last cause is one of the commonest sources of diagnostic error. The bony structures which most often give trouble are the transverse processes of the lumbar vertebrae and the sacrum. Careful inspection is required to avoid overlooking stones in these areas (Figs. 6–109 through 6–115). Another cause of difficulty is a technically poor roentgenogram due to overexposure or underexposure or to movement of the patient. It is not unusual to see a poorly made roentgenogram in which no shadow is present. However, a good roentgenogram immediately afterward may show the stone clearly (Fig. 6–116).

Phleboliths have been discussed previously (see Fig. 3–21). In most cases they may be recognized by their location, characteristic circular shape, and the difference in degree of density of the center and periphery. In some cases, however, ureteral stones may simulate phleboliths, and their differentiation by means of a urogram or plain film with an opaque catheter in place becomes necessary (Figs. 6–117, 6–118, and 6–119).

Opaque Stones

METHODS OF IDENTIFICATION AND LOCALIZATION

Use of Opaque Catheter and Additional Plain Films

When one employs an opaque catheter only for identification of shadows over the ureteral areas, errors in interpretation are likely to occur unless the physician keeps in mind the limitations of this particular examination. The fact that a shadow is in line with a ureteral catheter in the anteroposterior view is not sufficient evidence to make a diagnosis of stone. *Oblique* and even *lateral views* should be used to try to "throw out" or exclude the shadow. If, after these procedures, the shadow is still adjacent to or seemingly well removed from the catheter, there is still a possibility of error. A phlebolith or other extraureteral shadow may lie so close to the wall of the ureter that only the thickness of the ureteral wall separates it from the lead catheter. In such a case it might be erroneously interpreted as being a ureteral stone. On the other hand, a stone in a dilated ureter or ureteral diverticulum might be so far removed from the opaque catheter as to be considered excluded from the ureter. There is no doubt that a ureterogram is the more accurate procedure (Figs. 6–120 through 6–123). When in doubt, stereoscopic roentgenograms may be helpful. In occasional cases a lead catheter may completely obscure a small ureteral stone (Fig. 6–124).

Urograms

As mentioned in the preceding paragraph, urograms provide the most reliable means of identifying ureteral calculi. In some cases, when there is moderate obstruction but good function, the dilated ureter is well visualized by *excretory urography* down to and including the stone, so that a definite diagnosis may be made with an anteroposterior view only (Figs. 6–125 through 6–129). On the other hand, the excretory urogram may yield too fractional visualization for diagnosis, so that *retrograde pyelography* is necessary.

(Text continued on page 697.)

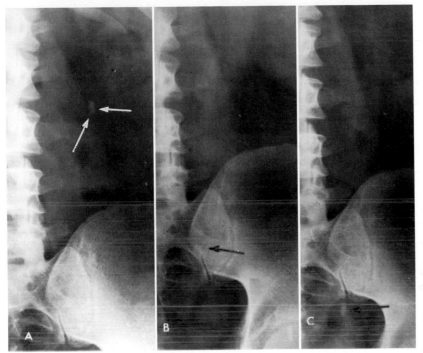

Figure 6–109.   Difficulty visualizing stones which overlie bone. A, *Plain film*. Shadow of stone in upper third of left ureter, well visualized. **B,** *Plain film* 1 month later. Could easily be read as normal, since stone is overlying left wing of sacrum (*arrow*). Indefinite shadow could be mistaken for minimal changes in bone. C, *Plain film* 1 week later than B. Stone has now descended below left sacro-iliac joint and is easily visualized.

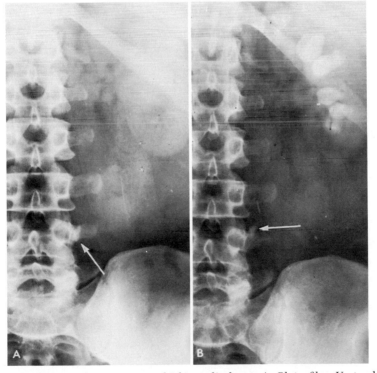

Figure 6–110.   Difficulty visualizing stones which overlie bone. A, *Plain film*. Ureteral stone overlying fourth left lumbar transverse process; could easily be overlooked as it appears to be part of bony structure (*arrow*). **B,** *Excretory urogram*. In this urogram, position of x-ray tube shifted enough to throw shadow above transverse process, where it can easily be seen. Pyeloureterectasis above.

Fig. 6–111

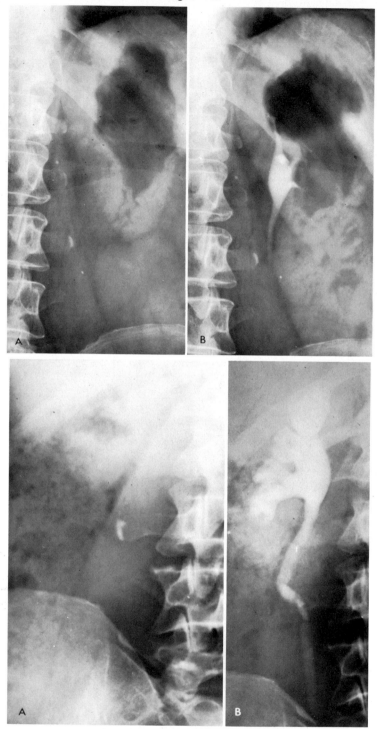

Fig. 6–112

Figure 6–111. Tip of transverse process simulates ureteral stone. **A,** *Plain film.* Increased density of tip of left transverse process of third lumbar vertebra. Might easily be mistaken for ureteral stone. **B,** *Excretory urogram.* Ureter outlined and is 1 cm lateral to shadow, excluding it from ureter.

Figure 6–112. Difficulty visualizing stones which overlie tip of transverse process. **A,** *Plain film.* Shadow overlying tip of right transverse process of third lumbar vertebra. Impossible to say whether shadow represents ureteral stone or increased density of tip of transverse process. **B,** *Excretory urogram.* Shadow is ureteral stone included in outline of ureter.

Fig. 6–113

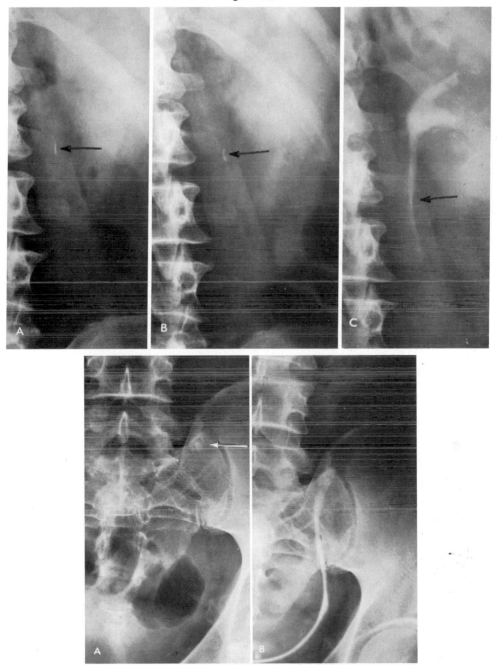

Fig. 6–114

Figure 6–113.   Difficulty visualizing stones which overlie tip of transverse process. A, *Plain film.* Shadow overlying tip of left transverse process of second lumbar vertebra; appears to be increased density of tip of transverse process. B, *Plain film.* Position of patient in relation to x-ray tube has been changed. Shadow slightly lateral to tip of transverse process, suggesting that it is ureteral stone. C, *Excretory urogram.* Shadow shown to be stone included in upper third of left ureter.

    Figure 6–114.   Difficulty visualizing stones which overlie bone. A, *Plain film.* Indefinite, irregular shadow over left upper margin of sacrum, which appears to be part of bony structure. B, *Left retrograde pyeloureterogram.* Shadow is large irregular stone which completely obstructs left ureter.

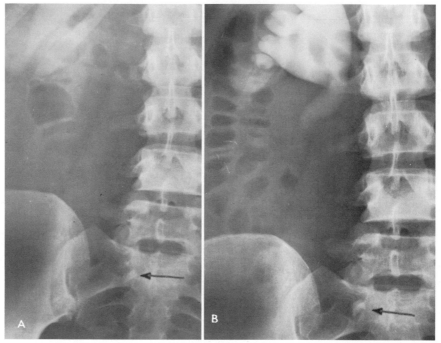

Figure 6–115. Difficulty visualizing stones which overlie bone. **A,** *Plain film.* Indefinite shadow over right wing of sacrum. Might easily be regarded as part of bony structure. **B,** *Excretory urogram.* Shadow is now more definite and is seen to represent large ureteral stone producing pyeloureterectasis above obstruction.

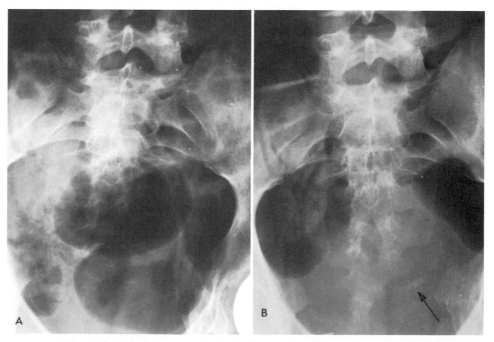

Figure 6–116. Illustration of manner in which calculi are missed because of poor roentgenograms or gas in bowel. **A,** *Plain film.* Gas obscures both lower ureteral areas. No definite shadow of ureteral stone apparent **B,** *Roentgenogram* made 1 day later, with better preparation. Shadow of ureteral calculus now visible in lower third of left ureter opposite left ischial spine.

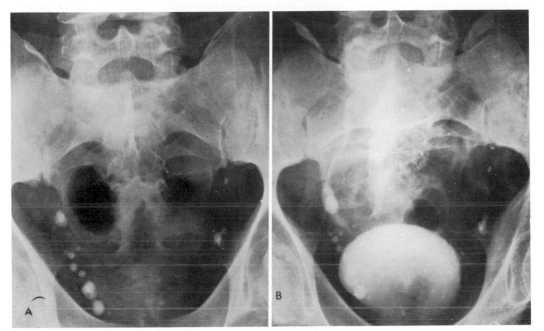

Figure 6–117. Difficulty distinguishing phleboliths and ureteral calculi. A, *Plain film*. Multiple shadows on both sides of bony pelvis which appear to be phleboliths, and fragmentary calcification of iliac vessels. B, *Excretory urogram*. Right ureter visualized and shows uppermost shadow on right to be large calculus included in ureter. Remainder of shadows are phleboliths.

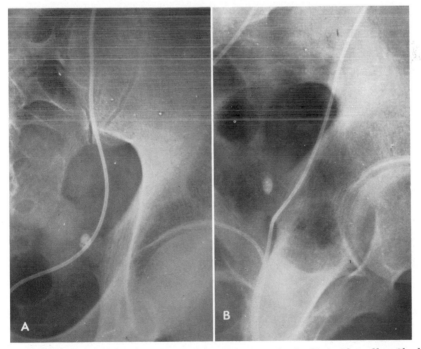

Figure 6–118. Difficulty distinguishing phleboliths and ureteral calculi. A, *Plain film*. Shadow opposite left ischial spine, with typical oval shape and center of poor density. Suggests phlebolith but is adjacent to lead catheter in left ureter. B, *Lateral view*. Shadow displaced away from ureteral catheter, indicating that it is phlebolith.

Fig. 6–119

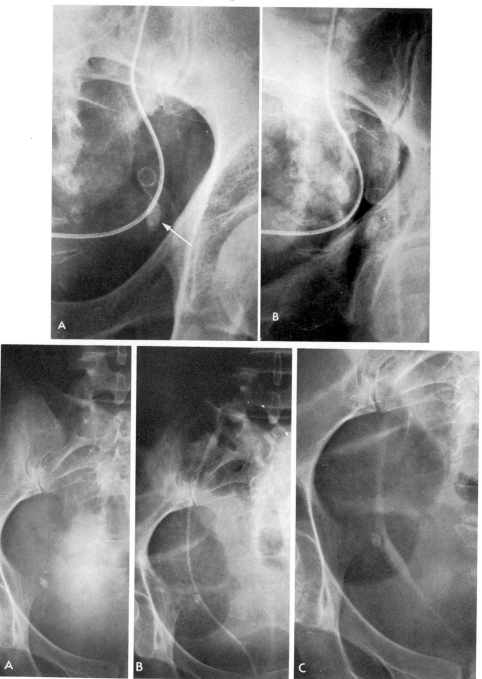

Fig. 6–120

Figure 6–119. **Phleboliths versus ureteral calculi. A,** *Plain film.* Large calcific shadow opposite left ischial spine, adjacent to calcified pelvic vessel and ureteral catheter. Identity cannot be accurately determined from this view. **B,** *Oblique view.* Shadow now appears well removed from ureteral catheter, **indicating that it is large phlebolith.**

Figure 6–120. **Extraureteral shadow simulating stone. Opaque catheter inadequate for diagnosis. A,** *Plain film.* Calcific shadow opposite right ischial spine. Could be either ureteral stone or phlebolith. **B,** *Plain film* with opaque catheter in right ureter. Shadow adjacent to catheter and might erroneously be considered ureteral stone. Oblique roentgenogram or urogram would be necessary for accurate diagnosis. **C,** *Right retrograde ureterogram.* Ureter outlined and is adjacent to shadow, but contrast medium is definitely removed from shadow and does not include it, **indicating that shadow is extraureteral.**

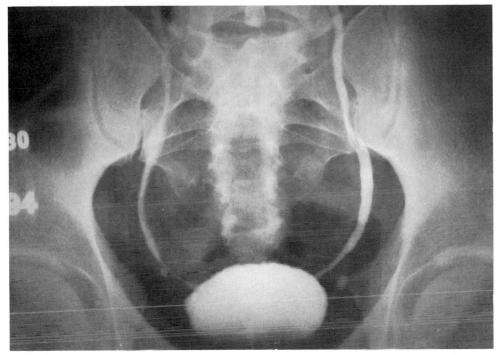

Figure 6–121. Extraureteral shadows identified with ureterogram. *Bilateral retrograde pyelogram.* Calcific shadows in region of lower portions of both ureters, excluded by retrograde pyelography. Although shadow on right is very close to ureter, it can be seen that urographic medium does not include it. Oblique view not necessary in this case.

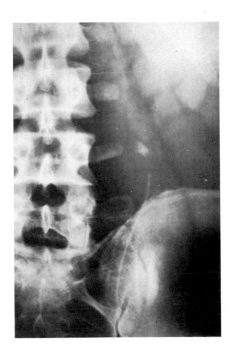

Figure 6–122. Ureteral stone obstructing midureter. Identification with opaque catheter. *Plain film.* Large irregular shadow in upper part of left ureter, opposite transverse process of fourth lumbar vertebra. **No function is evident from excretory urogram.** Catheter met obstruction in region of stone. Typical appearance of tip of catheter 1 to 2 cm below shadow of stone. This type of picture is commonly seen in cases of ureteral stone completely obstructing ureter.

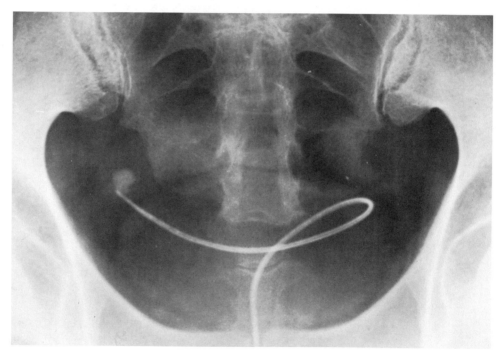

Figure 6–123. *Plain film.* Large stone in intramural portion of right ureter. Tip of catheter adjacent to stone. Oblique view or stereoscopic view would be necessary for accurate urographic diagnosis. However, on cystoscopic examination grating was felt and catheter would not pass by stone. With these additional clinical data, no further roentgenograms were necessary.

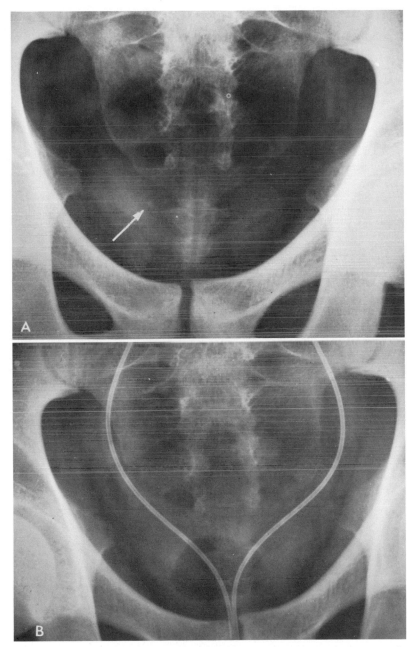

Figure 6–124.   Danger of opaque catheter completely obscuring small ureteral stone. **A,** *Plain film.* Minute indistinct shadow overlying lower right ureteral area. **B,** *Plain film* with opaque catheter in each ureter. Catheter in right ureter completely obscures small stone in lower part of right ureter.

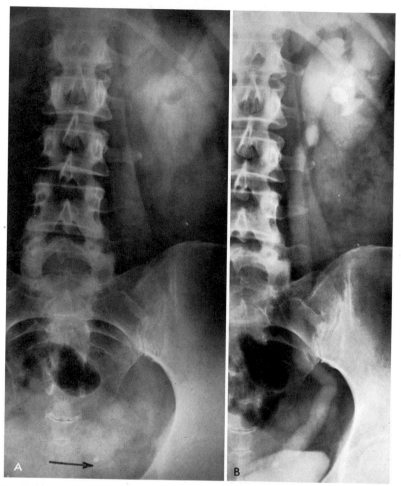

Figure 6–125. Ureteral stone identified with anteroposterior urogram only. **A,** *Plain film.* Calcific shadow over left lower ureteral area, not identified. **B,** *Excretory urogram.* Marked dilatation of ureter above shadow. Outline of dilated ureter ends abruptly above shadow, which is sufficient evidence that shadow represents stone in terminal portion of left ureter. Further urographic studies would be unnecessary.

Fig. 6-126

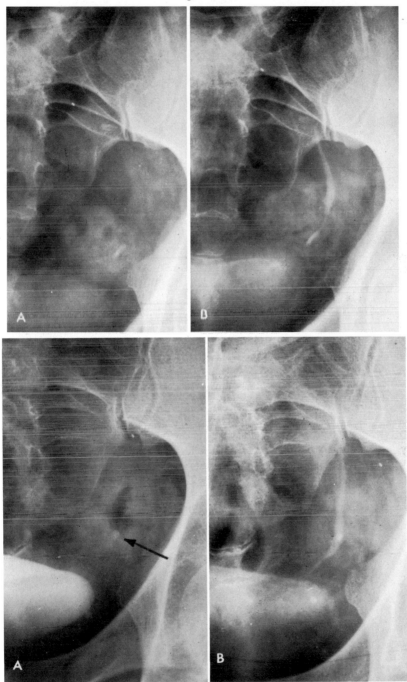

Fig. 6-127

Figure 6-126. Ureteral stone identified with anteroposterior urogram only. **A,** *Plain film.* Linear calcific shadow opposite left ischial spine, not identified. **B,** *Excretory urogram.* Ureter outlined; it is not dilated but is in line with shadow, and medium has collected around shadow, increasing its density, and indicating that it is stone in ureter. Necessity of further roentgenograms for diagnosis would seem questionable.

Figure 6-127. Ureteral stone identified with anteroposterior urogram only. **A,** *Excretory urogram.* Shadow over left lower ureteral area which was also present in plain film. Not identified. **B,** *Excretory urogram* (later film). Left ureter outlined and in line with shadow. However, absence of dilatation or other findings would still leave diagnosis in doubt. Oblique views would be necessary for accurate interpretation. This was proved to be stone.

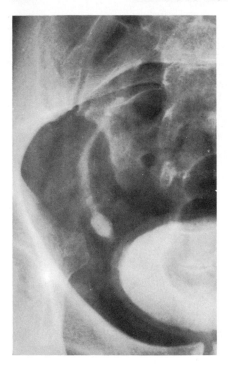

Figure 6–128. Ureteral stone not completely identified with anteroposterior urogram. *Excretory urogram.* Large calcific shadow overlying lower right ureteral area. It is in line with ureter and suggests that shadow may be stone in ureter. However, in absence of deformity, dilatation, or other pathologic changes in region of stone, other diagnostic procedures would be necessary for accurate interpretation. **Shadow was proved to be ureteral stone.**

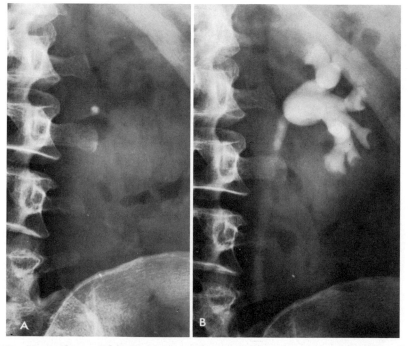

Figure 6–129. Ureteral stone identified with anteroposterior urogram only. **A,** *Plain film.* Calcific shadow above left third lumbar transverse process. **B,** *Excretory urogram.* Shadow identified as stone in upper part of ureter. Pelvis and ureter dilated above stone and contrast medium surrounds it.

The Excretory Urogram That Demonstrates Temporary Absence of Function. A rather unusual finding peculiar to excretory urography is the situation in which there is *failure of a kidney to excrete urographic medium because of an obstruction from a ureteral stone.* Apparently this situation may prevail almost immediately after obstruction occurs. The inability of the kidney to function (as far as excretion of urographic medium is concerned) is a temporary phenomenon, for as soon as the stone is removed the excretory ability of the kidney returns in a matter of hours following relief of the obstruction (Figs. 6-130 and 6-131).

The Obstructive Nephrogram. Opacification of the renal parenchyma from ureteral obstruction (renal colic from stone) was noted in 1932 by Wesson and Fulmer. From this original observation have emerged the diagnostic procedures of renal parenchymal opacification, namely nephrography and nephrotomography. (See discussion of technique and explanation of mechanics of nephrography in Chapter 1, page 54.) The consensus has been that although contrast medium in the intrarenal arteries and veins plays some part, most of the parenchymal opacification is from contrast medium in the renal tubules, in the renal tubular cells, and possibly in the interstitial tissues. Absorption of water from the tubules may further concentrate the intratubular contrast medium.

The peculiar phenomenon of renal opacification during acute obstruction (obstructive nephrography) has proved of diagnostic value in acute or subacute obstruction, especially that caused by ureteral calculi. Small ureteral calculi are notoriously difficult to demonstrate radiographically, in which event the presence of parenchymal opacification, in the absence of visualization of the collecting system (calyces, pelvis, and ureter), may help confirm the diagnosis (Fig. 6-132). Later films (from one to several hours) may also reveal opacification of the collecting system (Figs. 6-133 and 6-134).

The explanation of the obstructive nephrogram is not entirely clear. Excretion of urine is considered to be a process of ultrafiltration by the glomerulus. The rate of filtration or clearance of the renal plasma depends on the glomerular capillary pressure minus the sum of the osmotic pressure of the plasma and the intratubular (back) pressure.

One theory (Brenes and associates) suggests that glomerular filtration ceases because of back pressure from the obstruction, but secretion of contrast medium by the tubules continues because it is a process of active (vital) transport rather than simple ultrafiltration. The tubules filled with contrast medium provide the nephrographic effect.

Another theory suggests that glomerular filtration continues despite obstruction but the filtrate is reabsorbed and concentrated by the tubules. Jungmann's animal experiments support the latter view and he even goes so far as to suggest that there may be a correlation between the intensity of the nephrogram and the duration of the obstruction and intrarenal pressure.

The Hypotensive (Stasis) Nephrogram. It may be in order here to mention the nephrogram obtained during a sharp drop in blood pressure, as in surgical shock or in circulatory collapse during excretory urography. Investigations by Edling, Helander, and Renck suggest that hypotension causes glomerular capillary pressure to fall so low that glomerular filtration ceases. As glomerular filtration slows or ceases, urine formation likewise slows or ceases and contrast medium present in already formed glomerular filtrate remains in the tubules. A nephrogram is produced by this medium which persists until the hypotension is corrected and urine formation resumes.

(Text continued on page 702.)

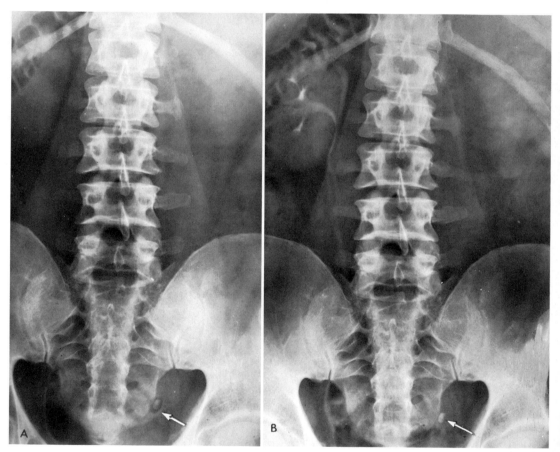

Figure 6–130. Obstructive ureteral stone (left) causing transient nonvisualization of kidney. **A,** *Plain film.* Calcific shadow over left lower ureteral area, not identified. **B,** *Excretory urogram.* Shadow is ureteral stone producing temporary absence of excretion of contrast medium from left kidney. Function returned promptly after removal of stone. Duplication on right, otherwise normal.

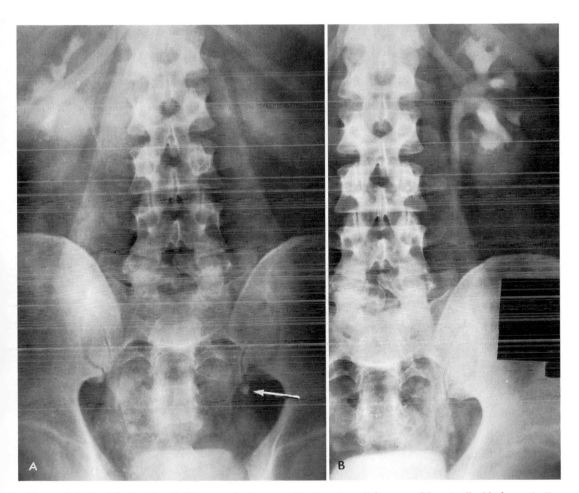

Figure 6–131.   Obstructive (left) ureteral stone causing transient "absence of function" of kidney. **A,** *Excretory urogram.* Stone in lower third of left ureter just below left sacro-iliac joint, which has caused temporary absence of function of left kidney. Right kidney normal. **B,** *Excretory urogram* 2 weeks later following ureterolithotomy. Function has returned to left kidney. Residual pyeloureterectasis present.

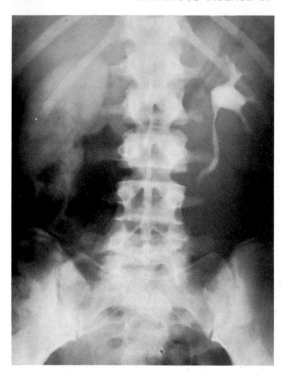

Figure 6–132. *Excretory urogram.* Small poorly opaque (cystine) **ureteral stone** (right) obscured by gas in bowel. **Renal colic with obstruction causing increased nephrographic effect** but poor filling of pelvis and calyces. Left kidney normal.

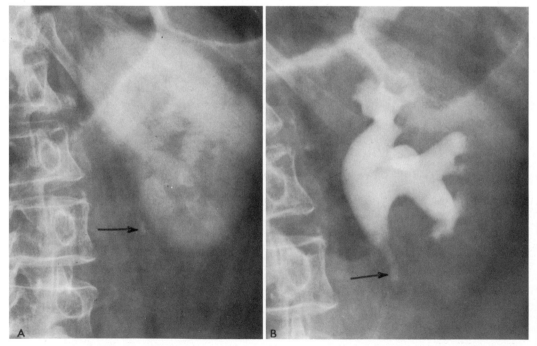

Figure 6–133. **A,** *Excretory urogram, 45-minute film.* Obstructive nephrogram from ureteral stone in upper third of ureter. **B,** *Excretory urogram, 6-hour film.* Collecting system now filled with contrast medium. Moderate pyelectasis. Note that intensity of nephrogram has now diminished.

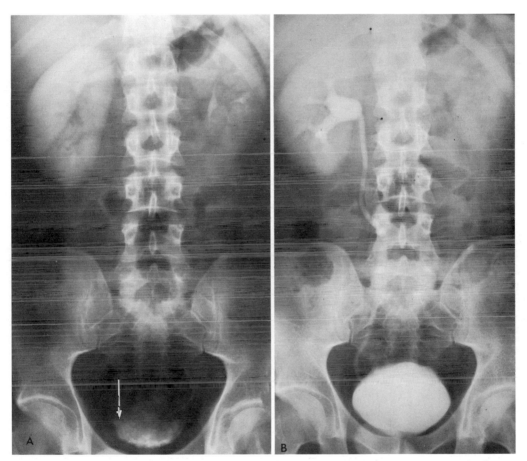

Figure 6–134.   A, *Excretory urogram, 2-hour film.* **Obstructive nephrogram** in patient with obstruction by stone in intramural ureter (*arrow*). Only small amount of contrast medium remains in normal left kidney. **B,** *Excretory urogram, 5½-hour film.* Collecting system now filled with contrast medium and nephrogram is of less density.

Oblique and Lateral Views: Pyeloureterectasis. Identification of ureteral stones by means of urographic medium presents problems almost identical with those encountered with renal stones. The mere demonstration that the shadow in question and the outline of the ureter coincide in the anteroposterior view may not be sufficient for diagnosis. The use of the *oblique and lateral views* (as explained previously in connection with diagnosis by means of an opaque catheter) also applies here. Other factors may be most helpful in interpretation, such as a *localized region of dilatation of the ureter* in the region where the stone is lodged (Figs. 6–135 through 6–138), or a *collection of medium around the stone,* increasing its density (Figs. 6–139, 6–140, and 6–141). *Ureteral dilatation just above or below the stone* or in both locations may be telltale evidence (Fig. 6–142). In some cases the ureter becomes spastic in the region of the stone, so that urographic medium seems to end abruptly a few millimeters above and below the stone. This phenomenon is observed when the stone is lodged in the intramural portion of the ureter (Figs. 6–143 through 6–147).

Pyeloureterectasis above a shadow is excellent supportive evidence that the shadow represents a calculus. Not uncommonly, however, considerable pyelectasis may be present, yet the ureter above the stone may appear to be only minimally dilated. In some cases the ureter may not be outlined with contrast medium, because contrast medium diffuses very slowly into the stagnant urine in the dilated part above the obstruction (Figs. 6–148 through 6–152). The use of reinjection, infusion technique, or delayed films (1 to 2 hours) may overcome this problem and provide adequate filling and visualization. If these methods are not successful, additional data may be obtained by means of an opaque ureteral catheter. *The retrograde introduction of urographic medium above an obstructing ureteral stone should be avoided when possible, as it may result in an acute renal infection.*

Nonopaque Stones and Stones of Poor Density

Stones of poor density and nonopaque stones may be most difficult to recognize. Often the only method available is to elicit "grating" or obstruction on passage of a ureteral catheter. Ureterectasis or ureteral spasm may suggest the presence of a stone. Collections of urographic medium around a nonopaque stone in an excretory urogram may point to its presence. The classic finding, of course, is a "negative" shadow or filling defect in the urographic medium (Fig. 6–153). A nonopaque stone may suggest ureteral obstruction from a stricture or a primary ureteral tumor (Fig. 6–154). Various degrees of density of a stone, such as an opaque center and nonopaque periphery, or vice versa, may produce unusual varieties of urograms (Fig. 6–155).

(Text continued on page 713.)

Fig. 6-135

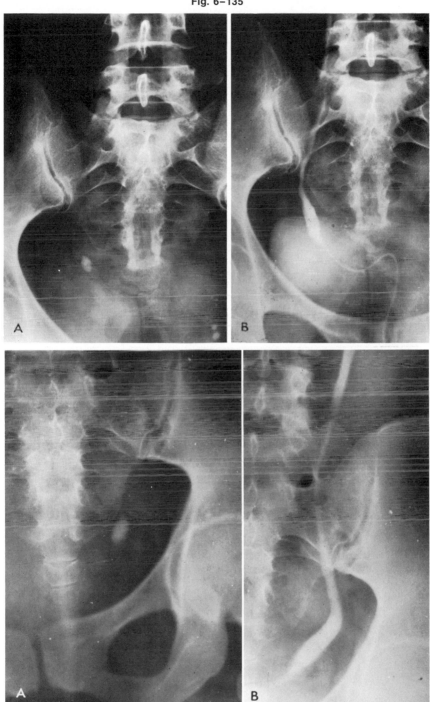

Fig. 6-136

Figure 6-135.   Ureteral stone. **A,** *Plain film.* Oval shadow in region of lower portion of right ureter, not identified. **B,** *Right retrograde pyelogram.* Shadow is shown to be in line with ureter but, in addition, there is **localized dilatation of ureter in region of stone,** which casts negative shadow, thereby offering definite proof that shadow represents stone in lower part of ureter.

Figure 6-136.   Ureteral stone. **A,** *Plain film.* Large oval shadow in region of lower portion of left ureter. **B,** *Left retrograde pyelogram.* Shadow is in line with ureter and **ureter is dilated in this area, furnishing** reasonably good evidence that shadow represents stone in ureter.

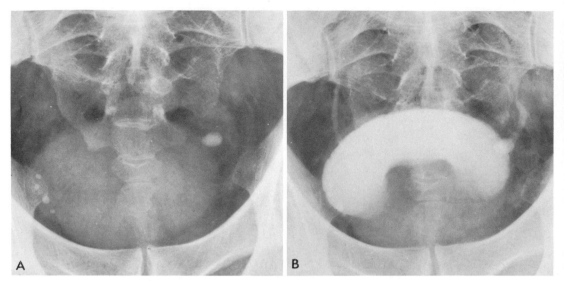

Figure 6–137. Ureteral stone and enlarged prostate. **A,** *Plain film.* Shadow over lower left ureteral area. **B,** *Excretory urogram.* Hyperplasia of prostate with filling defect in base of bladder and beginning "hook-shape" terminal ureters caused by prostatic enlargement. Shadow is stone in terminal "hook" of ureter.

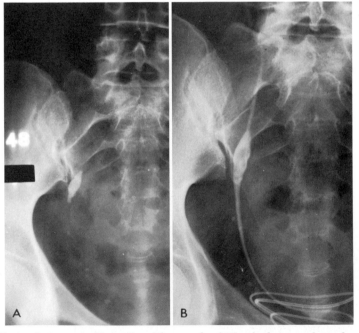

Figure 6–138. Ureteral stone. **A,** *Plain film.* Elongated calcific shadow overlying lower margin of right sacro-iliac joint. **B,** *Right retrograde ureterogram.* Shadow is identified as representing large ureteral stone, since there is **localized dilatation of ureter and stone casts negative shadow.**

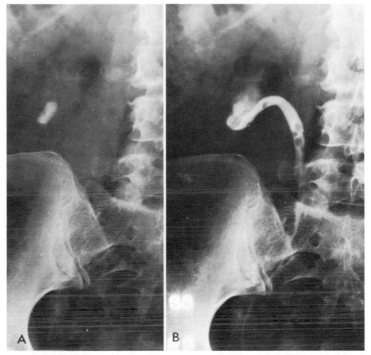

Figure 6–139.   Ureteral stone. **A,** *Plain film.* Calcific shadow just above ilium, to right of fourth lumbar vertebra. **B,** *Right retrograde pyelogram.* Shadow is proved to represent stone obstructing ureter just below ureteropelvic juncture. Ureter is angulated at this point and **medium collects around and includes shadow, permitting positive identification of stone.** Negative shadows in upper part of ureter from air bubbles.

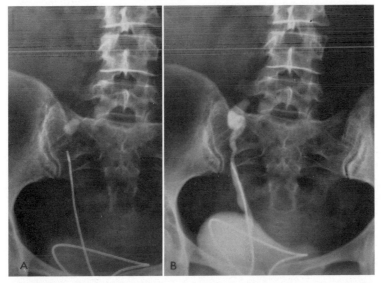

Figure 6–140.   Ureteral stone. **A,** *Plain film.* Large calcific shadow in course of right ureter, at upper margin of sacrum. Tip of lead catheter lies just beneath shadow. Shadow not identified. **B,** *Right ureterogram.* **Contrast medium surrounds shadow and ureter is dilated at this point, giving positive evidence that shadow represents stone in ureter.**

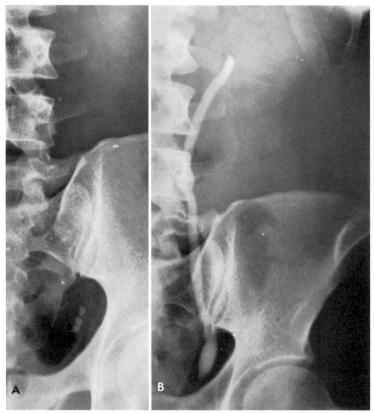

Figure 6–141. Multiple ureteral calculi in stump of ureter (previous nephrectomy). **A,** *Plain film.* Multiple calcific shadows in region of lower third of left ureter, in patient who had previously undergone left nephrectomy. **B,** *Left retrograde ureterogram.* Entire ureter dilated grade 2, but **ureter in region of shadows is dilated grade 3, indicating that they represent ureteral calculi** in terminal portion of ureter. Ureter ends abruptly at level of second transverse process, where it was ligated at previous nephrectomy.

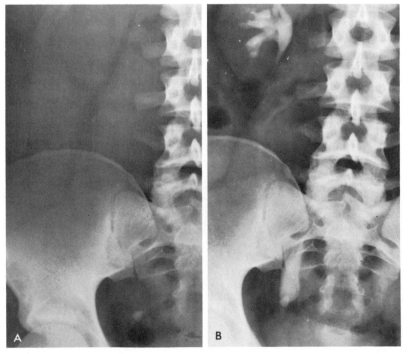

Figure 6–142. Ureteral stone with ureterectasis above. **A,** *Plain film.* Triangular shadow over lower right ureteral area. **B,** *Excretory urogram.* Outline of dilated ureter above shadow demonstrates shadow to be stone in ureter.

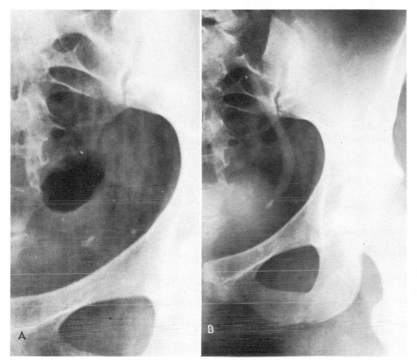

Figure 6–143. Ureteral stone. A, *Plain film.* Calcific shadow over left lower ureteral area. B, *Excretory urogram.* Dilatation of ureter above shadow with abrupt termination a few millimeters above stone. Typical finding with ureteral stone which is tightly grasped by spastic ureter.

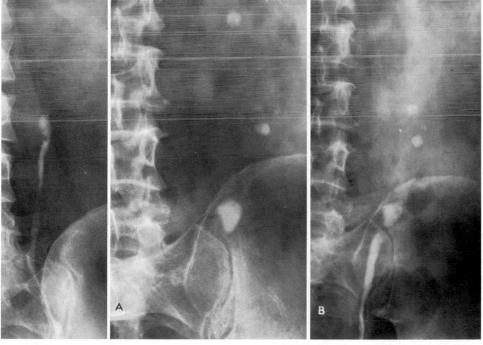

Fig. 6–144   Fig. 6–145

Figure 6–144. Ureteral stone. *Left retrograde pyelogram.* Large oval stone in upper portion of left ureter. Characteristic abrupt termination of contrast medium, which appears to end almost 0.5 cm below stone.
   Figure 6–145. Ureteral and renal calculi. A, *Plain film.* Large stone in middle portion of left ureter, with multiple stones in left kidney. B, *Left retrograde ureterogram.* Stone completely obstructing ureter. No contrast medium above obstruction. Characteristic abrupt termination of medium, which ends almost 1 cm below level of stone.

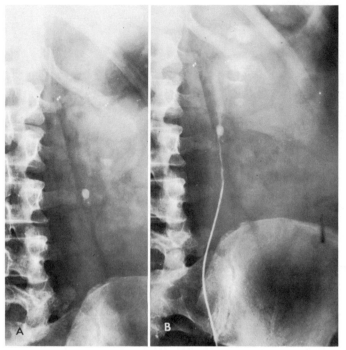

Figure 6–146.   Ureteral stone. **A,** *Plain film.* Stone in upper portion of left ureter and in lower pole of left kidney. **B,** *Left pyeloureterogram.* Stone in line with ureter. **Spasticity and narrowing of ureter in region of, and immediately below, stone.**

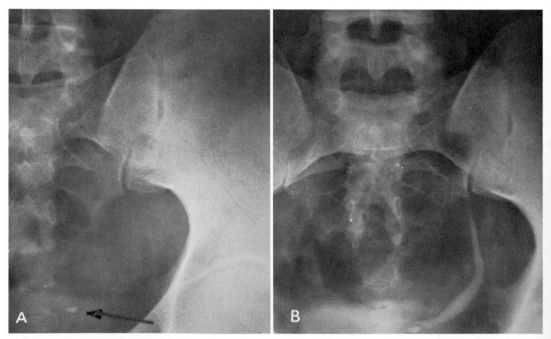

Figure 6–147.   Ureteral stone. **A,** *Plain film.* Stone in terminal portion of left ureter. **B,** *Excretory urogram.* **Characteristic abrupt termination of medium above stone,** with apparently none surrounding it. This form of visualization occurs commonly when stone is located in terminal portion of ureter.

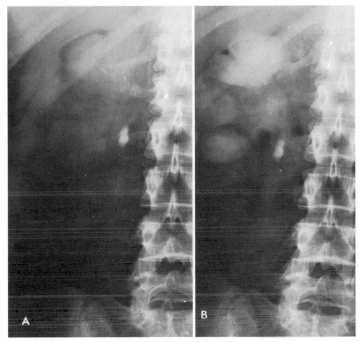

Figure 6–148. Obstructing ureteral stone causing pyeloureterectasis. **A,** *Plain film.* Irregular, elongated calcific shadow overlying tip of right transverse process of second lumbar vertebra. **B,** *Excretory urogram.* Shadow is in line with ureter. In addition, there is marked pyeloureterectasis above shadow, furnishing proof that there is stone obstructing upper third of right ureter.

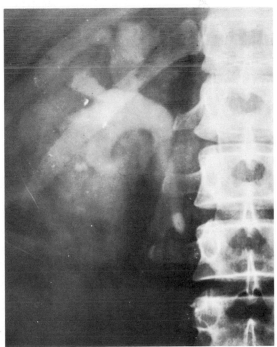

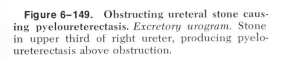

Figure 6–149. Obstructing ureteral stone causing pyeloureterectasis. *Excretory urogram.* Stone in upper third of right ureter, producing pyeloureterectasis above obstruction.

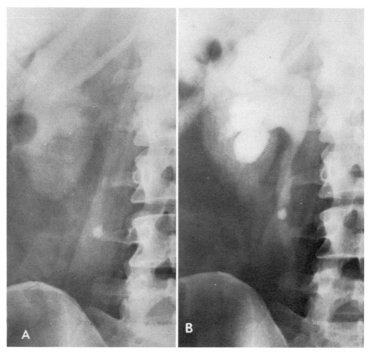

Figure 6–150. Obstructing ureteral stone causing moderate pyeloureterectasis. **A,** *Plain film.* Right ureteral shadow. **B,** *Excretory urogram.* Moderate pyeloureterectasis above stone. Characteristic abrupt termination of contrast medium just above and below stone.

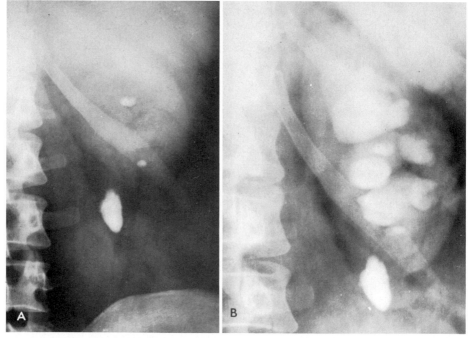

Figure 6–151. Large ureteral calculus causing pyeloureterectasis. Small renal calculi. **A,** *Plain film.* Large calcific shadow opposite transverse process of third lumbar vertebra with two smaller shadows overlying left renal area, which suggests large ureteral calculus and smaller renal calculi. **B,** *Excretory urogram.* Marked calycectasis with two small shadows included in dilated calyces. Although ureter is not outlined, it might be reasonably safe to surmise that large shadow represents ureteral stone which is cause of obstruction.

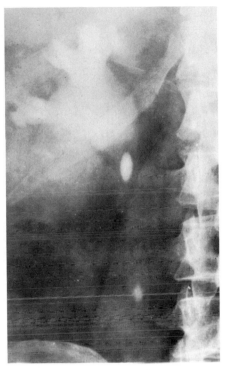

Figure 6–152. Ureteral stones causing pyeloureterectasis. **Ureter not outlined.** *Excretory urogram.* Ureteral stones, one just below ureteropelvic juncture, other in middle portion of ureter. Although ureter is not well outlined, from position of stones and pyelectasis above them, it would seem reasonable to assume that diagnosis of ureteral stones is correct.

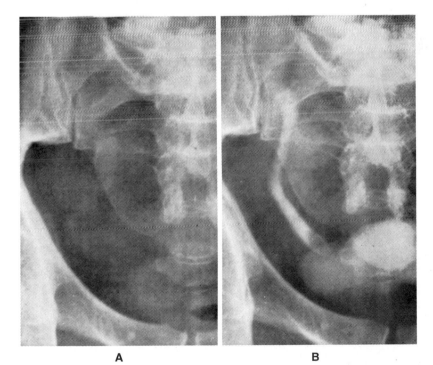

A   B

Figure 6–153. Nonopaque ureteral stone. **A,** *Plain film.* No ureteral stones visible. **B,** *Right retrograde ureterogram.* Filling defect in terminal portion of ureter from nonopaque stone.

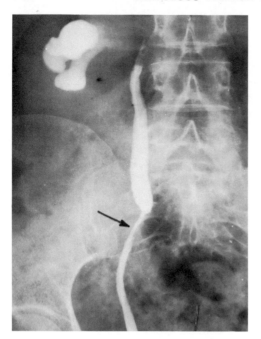

Figure 6–154. Nonopaque ureteral stone simulating either solid infiltrating ureteral tumor or ureteral stricture. *Right retrograde pyelogram.* Obstruction in middle portion of ureter over sacral promontory. Pyeloureterectasis above obstruction. Area just below dilatation impossible to fill with contrast medium. Plain film showed no shadow. Diagnosis rested between ureteral tumor, ureteral stricture, and nonopaque stone. Exploration revealed nonopaque ureteral stone.

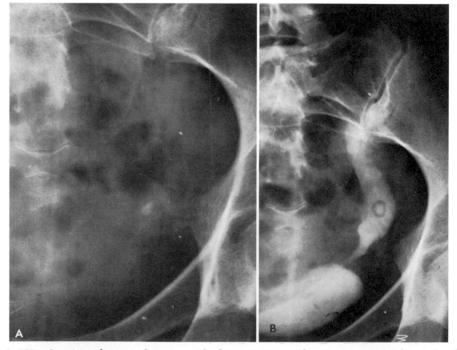

Figure 6–155. Laminated ureteral stone with dense center and nonopaque periphery. **A,** *Plain film.* Small calcific shadow opposite left ischial spine. **B,** *Excretory urogram.* Moderate dilatation of lower portion of left ureter. Nonopaque periphery of stone forms negative shadow, while center of shadow is of same density as urographic medium.

Miscellaneous Types, Locations, and Problems

STONES IN DILATED URETERS: LARGE URETERAL STONES

In advanced ureterectasis, single or multiple stones may move around freely in the ureter and by so doing change their appearance and location from film to film. The degree of dilatation and tortuosity of the ureters may be so great also that the shadows observed in the plain film would suggest that they were extraureteral.* Occasionally ureteral calculi can assume enormous proportions (Figs. 6–156 through 6–161).

URETERAL CALCULI IN ANOMALIES

The problem of ureteral stone in congenital anomalies is chiefly that of ureteral reduplication. (This condition will be discussed in Chapter 12.) It is not difficult to realize the errors that would be possible in such a situation. If the duplication were not recognized, a stone in one ureter obstructing one segment of a kidney might be called an extraurinary shadow if the other ureter only were visualized. Diagnosis may be most difficult in cases of incomplete duplication. In such cases the ureteral catheter usually will pass up only one branch of the ureter because of the anatomic arrangement at the site of bifurcation. In such a case it might be impossible to introduce an opaque catheter or medium up the other branch of the ureter where the stone was lodged. If the renal segment serving this branch of the ureter were temporarily functionless (to excretory urography), diagnosis would be difficult (Fig. 6–162).

---

*Stones associated with ureteroceles will be described in Chapter 12 (see Figs. 12–246 and 12–247).

MIGRATORY STONES

In most cases a ureteral stone moves only one way (down) in a ureter. In the occasional case, however, stones seem to change position and move up and down the ureter freely. In one film they may be in the lower part of the ureter, while in a later film they may be in the upper part or even in the renal pelvis. Although in most cases this means a dilated ureter, cases are encountered in which there appears to be little or no ureterectasis (Fig. 6–163).

STONES IN INTRAMURAL PART OF URETER

Mention has been made previously (Chapter 4) of the normal urographic relationship between the interureteric ridge and the intramural ureters (see Figs. 4–169, 4–170, and 4–172). Edling demonstrated that in cases of stone, tumor, or other lesions of the intramural ureter, alteration of this normal relationship could be helpful in diagnosis. All urologists are aware of the tremendous amount of edema that may be present in some cases when a stone is impacted in the intramural ureter. Cystoscopically it appears as a red granular areola often associated with bullous edema, which may reach such proportions that it may be mistaken for an infiltrating carcinoma of the bladder.

Edema of the intramural ureter increases the distance between the ureteral lumen and the interureteric ridge. When edema is minimal, the condition may be recognized only by comparing the two sides, which normally are symmetrical. The normal distance between the ureteral lumen and interureteric ridge is about 2 to 3 mm; when mild edema due to a stone is present, a slight increase in this distance (plus the presence of a small calcific shadow) may indicate the correct diagnosis of ureteral stone. In a recent communication on this subject Camiel emphasized the importance of this urographic observation and pointed out large radiolucent shadows or filling defects that may result from extensive periureteral edema. The edema may involve just the area of the ureteral orifice, or it may include the entire intramural ureter, which will appear as a radiolucent shadow which may be cylindrical, tulip-shaped, oval, or round or may even appear as a "halo" or "cobra head" effect around the stone or dilated ureter similar to that seen in cases of ureterocele. The contour of the interureteric ridge may also be altered by the edema (Figs. 6–164, 6–165, and 6–166).

The edema may be so extensive, diffuse, and poorly defined that the shadow does not appear to be confined strictly to the region of the ureteral orifice and intramural ureter. In some cases irritation around the intramural ureter may cause spastic ipsilateral contraction of the bladder with its typical urographic appearance (Fig. 6–167).

It should be appreciated that all of the findings enumerated may be present for a short time after the stone has passed or may be the result of traumatic edema from manipulation for a ureteral stone (see Fig. 6–172). It is important to remember also that even though the kidney on the involved side is not functioning (temporarily), the cystogram produced by contrast medium from the opposite kidney will demonstrate the radiolucent filling defects; it is not necessary for the involved ureter to be outlined with contrast medium before making the correct diagnosis.

TRANSURETHRAL MANIPULATION OF URETERAL CALCULI

The transurethral manipulation of ureteral stones presents urographic problems that are usually not too difficult of evaluation. Occasionally a stone may be engaged in an Ellik looped catheter or a Councill or Johnson (wire basket) stone extractor and held up in the ureter so that it cannot be withdrawn. In such a case a plain film may reveal the position of the stone in relation to the extractor so that suitable means may be employed to dislodge it (Figs. 6–168, 1–169, and 6–170). Edema of the ureter and ureteral orifice following traumatic manipulation may cause obstruction and temporary cessation of the ability of the kidney to excrete urographic medium. The edema may be so marked in the region of the ureteral orifice as to cause a filling defect in the cystogram which suggests a vesical tumor (Figs. 6–171 and 6–172).

(Text continued on page 726.)

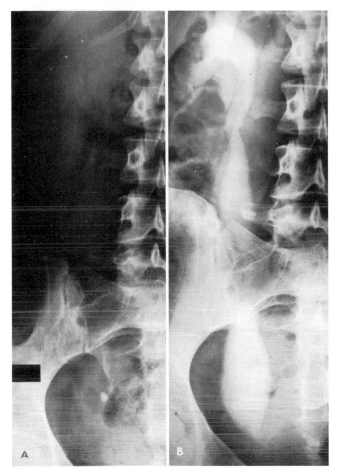

Figure 6–156. Ureteral stone in megaloureter. A, *Plain film*. Triangular ureteral stone in lower third of right ureter. B, *Right retrograde pyelogram (10-minute delayed pyelogram)*. Congenital (?) megaloureter with greatest amount of dilatation in lower third. Stone is included in ureter and apparently moves around considerably. Patient has recurring colic.

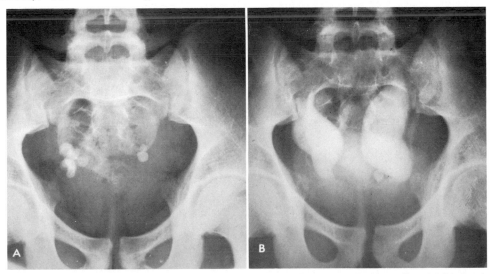

Figure 6–157. Ureteral calculi in bilateral congenital megaloureters. A, *Plain film*. Multiple shadows over both ureteral areas. B, *Excretory urogram*. Marked congenital (?) dilatation of lower third of each ureter. Shadows of ureteral calculi move around freely in dilated lower portions of ureters. Large shadow on left appears to be excluded from ureter, but in other roentgenograms it was shown to be definitely included. Unusual appearance is evidently result of incomplete filling of ureter.

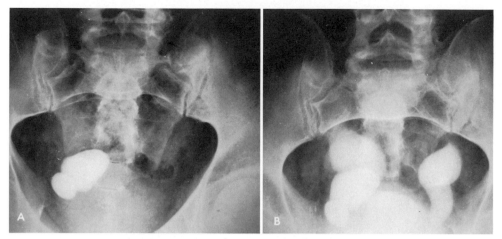

Figure 6–158. Ureteral calculi in dilated ureters suggest vesical calculi. A, *Plain film.* Impossible to tell from this roentgenogram whether large calcific shadows are in bladder or in ureter. **B,** *Excretory urogram.* Shadows are demonstrated to be stones in dilated lower portion of right ureter.

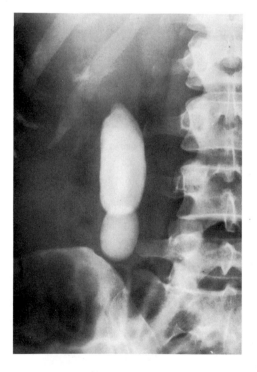

Figure 6–159. *Excretory urogram.* Large ureteral calculi, with poor renal function.

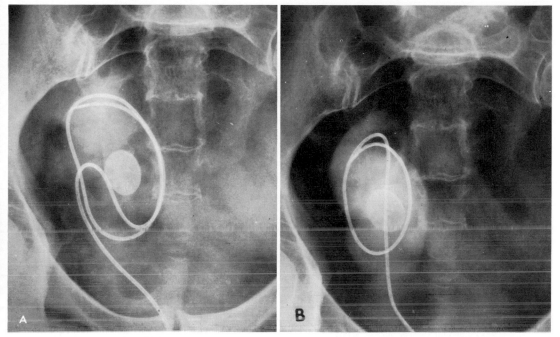

Figure 6–160. Ureteral calculus in dilated ureter suggests vesical calculus. A, *Plain film.* Large oval calculus overlying right vesical area. Lead catheter coiled around it. It is impossible to tell from this roentgenogram whether calculus is in vesical diverticulum or in dilated lower portion of ureter. B, *Right retrograde ureterogram.* Stone shown definitely to be in hugely dilated lower portion of right ureter.

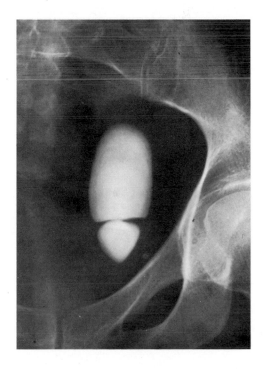

Figure 6–161. *Plain film.* Huge ureteral stone. Lower portion of stone still retains shape of minor calyx from which it apparently originated.

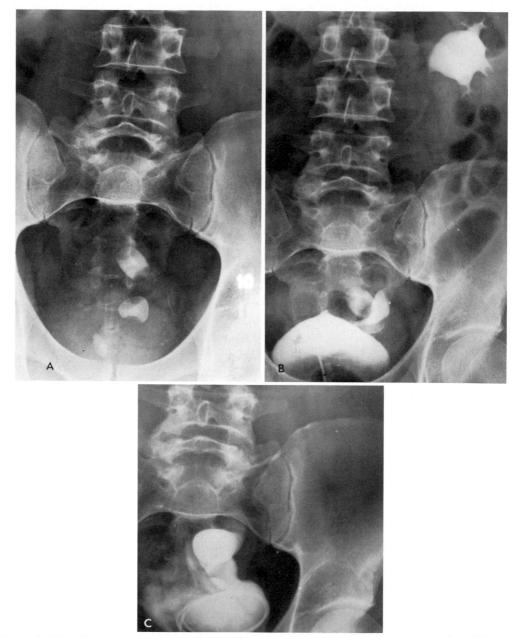

Figure 6–162. Large calculi in ectopic (duplicated) upper-pole ureter of a man. **A,** *Plain film.* Three large calcific shadows over middle and left vesical area. **B,** *Excretory urogram.* Pyelectasis, grade 1+, of lower half of duplicated left kidney. Calyces within normal limits. Ureter normal except lower third, where there is localized ureterectasis which overlies but does not include calcific shadows. **C,** *Left ureterogram.* Catheter introduced into ectopic ureteral orifice situated at 6 o'clock position in vesical neck. This ureter served "functionless" upper segment of left kidney. Dilated terminal portion of ectopic ureter included three calculi seen in **A.**

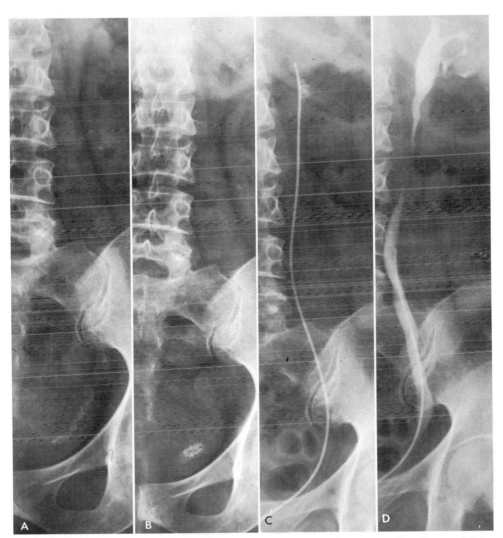

Figure 6–163. Migratory ureteral calculi. **A** and **B**, *Plain films* made on same day show multiple calculi low in left ureter with different distribution in each film. **C**, *Plain film* with opaque catheter in ureter (made 2 days later). Calculi are now in upper part of ureter and renal pelvis. **D**, *Retrograde pyelogram* shows atrophic kidney with typical vertical pelvis. Calculi are in pelvis.

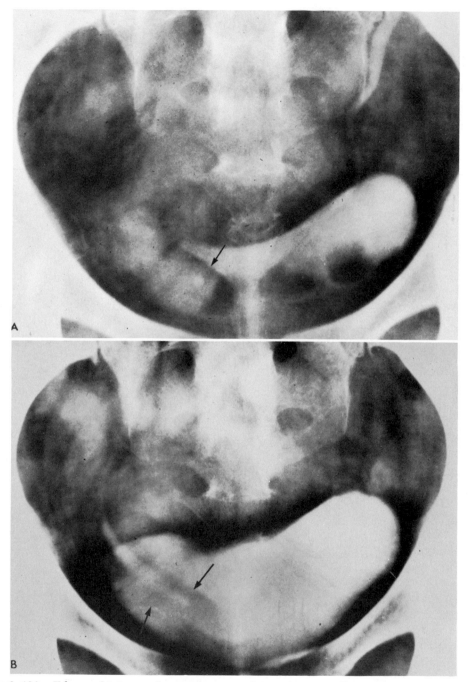

Figure 6–164. Edema of intramural ureter because of stone increases distance between ureteral lumen (and stone) and interureteric ridge. *Excretory urograms.* **A,** *Early film.* Small calculus in terminal right ureter. No medium has yet appeared in right ureter, but cystogram (from contrast medium from left kidney) shows spasm of right half of bladder and increased distance between stone and interureteric ridge (*arrow*). **B,** *Sixty-minute film.* Right ureter now outlined. "Sleeve-like" radiolucent area (*arrows*) surrounds intramural ureter. **C** (*on next page*), *Ninety-minute film*; patient erect. Radiolucent area appears V-shaped (*arrows*). (From Camiel, M. R.)

Fig. 6–164C

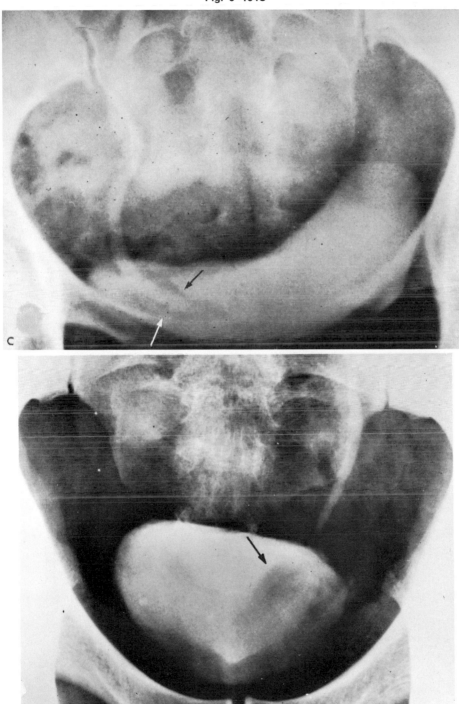

Fig. 6–165

Figure 6–165. Edema of intramural ureter because of recently passed stone. *Excretory urogram.* Left ureteral stone has recently passed but edema, still present, results in radiolucent filling defect with medial compression of interureteric ridge (*arrow*). (From Camiel, M. R.)

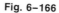

Fig. 6–166

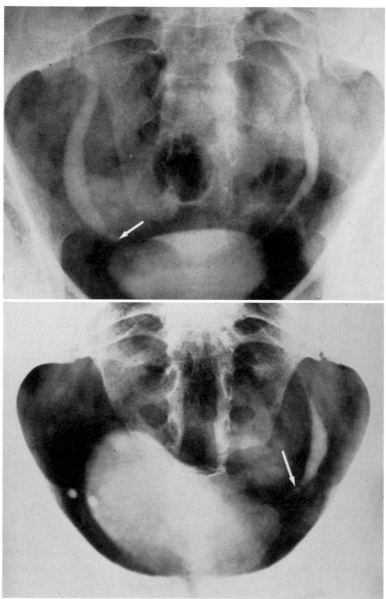

Fig. 6–167

Figure 6–166.   Edema of intramural ureter because of stone. *Excretory urogram.* Small stone (*arrow*) in right ureter at point where ureter enters bladder. Tulip-shaped radiolucent filling defect distal to stone with medial compression of interureteric ridge from edema of intramural ureter. (From Camiel, M. R.)

Figure 6–167.   *Excretory urogram.* Left ureteral stone just above bladder (*arrow*), causing spastic contraction of left wall. (From Camiel, M. R.)

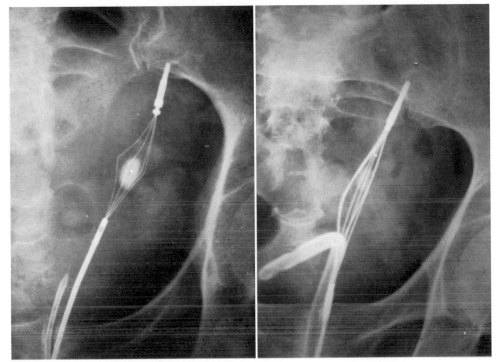

Fig. 6–168   Fig. 6–169

Figure 6–168. *Plain film.* Ureteral stone engaged in Johnson extractor. Twenty-four hours later, stone and extractor were withdrawn.

Figure 6–169. *Plain film.* Ureteral stone engaged in Councill extractor. Since it could not be withdrawn, extractor was left in place with urethral catheter alongside. Extractor with stone withdrawn successfully 48 hours later.

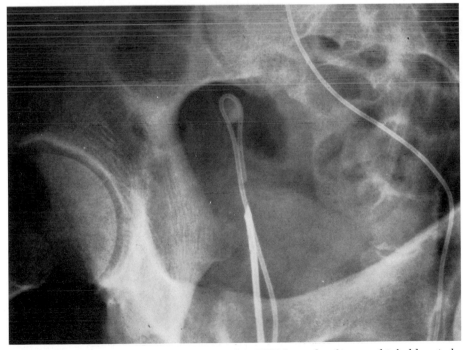

Figure 6–170. *Plain film.* Ureteral stone is engaged in Ellik looped catheter and is held up in lower third of ureter.

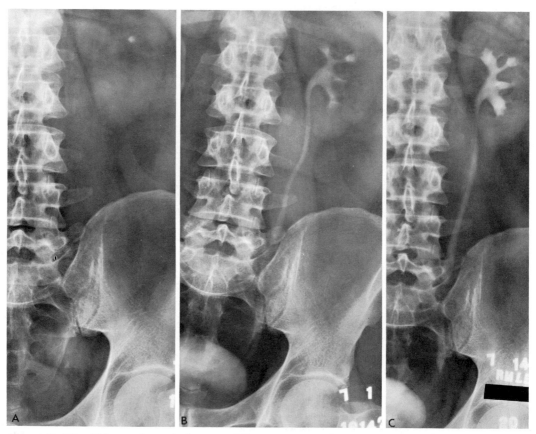

Figure 6–171.   Edema of terminal ureter following transurethral manipulation and removal of stone. **A,** *Plain film.* Shadow of ureteral calculus in lower third of left ureter; also one in left kidney. **B,** *Excretory urogram.* Moderate dilatation of ureter down to and including ureteral stone in lower third of ureter. Shadow in kidney is included in branch of upper calyx. **C,** *Excretory urogram* made several days after transurethral manipulation and removal of ureteral calculus. **Residual edema of lower third of left ureter prevents normal filling of ureter in this region.**

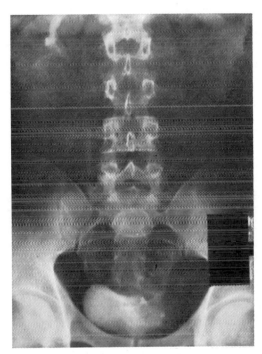

Figure 6–172. *Excretory urogram.* Temporary absence of function of left kidney, with filling defect in left half of bladder from edema secondary to unsuccessful transurethral manipulation of ureteral calculus impacted in intramural portion of left ureter. Stone subsequently passed and renal function returned to normal.

VESICAL CALCULI

Poor Radiopacity of Most Vesical Calculi

Of all urinary calculi, those situated in the urinary bladder are most often overlooked when one is examining the plain film. In many cases this is due to the fact that the physician examining the roentgenograms does not scrutinize the vesical area thoroughly. On the other hand, even if the roentgenograms are most carefully examined, a large number of vesical calculi will be missed. Primarily responsible for this situation is the fact that *many vesical calculi are composed of uric acid or urates and are either radiolucent or cast shadows of poor density.* Also, these calculi usually lie over bone (sacrum) which further increases the difficulty of roentgen visualization. Incomplete preparation of the patient's bowel often results in various rounded, indefinite shadows in the bony pelvis produced by fecal material in the rectosigmoid that may simulate the faint outlines of poorly visualized vesical calculi.

It is estimated that in 50 to 60% of cases vesical calculus cannot be diagnosed roentgenographically. For this reason one should never make the statement that vesical calculi are not present until the bladder has been thoroughly examined with the cystoscope. Some nonopaque calculi can be seen as negative shadows in either an excretory or retrograde cystogram (Figs. 6–173 through 6–176).

Roentgenographic Characteristics

Vesical calculi vary in number from a single calculus to large numbers of calculi and in size from sand to calculi of enormous proportions. Usually the calculi are circular or oval in outline, but almost any shape may be encountered (Figs. 6–177 through 6–183). One of the most unusual appearing types of stone is the hard burr or jackstone variety (Figs. 6–184 and 6–185), which gets its name from the many irregular prongs that project from its surface. This stone usually is composed of calcium oxalate. The commonest position of vesical calculi is in the center of the bony pelvis, well above the symphysis pubis. Intravesical protrusion of enlarged prostatic lobes may cause a rather odd configuration of vesical calculi, since they tend to arrange themselves around the intravesical encroachment of the enlarged prostate gland (Figs. 6–186, 6–187, and 6–188).

Stones Situated Partially or Entirely Within Vesical Diverticula

Stones situated either partially or entirely within vesical diverticula may present a rather bizarre appearance both as to location and as to shape. In such a situation they may be confused with large ureteral stones in a hugely dilated ureter. **Dumbbell-shaped stones**, with one end lodged in a diverticulum and the other projecting into the bladder, are not uncommonly seen (Figs. 6–189 and 6–190). Figure 6–191 illustrates a rather unusual case of dumbbell-shaped calculus in the bladder of a woman. One part of the stone was fixed in an area where a vesicovaginal fistula had been repaired previously. Vesical calculi are uncommon in women but do occur (Fig. 6–192). Multiple calculi situated in vesical diverticula may produce roentgenograms of unusual appearance (Figs. 6–193 and 6–194A, B, and C).

Differential Diagnosis From Encrusted Lesions in Bladder and Extravesical Shadows

Incrustations in the bladder caused by *incrusted cystitis* (Chapter 7), *vesical tumor* (see Figs. 10–317, 10–318, and 10–320), or a *postradium slough* may simulate true vesical calculi. Extraurinary calcification in the vesical region may simulate vesical stone and be excluded only by means of cystoscopic examination. Most such shadows are in the genital organs in women, although frequently they are seen in men, in which case their accurate identification is most difficult (Figs. 6–195, 6–196, and 6–197; see also Figs. 3–95 through 3–99).

(*Text continued on page 736.*)

Fig. 6–173

Fig. 6–174

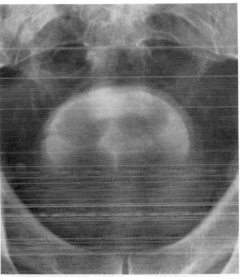

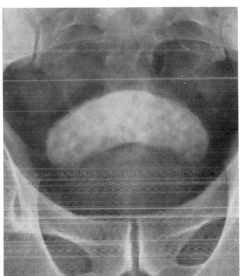

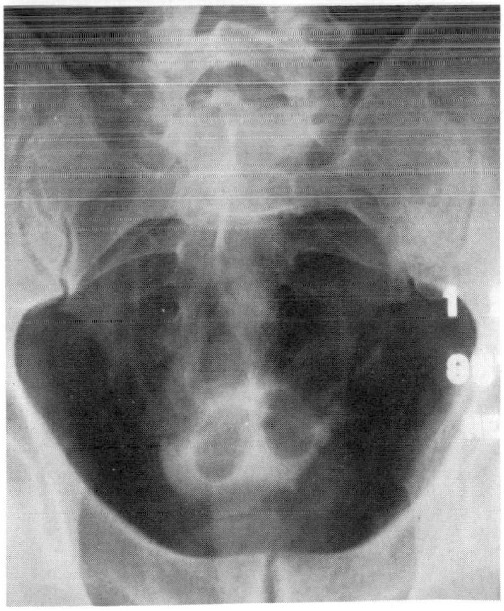

Figure 6–173. *Excretory cystogram.* Nonopaque vesical calculi producing negative shadows. Hypertrophy of prostate, producing negative filling defect in base of bladder. Plain film was negative.

Figure 6–174. *Excretory cystogram.* Multiple negative shadows from many small, round, nonopaque calculi in bladder. Note filling defect in base of bladder from hypertrophy of prostate. Plain film was negative.

Figure 6–175. *Excretory cystogram.* Nonopaque calculi in bladder produce large oval negative shadows. Plain film was negative.

Fig. 6–175

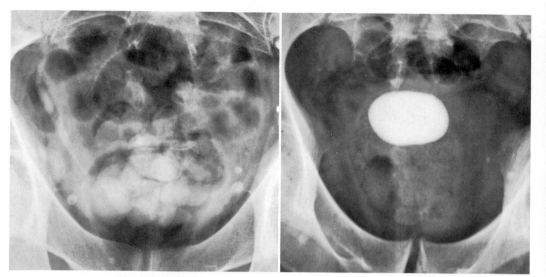

Fig. 6–176   Fig. 6–177

Figure 6–176. *Excretory urogram.* Fecal material in rectum suggests multiple vesical calculi of poor density.
Figure 6–177. *Plain film.* Vesical calculus.

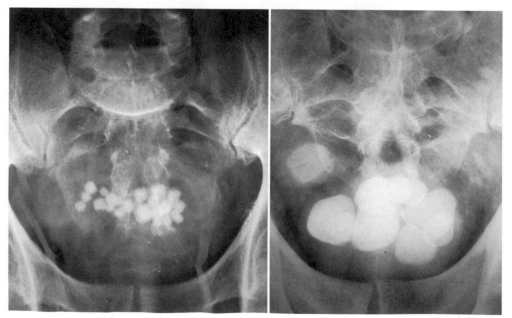

Fig. 6–178   Fig. 6–179
Figures 6–178 and 6–179. *Plain films.* Multiple radiopaque vesical calculi.

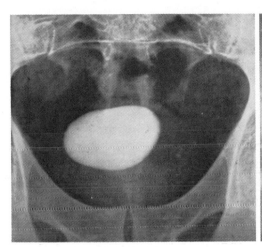
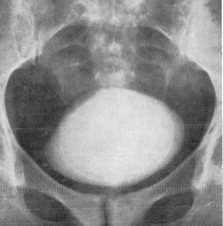

Fig. 6–180   **Fig. 6–181**

Figure 6–180. *Plain film.* Large vesical calculus.
Figure 6–181. *Plain film.* Huge vesical calculus removed suprapubically. Obstetrical forceps used to deliver stone from bladder. (Courtesy of Dr. W. N. Wishard.)

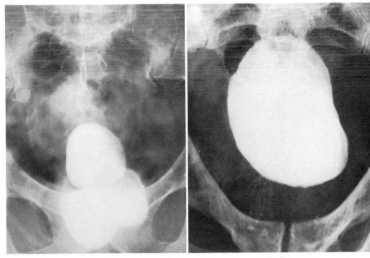

Fig. 6–182   **Fig. 6–183**

Figure 6–182. *Excretory urogram.* Multiple large vesical calculi.
Figure 6–183. *Plain film.* Large vesical calculus. Multiple small prostatic calculi.

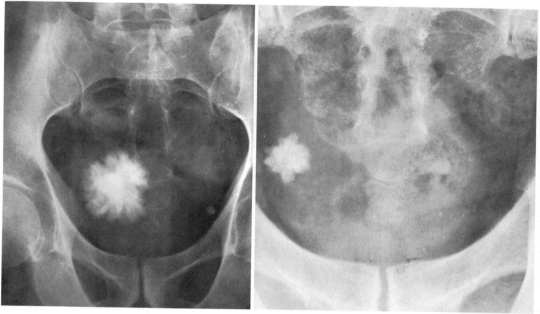

Fig. 6–184   Fig. 6–185

Figure 6–184. *Plain film.* Vesical calculus of burr-like type.
Figure 6–185. *Plain film.* Jackstone variety of stone in bladder of patient with hypertrophy of prostate.

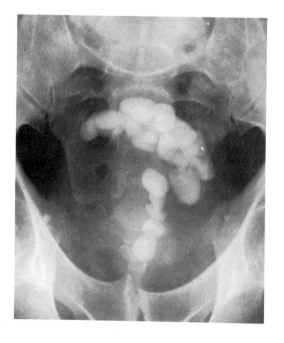

Figure 6–186. *Plain film.* Multiple vesical calculi in male patient with hypertrophy of prostate gland. Calculi are arranged around intravesical projection of enlarged prostate.

Fig. 6-187

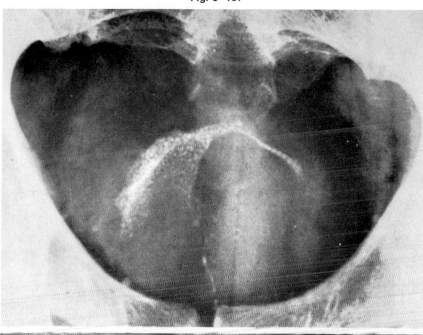

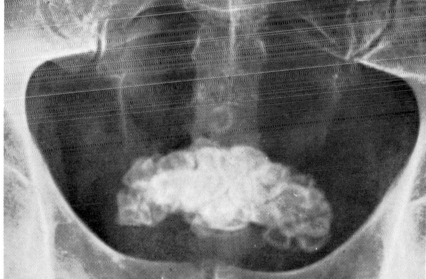

Fig. 6-188

Figure 6-187. *Plain film.* Large number of very small vesical calculi distributed around intravesical projection of enlarged prostatic lobes.
Figure 6-188. *Plain film.* Large number of small calculi in bladder distributed around intravesical projection of prostate.

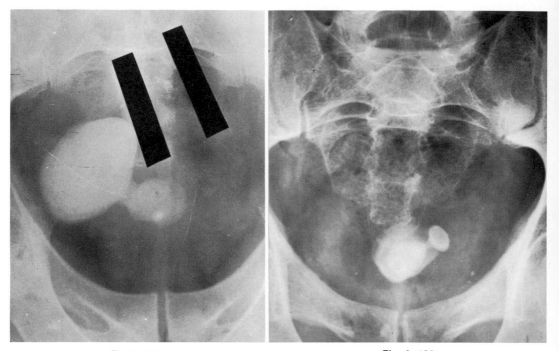

Fig. 6–189   Fig. 6–190

Figures 6–189 and 6–190. *Plain films.* Vesical calculus, dumbbell shape, with one portion of stone in diverticulum and other free in bladder.

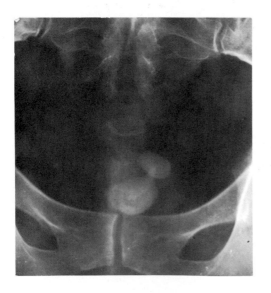

Figure 6–191. *Plain film.* Dumbbell vesical calculus at site of repair of vesicovaginal fistula. (From Cristol D. S., and Greene, L. F.: Vesical Calculi in Women. S. Clin. North America, Aug., 1945, pp. 987–992.)

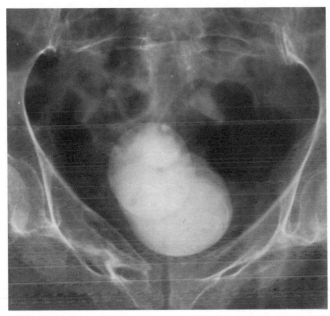

Figure 6-192. *Plain film.* Large vesical calculi in woman aged 61.

Figure 6-193. *Plain film.* Multiple vesical calculi filling large vesical diverticulum, which arises from right wall of bladder. There are few stones free in bladder adjacent to diverticulum. Urethral catheter in bladder.

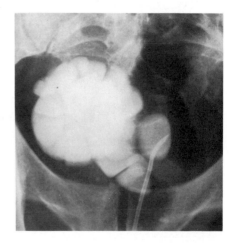

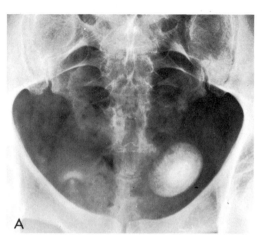

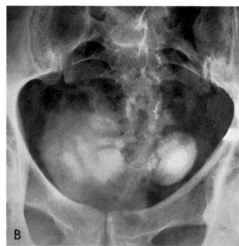

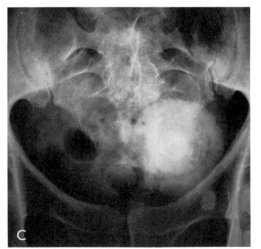

Figure 6–194. Laminated calculus in vesical diverticulum. **A,** *Plain film.* Large laminated vesical calculus overlying left half of bladder. **B,** *Excretory cystogram.* Medium partially fills right half of bladder, which is trabeculated and contains multiple cellules. Stone appears to be extravesical in this cystogram because contrast medium has not entered diverticulum. **C,** *Plain film* made 24 hours later. Residual contrast medium in large vesical diverticulum in which calculus is situated.

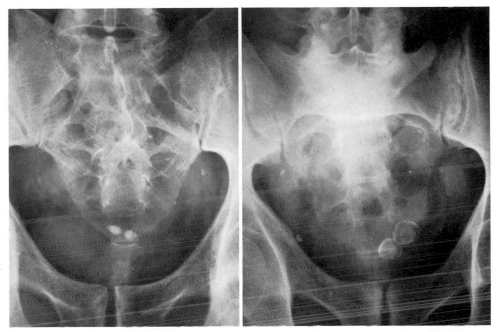

Fig. 6–195   Fig. 6–196

Figures 6–195 and 6–196. Extravesical calcifications look like vesical calculi. *Plain films.* Multiple calcific shadows over vesical region, which suggest vesical calculi. Cystoscopy showed no stones in bladder.

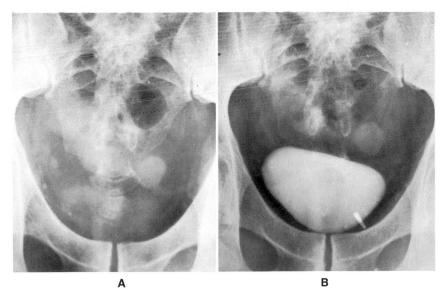

A   B

Figure 6–197. Extravesical shadow (fecal material in sigmoid?) mimics vesical calculus. A, *Plain film.* Circular shadow over left side of bony pelvis, overlying vesical region in a man. Suggests vesical calculus. B, *Retrograde cystogram.* Shadow definitely excluded; is not in urinary tract.

PROSTATIC CALCULI

Prostatic calculi may be divided into two groups; namely, *primary* and *secondary.* By primary is meant that the calculi were formed originally within the substance of the prostate gland. Secondary calculi are those which have formed elsewhere in the urinary tract and have become lodged in the prostatic urethra. Prostatic calculi often are missed because the plain film is not exposed low enough to show the prostatic region (see Fig. 3–4).

Primary Calculi

Primary prostatic calculi usually are multiple and relatively small, varying from 1 to 10 mm in diameter. In occasional cases, however, the calculi are very large and numerous and may almost completely replace the substance of the prostate gland. Diagnosis usually can be made on the basis of the typical appearance and location of the shadows of the calculi seen in the plain film. The shadows are situated in the region of the symphysis pubis, may be approximately 1 to 3 cm to either side (depending on the size of the gland), and may be above or below the level of the symphysis, depending on the length of the prostate, their location in the prostate, and the angle at which the film is exposed. When the shadows are projected a considerable distance above the symphysis, it may be difficult to decide whether they are vesical or prostatic calculi (Figs. 6–198 through 6–205; see also Fig. 3–4).

Secondary Calculi

Secondary calculi usually are larger and fewer than primary calculi. It is not always possible to distinguish roentgenographically between primary and secondary stones, so that the patient's history and the results of other urologic investigation, especially cystoscopic examination, may be necessary to enable one to make a decision (Figs. 6–206 through 6–210).

URETHRAL CALCULI

In most instances urethral calculi are relatively small ureteral or vesical calculi which, during the act of micturition, have passed into the urethra and have become lodged there. Occasionally, however, it is possible for a stone to form primarily in the urethra in a region where there is stasis of urine, owing to some pathologic change such as *urethral stricture* or *urethral diverticulum.* Diagnosis in such cases usually is made most easily by means of cystoscopy and urethral instrumentation of various types, although at times roentgenography and urethrography are helpful (Figs. 6–211 through 6–215).

(References begin on page 745.)

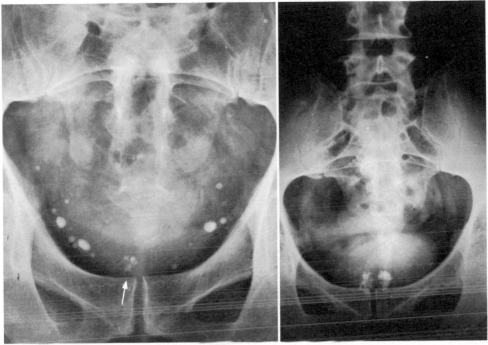

Fig. 6-198   Fig. 6-199

Figure 6-198. *Plain film.* Phleboliths on both sides of bony pelvis. Multiple minute prostatic calculi to right of midline.

Figure 6-199. *Plain film.* Multiple prostatic calculi.

Figure 6-200. *Plain film.* Multiple prostatic calculi.

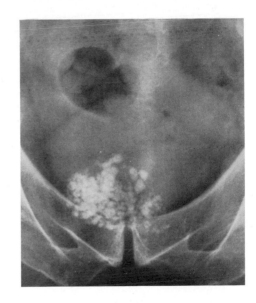

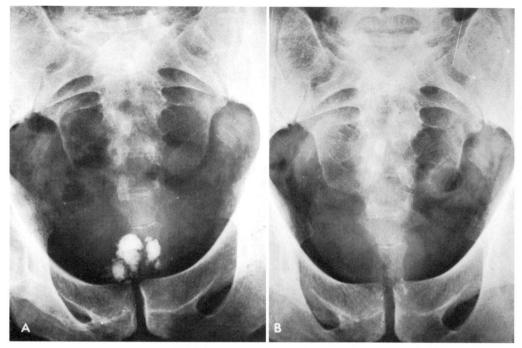

Figure 6–201. A, *Plain film.* Multiple prostatic calculi removed by transurethral prostatic resection.
B, *Plain film* (postoperative). A few minute calculi remaining after transurethral removal of prostatic calculi.

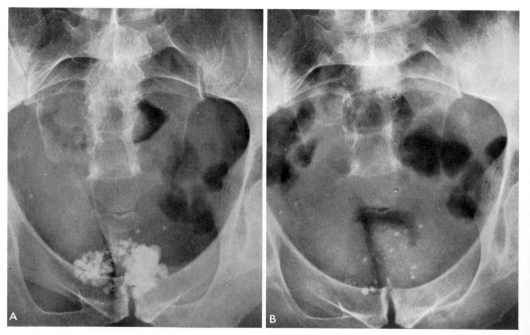

Figure 6–202. Multiple prostatic calculi removed by transurethral prostatic resection. A, *Plain film.*
B, *Plain film* (postoperative). A few minute calculi remaining after transurethral removal of prostatic calculi.

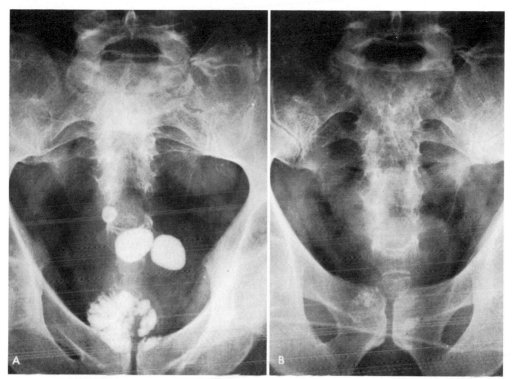

Figure 6–203. A, *Plain film.* Multiple prostatic calculi forming almost complete replacement of prostate gland. Multiple vesical calculi. B, *Plain film* (postoperative) A few prostatic calculi remaining after litholapaxy for vesical calculi and transurethral removal of prostatic calculi.

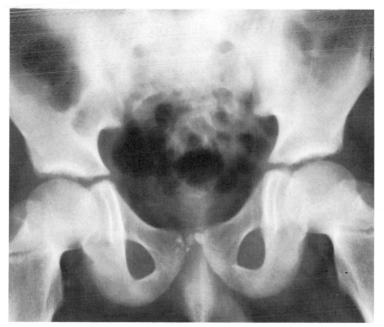

Figure 6–204. *Plain film.* Prostatic calculi in boy aged 11 years. (Calculi known to have been present since age 6.) (Courtesy of Dr. Robert Payne.)

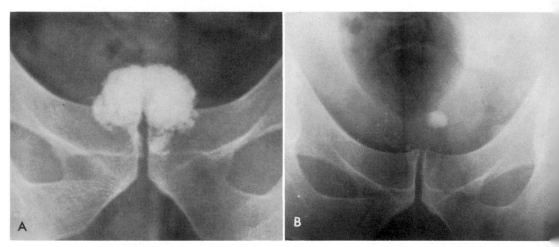

Figure 6–205. *Plain films.* **Spontaneous evacuation of prostatic calculi. A,** Extensive replacement o prostate with multiple prostatic calculi which could be palpated easily on digital rectal examination. **B,** Seve months later. Patient had spontaneously passed large number of calculi. A few had caught in urethral meatus requiring extraction with forceps. One large calculus and a few small calculi remain.

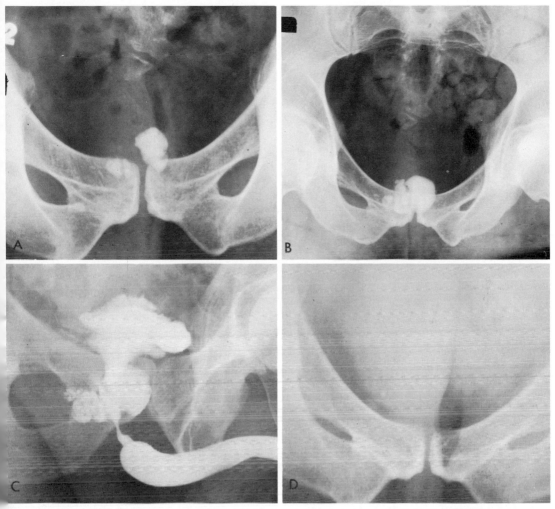

Figure 6–206. "Secondary" prostatic calculi. Cord bladder and incontinence due to myelodysplasia in a man, 24 years of age. Patient wears penile incontinence clip and has chronic pyuria. **A,** *Plain film,* April 1952. Prostatic calculi of moderate size. **B,** *Plain film,* January 1961. Considerable increase in size of calculi. **C,** *Retrograde urethrogram,* February 1961. Suggests stones have originated in old prostatic abscess cavities. **D,** *Plain film* following transurethral removal of stones. No stones are present.

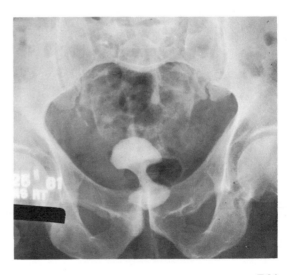

Figure 6–207. *Plain film.* Secondary dumbbell stone in prostatic urethra and bladder following suprapubic prostatectomy and removal of vesical calculi.

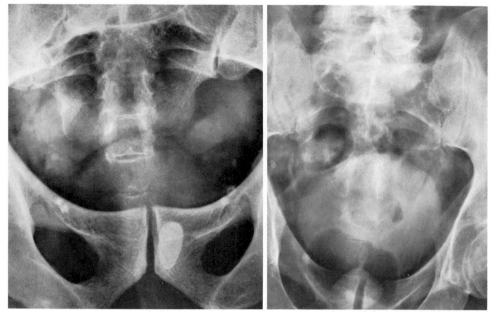

Fig. 6–208   Fig. 6–209

Figure 6–208. *Plain film.* **Secondary prostatic calculus** which has formed in prostatic urethra following suprapubic prostatectomy done 1 year previously. Stone was dislodged into bladder with cystoscope and litholapaxy was performed.

Figure 6–209. *Excretory cystogram.* **Secondary prostatic calculus** which has formed in prostatic urethra following transurethral prostatic resection. (Courtesy of Dr. J. K. Palmer.)

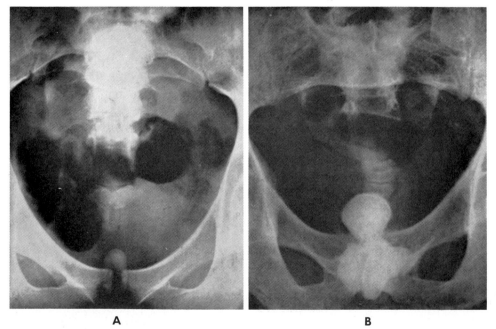

A   B

Figure 6–210. *Plain films.* **Examples of "secondary" prostatic calculi. A,** Stone formed in bladder and dropped into prostatic urethra. **Neurogenic bladder.** Stone was pushed into bladder with cystoscope and litholapaxy was performed. **B,** Another case. Secondary prostatic stone. Dumbbell calculus which formed in prostatic urethra following perineal prostatectomy several years previously. Large portion of stone projected into bladder. Suprapubic removal.

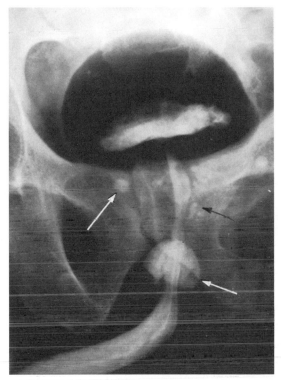

Figure 6–211. Calculi in diverticulum of bulbous urethra. Multiple prostatic calculi. *Urethrogram.* Two large calculi superimposed on each other, situated in diverticulum of bulbous urethra. Also multiple prostatic calculi. These stones were removed through external urethrotomy incision.

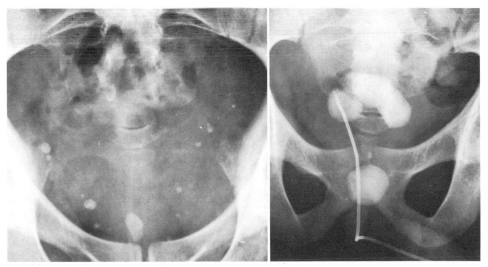

| Fig. 6–212 | Fig. 6–213 |

Figure 6–212. "Secondary" prostatic calculus. *Plain film.* Patient with **cord bladder.** Stone lodged in prostatic urethra, no doubt originating in bladder. Stone was dislodged with cystoscope and removed.

Figure 6–213. **Multiple vesical calculi. One has been passed into prostatic urethra.** *Plain film.* Patient with **neurogenic vesical dysfunction.** Multiple vesical calculi. Stone caught in prostatic urethra. This stone was dislodged into bladder with cystoscope and litholapaxy was performed.

Fig. 6–214

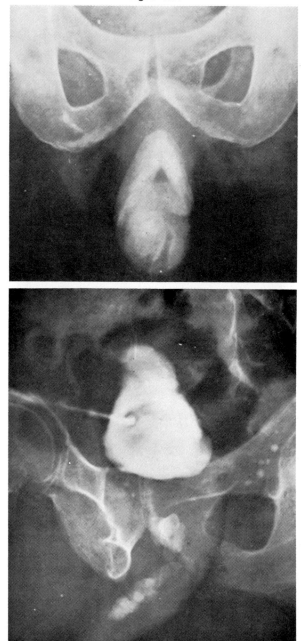

Fig. 6–215

Figure 6–214. *Retrograde cystogram,* made through suprapubic tube. **Multiple urethral calculi occupying almost entire perineal urethra.** They formed as **result of urethral stricture.** (Courtesy of Dr. Gordon W. Strom.)

Figure 6–215. *Plain film.* **Large urethral calculus forming cast of scrotal and perineal fistula,** associated with diverticulum, **in case of long-standing urethral stricture.** At operation, scrotal fistula was opened and scrotum was divided. Fistulous tract entered large diverticulum completely filled with calculus, which was removed in one piece. Diverticulum excised. (Courtesy of Dr. Gordon W. Strom.)

REFERENCES

Albright, F., Aub, J. C., and Bauer, W.: Hyperparathyroidism: A Common and Pleomorphic Condition as Illustrated by Seventeen Proved Cases From One Clinic. J.A.M.A. 102:1276-1287 (Apr. 21) 1934.

Albright, F., Baird, P. C., Cope, O., and Bloomberg, E.: Studies on the Physiology of the Parathyroid Glands. IV. Renal Complications of Hyperparathyroidism. Am. J. M. Sc. 187:49-65, 1934.

Albright, F., Dienes, L., and Sulkowitch, H. W.: Pyelonephritis With Nephrocalcinosis: Caused by Haemophilus influenzae and Alleviated by Sulfanilamide; Report of Two Cases. J.A.M.A. 110:357-360 (Jan. 29) 1938.

Alexander, S., and Brendler, H.: Treatment of Uric Acid Urolithiasis With Allopurinol: A Xanthine Oxidase Inhibitor. J. Urol. 97:340-343 (Feb.) 1967.

Arcelin: L'exploration radiologique des voies urinaires. In: Encyclopédie française d'urologie. Paris, Octave Doin et Fils, 1914, vol. 2, pp. 99-184.

Arons, W. L., Christensen, W. R., and Sosman, M. C.: Nephrocalcinosis Visible by X-ray, Associated With Chronic Glomerulonephritis. Ann. Int. Med. 42:260-282 (Feb.) 1955.

Bauld, W. S., MacDonald, S. A., and Hill, Mary C.: Effect of Renal Tubular Acidosis on Calcium Excretion. Brit. J. Urol. 30:285-291, 1958.

Beeson, P. B., Rocha, H., and Guez, L. B.: Experimental Pyelonephritis: Influence of Localized Injury in Different Parts of the Kidney on Susceptibility to Hematogenous Infection. Tr. A. Am. Physicians 70:120-126, 1957.

Benendo, B., and Litwak, A.: "Milk of Calcium" in Renal Cyst. Brit. J. Radiol. 37:70-71 (Jan.) 1964.

Berson, S. A., and Yalow, Rosalyn S.: Parathyroid Hormone in Plasma in Adenomatous Hyperparathyroidism, Uremia, and Bronchogenic Carcinoma. Science 154:907-909 (Nov. 18) 1966.

Black, B. M., and Zimmer, J. F.: Hyperparathyroidism, With Particular Reference to Treatment: Review of Two Hundred Seven Proved Cases. A.M.A. Arch. Surg. 72:830-837, 1956.

Boyce, W. H.: Radiology in the Diagnosis and Surgery of Renal Calculi. R. Clin. North America 3:89-102 (Apr.) 1965.

Boyce, W. H., Pool, C. S., Meschan, I., and King, J. S., Jr.: Organic Matrix of Urinary Calculi: Microradiographic Comparison of Crystalline Structure With Microscopic and Histochemical Studies. Acta radiol. 50:543-560, 1958.

Brenes, L. G., Stauffer, H. M., Forlano, R., and Koutouratsas, N.: Mechanism of Formation of the Obstructive Nephrogram. (Abstr.) Clin. Res. 10:405, 1962.

Burnett, C. H., Commons, R. R., Albright, F., and Howard, J. E.: Hypercalcemia Without Hypercalcinuria or Hypophosphatemia, Calcinosis and Renal Insufficiency: A Syndrome Following Prolonged Intake of Milk and Alkali. New England J. Med. 240:787-794 (May 19) 1949.

Camiel, M. R.: Stone in the Intramural Bladder Portion of the Ureter: Urographic Observations. Radiology 78:959-962 (June) 1962.

Camp, J. D.: Osseous Changes in Hyperparathyroidism: A Roentgenologic Study. J.A.M.A. 99:1913-1917 (Dec. 3) 1932.

Collini, W. R., Mattern, Susan R., Shapiro, Phyllis, Harris, Ruth C., and Zinsser, H. H.: Methods of Diminishing Cystine Excretion in Cystinuria. J. Urol. 93:729-734 (June) 1965.

Condon, R. E., Granville, G. E., Jordan, P. H., Jr., and Helgason, A. H.: Hypercalcemic Crisis and Intractable Gastrointestinal Ulceration in a Patient With Endocrine Polyglandular Syndrome. Ann. Surg. 167:185-190 (Feb.) 1968.

Crawhall, J. C., Scowen, E. F., and Watts, R. W. E.: Effect of Penicillamine on Cystinuria. Brit. M. J. 1:588-590 (Mar. 2) 1963.

Dent, C. E.: Some Problems of Hyperparathyroidism. Brit. M. J. 2:1495-1500 (Dec. 8) 1962.

Edling, N. P. G.: Further Studies of the Intraureteric Ridge of the Bladder. Acta radiol. 30:69-75, 1948.

Edling, N. P. G., Edvall, C. A., and Helander, C. G.: Correlation of Roentgen-Anatomic Changes and Functional Tests of the Kidneys in Hyperparathyroidism. Acta radiol. 55:43-48 (Jan.) 1961.

Edling, N. P. G., Helander, C. G., and Renck, L.: The Correlation Between Contrast Excretion and Arterial and Intrapelvic Pressures in Urography: An Experimental Study in Rabbits. Acta radiol. 42:442-450, 1954.

Elkin, M., Boyarsky, S., Martinez, J., and Kaplan, N.: Physiology of Ureteral Obstruction as Determined by Roentgenologic Studies. Am. J. Roentgenol. 92:291-301 (Aug.) 1964.

Engel, W. J.: Nephrocalcinosis. J.A.M.A. 145:288-294 (Feb. 3) 1951.

Epstein, F. H., Freedman, L. R., and Levitin, H.: Hypercalcemia, Nephrocalcinosis and Reversible Renal Insufficiency Associated With Hyperthyroidism. New England J. Med. 258:782-785 (Apr. 17) 1958.

Esposito, W. L.: Specific Nephrocalcinosis of Chronic Glomerulonephritis. Am. J. Roentgenol. 101:688-691 (Nov.) 1967.

Faconi, G.: Calcium and Phosphorus Metabolism. South African M. J. 34:769-772 (Sept. 10) 1960.

Foster, G. V., Baghdiantz, A., Kumar, M. A., Slack, E., Soliman, H. A., and MacIntyre, I.: Thyroid Origin of Calcitonin. Nature (London) 202:1303-1305 (June 27) 1964.

Geraci, J. E., Harris, H. W., and Keith, N. M.: Bilateral Diffuse Nephrocalcinosis: Report of Two Cases. Proc. Staff Meet., Mayo Clin. 25:305-315 (June 7) 1950.

Hellström, J., and Ivemark, B. I.: Primary Hyperparathyroidism: Clinical and Structural Findings in 138 Cases. Acta chir. scandinav., Suppl. 294, 1962, pp. 1-112.

Henken, E. M.: "Milk of Calcium" in a Renal Cyst: Report of a Case. Radiology 84:276-278 (Feb.) 1965.

Herskovic, T., Keating, F. R., Jr., and Gross, J. B.: Coexistent Pancreatitis and Hyperparathyroidism: Observations on 15 Cases. (Abstr.) Gastroenterology 52:1093 (June) 1967.

Hirsch, P. F., Gauthier, Geraldine F., and Munson, P. L.: Thyroid Hypocalcemic Principle and Recurrent Laryngeal Nerve Injury as Factors Affecting the Response to Parathyroidectomy in Rats. Endocrinology 73:244-252 (Aug.) 1963.

Howell, R. D.: Milk of Calcium Renal Stone. J. Urol. 82:197-199 (Aug.) 1959.

Huth, E. J.: Nephrolithiasis and Nephrocalcinosis. In Black, D. A. K.: Renal Disease. Ed. 2, Oxford, Blackwell Scientific Publications, 1967, pp. 421-445.

Irvine, W. T.: The Scientific Basis of Surgery. London, J. & A. Churchill, Ltd., chapter 18, 1965, 571 pp.

Jungmann, K.: Das Kolikurogramm (Ausscheidungsurographie während der Nierenkolik). Zentralbl. Chir. 93:426-432 (Mar. 23) 1968.

Keating, F. R.: Diagnosis of Primary Hyperparathyroidism: Clinical and Laboratory Aspects. J.A.M.A. 178:547-555 (Nov. 11) 1961.

Lagergren, C.: Biophysical Investigations of Urinary Calculi: An X-ray Crystallographic and Microradiographic Study. Acta radiol., Suppl. 133, 1956, pp. 1-71.

Lagergren, C., and Öhrling, H.: Urinary Calculi Composed of Pure Calcium Phosphate: Roentgen Crystallographic Analysis and Its Diagnostic Value. Acta chir. scandinav. 117:335-341, 1959.

Levinson, M. P., and Cooper, J. F.: Urological Findings in 58 Surgically Verified Cases of Parathyroid Adenoma. J. Urol. 96:1-5 (July) 1966.

Lightwood, R., and Payne, W. W.: British Pediatric Association: Proceedings of the Twenty-third General Meeting. A.M.A. Arch. Dis. Child. 27:302-303 (June) 1952.

Lloyd, H. M.: Primary Hyperparathyroidism: An Analysis of the Role of the Parathyroid Tumor. Medicine 47:53-71 (Jan.) 1968.

MacDonald, W. B., and Fellers, F. X.: Penicillamine in the Treatment of Patients with Cystinuria. J.A.M.A. 197:396-402 (Aug. 8) 1966.

Maurer, R. M., and Wildin, R. E.: Milk-of-Calcium Renal Stone: Report of a Case. Radiology 84:274-275 (Feb.) 1965.

McGeown, Mary G.: The Value of Specific Tests of Parathyroid Function. Proc. A. Clin. Biochem. 1:46, 1961.

McIntosh, D. A., Peterson, E. W., and McPhaul, J. J.: Autonomy of Parathyroid Function After Renal Homotransplantation. Ann. Int. Med. 65:900-907 (Nov.) 1966.

Moldawer, M. P., Nardi, G. L., and Raker, J. W.: Concomitance of Multiple Adenomas of the Parathyroids and Pancreatic Islets With Tumor of the Pituitary: A Syndrome With Familial Incidence. Am. J. M. Sc. 228:190-206 (Aug.) 1954.

Mortensen, JD: Nephrocalcinosis: A Collective Clinicopathologic Study. Thesis, Graduate School, University of Minnesota, 1953.

Mortensen, JD, and Emmett, J. L.: Nephrocalcinosis: A Collective and Clinicopathologic Study. J. Urol. 71:398-406 (Apr.) 1954.

Plimpton, C. H., and Gellhorn, A.: Hypercalcemia in Malignant Disease Without Evidence of Bone Destruction. Am. J. Med. 21:750-759 (Nov.) 1956.

Potter, W. M., Greene, L. F., and Keating, F. R., Jr.: Vesical Calculi and Hyperparathyroidism. J. Urol. 96:203-206 (Aug.) 1966.

Prien, E. L., and Frondel, C.: Studies in Urolithiasis. I. The Composition of Urinary Calculi. J. Urol. 57:949-991 (June) 1947.

Pugh, D. G.: Subperiosteal Resorption of Bone: A Roentgenologic Manifestation of Primary Hyperparathyroidism and Renal Osteodystrophy. Am. J. Roentgenol. 66:577-586 (Oct.) 1951.

Pullman, R. A. W., and King, R. J.: Milk of Calcium Renal Stone. Am. J. Roentgenol. 87:760-763 (Apr.) 1962.

Pyrah, L. N., Anderson, C. K., Hodgkinson, A., and Zarembsky, P. M.: A Case of Oxalate Nephrocalcinosis and Primary Hyperoxaluria. Brit. J. Urol. 31:235-248 (Sept.) 1959.

Pyrah, L. N., and Hodgkinson, A.: Nephrocalcinosis. Brit. J. Urol. 32:361-373, 1960.

Randall, R. E., Jr., Strauss, M. B., and McNeely, W. F.: The Milk-Alkali Syndrome. Arch. Int. Med. 107:163-181 (Feb.) 1961.

Richtsmeier, A. J.: The Symptoms of Hypercalcemia Associated With Sarcoidosis Masquerading as Peptic Ulcer. Ann. Int. Med. 51:1371-1378 (Dec.) 1959.

Riesz, P. B., and Wagner, C. W., Jr.: Unusual Renal Calcification Following Acute Bilateral Renal Cortical Necrosis: A Case Report. Am. J. Roentgenol. 101:705-707 (Nov.) 1967.

Rosenberg, M. A.: Milk of Calcium in a Renal Calyceal Diverticulum: Case Report and Review of Literature. Am. J. Roentgenol. 101:714-718 (Nov.) 1967.

Sallin, O.: Hypercalcemic Nephropathy in Thyrotoxicosis. Acta endocrinol. 29:425-434 (Nov.) 1958.

Scholz, D. A., and Keating, F. R., Jr.: Milk Alkali Syndrome: Review of Eight Cases. A.M.A. Arch. Int. Med. 95:460-468, 1955.

Schreiner, G. E., Smith, L. H., and Kyle, L. H.: Renal Hyperchloremic Acidosis: Familial Occurrence of Nephrocalcinosis With Hyperchloremia and Low Serum Bicarbonate. Am. J. Med. 15:122-129 (July) 1953.

Shanks, R. A., and MacDonald, A. M.: Nephrocalcinosis Infantum. A.M.A. Arch. Dis. Child. 34:115-119 (Apr.) 1959.

Shaw, M. T., and Davies, M.: Primary Hyperparathyroidism Presenting as Spinal Cord Compression. Brit. M. J. 4:230-231 (Oct. 26) 1968.

Snyder, C. H.: Idiopathic Hypercalcemia of Infancy. Am. J. Dis. Child. 96:376-380 (Sept.) 1958.

Stanbury, S. W.: Bone Disease in Uremia. Am. J. Med. 44:714-724 (May) 1968.

Talmage, R. V., and Kraintz, F. W.: Progressive Changes in Renal Phosphate and Calcium Excretion in Rats Following Parathyroidectomy or Parathyroid Administration. Proc. Soc. Exper. Biol. & Med. 87:263-267 (Nov.) 1954.

Thomas, W. C., Jr., Connor, T. B., and Morgan, H. G.: Some Observations on Patients With Hypercalcemia Exemplifying Problems in Differential Diagnosis, Especially in Hyperparathyroidism. J. Lab. & Clin. Med. 52:11-19 (July) 1958.

Underdahl, L. O., Woolner, L. B., and Black, B. M.: Multiple Endocrine Adenomas: Report of 8 Case in Which the Parathyroids, Pituitary and Pancreatic Islets Were Involved. J. Clin. Endocrinol. 13:20-47 (Jan.) 1953.

Vermooten, V.: Congenital Cystic Dilatation of the Renal Collecting Tubules: A New Disease Entity. Yale J. Biol. & Med. 23:450-453 (June) 1950-1951.

Walker, W. H., Pearson, R. E., and Johnson, N. R.: Milk-of-Calcium Renal Stone: Case Report. J. Urol. 84:517-520 (Oct.) 1960.

Walls, J., Schorr, W. J., and Kerr, D. N. S.: Prolonged Oliguria With Survival in Acute Bilateral Cortical Necrosis. Brit. M. J. 4:220-222 (Oct. 26) 1968.

Welbourn, R. B., and Sellwood, R. A.: Endocrine System. In Wells, C., and Kyle, J.: Scientific Foundations of Surgery. New York, American Elsevier Publishing Company, Inc., 1967, pp. 299-336.

Wesson, M. B., and Fulmer, C. C.: Influence of Ureteral Stones on Intravenous Urograms. Am. J. Roentgenol. 28;27-33 (July) 1932.

Widrow, S. H., and Levinsky, N. G.: The Effect of Parathyroid Extract on Renal Tubular Calcium Reabsorption in the Dog. J. Clin. Invest. 41:2151-2159 (Dec.) 1962.

Williams, R. H.: Textbook of Endocrinology. Ed. 4, Philadelphia, W. B. Saunders Company, chapter 11, 1968, 1259 pp.

Wilson, J. K. V., and Brown, W. H.: Nephrocalcinosis Associated With Sarcoidosis. Radiology 62:203-214 (Feb.) 1954.

Wing, A. J., Curtis, J. R., Eastwood, J. B., Smith, E. K. M., and de Wardener, H. E.: Transient and Persistent Hypercalcaemia in Patients Treated by Maintenance Haemodialysis. Brit. M. J. 4:150-152 (Oct. 19) 1968.

Winsbury-White, H. P.: Stone in the Urinary Tract. St. Louis, The C. V. Mosby Company, 1954, 328 pp.

Sarcoidosis

Anderson, J., Harper, C., Dent, C. E., and Philpot, C. R.: Effect of Cortisone on Calcium Metabolism in Sarcoidosis With Hypercalcemia: Possible Antagonistic Actions of Cortisone and Vitamin D. Lancet 2:720-724 (Oct. 9) 1954.

Burr, J. M., Farrell, J. J., and Hills, A. G.: Sarcoidosis and Hyperparathyroidism With Hypercalcemia: Special Usefulness of the Cortisone Test. New England J. Med. 261:1271-1275 (Dec. 17) 1959.

Davidson, C. N., Dennis, J. M., McNinch, E. R., Willson, J. K. V., and Brown, W. H.: Nephrocalcinosis Associated With Sarcoidosis: A Presentation and Discussion of Seven Cases. Radiology 62:203-214 (Feb.) 1954.

Goetz, A. A.: Effect of Cortisone on Hypercalcemia in Sarcoidosis: Relief of Gastrointestinal, Dermatological, and Renal Symptoms With Steroid Therapy. J.A.M.A. 174:380-384 (Sept. 24) 1960.

Goldenberg, G. J., and Greenspan, R. H.: Middle-Lobe Atelectasis due to Endobronchial Sarcoidosis: With Hypercalcemia and Renal Impairment. New England J. Med. 262:1112-1116 (June 2) 1960.

Harrell, G. T., and Fisher, S.: Blood Chemical Changes in Boeck's Sarcoid With Particular Reference to Protein, Calcium and Phosphatase Values. J. Clin. Invest. 18:687-693 (Nov.) 1939.

Jackson, W. P. U., and Dancaster, C.: A Consideration of the Hypercalciuria in Sarcoidosis, Idiopathic Hypercalciuria, and That Produced by Vitamin D: A New Suggestion Regarding Calcium Metabolism. J. Clin. Endocrinol. 19:658-680 (June) 1959.

Kirklin, B. R. and Morton, S. A.: Roentgenographic Changes in Sarcoid and Related Lesions. Radiology 16:328-333 (Mar.) 1931.

Klatskin, G., and Gordon, M.: Renal Complications of Sarcoidosis and Their Relationship to Hypercalcemia: With a Report of Two Cases Simulating Hyperparathyroidism. Am. J. Med. 15:484-498 (Oct.) 1953.

Lorincz, A. L., Malkinson, F. D., and Rothman, S.: Cutaneous Manifestations of Incipient Systemic Disease. M. Clin. North America 44:249-274 (Jan.) 1960.

Mather, G.: Calcium Metabolism and Bone Changes in Sarcoidosis. Brit. M. J. 1:248-253 (Feb. 2) 1957.

Scholz, D. A., and Keating, F. R., Jr.: Renal Insufficiency, Renal Calculi and Nephrocalcinosis in Sarcoidosis: Report of Eight Cases. Am. J. Med. 21:75-84 (July) 1956.

Snapper, I., and Gechman, E.: Calcium and Phosphorus Metabolism and Its Relationship to Nephrolithiasis. In Butt, A. J.: Etiologic Factors in Renal Lithiasis. Springfield, Illinois, Charles C Thomas, Publisher, 1956, pp. 53-88.

Solomon, R. B., and Channick, B. J.: Boeck's Sarcoidosis Simulating Hyperparathyroidism. Ann. Int. Med. 53:1232-1238 (Dec.) 1960.

Utz, J. P., Van Scott, E., Bernton, H. W., Edgcomb, J. H., Bunim, J. J., Bell, N. H., and Kaufman, H. E.: Sarcoidosis. Clinical Staff Conference at the National Institutes of Health. Ann. Int. Med. 51.1356-1370 (Dec.) 1959.

Primary Hyperoxaluria

Cochran, M., Hodgkinson, A., Zarembski, P. M., and Anderson, C. K.: Hyperoxaluria in Adults. Brit. J. Surg. 55:121-128 (Feb.) 1968.

Hockaday, T. D. R., Clayton, Joan E., Frederick, Elizabeth W., and Smith, L. H., Jr.: Primary Hyperoxaluria. Medicine 43:315-345 (May) 1964.

Smith, L. H., Jones, J. D., and Keating, F. R., Jr.: Primary Hyperoxaluria. Read at the International Symposium on Renal Stone Research, Leeds, England, April 17 to 20, 1968.

Williams, H. E., and Smith, L. H., Jr.: Disorders of Oxalate Metabolism. Am. J. Med. 45:715-735 (Nov.) 1968.

Wyngaarden, J. B., and Elder, T. D.: Primary Hyperoxaluria and Oxalosis. In Stanbury, J. B., Wyngaarden, J. B., and Fredrickson, D. S.: The Metabolic Basis of Inherited Disease. Ed. 2, New York, McGraw-Hill Book Company, Inc., 1966, pp. 189-212.

CHAPTER 7

Nontuberculous Infections of the Genitourinary Tract

Section 1

by
Glen W. Hartman

ACUTE PYELONEPHRITIS

Urography has little to offer in the diagnosis of acute pyelonephritis, namely, the clinical syndrome of sudden onset of fever, costovertebral angle tenderness, dysuria, and frequency. It is indicated, however, to exclude possible underlying lesions such as obstruction or stone that may have precipitated the infection. Urography may be performed without added risk during the acute febrile episode; often, however, it may be better clinical practice to wait until acute infection is under control before subjecting the patient to urography.

CHRONIC PYELONEPHRITIS

The term "chronic pyelonephritis" has been loosely applied to various renal conditions regardless of their etiology. Recently, however, it has been suggested that the term should apply only when bacterial infection causes renal damage; Beeson lists the following as the most reliable criteria in establishing the clinical diagnosis: (1) repeated episodes of febrile illness associated with pain and tenderness in the region of the kidney, pyuria, and bacteriuria; (2) presence of a pathologic condition known to predispose to urinary tract infection such as vesicoureteral reflux or obstruction; (3) impaired renal function; and (4) characteristic urographic findings. If one accepts this definition, it is also necessary to limit the radiographic diagnosis of chronic pyelonephritis to renal changes that result only from bacterial infections of the kidney and to avoid using the term for various nonspecific renal abnormalities of unknown etiology.

ROUTES OF INFECTION

Bacteria are thought to reach the kidney by three separate routes, namely (1) hematogenous, (2) ascending via the ureter, and (3) lymphatic.

The **hematogenous** route has been studied by the intravenous injection of bacteria into experimental animals. Renal infection occurs consistently with the intravenous injection of cocci but bacillary pyelonephritis does not result experimentally unless special conditions prevail such as previous scarring of the kidney produced by infection or fulguration, or urinary stasis produced by ureteral ligation (Beeson, Rocha, and Guze; de Navasquez, 1950; 1956). Because the great majority of urinary tract infections in humans are caused by bacilli, it has appeared unlikely that the hematogenous route is the primary one. However, Shopfner expressed a different view. He studied 69 infants suffering from sepsis and found that 33% had radiographic evidence of urinary tract infection, as evidenced by such findings as ileus and atony of the calyces, pelves, and ureters, vesicoureteral reflux, and "nonobstructive" hydronephrosis. He concluded that the hematogenous route of renal infection is the common one and that the ureters and bladder are infected simultaneously.

It is generally accepted that severe parenchymal infections such as solitary abscess (renal carbuncle), multiple cortical abscesses, diffuse cortical infection, and perinephritic abscess are blood-borne. These are usually coccal infections (frequently *Staphylococcus aureus*) initiated by foci of infection elsewhere in the body.

The **ascending route** (via the ureter) is generally thought to be responsible for the large majority of renal infections, both acute and chronic. Responsible organisms are usually normal fecal flora such as gram-negative bacilli or *Streptococcus faecalis*. In the past, the ascending theory was opposed because it was thought to depend in part on the "swimming upstream" concept, but since vesicoureteral reflux has been demonstrated to occur in 50% to 80% of children with chronic pyelonephritis a method of transport of bacteria from bladder to kidney is apparent (Hinman and Hutch; Hodson and Edwards).

The **lymphatic route** is probably rare, but theoretically it is possible for bacteria to reach the kidneys via lymphatics draining the bladder, sigmoid, or rectum.

PATHOLOGY

The term "chronic pyelonephritis" has been used so loosely in the past that Hodson (1967b) says it is essential that it be defined specifically as "those changes in the kidney which result directly from bacterial infection." **Gross pathologic changes** are localized and in the chronic stage consist of a large area of fibrosis or scar which involves the entire thickness of the kidney. The scars are irregular in distribution and the underlying calyx is blunted, but the corresponding papillae, although fibrosed and retracted, are not excavated or sloughed as in papillary necrosis. The involved kidney is small (atrophied) while the collecting system may be dilated and have a thickened fibrosed wall. It is important to the physician to appreciate that all gross renal changes resulting from chronic pyelonephritis are easily demonstrated on good-quality excretory urograms in which the renal parenchyma is clearly visualized. Hodson (1959) must be credited with bringing these facts emphatically to the attention of the profession.

Microscopically, pyelonephritis is often difficult or impossible to differentiate from other renal abnormalities, especially the sequelae of renal vascular disease and interstitial nephritis, as indicated by Kimmelstiel and colleagues and Heptinstall,[*] who stress the focal nature of chronic pyelonephritis which limits the usefulness of renal biopsy for diagnosis. Heptinstall is "doubtful that renal biopsy can be used for making the diagnosis of chronic pyelonephritis unless use is made of information from the radiologist on the status of the calyceal system and from the clinician on the presence of urinary tract infection." This supports Hodson's thesis that the gross renal changes detectable on urograms are extremely important.

---

[*]For a complete review of the pathology of chronic pyelonephritis the reader is referred to both of these articles.

UROGRAPHY IN DIAGNOSIS
(Figs. 7-1 through 7-26)

Technique adequate to demonstrate renal parenchyma clearly is essential for the urographic diagnosis of chronic pyelonephritis; retrograde pyelography is rarely required or indicated, and then only to supplement excretory urography in instances of markedly impaired or absent renal function. Even when renal function is markedly impaired, the renal parenchyma and collecting system may be satisfactorily visualized by relatively simple adjustment of techniques such as reinjection, large initial dose of medium, ureteral compression, and tomography (see Fig. 7-22). (See also discussion in Chapter 1, pages 19–20.)

Minimal urographic changes of chronic pyelonephritis may be confined to the collecting system. **Linear striations of the mucosa** of the pelvis and upper ureter (see Fig. 7-35) are occasionally present during active infection and probably represent mucosal edema (Gwinn and Barnes). The pelviocalyceal system and ureters may be slightly dilated or unduly distensible if ureteral compression is employed. Minimal calyceal blunting may be evident.

The hallmark of the urographic diagnosis of chronic pyelonephritis, however, is the **coarse localized renal scar with clubbing of the underlying calyx** (Figs. 7-1 through 7-26). Being focal, these scars can be either unilateral or bilateral, and, although no constant pattern of distribution can be described, the poles are most commonly involved (Hodson, 1967b). The scars may be so extensive that the blunted calyx appears to lie directly beneath the renal capsule, and marked atrophy occurs commonly in advanced stages of the disease.

Less prominent scarring and blunting may be difficult to detect, but Hodson (1959) has emphasized that careful comparison of the relationship of the calyces to the renal outline will reveal minor pathologic changes. He has devised a diagrammatic method of demonstrating this relationship (Fig. 7-1A). The dotted line drawn through the calyceal tips is designated the "interpapillary line." In the normal kidney it bears a constant relationship to the surface outline of the kidney except possibly the upper lateral border of the left kidney, which may be narrowed by "splenic impression." (See Figs. 4-133 and 4-134.) The parenchymal zones are often thicker at the two poles than elsewhere in the kidney but they are **equally** thick at the poles; and if the collecting systems are bilaterally symmetrical, the parenchymal zones are equally thick at all four poles. (See discussion, Chapter 12, page 1436.) Abnormalities due to parenchymal scarring are illustrated in Figures 7-1B through 7-4.

Localized areas of normal parenchyma remaining in grossly scarred kidneys may undergo compensatory hypertrophy resulting in a **pseudotumor**[*] (King, Friedenberg, and Tena). It is extremely important to recognize the nature of the pseudotumor because it may resemble a solid renal tumor on either urography, nephrotomography, or angiography, and misdiagnosis may result in unnecessary nephrectomy. The absence of tumor vessels on vascular studies and awareness of the possibility of localized hypertrophy help prevent this error (Figs. 7-19 and 7-20).

Severe cicatricial changes of the calyces and pelvis occur uncommonly in nontuberculous infection, but may cause bizarre deformities or obliteration of the collecting system (Figs. 7-24 and 7-25).

Chronic Pyelonephritis in Children

Chronic atrophic pyelonephritis is primarily a disease of children, but the resultant scarring persists and may not be demonstrated until adulthood. This concept is supported by the demonstration of a high incidence of **associated vesicoureteral reflux** in patients of this age

[*]See also discussion, Chapter 12, page 1436, and Figs. 12-150 and 12-151.

group. The characteristic urographic findings of chronic pyelonephritis are virtually diagnostic during childhood, but in adults the scars resulting from segmental infarction may at times be indistinguishable. Chronic pyelonephritis may interfere with renal growth during childhood, and Hodson (1967b) emphasizes that renal growth is a very sensitive method of detecting or excluding renal damage. He has established a clinical scale that correlates the relationship between normal kidney length and child height, which is very helpful in the clinical follow-up of children who have chronic pyelonephritis (Hodson, 1967a). **The association of reflux and urinary tract infection in children makes the voiding cystogram as essential as the excretory urogram in evaluating children who have urinary tract infection.**

DIFFERENTIAL DIAGNOSIS

Segmental renal infarction resulting in a gross renal scar may at times be impossible to differentiate from chronic pyelonephritis. In most instances, however, the papilla underlying an infarct undergoes less scarring and retraction and therefore the calyx retains normal cupping. This is very helpful since calyceal blunting is a constant feature of chronic pyelonephritis. **Total renal infarction** causes smooth overall renal atrophy with nonfunction and a normal collecting system when examined by retrograde pyelography. Excretion of contrast medium may be reestablished later, provided adequate collateral circulation develops.

Back pressure renal atrophy (hydronephrotic atrophy) is a relatively common manifestation of temporary obstruction of the collecting system and has been recently described in detail (Hodson and Craven). (See Fig. 5-7.) Obstruction of the ureteropelvic junction or ureter may cause no permanent renal abnormality, but may result in diffuse calyceal blunting

associated with generalized thinning of the renal cortex if relief of the obstruction is delayed. Obstruction of a single major calyx or infundibulum causes similar changes in the related calyceal tips and localized scarring. In the latter instance the changes closely resemble the scar of chronic pyelonephritis.

Renal atrophy from various causes, including chronic pyelonephritis, may result in **fibrolipomatosis** (Fig. 7-26). (See also Figs. 4-86 through 4-91.) In this condition a substantial amount of fat is deposited in the renal sinus, replacing atrophied renal parenchyma. Urography reveals attenuation, elongation, compression, and distortion of the infundibula suggesting peripelvic masses. Slight calyceal blunting is usually present. Nephrotomography is diagnostic because the large accumulation of radiolucent peripelvic fat is well demonstrated in contrast to the opacified atrophied renal parenchyma.

Irregularity of the parenchyma related to **persistent fetal lobulation** should not be confused with chronic pyelonephritis. In this situation the calyces are normal and the indentations of the cortex representing the partitions of Bertin lie between the calyces. (See Figs. 4-135 and 4-136.)

Atrophy of the kidney may result from numerous other noninflammatory conditions, but rarely is calyceal blunting a predominant feature. **Nephrosclerosis** and **chronic glomerulonephritis** result in bilateral, symmetrical small kidneys with anatomically normal collecting systems. **Radiation nephritis** is usually unilateral, and at times may closely resemble chronic pyelonephritis. The urographic picture of **tuberculosis** or **papillary necrosis** usually has little in common with that of chronic pyelonephritis because cortical scarring is not a salient feature of these conditions.

Congenital hypoplasia of the kidney is relatively uncommon and should be considered only if the renal collecting system is anatomically normal. Even the small kidney with normal gross architecture noted in infancy may be the result of intrauterine vascular occlusion, neonatal thrombosis, or vesicoureteral reflux. Pathologic examination of the kidney is usually of no value in detecting the etiology of a diminutive kidney (Emmett, Alvarez-Ierena, and McDonald).

TUMEFACTIVE XANTHOGRANULOMATOUS PYELONEPHRITIS
(Figs. 7-27, 7-28, and 7-29)

Xanthogranulomatous pyelonephritis is an uncommon manifestation of chronic renal infection. Symptoms are similar to those seen in other chronic renal infections although chills and fever are not always present. **Grossly** a yellow tumefactive mass is found to replace a portion of the kidney. It may extend into perinephric tissues and may closely resemble hypernephroma. The characteristic yellow color results from lipid-laden foam cells which microscopically resemble the clear cells of hypernephroma.

The **basic urographic finding** is the presence of an intrarenal mass which is usually indistinguishable from other renal tumors. The mass occasionally contains amorphous calcification, and renal calculi frequently coexist. Pyelocaliectasis may be present without evidence of obstruction, and if the process is far advanced the kidney may fail to function (Clark, McAllister, and Harrell). Angiography and nephrotomography reveal a solid renal mass without evidence of malignant tumor vascularity.

(Text continued on page 775.)

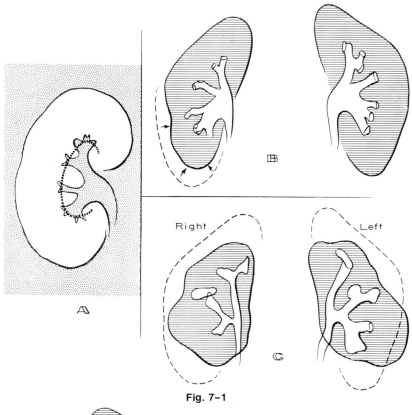

Fig. 7–1

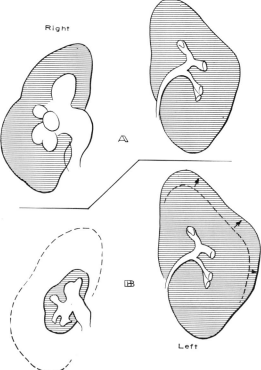

Fig. 7–2

Figure 7–1. A, Normal kidney showing interpapillary line used for measurement of thickness of renal substance. **B,** Tracing of excretory pyelogram of woman, 21 years of age. In two regions of lower half of right kidney there is localized narrowing of renal substance and clubbing of adjacent calyces. **Early focal pyelonephritis.** Left kidney is normal. **C,** Tracing of excretory pyelogram of woman, 29 years of age. **Advanced bilateral chronic pyelonephritis.** Note small size of kidneys, irregular outlines, and marked variations of thickness of renal substance with calyceal clubbing. Dotted lines indicate normal contour of kidney. (Modified from Hodson, C. J., 1959.)

Figure 7–2. Diagrammatic presentation of **chronic atrophic pyelonephritis of right kidney** following transvesical meatotomy for removal of ureteral stone. A, Preoperative condition. Right pyelocaliectasis caused by obstruction from ureteral stone. **B,** Same case, 11 years after meatotomy. Atrophy of right kidney and compensatory hyperplasia of left kidney. Dotted lines indicate contour of kidneys in their normal state. (Modified from Hodson, C. J., and Edwards, D., 1960.)

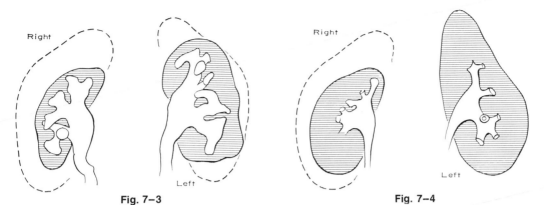

Fig. 7–3   **Fig. 7–4**

Figure 7–3. Diagrammatic presentation of **bilateral atrophic pyelonephritis** in girl, 7 years of age, with bilateral vesicoureteral reflux. Dotted lines indicate contour of kidneys in their normal state. (Modified from Hodson, C. J., and Edwards, D., 1960.)

Figure 7–4. Diagrammatic presentation of **unilateral (right) atrophic pyelonephritis** in girl, 10 years of age, who had 6-year history of recurring infection. (Modified from Hodson, C. J., and Edwards, D., 1960.)

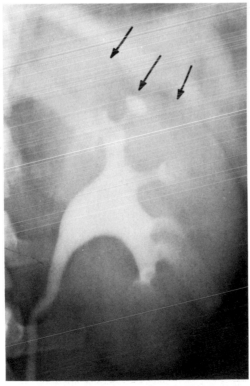

Figure 7–5. *Excretory urogram.* **Minimal chronic pyelonephritis.** Localized parenchymal scar (*arrows*) with underlying calyceal blunting. Far-advanced atrophic pyelonephritis was present in right kidney.

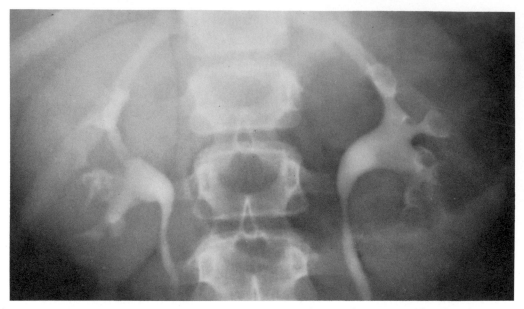

Figure 7–6. *Excretory urogram.* **Minimal chronic pyelonephritis.** Eleven-year-old girl with scarring of lower pole of right kidney and blunting of underlying calyces. Upper pole of right kidney and both poles of left kidney are approximately equally thick.

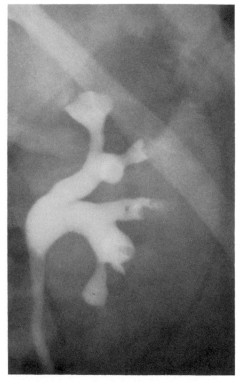

Figure 7–7. *Excretory urogram.* **Unilateral chronic pyelonephritis.** Blunting involving only lower-pole calyx with thinning of parenchyma of medial aspect of lower pole of left kidney.

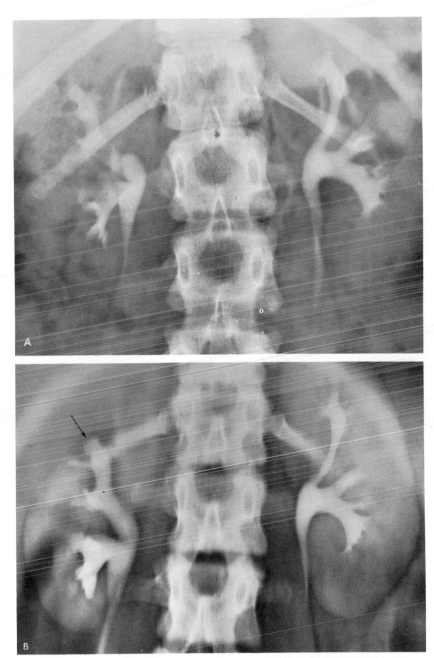

Figure 7-8. Chronic pyelonephritis of right kidney. History of recurring urinary infection since child-hood in girl, 15 years of age. **A,** *Excretory urogram.* Suggestion of atrophy of cortex of upper pole of right kidney, but renal outline indistinct. **B,** *Nephrotomogram.* Excellent visualization of both renal outlines. Gross cortical scar of upper pole with blunting of underlying calyces (*arrow*). Less marked changes are present in lower pole. Compensatory hypertrophy, left kidney.

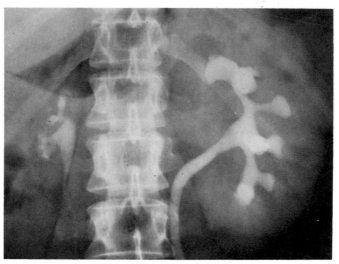

Figure 7–9.   *Excretory urogram.* **Chronic pyelonephritis.** Marked atrophy of right kidney and compensatory hypertrophy of left kidney with minimal calyceal blunting.

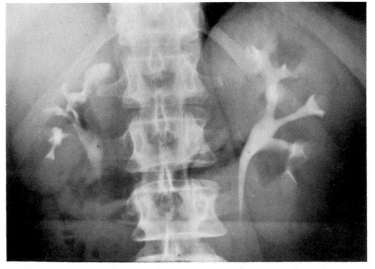

Figure 7–10.   *Excretory urogram.* **Advanced chronic pyelonephritis** of right kidney. Compensatory hypertrophy of left kidney.

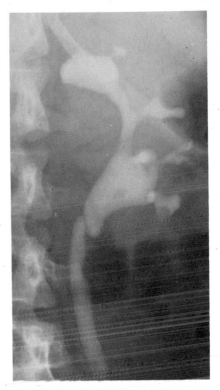

Figure 7–11. *Excretory urogram.* Advanced chronic pyelonephritis of left kidney.

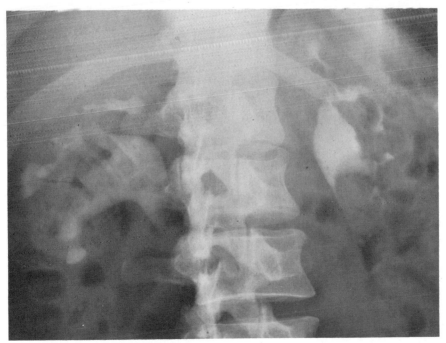

Figure 7–12. *Excretory urogram.* **Bilateral chronic pyelonephritis.** Calyceal blunting, right kidney with gross renal scars. Cicatricial changes of left calyceal system.

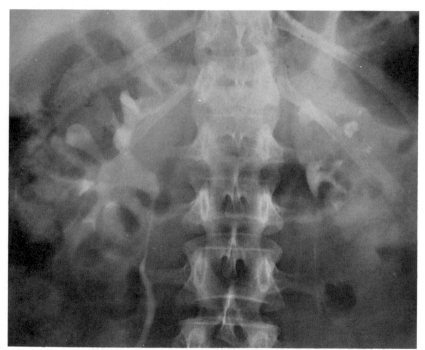

Figure 7–13. *Excretory urogram.* **Bilateral chronic pyelonephritis.** Calyceal blunting and parenchymal scarring on right. Advanced atrophy on left.

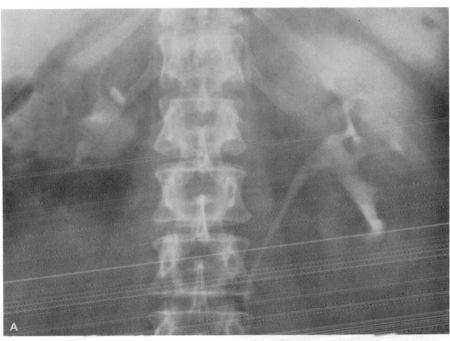

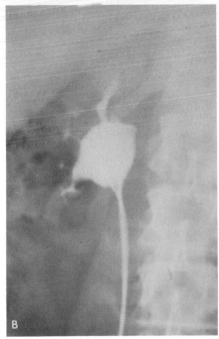

Figure 7-14. Bilateral chronic pyelonephritis complicated by nephrolithiasis and
right renal atrophy. **A,** *Excretory urogram.*
Poorly visualized atrophic right kidney
with stone forming a cast of lower calyx.
Compensatory hypertrophy of left kidney.

B, *Right retrograde pyelogram.*

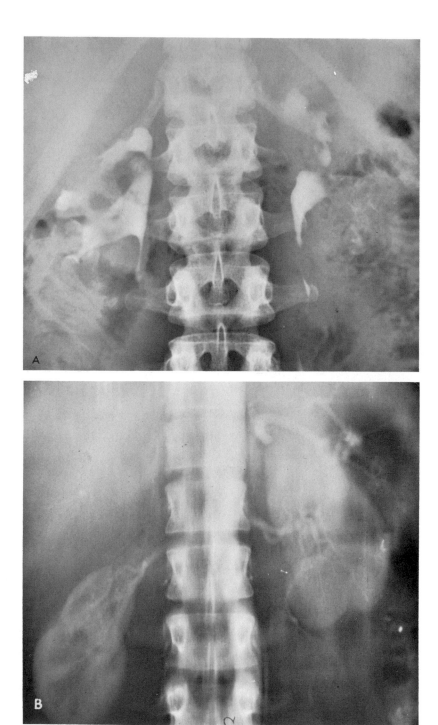

Figure 7–15. *See opposite page for legend.*

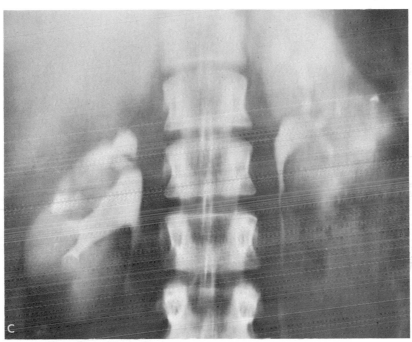

Figure 7–15. Chronic bilateral atrophic pyelonephritis. Thirty-six-year-old woman with long-standing history of urinary tract infection and hypertension for 10 years. **A,** *Excretory urogram.* Calyceal clubbing and deformity, but renal outlines not demonstrated. **B,** *Arterial phase of nephrotomogram.* Scarring of upper pole of right kidney and lower pole of left kidney. **C,** *Nephrographic phase of nephrotomogram.* Entire right kidney in "focus" at this level. Typical findings of calyceal blunting associated with cortical atrophy are well demonstrated.

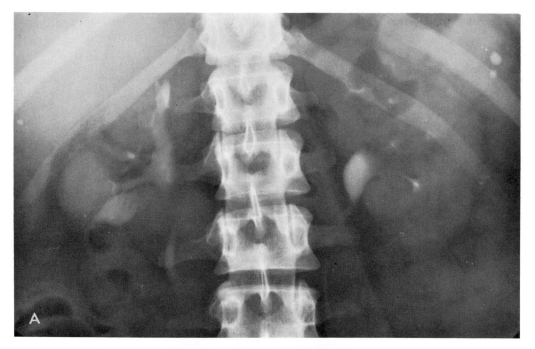

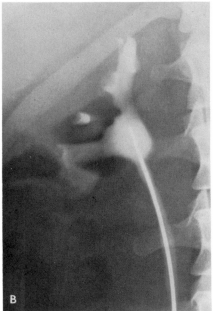

Figure 7–16. *See opposite page for legend.*

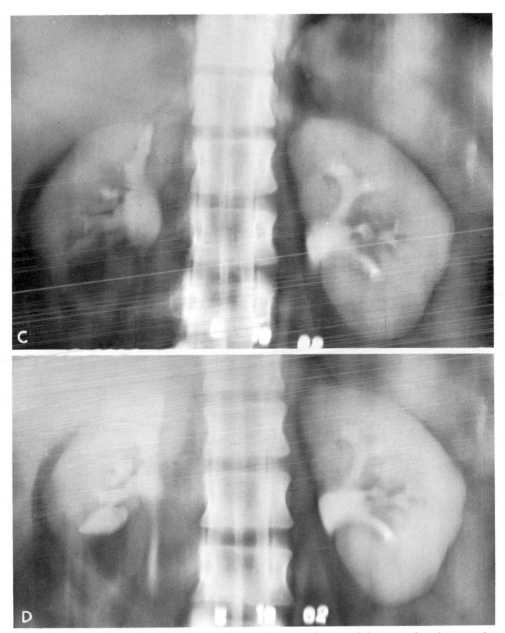

Figure 7–16.   Right chronic pyelonephritis. Woman 39 years of age with long-standing history of urinary tract infection and hypertension. **A,** *Excretory urogram.* Renal outlines only partially demonstrated. Marked deformity of lower pole calyx of right kidney. **B,** *Right retrograde pyelogram.* **C** and **D,** *Nephrotomograms at 6-cm and 8-cm levels respectively.* Cortical scarring of upper pole of right kidney is well shown at 6 cm. Lower pole is best seen at 8 cm.

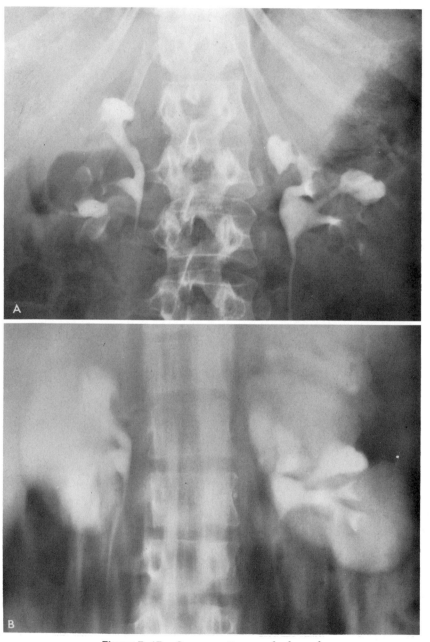

Figure 7–17. *See opposite page for legend.*

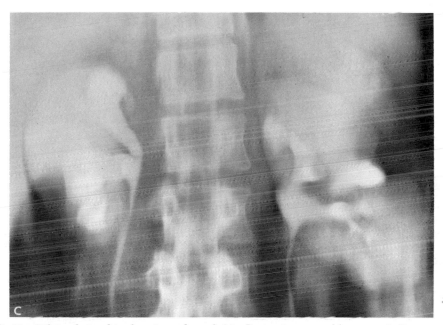

Figure 7–17.   Bilateral atrophic chronic pyelonephritis. Forty-nine year-old woman. A, *Excretory urogram.* Marked calyceal blunting, but renal cortex not outlined. B, *Nephrotomogram (5-cm "cut").* Left kidney best seen at this level, with marked localized scarring. C, *Nephrotomogram (7-cm "cut").* Right kidney shows best in this "cut." Abnormal irregular dilated calyces with complete loss of cortex above upper calyx and marked atrophy of lower pole of kidney.

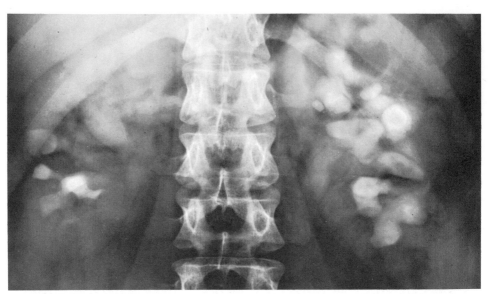

Figure 7–18. *Excretory urogram (20-minute film).* **Bilateral chronic pyelonephritis.** Reduced function of both kidneys, more marked on right. Calyces irregular, dilated, and deformed. Marked cortical thinning.

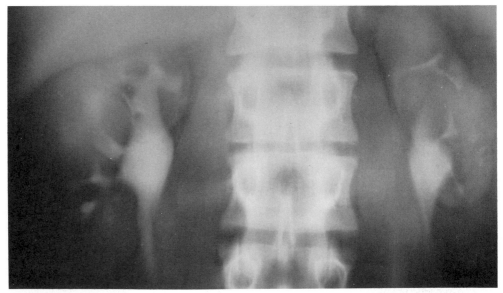

Figure 7–19. *Infusion tomogram.* **Bilateral chronic pyelonephritis.** Thirty-one-year-old man with hypertension. Marked atrophy of left kidney and upper pole of right kidney. Compensatory hypertrophy of remaining normal tissue in lateral portion of both kidneys simulates intrarenal mass lesions.

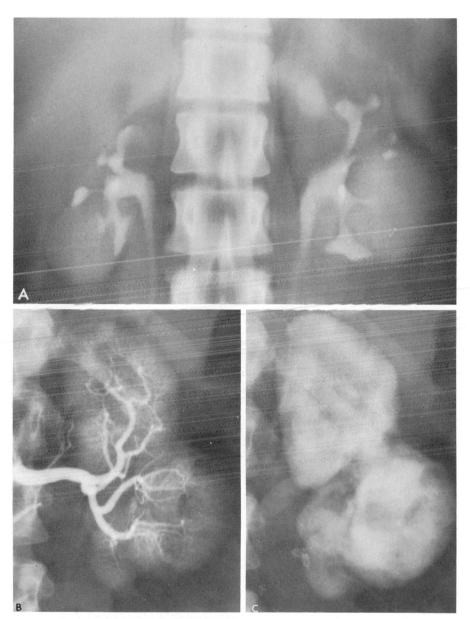

Figure 7–20. Bilateral atrophic pyelonephritis. "Pseudotumor." **A,** *Excretory urogram*. Marked parenchymal scarring with associated calyceal blunting. Prominent lower poles bilaterally raise question of intrarenal mass lesions. **B,** *Selective left renal arteriogram*. Island of normal parenchyma in left lower pole has undergone compensatory hypertrophy (pseudotumor). **C,** *Arteriogram, nephrographic phase.*

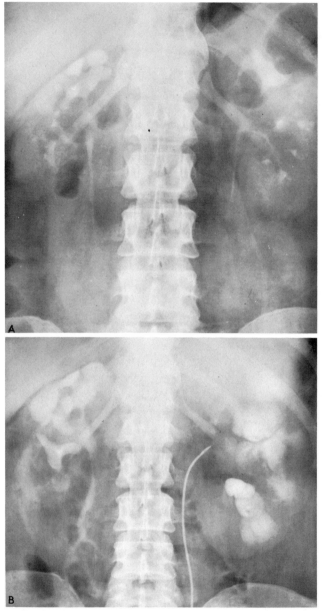

Figure 7-21. Bilateral chronic pyelonephritis of many years' standing, with progression. **A,** *Excretory urogram.* Most advanced changes appear to be in right kidney. **B,** *Retrograde pyelograms* made 14 years later. Progressive parenchymal atrophy and calycectasis of right kidney. Extensive pyonephrosis of left kidney. Left nephrectomy. *Pathologic diagnosis:* Inflammatory stenosis of ureteropelvic juncture with advanced cortical destruction.

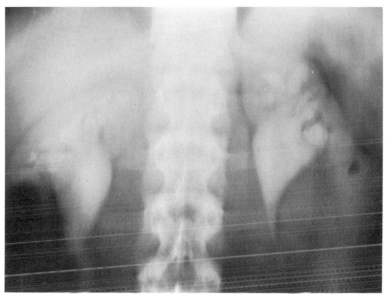

Figure 7–22. *Infusion with tomography.* **Bilateral pyelonephritis and chronic renal failure.** Twenty-two-year-old male with repeated urinary tract infections and gross bilateral reflux. Blood urea, 105 mg/100 ml; serum creatinine, 4.85 mg/100 ml. High-dose excretory urography adequately demonstrates advanced renal disease despite renal failure.

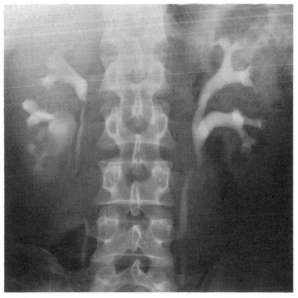

Figure 7–23. *Excretory urogram.* **Complete duplication of right collecting system with pyelonephritis** involving lower segment. (Vesicoureteral reflux was present in lower-pole ureter.)

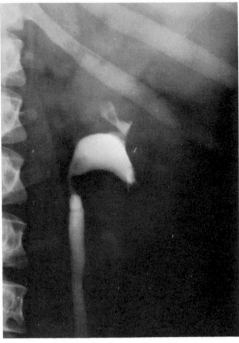

Figure 7–24. *Left retrograde pyelogram.* **Obliterative chronic pyelonephritis.** Moderately advanced cicatricial changes involving calyces and upper ureter.

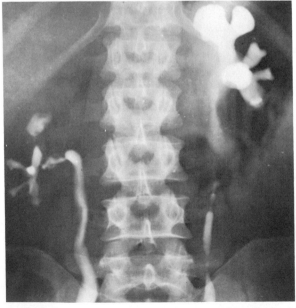

Figure 7–25. *Bilateral retrograde pyelogram.* **Bilateral chronic pyelonephritis.** Marked cicatricial change of right renal pelvis and calyces. Dilatation of upper right ureter. Calycectasis and calyceal blunting of left kidney with strictures of left ureter.

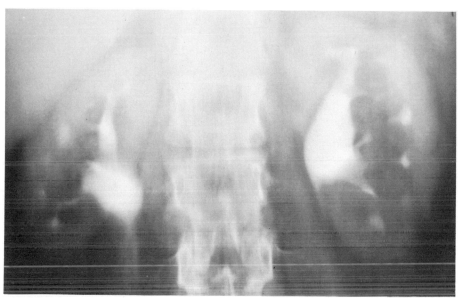

Figure 7-26. *Nephrotomogram.* **Fibrolipomatosis associated with chronic pyelonephritis.** Typical findings of diffuse cortical thinning, calyceal blunting, attenuation of infundibula, and fatty replacement in renal sinus. Fatty tissue is radiolucent.

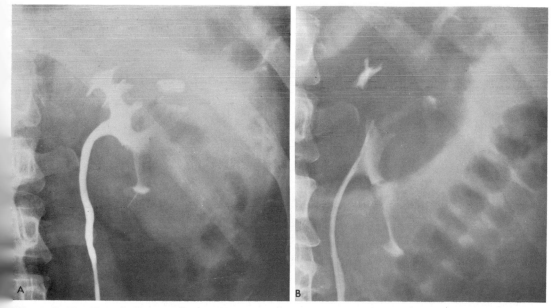

Figure 7-27. **Tumefactive xanthogranulomatous pyelonephritis. A,** *Retrograde pyelogram.* Mass lesion of lower pole of left kidney, **B,** *Three months later.* Enlargement of mass with greater compression and deformity of calyces, and kidney displaced against spinal column. Nephrectomy done at this time.

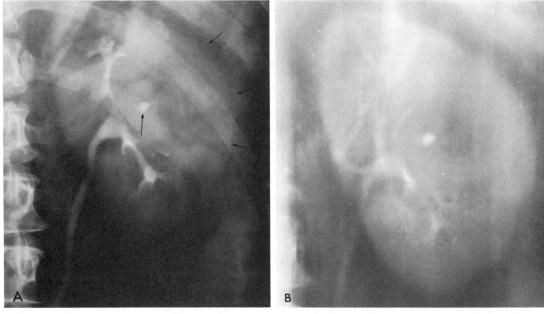

Figure 7–28. Tumefactive xanthogranulomatous pyelonephritis. **A,** *Excretory urogram.* Mass lesion of left kidney with calyceal deformity and renal calculus (*vertical arrow*). **B,** *Nephrotomogram.* This delineates outline of mass better than does **A** and demonstrates that the mass is solid. Preoperative diagnosis: hypernephroma.

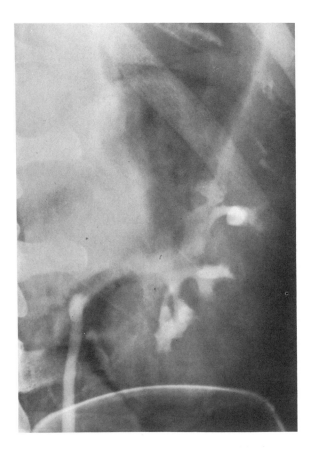

Figure 7–29. *Excretory urogram.* Tumefactive xanthogranulomatous pyelonephritis. Large mass occupying upper pole of left kidney. Underlying calyces distorted and blunted. Urine culture revealed *Proteus* organisms. Resected specimen: xanthogranulomatous pyelonephritis.

PYELOURETERECTASIS AND PYELONEPHRITIS OF PREGNANCY

(Figs. 7-30 through 7-34)

Pyeloureterectasis during and following pregnancy has been commonly observed urographically for decades, but the cause of the dilatation remains unsettled and controversial. Some degree of dilatation occurs during every pregnancy and it usually subsides within 2 months following delivery. The right side is more commonly dilated and usually to a greater degree than the left. The dilatation typically ends at the level of the pelvic inlet.

Two factors have been considered to play a role in development of dilatation during normal pregnancies; namely (1) physiologic changes and (2) obstruction. **Physiologic alterations** affect the entire urinary collecting system and result from changes in circulating levels of hormones. Hodson believes that primary effects are due to decreased muscle tone and activity which result in a slower flow rate of urine. A recent report (Marshall, Lyon, and Minkler) of pyeloureterectasis developing in a woman while she was taking an oral contraceptive appears to support the theory of physiologic pyeloureterectasis.

However, hormonal effects cannot explain the predilection for involvement of the right collecting system, and the characteristic termination of ureteral dilatation at the pelvic inlet suggests **obstruction** at this level. During the second trimester the uterus would be expected to cause some compression of the ureters at the level of the pelvic inlet, especially when the patient is supine (Harrow, Sloane, and Salhanick). It has been thought that the sigmoid colon protects the left ureter from such compression. Recently, however, Dure-Smith studied several cadavers with opaque catheters or medium in the ureters and iliac vessels and concluded that differences in anatomic rela-

tionships of the ureters and iliac arteries on the two sides predisposed the right ureter to partial obstruction at the pelvic inlet.

Pyelitis or pyelonephritis of pregnancy is a clinical diagnosis which is made in 1% or 2% of all pregnancies. The clinical findings of fever, flank tenderness associated with chills, nausea, and vomiting are well known. Infection is much more common during the last two trimesters and the right side is more commonly affected (Kincaid-Smith). Bacteriuria during the first trimester has been found in two thirds of all patients in whom pyelonephritis of pregnancy subsequently develops (Kincaid-Smith and Bullen). The mechanism by which the upper urinary tract is predisposed to the development of infection can be explained either by a slow flow rate resulting from hormonally induced physiologic changes or by partial ureteral obstruction by the gravid uterus. The latter explanation appears more likely.

Ureteral reflux must be considered a possible predisposing factor in the development of pyelonephritis of pregnancy. Hutch, Ayres, and Noll demonstrated vesicoureteral reflux in 5 of 12 patients whose pregnancy was complicated by pyelonephritis, while Heidrick, Mattingly, and Amberg made single-film voiding cystograms on 200 randomly selected patients during their last trimester and found that only 7 (3.5%) had reflux. Although these findings suggest that infection of the upper urinary tract may result from reflux of infected urine from the bladder, cystography is not indicated during pregnancy.

Urography can be delayed in most instances until the postpartum period. It is indicated during pregnancy only in cases of multiple severe recurrences of infection that are refractory to drug or antibiotic therapy and require urography to exclude some underlying organic lesions which may require urgent surgical correction. *In these instances the urographic technique must be modified to reduce the radiation dose to the fetus.*

Occasionally pyelocaliectasis does not subside after pregnancy and the characteristic dilatation may then be observed years after the last pregnancy (Fig. 7-34). This is a frequent incidental finding and usually of no clinical significance. It has been demonstrated, however, that persistent dilatation is much more common in women with a history of pyelonephritis of pregnancy (Fry and Spiro). Clark (see Chapter 18) attributes this chronic ureterectasis to pressure and obstruction from a dilated right ovarian vein.

(Text continued on page 779.)

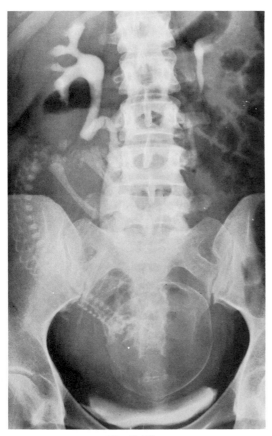
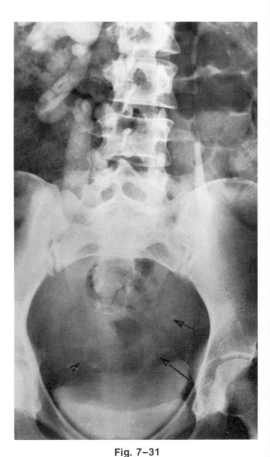

Fig. 7–30   **Fig. 7–31**

Figure 7–30. *Excretory urogram.* **Pyeloureterectasis of pregnancy.** Characteristic pyeloureterectasis on right side. Fetal parts visible.

Figure 7–31. *Excretory urogram.* **Pyeloureterectasis of pregnancy** which is more advanced. Fetal parts faintly visible in pelvis (*arrows*).

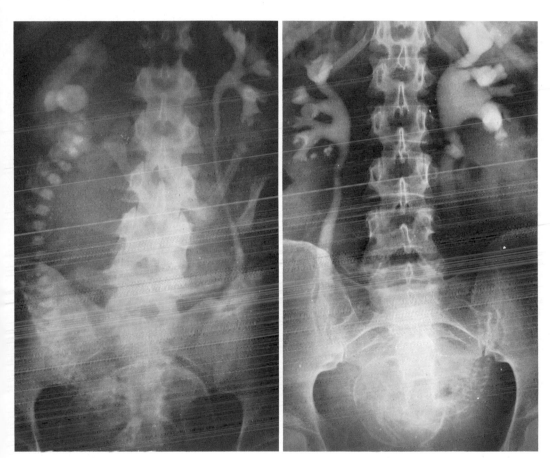

Fig. 7–32   Fig. 7–33

Figure 7–32. *Excretory urogram.* **Far-advanced pyeloureterectasis of pregnancy.** Obstruction of right ureter, with poorly functioning right kidney and marked calycectasis. Fetal parts well visualized. Left kidney normal.

Figure 7–33. *Excretory urogram.* **Bilateral pyeloureterectasis of pregnancy.** Atypical in that left kidney is site of greater obstruction than right. Fetal parts visible in pelvis.

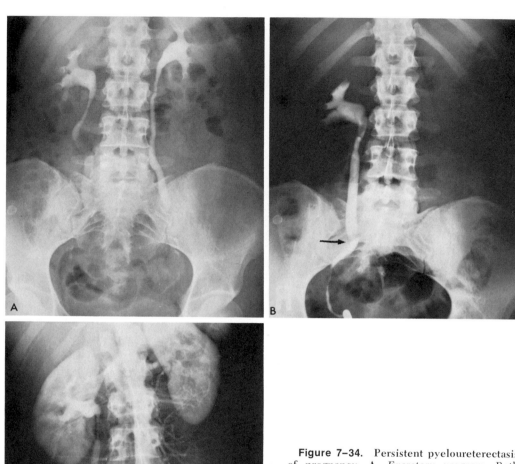

Figure 7–34. Persistent pyeloureterectasis of pregnancy. **A,** *Excretory urogram.* Both ureters slightly dilated to level of pelvic inlet. **B,** *Right retrograde pyelogram.* "Vascular impression" at level of pelvic inlet (*arrow*). **C,** *Intravenous aortogram.* Normal right iliac artery crosses ureter at point of vascular impression (*arrow*).

URETERITIS; URETERAL STRICTURES; VESICOURETERAL REFLUX

(Figs. 7-35 through 7-50)

Ureteral infection is usually associated with chronic pyelonephritis in children, but the resulting urographic changes received little attention until cystography was performed under fluoroscopic control. Dynamic factors such as **atony, abnormal peristalsis, and dilatation** were then observed in patients with vesicoureteral reflux and attributed to active ureteral infection. Following successful antibiotic therapy the ureteral dilatation may disappear and normal peristalsis may return (Shopfner). Improvement is less likely if the infection is chronic and neglected or inadequately treated.

Vesicoureteral reflux accentuates the degree of ureteral dilatation and therefore ureters that appear normal on excretory urograms may be found to be grossly dilated during voiding cystography (see Fig. 7-41). The lower one third of the ureter is frequently dilated on the urogram when reflux is present. Ureteral compression is a helpful adjunct during excretory urography because undue distensibility of the upper ureter may then be demonstrated. Linear striations of the ureter (Fig. 7-35) resulting from mucosal edema are occasionally associated with chronic pyelonephritis.

The most common findings are irregular areas of alternate dilatation and constriction associated with tortuosity (Figs. 7-36 through 7-40). **Inflammatory ureteral strictures** are relatively uncommon (Figs. 7-42 through 7-49) in nontuberculous infections. The diagnosis of stricture can be established by urography only when the collecting system is definitely dilated above the area in question. Urographic demonstration of a narrowed ureteral segment and inability to pass a ureteral catheter are not sufficient findings in themselves to warrant a diagnosis of stricture since either may result from spasm or ureteral peristalsis. Retroperitoneal abscess formation secondary to **regional enteritis** may be the cause of an inflammatory stricture of the right ureter (Fig. 7-50). Although this condition is relatively uncommon, it should be thought of in patients with this chronic disabling intestinal disease.

(Text continued on page 787.)

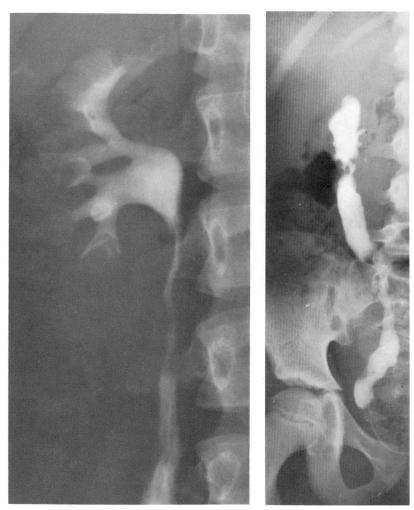

Fig. 7–35   Fig. 7–36

Figure 7–35. *Excretory urogram.* **Inflammatory linear striations,** upper right ureter. Twenty-two-year-old woman with active urinary tract infection. After 6 weeks of antibiotic therapy, striations were no longer evident.

Figure 7–36. *Right retrograde pyelogram.* **Advanced chronic pyelonephritis and ureteritis.** Malrotation with obliteration and cicatrization of many calyces, with marked changes in ureter.

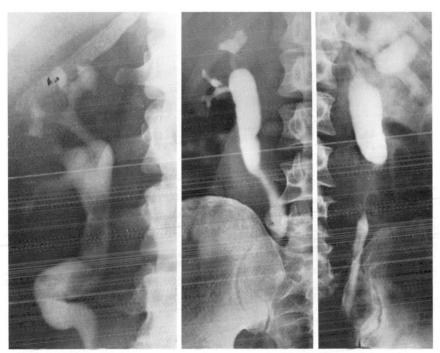

| Fig. 7–37 | Fig. 7–38 | Fig. 7–39 |

Figure 7–37. *Right retrograde pyelogram.* **Chronic pyelonephritis and ureteritis.** Irregular dilatation of pelvis and ureter, with alternate regions of dilatation and constriction. Filling defect in ureter from blood clots, might be confused with primary ureteral tumor.

Figure 7–38. *Right retrograde pyelogram.* **Chronic pyelonephritis and ureteritis.** Urographic evidence of inflammatory change confined almost solely to ureter, upper half of which is irregularly dilated, grade 2. Possible stricture in midportion of ureter.

Figure 7–39. *Left retrograde pyelogram.* **Advanced chronic pyelonephritis with ureteral stricture.** Marked inflammatory changes in ureter associated with stricture of middle portion of ureter and dilatation above and below. Advanced calycectasis.

Fig. 7–40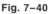

Fig. 7–41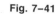

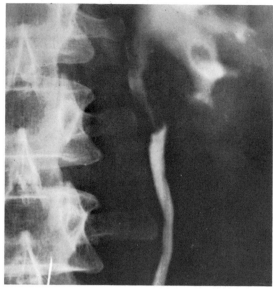

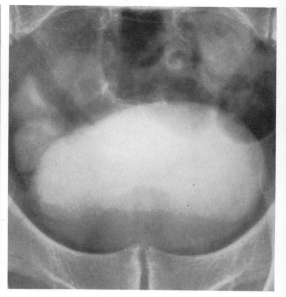

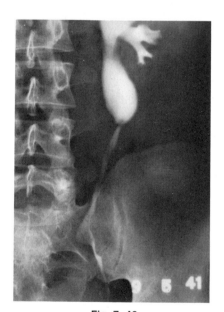

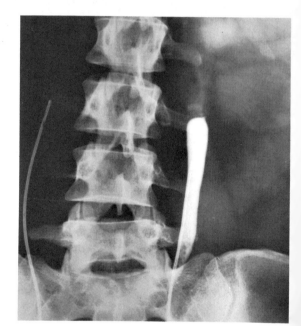

Fig. 7–42

Fig. 7–43

Figure 7–40. *Retrograde pyelogram.* **Chronic pyelonephritis with ureteral stricture.** Marked inflammatory changes in upper third of ureter, with area of narrowing 3 cm below ureteropelvic juncture. Left nephrectomy: definite thickening of ureter below ureteropelvic juncture.

Figure 7–41. *Excretory urogram.* **Reflux into right ureteral stump.** Prior right nephrectomy and partial ureterectomy for atrophic pyelonephritis. Tortuous, dilated ureteral stump provided reservoir for residual urine and continuing infections.

Figure 7–42. *Retrograde pyelogram.* **Ureteral stricture.** Plastic operation done on ureter for stricture.

Figure 7–43. *Retrograde pyelogram.* **Ureteral stricture.** Left nephrectomy. *Pathologic diagnosis:* chronic pyelonephritis with dilatation of pelvis due to stricture of ureter.

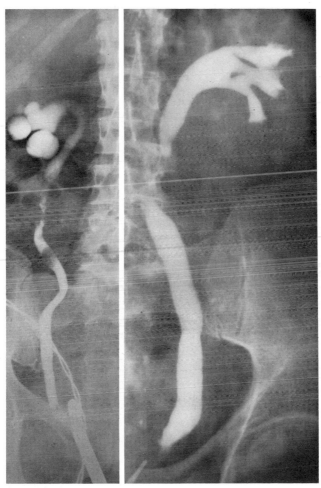

Fig. 7–44   **Fig. 7–45**

Figure 7–44.   *Retrograde pyelogram.* **Ureteral stricture.** Obstruction 2.5 cm below ureteropelvic juncture. Pyelocaliectasis.

Figure 7–45.   *Retrograde pyelogram.* **Multiple inflammatory strictures** of left ureter: one **opposite fourth lumbar vertebra** at junction of upper and middle thirds, which does not fill, and other in terminal portion of left ureter, with marked ureterectasis.

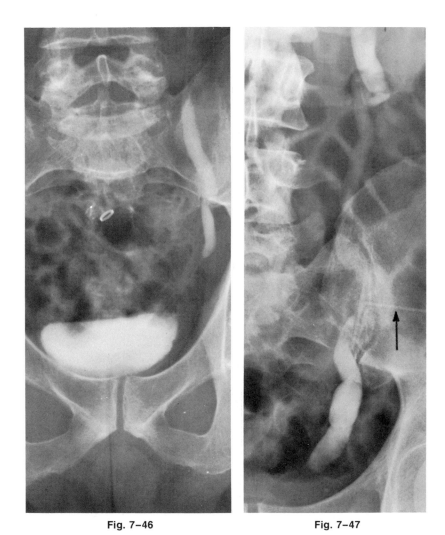

Fig. 7–46   Fig. 7–47

Figure 7–46. *Excretory urogram.* Inflammatory ureteral stricture, lower left ureter.

Figure 7–47. **Stricture of terminal portion of ureter**; may or may not have been complication of trans-urethral surgical procedure. *Left retrograde pyelogram* made through **T** tube (*arrow*) after ureter had been opened. Impossible to pass catheter through stricture from either above or below.

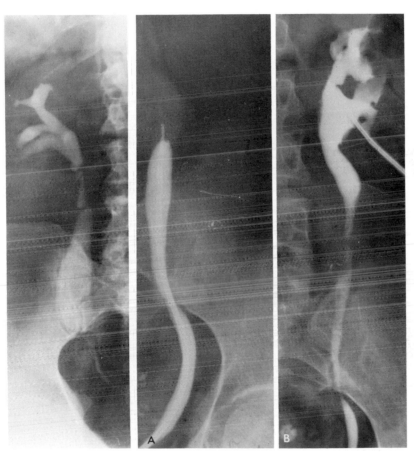

Fig. 7–48   Fig. 7–49

Figure 7–48. *Retrograde pyelogram.* **Inflammatory ureteral stricture.** Localized dilatation of right mid-ureter, with little or no dilatation above or below. Operation disclosed definite stricture 4 cm long beginning at brim of pelvis and extending distally.

Figure 7–49.   Results of end-to-end anastomosis of ureter following excision of impassable stricture. **A,** *Preoperative left retrograde pyelogram.* **Complete obstruction from stricture in midureter. B,** *Postoperative left pyelogram* through nephrostomy tube. Ureter patent. Contrast medium flows easily into bladder. (Courtesy of Dr. T. D. Moore.)

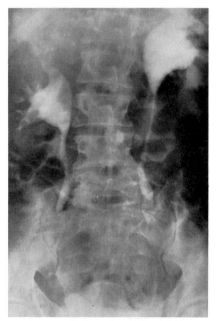

Figure 7–50.   *Excretory urogram.* **Regional ileitis** (Crohn's disease) with infiltration in the retroperitoneum resulting in bilateral partial ureteral obstruction. (From Schofield, P. F., Staff, W. G., and Moore, T.)

PYELITIS AND URETERITIS CYSTICA
(Figs. 7-51 through 7-56)

Pyelitis cystica and ureteritis cystica are identical lesions and frequently co-exist. The cysts result from chronic inflammation and are located immediately beneath the mucosa. They range from microscopic dimensions to 2 cm in diameter (Loitman and Chiat). The entire ureter may be involved, but the upper one third is most frequently affected.

Urographic findings are usually diagnostic. The subepithelial location allows the cysts to project into the lumen, creating sharply defined radiolucent filling defects. A characteristic "scalloping" of the ureter is evident when the cysts are seen in profile. Air bubbles introduced during retrograde pyelography may be confused with pyeloureteritis cystica, but air bubbles are inconsistent in location, are perfectly smooth, and do not produce scalloping of the margins of the ureter. Other causes of filling defects such as blood clots, radiopaque calculi, and epithelial tumors are easily distinguishable.

MALACOPLAKIA OF THE URINARY TRACT
(Figs. 7-57 through 7-60)

Malacoplakia is essentially a granulomatous disease of the urinary tract but it has also been reported in the prostate (Goldman; Hoffmann and Garrido) and testes (Brown and Smith; Haukohl and Chinchinian). It is most commonly encountered in the bladder but also occurs in both the ureters and the renal pelvis. It was first reported in 1902 by Michaelis and Gutmann and was named in 1903 by von Hansemann who combined two Greek words malakos (soft) and plakos (plaque), which describe its gross appearance. Melicow found 68 cases in 1957; reports of almost 100 are now in the literature.

Clinically the disease presents as a persistent chronic urinary infection which will not respond to treatment. Diagnosis is usually made by cystoscopy and cystoscopic biopsy. Grossly the lesions appear as multiple, pale yellowish or yellowish gray, soft, slightly raised discrete plaques that vary in diameter from minute to 2 or 3 cm; some may become confluent. Often the plaques are circumscribed by a thin areola of hyperemia.

If the upper urinary tract is not involved, the *excretory urogram* is usually normal. If the lesions involve the ureter they may cause obstruction with a defect simulating a primary ureteral tumor or stricture (Schneiderman and Simon) or generalized dilatation with multiple filling defects or a scalloping appearance or both (Kolodny) (Figs. 7-57 and 7-58). In patients with extensive involvement of the bladder the cystogram may show multiple filling defects which cannot be distinguished from cystitis glandularis or carcinoma. In most cases, however, bladder diagnosis is made by cystoscopic examination and biopsy.

Pathology: The gross appearance of the lesions has already been described. **Microscopic diagnosis** is somewhat difficult and usually requires significant experience on the part of the pathologist. The usual description given is a "subepithelial infiltration" principally of histiocytes (Hansemann cells) within which are diagnostic round mineralized concretions called "Michaelis-Gutmann bodies" (Figs. 7-59 and 7-60).

GAS-PRODUCING INFECTIONS OF THE URINARY TRACT; RENAL AND PERIRENAL EMPHYSEMA; CYSTITIS EMPHYSEMATOSA
(Figs. 7-61 through 7-70)

Gas in the renal substance, perirenal areas, bladder wall, or lumen of the collecting system may result from infection, penetrating trauma, fistulous connection with the intestinal tract, penetrating posterior-wall duodenal ulcer, and various diagnostic and surgical procedures. The exact location of the gas is usually obvious because of its distribution.

Gas-producing infections of the urinary tract are usually a rare manifestation of ordinary urinary **aerobic** pathogens such as *Escherichia coli*. Bacterial generation of gas occurs more commonly in the severe diabetic patient, which promotes speculation that hyperglycemia may furnish a special situation in which excess glucose in the tissues may be fermented by the bacteria. The urinary tract and perirenal areas are rarely involved with **anaerobic** gangrenous infections caused by clostridia unless it is part of a generalized process.

Gas within the wall of the bladder or within the renal substance is seen only when infection involves the kidney or bladder, but large amounts of gas may also accumulate within the collecting system. Gas within the collecting system may result from small-intestine or colonic fistulas but gas is not then seen within the bladder wall or kidney substance because there is sufficient inflammatory reaction adjacent to the fistula to prevent air from dissecting along soft-tissue planes. Fistulas are usually secondary to carcinoma or diverticulitis of the colon with secondary involvement of the bladder.

Cystitis emphysematosa may be suspected from the cystoscopic appearance of the bladder. In most reported cases the vesical mucosa has been described by such terms as marked acute cystitis; bladder mucosa fiery red, velvety, granular, shaggy, and rough; mucosa thrown into folds or rugae, between which are hundreds of transparent silvery globules, vesicles, or cysts, having the appearance of air bubbles. These cysts may be easily ruptured by the heel of the cystoscope. The urographic diagnosis can be suspected on the plain film from the distribution of the gas bubbles in the region of the bladder. Excretory urography establishes the diagnosis by confirming the location of the gas in the bladder wall, especially if films are made with the bladder in various degrees of distention. In rare instances a severe urinary infection may generate sufficient gas to outline the bladder in a manner similar to that occurring in air cystography.

The most common causes for gas in the urinary collecting system are iatrogenic. Careless technique frequently results in the injection of air during retrograde pyelography or voiding cystourethrography, and gas occasionally accumulates in the renal pelvis and ureter in patients who have had a ureterosigmoidostomy (Fig. 7-62). In the latter instance the accumulation is accompanied by reflux of fecal material and infection ensues.

(Text continued on page 800.)

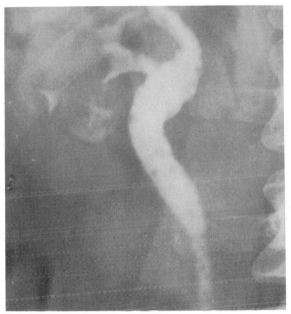

Figure 7–51. Pyelitis and ureteritis cystica. Marked inflammatory changes in calyces from long-standing infection, with pyelitis cystica involving pelvis and ureter. Cysts produce small negative shadows which suggest air bubbles. (Courtesy of Dr. E. D. Busby.)

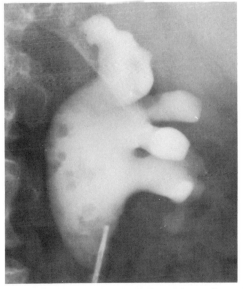

Figure 7–52. *Left retrograde pyelogram.* **Pyelitis cystica** and atrophic pyelonephritis.

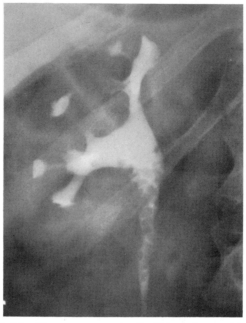

Figure 7–53.   *Excretory urogram.* Pyelitis and ureteritis cystica.

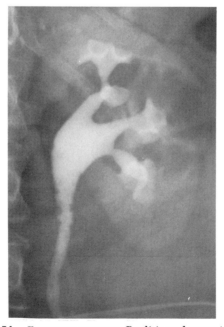

Figure 7–54.   *Excretory urogram.* Pyelitis and ureteritis cystica.

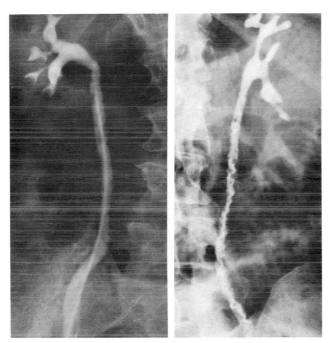

Fig. 7–55   Fig. 7–56

Figure 7–55. Ureteritis cystica. (Courtesy of Dr. G. F. Whitlock.)

Figure 7–56. **Advanced ureteritis cystica and renal cyst.** Calyceal blunting of left kidney. Renal cyst distorts lower-pole calyces. (From Loitman, B. S., and Chiat, H.)

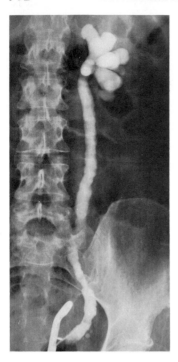

Figure 7-57. *Left retrograde pyelogram* in woman aged 48 with chronic urinary infection. **Malacoplakia of ureter** with filling defects, irregularity of entire left ureter, and associated ureterectasis and pyelocaliectasis. Surgical exploration and resection of lower ureter revealed extensive malacoplakia. (From Kolodny, G. M.)

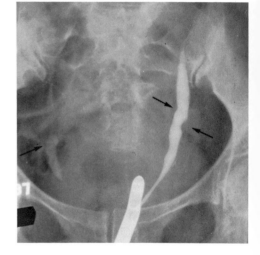

Figure 7-58. *Left retrograde ureterogram.* **Malacoplakic stump of left ureter** (left kidney and upper ureter had been removed previously elsewhere for malacoplakia of renal pelvis and upper ureter).

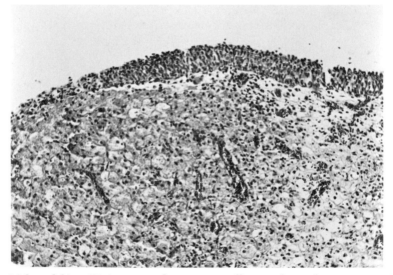

Figure 7-59. Malacoplakia. Histiocytic inflammatory collection beneath intact transitional mucosa. (Hematoxylin and eosin; ×140.)

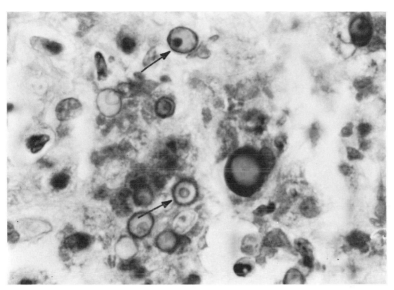

Figure 7–60. Malacoplakia. Michaelis-Gutmann bodies (*arrows*) within cytoplasm of histiocytes. Note characteristic internal structure. (Periodic acid Schiff stain; ×1070.)

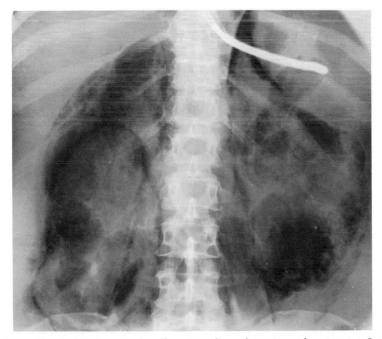

Figure 7–61. *Plain film.* **Extensive renal and perirenal emphysema** with urinary infection in diabetic patient. Kidneys and adrenal glands outlined on both sides. No gas could be seen within renal pelves. (From Gillies, C. L., and Flocks, R.)

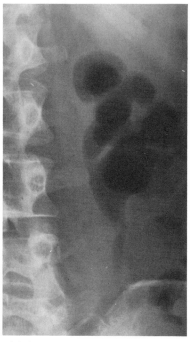

Figure 7–62. *Plain film.* **Gas-filled left ureter, pelvis, and calyces from ureterosigmoidostomy.** Forty-six-year-old female with previous left ureterosigmoidostomy. Left collecting system dilated. Left kidney failed to function on excretory urography.

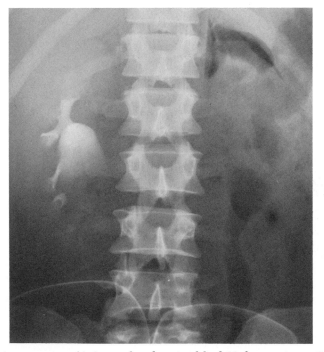

Figure 7–63. *Excretory urogram.* **Air in renal and ureteral bed** 11 days postoperative. Left nephrectomy and ureterectomy for hydronephrosis. Gas outlines ureter and upper portion of renal bed.

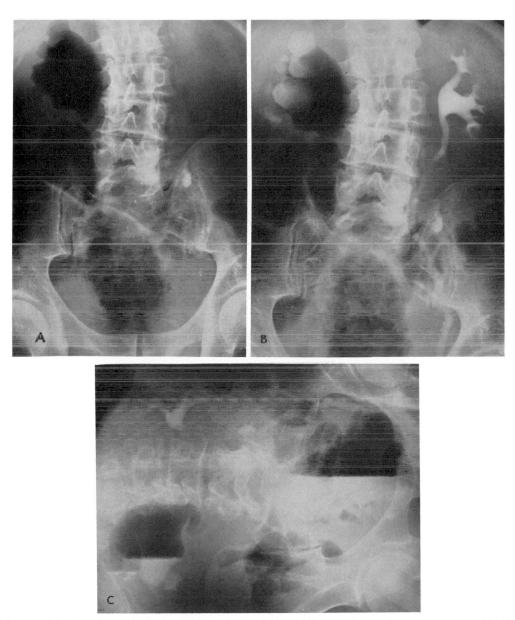

Figure 7–64. Emphysematous cystitis associated with gas filling of right collecting system and bladder. Nondiabetic man aged 70 years. Bilateral vesicoureteral reflux demonstrated on cystogram and *E. coli* isolated from urine. **A,** *Plain film.* Gas outlines dilated right pelviocalyceal system, ureter, and bladder. Multiple locules of gas within bladder wall. **B,** *Excretory urogram.* Both kidneys excrete medium. **C,** *Lateral decubitus view.* "Air-fluid" levels in right renal pelvis and in bladder.

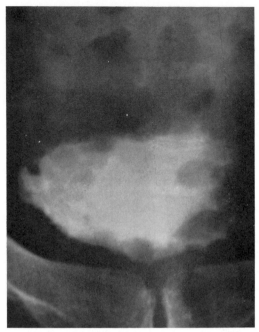

Figure 7–65. *Excretory cystogram.* **Bullous edema of vesical mucosa which could be mistaken for cystitis emphysematosa.** Man aged 66. Edema was caused by pelvic abscess which followed surgical resection of sigmoid colon for carcinoma.

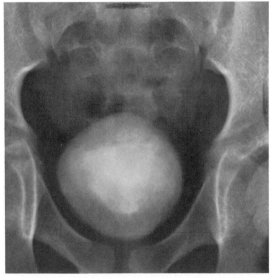

Figure 7–66. *Excretory urogram.* **Emphysematous cystitis.** Six-year-old girl with symptoms of urinary tract infection. Air throughout bladder wall creating a halo effect where seen in profile.

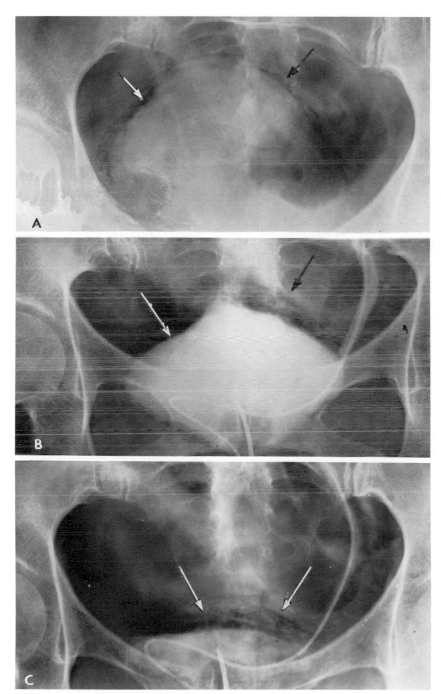

Figure 7–67. Cystitis emphysematosa in diabetic patient. A, *Excretory urogram.* Translucent ring of negative air or gas shadows surround bladder (*arrows*). B, *Retrograde cystogram.* Same (*arrows*). C, Bladder incompletely filled with contrast medium which has run back from making a left pyelogram. Ring of gas shadows seems to maintain same relation to collapsed wall of bladder. (From Teasley, G. H.)

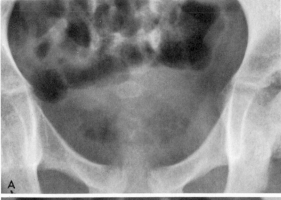
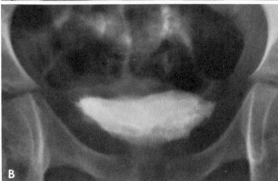

Figure 7–68. **Air in bladder** of 4-year-old girl with *E. coli* infection. **A,** *Plain film.* Multiple air bubbles in region of bladder. **B,** *Excretory urogram.* Multiple views demonstrated that bubbles of air were within bladder lumen.

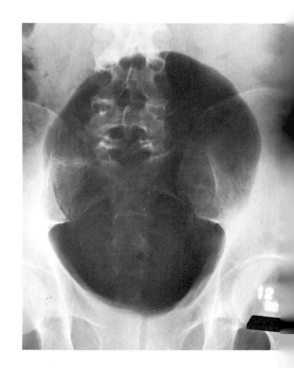

Figure 7–69. *Plain film.* Distention of bladder from spontaneous generation of gas in severely diabetic male aged 30. Severe urinary tract infection (*E. coli*) resulting in marked production and accumulation of gas.

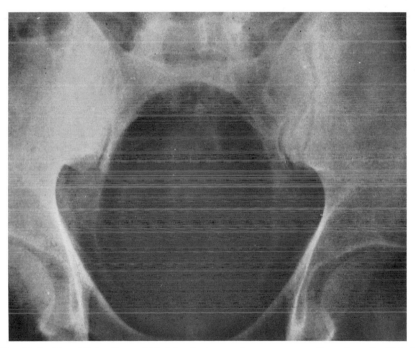

Figure 7–70. *Plain film.* Distention of bladder from spontaneous generation of gas in diabetic male with urinary infection. (From Kent, H. P.)

Section 2

RENAL PARENCHYMAL (CORTICAL) INFECTION – CORTICAL ABSCESS; RENAL "CARBUNCLE"; PERINEPHRITIS; PERINEPHRIC ABSCESS;* PYONEPHROSIS, AND SO FORTH

(Figs. 7-71 through 7-97)

The onset of cortical infection of a kidney may be acute and fulminating, simulating an acute abdominal emergency. The infection is usually seen, however, as an obscure, insidious, and gradually progressive disease with few localizing symptoms, associated with low-grade fever, general malaise, and loss of weight. Although in the majority of cases the condition is preceded by some pyogenic infection such as a furuncle, carbuncle, infected tooth, or infection of the upper part of the respiratory tract, the patient may have forgotten about the preceding infection unless carefully questioned. Unless the physician thinks of the possibility of cortical infection, diagnosis is usually not made until late in the course of the disease.

The distinction among cortical infection, multiple cortical abscesses, massive solitary cortical abscess (carbuncle), perinephritis, and perinephric abscess is not clear-cut. Infection may occur early in the loose fatty tissue surrounding a kidney and progress to an abscess of enormous size with few if any symptoms. It may or may not be associated with gross cortical abscesses of substantial proportions. The problems of diagnosis are chiefly clinical rather than urographic, and keen diagnostic acumen may be necessary to suspect the

diagnosis. If one waits for gross urographic changes to occur before making a diagnosis, valuable time may be lost. It is not within the province of this book to discuss in detail the clinical problem involved. Excellent articles on this subject (Beer; Cabot, 1930; 1936; Cabot and Montgomery) should be consulted for a discussion of this important problem.

UROGRAPHIC FINDINGS

One of the earliest changes seen is evidence of pressure on a calyx, which may be caused by either a perirenal accumulation of pus or a cortical abscess in the vicinity of the calyx. The calyx may fill incompletely during excretory urography, but if pressure on the calyx is minimal it may be possible to fill the calyx during retrograde pyelography. If such is accomplished, the calyx may appear almost normal or only slightly dilated and the finding may be dismissed as of no importance unless the physician is keenly aware of the possibilities. If the process is advanced, however, **incomplete calyceal filling** or even complete obliteration may be evident from the retrograde pyelogram (Figs. 7-71 through 7-74).

The sign of "fixation" or decrease in mobility of a kidney has been stressed by Mathé and is a fairly common and important finding. This can be demonstrated by exposing films during both phases of respiration or by obtaining a film with the patient upright. A normal kidney should have an excursion of the width of one lumbar vertebra. If the kidney is fixed in its position, perirenal inflammation should be suspected.

Haziness of the renal outline, poor visualization or complete **obliteration of the outline of the psoas muscle,** and **lumbar scoliosis** with the concavity toward the affected kidney are important and well-known findings (see Fig. 7-88). They may be of great help in diagnosis if properly correlated with the clinical data at hand.

---

*In former years this disease was relatively common and of great importance to the urologist. Since the advent of modern chemotherapy and antibiotics, however, its incidence has greatly diminished so that, like genitourinary tuberculosis, cases are relatively rare and are being missed. For this reason we are maintaining a generous number of illustrations of perinephric abscess in this edition.

It must not be forgotten, however, that these signs are present in a certain percentage of cases in which the kidney is normal.

Displacement of the kidney may be of great diagnostic importance. Depending on the position of the cortical or perinephric abscess, the kidney may be pushed medially against the spinal column, laterally, downward, or upward (see Fig. 7-91). Menville has also called attention to the anterior displacement of the kidney, which may be demonstrated by pyelograms made in the lateral position (see Fig. 7-90). If these findings are tempered with good clinical judgment and carefully considered with the available clinical findings, they may be of great diagnostic help. It must be remembered, however, that normal kidneys are subject to wide variation in position. The additional finding of a soft-tissue mass (representing an abscess situated in a position to cause the displacement) is valuable evidence that the renal displacement is due to a pathologic process.

Erosion of Abscess Into Collecting System or Contiguous Structures; Fistulas

A **cortical abscess** may erode into and **communicate with the collecting system** so that the resulting urogram will show irregular cavities and cortical necrosis simulating tuberculosis (Figs. 7-75 through 7-80; see also Fig. 7-89). A cortical abscess may also "point" toward the periphery and rupture through the renal capsule into the perinephric fat rather than into the pelviocalyceal system. In occasional cases this rupture can be seen in the plain film as a loss in continuity of the margin of the kidney.

When a **noncommunicating abscess** becomes sufficiently large, it may cause calyceal deformity typical of any "expanding" lesion of the kidney and may be difficult to distinguish from simple solitary cyst or cortical tumor. Nephrotomography and arteriography are then very helpful in excluding a cyst, **but angiographic changes may closely resemble hypernephroma because neovascularity simulating tumor vessels is a common finding in cortical abscesses** (Figs. 7-81 through 7-86).

The clinical manifestations of **pyonephrosis** are similar to those of cortical abscess. It is a separate pathologic entity, however, because the infection is predominantly within the pelvis and calyces. Obstruction is a constant feature and as a result exudate accumulates within a dilated pelviocalyceal system. The involved kidney fails to function during excretory urography, but the renal shadow may appear enlarged. Retrograde pyelography demonstrates either complete obstruction, usually at the ureteropelvic junction, or a peculiar pyelographic picture resulting from dispersion of the contrast medium throughout exudate that has accumulated in the dilated pelvis and calyces.

Complications of Parenchymal (Cortical) Infections (Psoas and Subphrenic Abscess; Nephrobronchial Fistula) (Figs. 7-87 through 7-97)

Complications of cortical and perinephric abscess usually are serious conditions. **Psoas abscess** may result as an advanced phase of involvement of the fascia of the psoas muscle. Pus may burrow down the fascial plane of this muscle and produce severe pain and painful flexion of the thigh. Occasionally the plain film may be helpful by demonstrating a soft-tissue mass in this area. **Subphrenic abscess** and extension of the process into a pleural cavity and lung are occasionally seen in severe cases. In cases in which there is elevation or limitation of excursion of the diaphragm or collection of fluid in a pleural cavity, one should always think of the possibility of a **perinephric abscess** as the source. In rare cases the infection may extend through the diaphragm into a **pleural cavity**, involve the corresponding lung, and perforate into a bronchus, producing a **nephrobronchial fistula** (Fig. 7-96) which may be demonstrated urographically. Rupture of the abscess through the skin in the loin may leave **chronic draining fistulas** that may be demonstrated with contrast medium.

Erosion with perforation of the proximal portion of a ureter, and rupture of the abscess into the gastrointestinal tract, are rare complications. Finally, in cases in which the condition has been neglected and the process is of long standing, complete or partial healing may occur with the deposition of a large amount of calcium in the renal region and complete obliteration of the kidney.

(Text continued on page 818.)

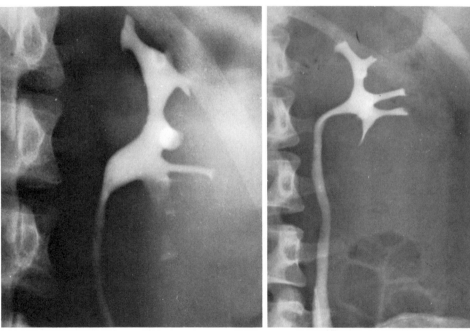

Fig. 7–71   Fig. 7–72

Figure 7–71. *Retrograde pyelogram.* **Cortical abscess,** lower pole of left kidney. Distortion and incomplete filling of the lower-pole calyx result.

Figure 7–72. *Left retrograde pyelogram.* **Cortical abscess** in lower pole of left kidney, causing crescentic deformity of lower calyces of left kidney, simulating tumor or cyst.

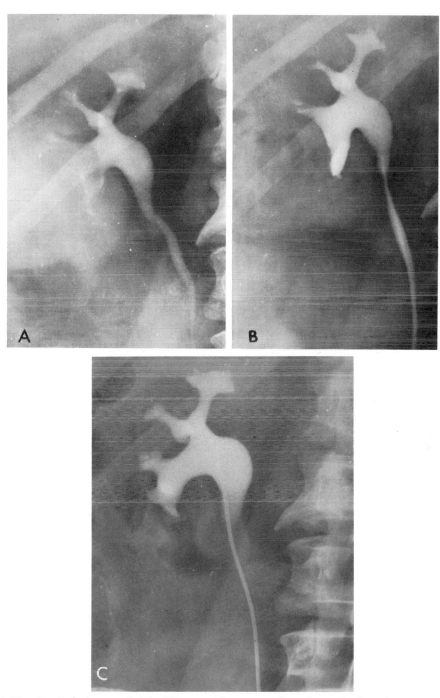

Figure 7–73.   **Cortical abscess of right kidney,** with progress films during healing. **A,** *Excretory urogram.* Cortical abscess in lower pole of right kidney, causing crescentic deformity of lower group of calyces, which ould be confused with cyst or tumor. **B,** *Right retrograde pyelogram,* made 2 days after **A. C,** *Right retrograde yelogram* made several months later, after inflammatory process had subsided. Lower group of calyces as returned to normal.

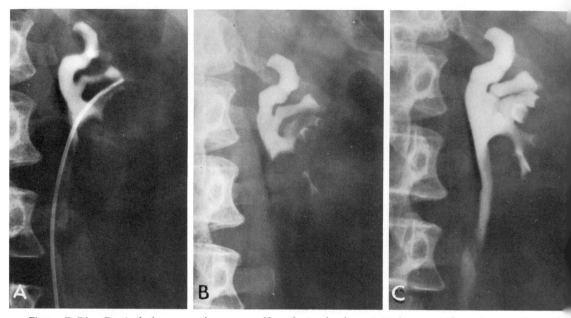

Figure 7–74.   **Cortical abscess** with progress films during healing. **A,** *Left retrograde pyelogram.* Cortical abscess in lower pole of left kidney, causing crescentic deformity of lower calyces, simulating cyst or tumor. **B,** *Left retrograde pyelogram* 2 weeks later, during which time antibiotics had been administered. Considerable improvement is shown by beginning return to normal of lower calyces. **C,** *Left retrograde pyelogram* 2 months after **B,** when inflammatory process had subsided. Kidney is now urographically normal, and lower calyces have returned to normal.

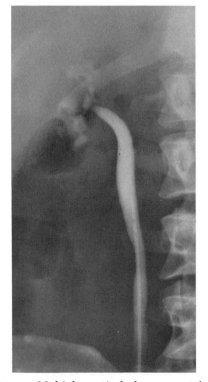

Figure 7–75.   *Retrograde pyelogram.* **Multiple cortical abscesses,** right kidney. Several abscesses have eroded into pelviocalyceal system and filled with medium during retrograde pyelography.

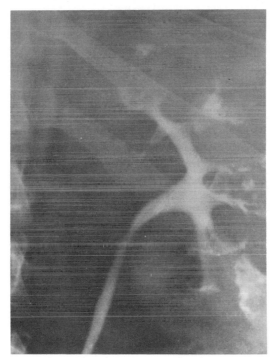

Figure 7–76. *Retrograde pyelogram.* **Cortical abscess,** left kidney. Left retrograde pyelogram demonstrates communication between abscesses and calyces, with marked calyceal deformity.

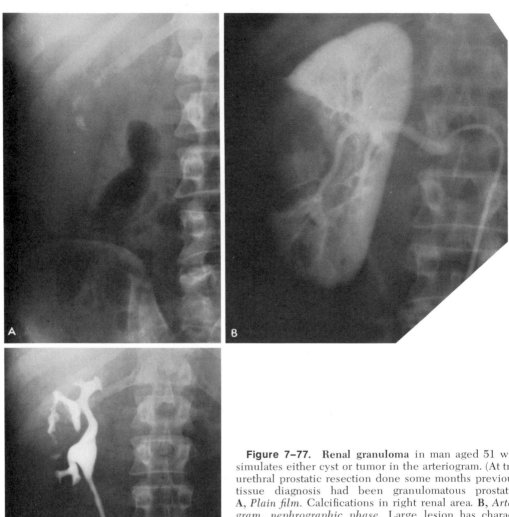

Figure 7–77. **Renal granuloma** in man aged 51 which simulates either cyst or tumor in the arteriogram. (At transurethral prostatic resection done some months previously, tissue diagnosis had been granulomatous prostatitis. **A,** *Plain film.* Calcifications in right renal area. **B,** *Arteriogram, nephrographic phase.* Large lesion has characteristics of either simple cyst or tumor. **C,** *Retrograde pyelogram.* Contrast medium enters mass, forming irregular cavity which communicates with upper calyx. *Operation:* Nephrectomy. Pathology: Large granuloma with necrotic area in central portion which communicates with upper calyx. (It was impossible to demonstrate tubercle bacilli in either urine or tissue.) (Courtesy of Dr. Clyde Blackard.)

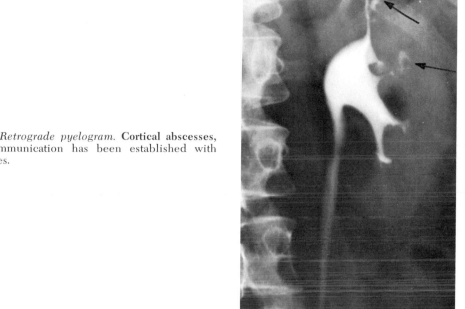

Figure 7–78. *Retrograde pyelogram.* **Cortical abscesses,** left kidney. Communication has been established with upper-pole calyces.

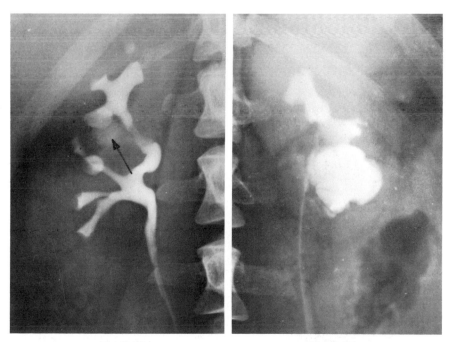

Fig. 7–79   Fig. 7–80

Figure 7–79. *Retrograde pyelogram.* **Cortical abscess** which has eroded through infundibulum of upper lyx and communicates with pelviocalyceal system.

Figure 7–80. *Retrograde pyelogram.* **Cortical abscess** involving lower pole of left kidney and communicating with lower group of calyces, causing marked deformity and cortical necrosis.

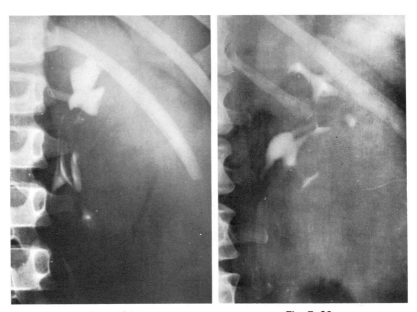

Fig. 7–81   Fig. 7–82

Figure 7–81. *Excretory urogram.* **Cortical abscess,** left kidney. Large, sharply outlined mass causing crescentic deformity of pelvis and lower-pole calyces.

Figure 7–82. *Excretory urogram.* **Large cortical abscess,** lower pole of left kidney. Ureter displaced medially and slight deformity of lower-pole calyces.

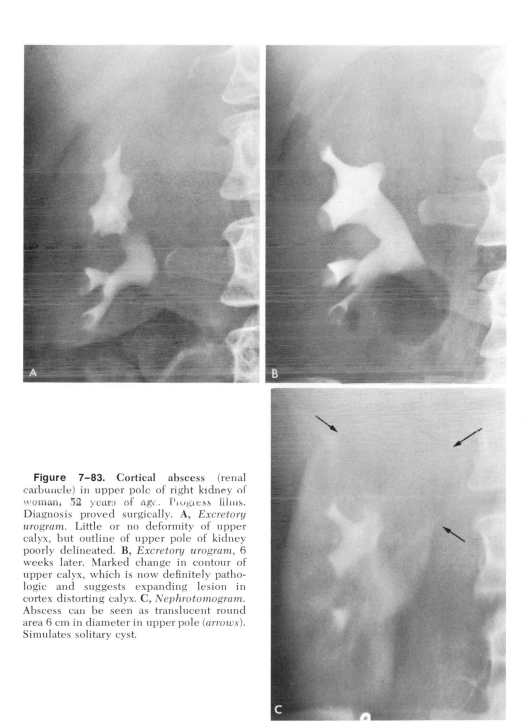

Figure 7–83. Cortical abscess (renal carbuncle) in upper pole of right kidney of woman, 52 years of age. Progress films. Diagnosis proved surgically. **A,** *Excretory urogram.* Little or no deformity of upper calyx, but outline of upper pole of kidney poorly delineated. **B,** *Excretory urogram,* 6 weeks later. Marked change in contour of upper calyx, which is now definitely pathologic and suggests expanding lesion in cortex distorting calyx. **C,** *Nephrotomogram.* Abscess can be seen as translucent round area 6 cm in diameter in upper pole (*arrows*). Simulates solitary cyst.

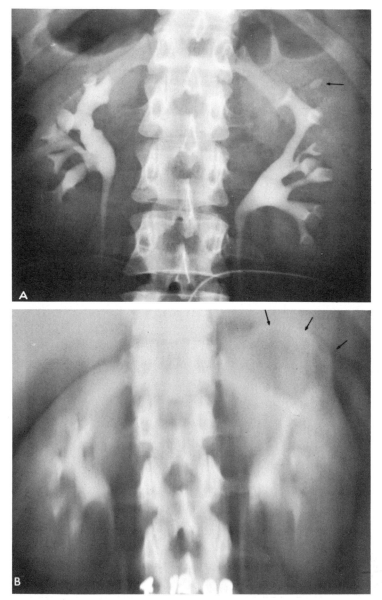

Figure 7–84.   Renal abscess, left kidney. A, *Excretory urogram.* Small parenchymal calculus (*arrow*) Renal outline of upper pole of left kidney is ill defined. **B,** *Nephrotomogram.* Thick-walled mass lesio (*arrows*) in upper pole of left kidney. Preoperative diagnosis: renal abscess versus necrotic hypernephrom;

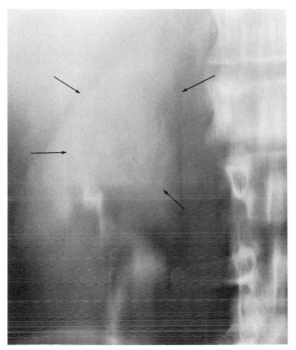

Figure 7–85. *Nephrotomogram.* **Cortical renal abscess.** Mass lesion, upper pole of right kidney. Margins of abscess (*arrows*) indistinct.

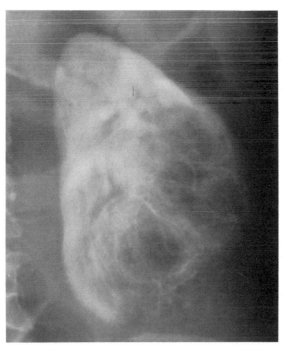

Figure 7–86. *Arteriogram.* **Renal abscess.** Highly vascular inflammatory mass occupying most of left kidney. Hypernephroma could produce similar picture. (From Becker, J. A., Fleming, R., Kanter, I., and Melicow, M.)

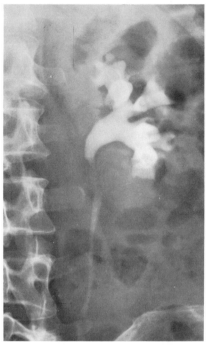

Figure 7–87. *Retrograde pyelogram.* **Solitary abscess** of lower pole of left kidney, which is compressing and obstructing 3 cm of ureter immediately below ureteropelvic juncture and causing calycectasis.

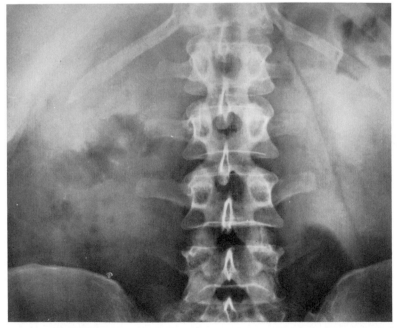

Figure 7–88. *Plain film.* **Perinephric abscess** involving right kidney. Note haziness of shadow on right with absence of normal outline of psoas muscle, which is considered characteristic of perinephric abscess.

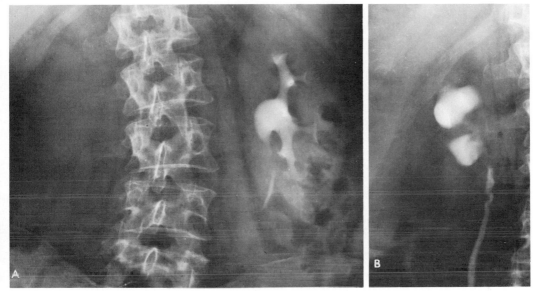

Figure 7-89.   Cortical abscess of right kidney **with perinephric abscess. A,** *Excretory urogram.* Large perinephric abscess of right kidney, which has no function. Scoliosis of lumbar portion of spinal column, with concavity toward right and absence of normal psoas outline. Left kidney normal. **B,** *Right retrograde pyelogram.* Cortical abscess has eroded into pelviocalyceal system.

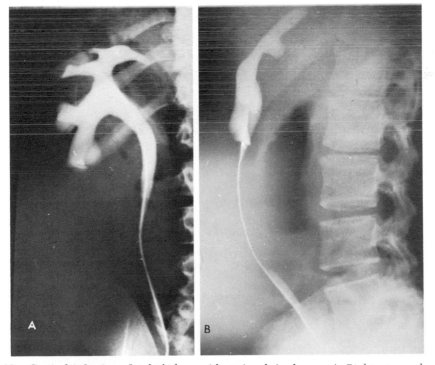

Figure 7-90.   Cortical infection of right kidney **with perinephric abscess. A,** *Right retrograde pyelogram, anteroposterior view.* Deformity of upper calyces, with flattening and crescentic outline, suggesting pressure from cortical abscess. **B,** *Lateral view.* Marked anterior displacement of kidney from perinephric abscess. (From Menville, J. G.)

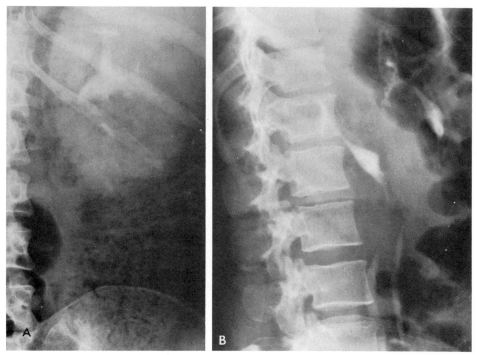

Figure 7–91. Perinephric abscess with displacement of kidney. **A,** *Excretory urogram.* Upward and lateral displacement of left kidney with poor filling. **B,** *Lateral view.* Marked anterior displacement of left kidney caused by perinephric abscess. (Courtesy of Dr. S. J. Arnold and Department of Urology and Radiology, Jewish Hospital of Brooklyn.)

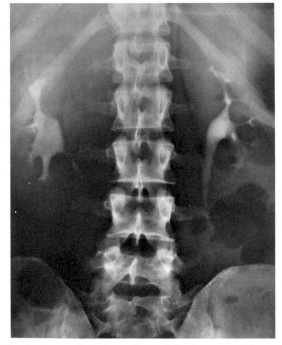

Figure 7–92. Perinephric abscess, right kidney. Lateral displacement of upper pole and absence of psoas shadow.

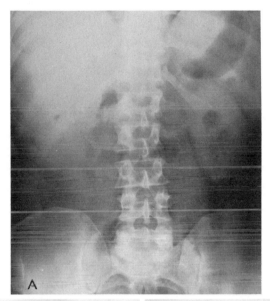

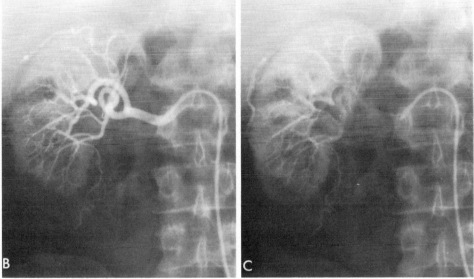

Figure 7–93. Perinephric abscess. Fifty-one-year-old man. **A,** *Plain film.* Absent right psoas shadow. Indistinct outline, right kidney. **B,** *Arteriogram.* Capsular arteries enlarged and tortuous, especially over lower pole. **C,** *Arteriogram, late arterial phase.* Capsular arteries supply tangle of vessels in abscess overlying lower pole.

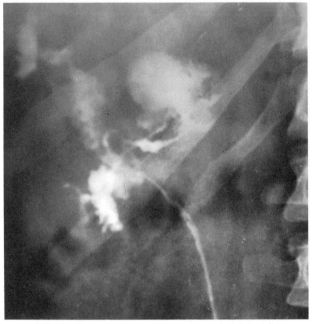

Figure 7–94. *Retrograde pyelogram.* **Multiple abscesses of kidney and perinephric abscess.** Abscess pockets communicate with pelviocalyceal system. Incision and drainage showed multilocular pockets in renal region filled with granulation tissue.

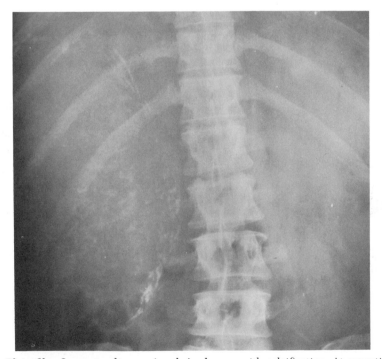

Figure 7–95. *Plain film.* Long-standing **perinephric abscess** with calcification. At operation no renal substance could be demonstrated. (Courtesy of Dr. J. M. Pace.)

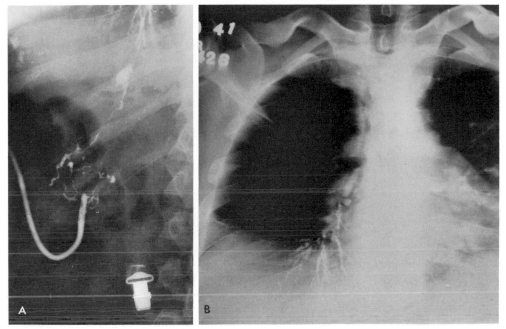

Figure 7–96.   Perinephric abscess with nephrobronchial fistula. **A,** Medium injected through catheter inserted in draining lumbar sinus outlines irregular cavity in right renal region with communication through diaphragm to lower part of bronchial tree. **B,** Film of chest shows contrast medium outlining lower small bronchi. Note: This condition originated from branched calculus in right kidney, complicated by multiple cortical abscesses and perinephric abscess. Subcapsular nephrectomy was done for this condition. Draining sinus continued and incision was explored about 1½ months later. A piece of stone and a fragment of renal pelvis were removed and sinus was curetted. These films were made 1 month after curettage.

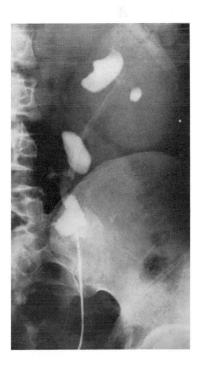

Figure 7–97.   *Retrograde pyelogram.* Cortical abscess of left kidney with perinephric abscess and erosion of upper half of left ureter, as evidenced by extravasation of medium along course of ureter. Marked lateral displacement of left kidney and obliteration of normal psoas outline.

CYSTITIS

The diagnosis of cystitis is provided by cystoscopy. In mild or moderate cases the mucosa of the bladder appears reddened in more or less discrete circumscribed areas, which has given rise to the term **areal cystitis**. In severe cases the entire mucosa may be involved, reddened, and bleeding easily on distention; this condition is termed **diffuse cystitis**.

AMICROBIC CYSTITIS

In most cases it is not possible to distinguish a bacillary from a coccal infection by the cystoscopic appearance of the bladder. An exception to this statement is a peculiar and rather unusual condition which in the past has been called "hemorrhagic amicrobial cystitis." This condition appears most commonly in women and is sudden in onset, the first symptoms being the passage of gross blood. Cystoscopically the entire bladder mucosa is the site of punctate hemorrhagic areas which are so acute they almost appear to be the result of trauma from some sharp instrument introduced into the bladder. Urine cultures are always negative but microscopic examination shows many pus cells and, of course, gross blood. The etiology of the condition has been thought to be a blood-borne infection with a sudden shower of cocci involving the bladder mucosa. The process is self-limiting and usually of relatively short (few days) duration. At the height of the disease the symptoms may be extremely severe, the patient suffering with frequency, dysuria, and stranguria. Vesical capacity may be reduced to almost zero and the extreme vesical irritability may act as an obstruction to the ureters resulting in temporary ureterectasis (Figs. 7-98 and 7-99).

Before the era of modern urinary antiseptics, neoarsphenamine or oxophenarsine (Mapharsen) was used to treat the condition, at times with seemingly brilliant results. At present the use of sulfonamide drugs seems to be as good as any treatment, as the condition subsides whether or not treatment is given.

TUBERCULOUS CYSTITIS

As emphasized in Chapter 8, tuberculosis may mimic almost any disease. Formerly, before the era of modern antituberculosis therapy, most experienced urologists could usually make a "snap" diagnosis of urinary tuberculosis simply by the cystoscopic appearance of the bladder. The areas of cystitis were more acute, "angry," granular, or ulcerated than in nontuberculous infections, and tended to collect on the same side of the bladder as the involved (or more involved) kidney, usually being most severe in the region of the ureteral orifice.

Today, owing to the excellent antimicrobial treatment for the disease, very few "typical" cases of tuberculous cystitis are encountered. In fact, a large proportion of cases now are not recognized even by most experienced cystoscopists. One must be alert and thinking of the condition to avoid errors. Unilateral lesions a little more acute and granular-appearing than in other infections and lying adjacent to one ureteral orifice should be suspect. Diagnosis of course depends on urography and identification of *Mycobacterium tuberculosis* (see Chapter 8).

INTERSTITIAL CYSTITIS (HUNNER'S ULCER; ELUSIVE ULCER; PANMURAL CYSTITIS, AND SO FORTH)

This condition is found almost exclusively in women and almost exclusively at or after the menopause. It is a most painful lesion and many distraught women with this painful disease go from one physician to another seeking relief, only to be told that they have crystal-clear uninfected urine and hence no "organic" reason for this complaint.

In untreated patients, cystoscopy shows one or more characteristic lesions almost always in the upper half (fundus) of the bladder. The untreated lesion appears as a well-circumscribed salmon colored "ulcer" that is almost translucent, like a stained-glass window. Often in the center of the lesion is a small superficial tag of mucosa which appears free except for an attachment of one edge to the lesion, the tag waving around from the currents of water from the cystoscope. If this lesion is touched with the heel of the cystoscope or a ureteral catheter the patient will cry out with severe pain and almost jump off the cystoscopic table. On the other hand if the normal-appearing areas of the bladder are touched no pain is elicited.

The lesions cause the bladder to lose its normal capacity. Distention of the bladder with water during cystoscopy can cause excruciating pain and cause the lesion to bleed. In cases of long-standing disease the bladder capacity may finally be reduced to less than an ounce so that the patient is practically incontinent and must wear pads to absorb the urine.

The cause of the disease has never been determined. Primary lesions of the blood vessels or trophic lesions of the nerves have been suggested. Microscopically all that can be seen is round cell infiltration in the submucosa with some extension into the detrusor muscle.

Treatment has been unsatisfactory. If the lesion or lesions are excised surgically, they promptly appear in some other area of the bladder (giving rise to the term "elusive ulcer"). The most prompt relief is obtained from cystoscopic overdistention of the bladder under general anesthesia, distending it with water until the mucosa over the lesions tears to a depth of at least 1/8 inch and bleeds sharply. Although relief is prompt, symptoms usually recur within a few months to a year and require further overdistention. One drawback to this type of treatment is that at each overdistention stellate scars are made in the lesion and the bladder appears to contract more as a result.

Office treatment using intermittent vesical lavage with dilute solutions of either oxychlorosene (Clorpactin) or silver nitrate is often quite effective and may keep the patient reasonably comfortable.

Urography is of little value in diagnosis except to demonstrate a bladder of reduced capacity and, for some unknown reason, occasionally unilateral vesicoureteral reflux.

EOSINOPHILIC CYSTITIS

In recent years a few cases of an unusual condition called "eosinophilic cystitis" have been reported. Most of these have been in children. Cystoscopically the condition has been described as "slightly elevated plaque-like lesions varying in size from 1/4 to 1/2 cm in diameter"; "bullous edema and clusters of glistening velvety-red globules which looked somewhat like botryoid sarcoma"; "a 1-cm red polypoid lesion on the interureteric ridge with a few cyst-like areas on the lateral wall of the bladder with an area in the dome of grape-like polyps." In all these cases, biopsies have revealed intense inflammatory infiltration of the mucosa and bladder muscle with eosinophils. The etiology of the condition has not been determined and treatment has been empirical. Urograms have shown irregular deformity of the bladder, both dilatation and contraction, and evidence of vesicoureteral reflux (Fig. 7-100).

CYSTITIS CYSTICA

Although this lesion is most common in the bladder it also involves the renal pelvis and ureters (see discussion above). Diagnosis is made cystoscopically, as the gross appearance of the lesions is typical and easily recognized. They appear as multiple small "cysts" which give the appearance of "cooked tapioca." The most common location is the trigone and region of the vesical neck; if the trigone is completely covered it has a "cobblestone" appearance and the ureteral orifices may be difficult to identify. The lesions may involve the entire bladder but when this is the case usually the "cysts" are more or less single, are rather sparsely distributed, and may be surrounded by a small halo of erythema. Erythema is not prominent in the dense trigonal mass of cysts.

It has always been considered that the disease is the result of or associated with chronic urinary infection either past or present, but it is also known that sparse microscopic lesions may be found in almost all bladders if carefully examined.

Pathogenesis

In a pathologic study in depth, Bothe and Cristol supported von Brunn's theory. Von Brunn described "epithelial buds" and "epithelial nests" which develop from downward proliferation of the normal transitional epithelium that lines the urinary tract. If the downward projection separates from the surface epithelium, it is called a "nest"; if it maintains a connection, it is called a "bud." These buds and nests then undergo central degeneration which gives them the appearance of cysts. Patch and Rhea also supported this theory. General opinion favors the theory that no secretory activity is present. These "cysts" remain small, are situated immediately beneath the mucosal lining, and elevate the lining into the lumen of the bladder, ureters, or renal pelvis to produce the characteristic appearance of the condition. Stirling and Ash postulated a somewhat different concept of pathogenesis. Their study suggested "glandular metaplasia" of the surface epithelium as the primary cause. The gland-like structures appear to be embedded in the stroma; hyperplastic inflammation elevates the surface of the vesical mucosa and throws it into folds with the formation of large branching-like crypts. If these are cut across in making microscopic sections, they appear

isolated (von Brunn's nests); however, in reality they are all connected with the mucosa above.

This brings up the problem of numerous conditions such as cystitis glandularis, cystitis granulosa, and cystitis folliculosa which Stirling and Ash choose to call "chronic proliferative lesions of the urinary tract." They point out that it is possible for "metaplasia" to change transitional cell epithelium to squamous epithelium (leukoplakia, squamous cell carcinoma, and so forth) or to glandular epithelium (benign hyperplasia of glands or adenocarcinoma). This subject will be discussed more fully below under Cystitis Glandularis.

Urography

Although urography is necessary for the diagnosis of pyelitis and ureteritis cystica, it is of limited value in cystitis cystica unless the condition is extensive. Diagnosis is so easily and accurately accomplished by cystoscopy that time and expense should not be incurred in urographic diagnosis.

CYSTITIS GLANDULARIS (OTHER TERMS: CYSTITIS GRANULOMA; BENIGN HYPERPLASIA OF GLANDS; HYPERPLASIA OF ALBARRAN'S GLANDS; CYSTIC ADENOMA; CHRONIC PROLIFERATIVE LESIONS OF THE URINARY TRACT)

This is a relatively uncommon lesion with larger cystic glands which may penetrate fairly deeply into the wall of the bladder. As in cystitis cystica, the lesions have a predilection for the trigone and region of the vesical neck. Grossly the lesions may appear as granuloma and often look like a solid infiltrating carcinoma of the bladder, the true diagnosis being made only by biopsy and microscopic examination of the tissue.

Histopathology

Two types of glands have been identified (Emmett and McDonald): (1) intestinal type glands (Fig. 7-101) and (2) subtrigonal glands of Albarran (Fig. 7-102). The intestinal-type glands are lined by a simple layer of columnar epithelium with small basally placed nuclei. The cells are filled with mucus, making them indistinguishable from goblet cells of the intestinal tract.

The subtrigonal type of gland is lined by multiple layers of cells. "Adjacent to the lumen of these glands was a single layer of columnar cells which had basally placed nuclei showing a free border of cytoplasm. The several layers of cells outside this single layer consisted of epithelium which suggested stratified squamous epithelium (although keratinization was not a prominent feature)." This type of gland also secretes mucus but of a definitely thinner consistency than that secreted by the intestinal type glands. It has been suggested that either type of gland could possibly be the origin of the occasional rare case of adenocarcinoma of the bladder, but it has been pointed out many times that adenocarcinoma of the bladder can arise from transitional epithelium of the bladder (without the intermediary formation of benign glands) by the process of metaplasia (Broders; Kettle).

Diagnosis

Diagnosis is made chiefly by cystoscopy and biopsy. Urography may be of help especially in severe cases where the ureters are obstructed by extensive lesions. Such a case is usually thought to be carcinoma of the trigone and base of the bladder until biopsy proves the true nature of the process. We have observed one case (Emmett and McDonald) in which the lesion was discrete, well circumscribed, about 3 cm in diameter, and located on the mid left lateral wall of the bladder with no connection with the region of the vesical neck or trigone. When the lesions are large they may be visualized as multiple filling defects in the cystogram which suggests bullous edema or multiple tumors (Fig. 7-103).

Treatment usually can be satisfactorily carried out by multiple transurethral resections or fulgurations. The bladder should be examined cystoscopically at least twice yearly for many years (as one would advise for a bona fide tumor) and any persistent or recurring lesions destroyed.

(Text continued on page 825.)

Fig. 7–98

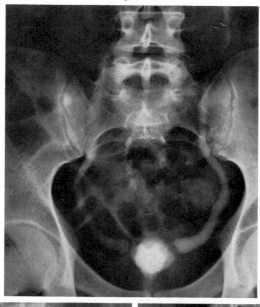

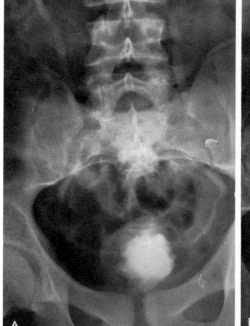 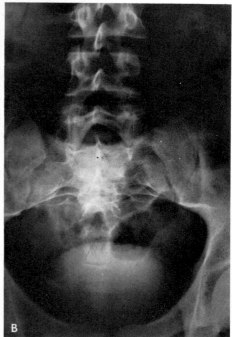

Fig. 7–99

Figure 7–98. *Excretory urogram.* "Amicrobic" cystitis with marked contraction of bladder, causing ob-struction of both ureters, with ureterectasis.

Figure 7–99. "Amicrobic" cystitis with marked contraction of bladder. A, *Excretory urogram.* Marked contraction of bladder, causing obstruction of both ureters, with moderate ureterectasis. B, *Excretory urogram* made after treatment. Vesical capacity has returned to normal. Normal vesical contour. Ureterectasis has disappeared.

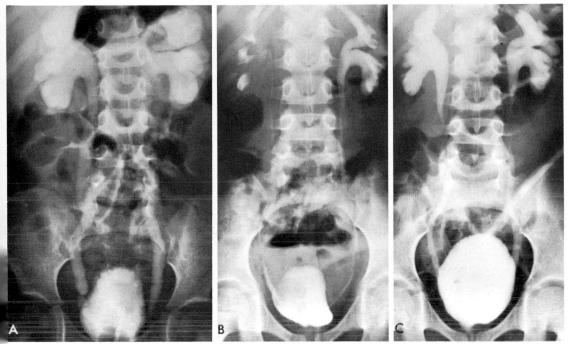

Figure 7–100. A, *Retrograde cystogram.* Eosinophilic cystitis in girl aged 2 years. Note irregularity and contraction of bladder with extensive bilateral vesicoureteral reflux. B, *Excretory urogram* following treatment (which included temporary supracystostomy). Marked improvement in kidneys and bladder. C, *Retrograde cystogram.* Bilateral reflux still present. (From Champion, R. H., and Ackles, R. C.)

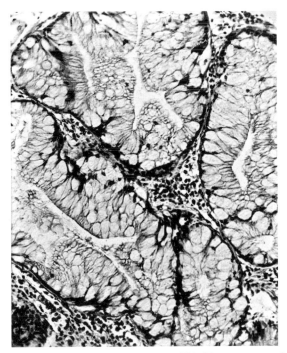

Figure 7–101. *Photomicrograph* from biopsy specimen of bladder in a case of **cystitis glandularis.** Intestinal type of glands with goblet cells (see text for explanation). (Hematoxylin and eosin; ×145.) (From Emmett, J. L., and McDonald, J. R.)

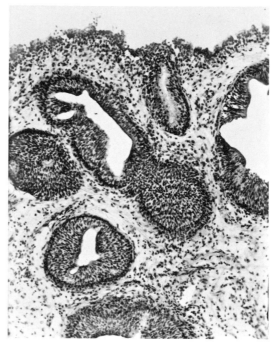

Figure 7–102. *Photomicrograph* from biopsy specimen of bladder in a case of **cystitis glandularis. Subtrigonal type of glands** lined by several layers of cells (see text for explanation). (Hematoxylin and eosin; reduced from ×95.) (From Emmett, J. L., and McDonald, J. R.)

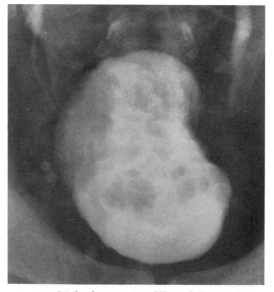

Figure 7–103. *Excretory urogram.* Multiple negative filling defects in cystogram from **extensive cystitis glandularis** in man aged 33.

BRUCELLOSIS OF THE URINARY TRACT

Sir David Bruce, working on the island of Malta, was the first (1886) to isolate and describe the organism responsible for the disease we now know as "brucellosis." He named the organism *Micrococcus melitensis*. In 1918 Alice Evans showed this organism to be similar to *Bacillus abortus* of Bang. She suggested the name "brucellosis" (in honor of Sir David Bruce) be used instead of the terms "Malta fever" or "undulant fever." The *Brucella* group of organisms now includes the *abortus*, *suis*, and *melitensis* species.

Infection with *Brucella* species has been shown to occur in almost every organ in the human body. It has been stated that in about 50% of cases the *Brucella* organisms may be found in the urine during some stage of the disease. There is a paucity of literature on the subject of brucellosis of the urinary tract. Most of the articles concern probable *Brucella* infections of the testes, epididymides, and prostate. Proved cases of brucellosis of the kidneys and bladder are rare.

Seven cases of brucellosis of the urinary tract have been reported from the Mayo Clinic (Greene and Albers; Greene, Weed, and Albers; Kelalis, Greene, and Weed). In these reports the similarity to tuberculosis was stressed. An amicrobic urinary infection associated with acute cystitis which is refractory to the ordinary types of treatment in a patient who has a past history of brucellosis, or who has worked as a butcher or in a meat-packing plant, should make one suspect the presence of the disease. The urine contains much pus, but no organisms are found with Gram's stain on routine cultures. It usually is necessary to employ special methods of culture for identification. Among those more commonly used is incubation at 37 C on hormone blood-agar plates in 10% carbon dioxide. Cystoscopically the severe, acute ulcerative cystitis suggests tuberculosis. Urine inoculated into guinea pigs shows no tuberculosis, but occasional lesions develop in the spleen, and these lesions on culture will show *Brucella* organisms. A positive agglutination reaction in a high titer (1:400 or more) is suggestive.

Urographic Findings (Figs. 7-104 through 7-107)

Little has been known or written about urographic changes that may occur in kidneys attacked by this disease. In the seven Mayo Clinic cases mentioned, the urograms showed varying degrees of cicatricial deformity and dilatation of the pelvis and calyces simulating advanced tuberculosis. In one case, cicatricial narrowing of the calyces was sufficient to isolate portions of a calyx so that, although it could be visualized in the excretory urogram, no medium entered it as seen in the retrograde urogram. One of the most interesting findings was calcification of the renal cortex. In one case the calcification was extensive and seemed to be "splashed" over all areas of the kidney without regard to the position of the pelvis and calyces or cortex and medulla. This is in contradistinction to the calcification seen in renal tuberculosis, which usually involves and outlines definite calyces or groups of calyces. The condition must also be differentiated from nephrocalcinosis, in which the calcification usually is limited to the pyramids. It is of interest that in two of the seven cases a granulomatous lesion of the kidney (proved by tissue culture to be a brucelloma) was incorrectly diagnosed as hypernephroma because the lesion presented as a space-occupying lesion (Fig. 7-107).

FUNGAL INFECTIONS OF THE KIDNEY; ACTINOMYCOSIS; MONILIASIS

(Figs. 7-108 and 7-109)

Fungal infections rarely involve the urinary tract. **Renal actinomycosis** occurs rarely as a secondary lesion, the kidney in most such cases becoming involved from the gastrointestinal tract or through the diaphragm from pulmonary disease. Urographically the lesion is impossible to differentiate from an ordinary renal carbuncle, cortical abscess, perinephric abscess, or renal tumor unless the diagnosis can be made from finding the *Actinomyces* organisms or "sulfur bodies" in the urine or pus draining from a wound or sinus.

Renal infection resulting from **moniliasis** is rare, but is more likely to occur in diabetics and in debilitated patients, especially if long-term antibiotic therapy has been employed. Destructive calyceal changes may result and the renal substance may be replaced by abscesses (Cowan and colleagues).

(Text continued on page 832.)

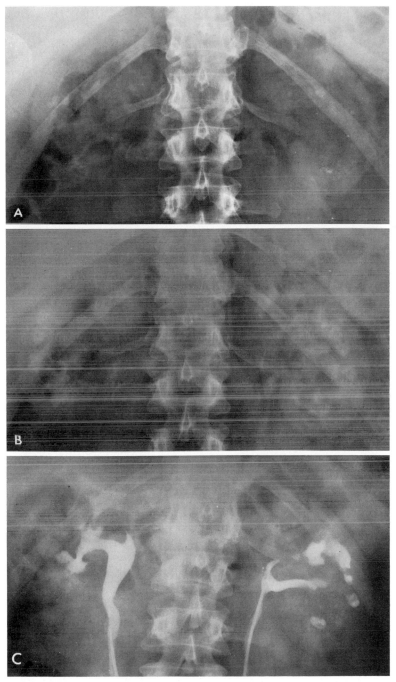

Figure 7–104. Brucellosis. **A,** *Plain film.* Multiple small irregular areas of calcification widely distributed over both renal areas. **B,** *Excretory urogram.* Marked calycectasis, with much cortical destruction. Difficult to localize calcification. Much of it is obscured by dilated calyces that appear irregular and moth-eaten and are suggestive of tuberculosis. **C,** *Bilateral retrograde pyelogram.* Note inability to fill upper group of calyces of either kidney, apparently due to cicatricial narrowing of infundibulum serving upper calyces. Note also extreme deformity of middle and lower calyces characterized by alternate areas of cicatrization and dilatation. (Courtesy of Dr. L. F. Greene.)

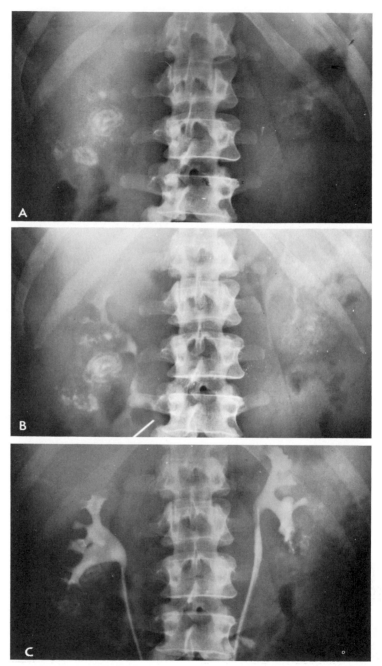

Figure 7–105. Brucellosis, **A,** *Plain film.* Calcific shadows of irregular size and shape "splashed" over both renal areas, most marked on right. **B,** *Excretory urogram.* Calcific shadows do not outline any definite calyces. Some overlie calyces, while others are well removed, suggesting cortical rather than calyceal or pyramidal involvement. **C,** *Bilateral retrograde pyelogram.* Very few, if any, changes in pelvis and calyces.

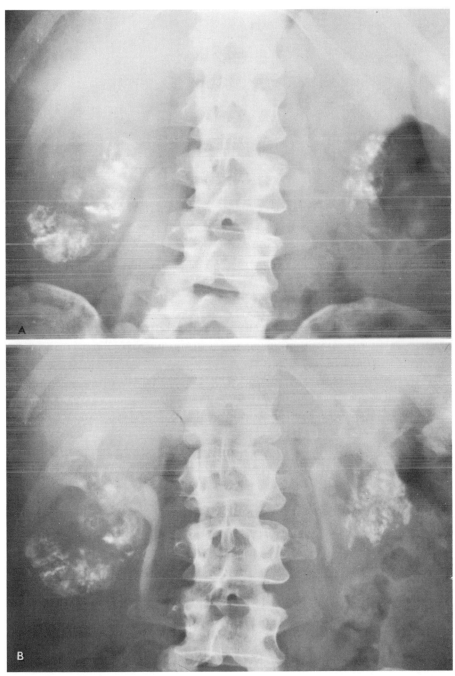

Figure 7–106. Brucellosis. Same case as Figure 7–105, 10 years later. Marked increase in degree of renal calcification. There is also calcific area in spleen. **A,** *Plain film.* **B,** *Excretory urogram.*

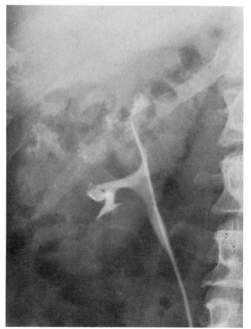

Figure 7–107.   **Brucelloma simulating hypernephroma.** *Retrograde pyelogram* shows space-occupying lesion in lateral aspect of right kidney containing calcium. Hypernephroma suspected. Nephrectomy. Granuloma typical of tuberculosis revealed by both gross and microscopic examination. Tissue culture was positive for *Brucella suis*. (From Kelalis, P. P., Greene, L. F., and Weed, L. A.)

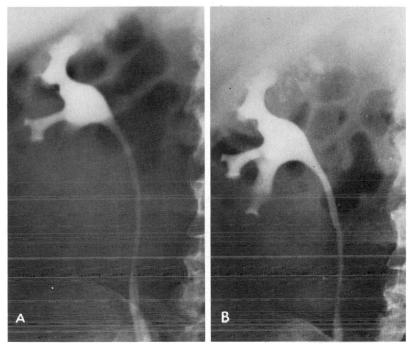

Figure 7–108. Renal actinomycosis. A, *Right retrograde pyelogram.* B, Second attempt at right retrograde pyelogram. Note difficulty in filling lower calyx because of pressure from lesion in lower pole. Similar to finding of ordinary renal carbuncle.

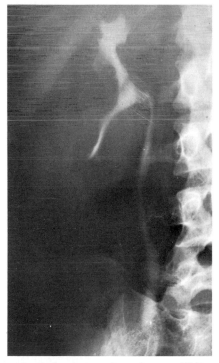

Figure 7–109. Renal actinomycosis. *Right retrograde pyelogram.* Obliteration of middle calyx and elongation of upper and lower calyces with abnormal terminations, suggesting renal tumor. (From Hunt, V. C., and Mayo, C. W.)

PROSTATITIS, PROSTATIC ABSCESS, AND CHRONIC DUCT ABSCESSES OF THE PROSTATE

Generally speaking, infection of the prostate gland does not lend itself well to urographic diagnosis. In *acute prostatitis* an elongated straight prostatic urethra is evident, which is also characteristic of prostatic carcinoma (see Fig. 5-285). After the acute process has subsided, the urethra returns to normal. An *acute prostatic abscess* willl occasionally reach such proportions that it will encroach on the base of the bladder and produce a filling defect (Fig. 7-110). The lesion most commonly demonstrated urographically is dilatation of multiple prostatic ducts which communicate with multiple old abscess cavities that have drained into the urethra (Figs. 7-111 and 7-112A and B).

GRANULOMATOUS PROSTATITIS

Granulomatous prostatitis is considered here because it is so often mistaken for carcinoma of the prostate. It occurs frequently enough that urologists should be familiar with the condition.

Nonspecific Granulomatous Prostatitis

The lesion was first described in a pathologic study from the Mayo Clinic by Tanner and McDonald. Its clinical importance was first discussed by Thompson and Albers who pointed out its clinical similarity to carcinoma of the prostate gland. They described 36 patients who had undergone transurethral resection for prostatic obstruction and in whom microscopic examination of the tissue showed "granulomatous prostatitis." In 20 of these patients the preoperative diagnosis had been carcinoma of the prostate while in the remainder it had been benign enlargement of the prostate. They pointed out that in the majority of patients, on digi-

tal rectal examination, the prostate was enlarged, indurated, fixed, and in some cases nodular, having all the characteristics of cancer of the prostate. They could detect no clinical data to help make the correct preoperative diagnosis except that some of the patients had had recurring febrile episodes which, however, were not infrequently observed in obstruction from benign enlargement of the prostate or carcinoma.

Further studies of this disease have been carried out by Kelalis, Greene, and Harrison; and Kelalis and Greene. In a study of 70 Mayo Clinic cases they noted that a preoperative diagnosis of carcinoma of the prostate had been made (on the basis of digital rectal examination) in 54 (77%). They emphasized the importance of a careful history, which will reveal previously recurring attacks of fever. This symptom plus dysuria and a hard gland on palpation comprise what they have called the pathognomonic "triad" of the disease. It must be appreciated, however, that this triad is also encountered in both benign and malignant enlargements of the prostate gland, so accurate diagnosis may be made only by biopsy. Microscopic examination of prostatic tissue removed either at transurethral resection or at open operation may provide the first clue to the true diagnosis. If operation is not required to relieve obstruction, needle biopsy by either the perineal or the transrectal route will provide the diagnosis. When there is any question of the diagnosis, needle biopsy should be done, as the condition is a self-resolving process which may be treated successfully nonsurgically with sulfonamide drugs, antibiotics, phenazopyridine (Pyridium), and sitz baths. Prognosis is good.

Roentgen Data

Radiographic examination is not rewarding. Prostatic calculi are visualized in 10% to 15% of cases and of course there are no metastatic lesions. Excretory urography usually gives negative results although ureteral obstruction has been demonstrated in the allergic variety.

Etiology

It has been postulated that the disease may be a reaction of the prostate gland to extravasated prostatic secretions from rupture of prostatic acini and ducts which have resulted from infection or obstruction.

Pathology

There is no characteristic gross appearance although small, yellow, nodular areas may be scattered throughout the gland.

Diagnosis is made on the typical microscopic appearance. It consists of "histiocytic granulomatous inflammation with abundant histiocytes having vacuolated cytoplasm due to lipid, intense lymphocytic infiltration, polymorphonuclear leukocytes, and occasional eosinophils and plasma cells (Fig. 7-113). Giant cells of the foreign-body type are scattered throughout the reaction, which exhibits no particular pattern of distribution. An extremely important feature is the complete absence of caseation. This serves to distinguish granulomatous prostatitis from other specific lesions of the prostate, particularly tuberculosis. Resolution of the lesion takes place by fibrosis."

Allergic Granulomatous Prostatitis (Allergic Granulomas of the Prostate)

In 1951 Melicow reported an asthmatic patient who underwent suprapubic prostatectomy for urinary obstruction, and pathologic examination of the prostate disclosed a peculiar granulomatous lesion. The microscopic appearance differed somewhat from that of the "nonspecific" type of granulomatous prostatitis in that it presented "numerous areas of a unique type of necrosis (fibrinoid) surrounded by eosinophils but free of epithelioid and giant cells" (Fig. 7-114). The differential count of the blood showed 26% eosinophils. The course was generally downhill and finally the patient died. At autopsy an "organizing necrotizing pneumonia" was present and "allergic granulomas" similar to the prostatic lesion were found in the bladder, rectum, seminal vesicles, esophagus, heart, voluntary muscle, and spleen.

The patient was classified in a category of patients "in whom asthma combined with a pronounced blood eosinophilia, eosinophilic infiltration in the lungs, and scattered granulomas with or without necrotizing arteritis (periarteritis nodosa) were manifestations of a complex vascular allergy or of a generalized vascular and connective tissue disturbance."

In contrast to the relatively benign nature of "nonspecific" granulomatous prostatitis, the "allergic" variety is a dangerous and lethal disease. Fortunately, however, it is relatively rare. It presents the same clinical problem as does the nonspecific variety in that on digital rectal examination this lesion also feels like carcinoma of the prostate. In 1964 Kelalis, Harrison, and Greene found four cases reported in the literature (which included Melicow's case) and reported an additional five cases from the records of the Mayo Clinic (two of which had been reported previously by Thompson and Albers). In 1966 Kelalis, Harrison, and Utz reported a 28-year-old man in whom the lesion was so extensive that it had caused bilateral ureteral obstruction (hydronephrosis on the right and nonfunctioning of the kidney on the left) (Fig. 7-115). There were also multiple nodules at the base of the penis. Dramatic regression of the disease was obtained with prednisone administered orally, first in a 10-mg dose four times daily and later in a 5-mg dose three times daily which the patient required as a maintenance dose to remain symptom-free.

(Text continued on page 837.)

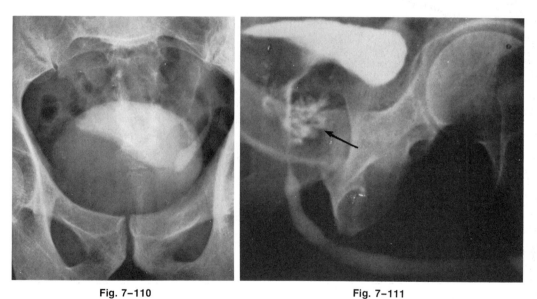

Fig. 7–110   **Fig. 7–111**

Figure 7–110. *Excretory urogram.* Acute prostatic abscess causing filling defect in right half of bladder.
Figure 7–111. *Cystourethrogram.* Chronic abscesses of prostatic ducts (*arrow*). Note width of normal anterior urethra.

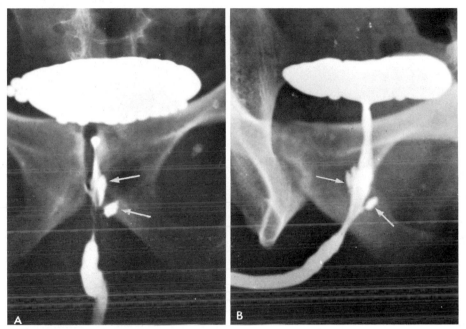

Figure 7–112. Chronic abscesses of prostatic ducts. A, *Cystourethrogram in anteroposterior position.* B, *Oblique view. Lower arrow (arrow* on patient's right) points to utricle.

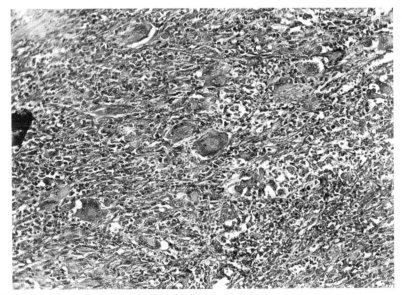

Figure 7–113. Granulomatous prostatitis with giant cells of foreign-body type scattered throughout reaction, which exhibits no particular pattern of distribution. Histiocytes and other inflammatory cells are also present. Note absence of caseation. (Hematoxylin and eosin; ×145.) (From Kelalis, P. P., and Greene, L. F.)

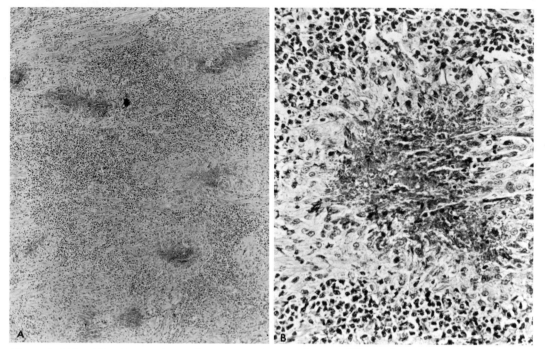

Figure 7–114. Allergic granuloma of prostate. **A,** Scattered areas of fibrinoid necrosis with intense infiltration of eosinophils. (Hematoxylin and eosin; ×50.) **B,** Area of fibrinoid necrosis surrounded by palisading histiocytes and abundant eosinophils. (Hematoxylin and eosin; ×200.) (From Kelalis, P. P., Harrison, E. G., Jr., and Utz, D. C.)

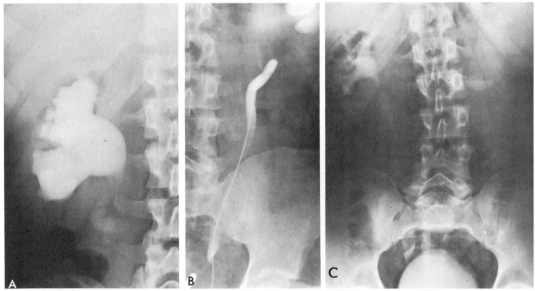

Figure 7–115. Bilateral ureteral obstruction from extensive allergic granulomatous prostatitis in male aged 28. Successful treatment with prednisone. **A,** *Excretory urogram* demonstrates hydronephrosis and hydroureter on right, nonfunction on left. **B,** *Left retrograde pyeloureterogram* reveals obstruction in distal pelvic ureter. **C,** *Excretory urogram* after 3 months of treatment with prednisone. Right kidney has returned almost to normal. Still no function on left. (From Kelalis, P. P., Harrison, E. G., Jr., and Utz, D. C.)

GENITOURINARY BILHARZIASIS (SCHISTOSOMIASIS)*

by
Kamal A. Hanash

Bilharziasis is probably one of the oldest diseases known to mankind. In 1910 Ruffer discovered bilharzial ova in the kidneys of mummies dating back to the 20th dynasty (1200 to 1090 B.C.) (Makar). In 1951 Theodore Bilharz was the first to discover the worms and their relationship to hematuria (Makar). In the past decade the disease has spread extensively and become endemic in different parts of the world, including most of Africa, the southern tips of Europe, Western Asia, the islands on the east coast of Africa, Japan, and even India and Pakistan (Faust and Russell). It is estimated that between 200,000,000 and 300,000,000 people are affected with this disease. Because so many American soldiers have been in these endemic areas and because of the great increase in foreign travel (due to easy access by air transportation), more cases of urinary bilharziasis are being seen in the offices of American urologists. For this reason it is important that the profession become acquainted with this disease.

Pathogenesis

Bilharziasis is a parasitic disease caused by a blood fluke. There are three forms of flukes responsible: (1) *Schistosoma japonicum*, (2) *S. mansoni*, and (3) *S. haematobium*.† *S. mansoni* involves chiefly the rectum and liver, while *S. japonicum* involves mainly the lungs and liver. *S. haematobium* involves primarily the urinary tract. Vermooten has given an excellent brief account of the life cycle of this parasite, from which the following description is taken: The egg is discharged with the urine (from human beings). When it comes in contact with water it swells, ruptures, and liberates a miracidium. This then penetrates a specific species of snail *(Physopsis africana)* and becomes a sporocyst. Each sporocyst gives rise to a second generation of sporocysts, from which tens of thousands of cercariae are produced. In 5 to 7 weeks they leave the snail and swim free in water for 1 to 7 days, when they die unless they can reach and penetrate the skin or mucous membrane of a human being. Here they enter the venous and lymphatic systems and are carried to the heart and then to the capillaries of the lung. From there they eventually reach the portal vein, where they grow into adult worms.

Approximately 3 weeks after entry through the skin the maturing worms migrate out of the portal vein, traveling against the bloodstream via the inferior and superior mesenteric veins and the hemorrhoidal, spermatic, and retrocecal veins into the vesical, pelvic, and ureteral plexuses, being especially abundant in the veins of the submucosa of the bladder (Makar).

Venous anastomoses between the portal system and the systemic circulation have also been demonstrated around the distal lower third of the pelvic ureter, the vesicoprostatic venous plexus, and the middle rectal veins, probably accounting for the presence of the worm in this region. In the vesical plexus the female worm leaves the male, and because of her smaller size is able to pass into smaller vessels (where the male cannot go) and deposits her ova or eggs in the venules beneath the mucous membrane of the bladder. The eggs are laid in a chain of approximately 20, positioned so that their spines engage the vessel wall; this helps their extrusion into the perivenous spaces. Aided by contrac-

---

*The authors are indebted to Dr. A. A. Z. Hanna, assistant professor of radiology, Cairo University, for valuable advice and suggestions in the preparation of the material on bilharziasis.

†The term "bilharziasis" should refer only to the disease produced by *S. haematobium*; however, in the literature it has been used loosely to include all three varieties.

tions of the muscular wall of the ureter or bladder or both, the ova reach the lumen of the viscus and are voided with the urine. It is also thought that rupture of the wall of the vein may be aided by a ferment excreted by the ova.

Pathology

Considerable reaction is initiated in the tissues surrounding the ova. Grossly and cystoscopically the early lesions appear as small areas of hyperemia associated with slight edema. When the ova break through the vesical mucosa, red granular bleeding areas result and account for the typical "endemic hematuria of Egypt," which is so common in the early stage of the disease.

As the lesions progress they appear as small, pale, yellowish granules with slightly raised shiny surfaces surrounded by a zone of hyperemia. The lesions simulate tubercles and are the result of proliferative changes in the tissues, associated with hyperplasia. As the process becomes chronic, lesions enlarge and become nodular. Groups of nodules may coalesce to form bilharzial nodes; these nodes may undergo necrosis and ulceration or become calcified. Chronic irritation often gives rise to papillomatous growths which predispose to carcinoma (14% to 47%) (Figs. 7-116 and 7-117).

Bladder

In some cases, because of nonvascularity of the involved bladder regions or the host's defense mechanism, atrophy of the mucous membrane occurs. In such a situation, old calcified bilharzial ova buried in the submucosal layer present the cystoscopic picture of a typical *sandy patch* (sand under water). If bilharzial ova are trapped in the vesical musculature, they may lead to muscular hyperplasia but more often to fibrosis and atrophy of the muscle bundles with subsequent con-

traction and deformity of the bladder wall (Makar). In the trigonal area the bilharzial ova lie in the muscular rather than the submucosal layer; hence they gradually lead to fibrosis of the bladder neck, atrophy of the trigonal muscle, and *clinical* obstruction of the vesical neck. The mechanism of the "obstruction" has been explained as an organic fibrosis of the internal sphincter; it has also been attributed to failure of the trigonal muscle to properly open the bladder neck (Wolstenholme and O'Connor). Other causes of obstruction include ball-valve action of a vesical papilloma at the vesical outlet, fibrosis of the entire prostatic urethra, and obstruction of the vesical neck secondary to bilharzial prostatitis or seminal vesiculitis (Makar).

Ureter

In the ureter, as in the bladder, the ova lying in the subepithelial layer produce hyperplasia of the epithelium with formation of papillomas or nodules (Fig. 7-117) which protrude into the lumen of the ureter. At times, however, the epithelial hyperplasia may invaginate into the submucosa to form pseudoglandular structures; obstruction of their necks will result in retention cysts. This cystic condition, termed "ureteritis cystica," may lead to "ureteritis calcinosa" secondary to calcification of the walls of the cysts. The hyperplastic process is followed by atrophy of the subepithelial and epithelial layers and ulceration of the mucosa with deposition of urate, phosphate, and oxalate crystals on the ulcers. The end result of ureteral bilharziasis is the formation of a granulomatous sclerosing reaction with dense fibrosis involving the entire wall of the ureter. The final result is scarring, stricture formation, loss of peristaltic activity and elasticity of the involved ureter, calcification of the dead ova in the ureteral wall, and secondary ureteral calculi. The lesions are usually bilateral and may occur in any part of the ureter. Most commonly they are found in the intramural urete-

(usually secondary to vesical bilharziasis), next in the distal part of the ureter, and least commonly in the lumbar portion of the ureter. The most common site of involvement in the lumbar ureter is the level of the third lumbar vertebra.

Ureteral stricture is an important complication of ureteral bilharziasis. Strictures are classified into three types: (1) annular, (2) spindle-shaped, and (3) the "third-lumbar ureteral stricture" or Makar's stricture (named after N. Makar of Egypt who first described it). There are usually advanced degrees of dilatation and tortuosity of the ureter proximal to the stricture; secondary ureteral and renal lithiasis, hydronephrosis, and atrophy of the kidney may ensue. Dilatation and tortuosity of the pelvic ureter associated with a normal lumbar ureter and normal upper urinary tracts were considered by Vermooten to be pathognomonic of bilharziasis.

Vesicoureteral reflux is a common complication of urinary bilharziasis (incidence of 44.3%). It usually results from a deformed, laterally displaced, and gaping ureteral orifice which is secondary to fibrosis and loss of elasticity of the intramural ureter and adjacent vesical musculature.

Genitalia

The genital organs may also be involved with the disease. Granulomatous sclerosis and fibrosis involve principally the urethra, prostate, and seminal vesicles; more rarely the epididymides, spermatic cords, and testicles may be affected.

Roentgen Diagnosis

THE PLAIN FILM

The bladder is involved in 85% and the ureter in 44% of all cases of urinary bilharziasis. The end stage of the bilharzial lesion is fibrosis often associated with calcification of the dead ova; these calcific lesions can be seen in the plain film, which probably represents the most important single diagnostic finding in this disease. Certain findings in the plain film strongly suggest *Bilharzia*. One of the earlier findings is a curvilinear line of calcification located in the suprapubic region. As the disease progresses, this calcified line extends until it may completely outline the periphery of the bladder (Fig. 7-118). Further deposition of calcium in the wall and epithelial lining of the bladder produces thick calcified bands within the bladder wall (Ragheb) (Figs. 7-119 and 7-120); the bladder may become so heavily calcified and contracted (Fig. 7-121) that it may give the appearance of a large vesical calculus. (True calculi occur frequently in vesical bilharziasis [incidence 39%] [Afifi] [Fig. 7-122].) When the vesical wall becomes diffusely calcified it may look like a cystogram made with contrast medium. In the case of extensive bilharzial tumors of the bladder, a pathognomonic finding is obliteration of one side of the bladder as though half of the bladder had been excised or "amputated"—leaving only an irregular serrated margin (see Figs. 10-299 and 10-302).

Ureteral bilharziasis is commonly associated with the bladder disease. Changes most frequently seen are linear calcifications involving the distal ureter (Fig. 7-118). As the disease progresses the whole ureter may become heavily calcified; if the ureter is greatly dilated from an associated stricture it may look like a calcified loop of intestine (Fig. 7-123). Calcification rarely involves the proximal ureter and the ureteropelvic junction. Calcified papillomas are commonly seen in the lower third of the ureter and may be difficult to differentiate from ureteral calculi (Fig. 7-122). Ureteritis calcinosa involving the lower third of the ureter appears as spotty, irregular calcifications, which are considered pathognomic (Fig. 7-124).

Ureteral calculi are common in urinary bilharziasis and evidence of them in the plain film should always lead one to suspect the possibility of distal ureteral stricture.

The kidney is less commonly involved because of the smaller venous anastomoses between the renal cortex and the portal system venous anastomoses which usually prevent passage of bilharzial ova to the kidney and upper urinary tract. A case of bilharzial calcification of the renal capsule has been recently reported (Atala and Zaher). Renal involvement, however, is usually secondary to vesicoureteral bilharziasis, and usually results in the formation of renal calculi and nephrocalcinosis (Fig. 7-125).

In **genital bilharziasis** the most common site of calcification is the seminal vesicles, which provide the typical appearance in a mulberry-shaped calcification seen in the plain film (Fig. 7-126).

THE UROGRAM

Bladder

The most common finding revealed by the excretory cystogram is a contracted irregular bladder wall; in some cases large, irregular filling defects produced by multiple bladder tumors are present; this may be considered as the end stage of this disease (Figs. 7-116, 7-117, and 7-127). Elevation of the base of the bladder from bilharzial infection of the prostate is frequently encountered; it is even occasionally seen in children. Vesical calculi are common and may mimic vesical neoplasms.

Ureter and Kidney

A "snake head" or spindle-shaped appearance of the terminal (pelvic) ureter is considered pathognomonic (Fig. 7-128); it

results from stricture of the intramural ureter. Multiple strictures usually located in the lower third of the ureter with their multiple spindle-shaped configurations can mimic ureteral tuberculosis (Fig. 7-124). Above the site of the stricture the ureters are often greatly dilated, tortuous, and kinked; vesicoureteral reflux is present in approximately one third of cases (Fig. 7-127). These changes are usually bilateral and involve principally the lower portion of the ureters, but as the disease progresses the pathologic process may extend proximally to involve the upper third of the ureter, the renal pelvis, and the renal calyces; hydronephrosis may result. *Renal calculi* are not uncommon; they may attain considerable size and form branched (staghorn) calculi (Figs. 7-125 and 7-129). Noncalcified papillomas in the ureter usually appear as smooth filling defects (Figs. 7-117 and 7-130) which may be differentiated from the defects of bilharzial ureteritis cystica by their greater size and smaller number (Fig. 7-131). The calcified honeycomb appearance of ureteritis calcinosa is considered pathognomonic of bilharziasis, but must be differentiated from ureteral tumors which occur only rarely in ureteral bilharziasis (Fig. 7-124). The third-lumbar stricture (Makar) with its associated dilatation of the ureter above and secondary hydronephrosis may mimic the urographic appearance of idiopathic retroperitoneal fibrosis (Figs. 7-132 and 7-133). The annular ureteral stricture is the commonest type encountered in this disease (Fig. 7-134), followed in incidence by the spindle-shaped type (Fig. 7-128) and then the third-lumbar stricture (or Makar's stricture). Secondary ureteral calculi are common findings in urinary bilharziasis (Fig. 7-135).

Obstruction at the ureteropelvic juncture is a rare finding in bilharziasis; results from fibrous compression and must be differentiated from hydronephrosis caused by vesicoureteral reflux. Scarring and thinning of the renal parenchyma with resultant deformed calyces may be the end result in chronic untreated disease.

The Bladder Neck

Micturition and retrograde cystourethrography are important aids in the diagnosis of bilharzial obstruction of the bladder neck (A. A. Z. Hanna). The retrograde cystourethrogram will reveal a shortened and sometimes sacculated prostatic urethra with elevation of its base and shelving of the posterior lip of the vesical neck, which appears stenosed and displaced forward.

The remainder of the prostatic urethra is usually normal except for possibly some hypertrophy of the verumontanum or an occasional extravasation of contrast medium into dilated prostatic ducts. The micturition cystourethrogram may be helpful for making the diagnosis of bilharzial obstruction of the vesical neck (Fig. 7-136). It helps visualize the degree of relaxation of the vesical neck during micturition as well as the degree of filling and dilatation of the prostatic urethra. Multiple anteroposterior, oblique, and lateral views may be required.

(References begin on page 851.)

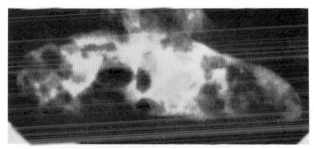

Figure 7–116. Bilharziasis. *Excretory urogram* showing "honeycomb-type" filling defects produced by diffuse involvement of bladder by granulomatous polypi. (From El-Badawi, A. A.)

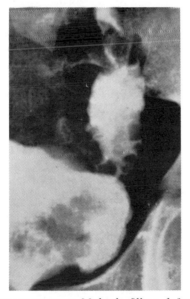

Figure 7–117. Bilharziasis. *Excretory urogram.* Multiple filling defects in bladder and honeycomb-like defects of distal part of pelvic ureter produced by granulomatous polyposis. (From El-Badawi, A. A.)

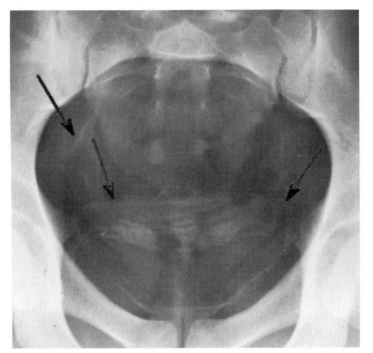

Figure 7–118.   Urinary bilharziasis. *Plain film.* Typical bilharzial calcification of bladder and lower part of ureters. Early manifestation. Note smooth, thin, curvilinear calcific line in suprapubic area outlining periphery of bladder. (Courtesy of Dr. F. Shehadeh.)

Fig. 7–119

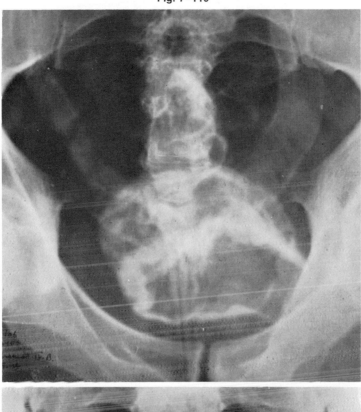

Fig. 7–120

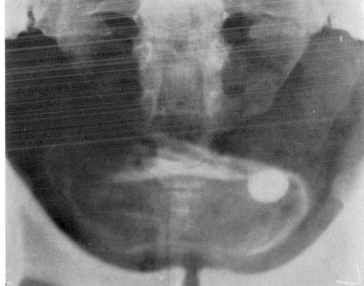

Figure 7–119. **Bilharziasis.** *Plain film.* Extensive calcification of bladder and both dilated ureters from bilharziasis. (Courtesy of Prof. J. Bitschai.)

Figure 7–120. **Bilharziasis.** *Plain film.* Calcification of wall of bladder caused by bilharziasis. Also stone in left ureter above ureteral stricture. (Courtesy of Prof. J. Bitschai.)

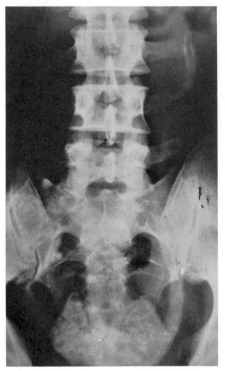

Figure 7–121.   Bilharziasis. *Plain film.* Extensive calcification of bladder, entire left ureter, and lower third of right ureter from bilharziasis. Film is unusual in that calcification of upper part of ureter in this disease is fairly rare. (Courtesy of Prof. J. Bitschai.)

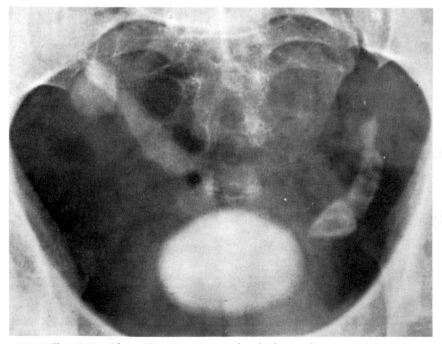

Figure 7–122.   Bilharziasis. *Plain film.* Large vesical calculus and primary bilateral ureteral calcul resulting from bilharziasis. (Courtesy of Prof. J. Bitschai.)

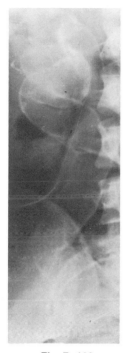

Fig. 7–123 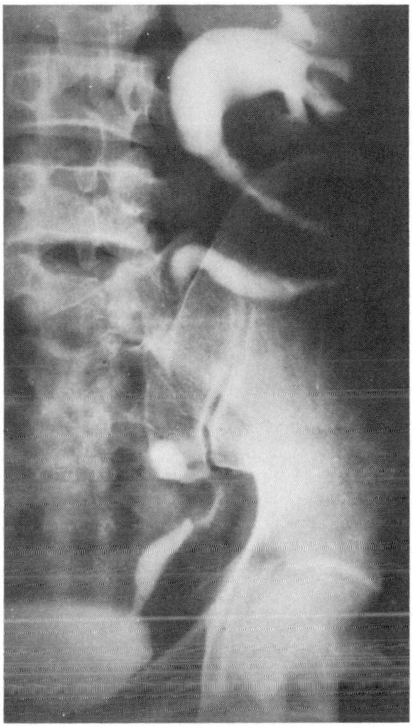   Fig. 7–124

Figure 7–123. Urinary bilharziasis. *Plain film.* Marked dilatation and tortuosity of entirely calcified right ureter in advanced untreated bilharziasis. (Courtesy of Dr. A. A. Z. Hanna.)

Figure 7–124. Urinary bilharziasis. *Excretory urogram.* Ureteritis calcinosa involving upper third of left ureter associated with tortuosity and multiple spindle-shaped dilatation of ureter secondary to ureteral strictures. (Courtesy of Dr. A. A. Z. Hanna.)

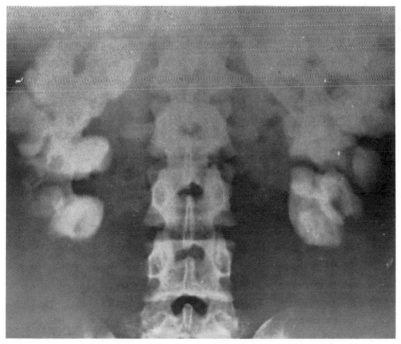

Figure 7–125. Bilharziasis. *Plain film.* Extensive bilateral branched calculi in young Egyptian man suffering from long-standing bilharziasis. (Courtesy of Prof. J. Bitschai.)

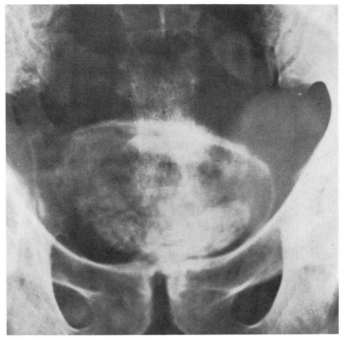

Figure 7–126.   **Bilharziasis.** *Plain film.* Calcification of bladder wall, seminal vesicles, and prostate gland from bilharziasis. (Courtesy of Prof. J. Bitschai.)

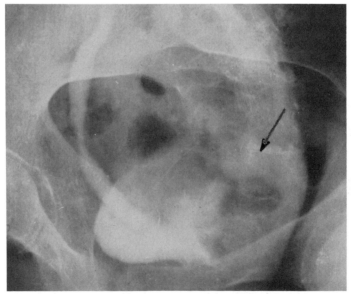

Figure 7–127.   **Urinary bilharziasis.** *Retrograde cystogram.* Right vesicoureteral reflux secondary to urinary bilharziasis. Note filling defect in bladder (*arrow*) suggestive of carcinoma. (Courtesy of Dr. A. A. Z Hanna.)

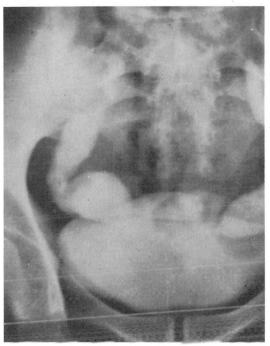

Figure 7-128. Urinary bilharziasis. *Excretory urogram.* Typical "snake head" spindle-shaped appearance of distal lower third of ureters secondary to stricture in intramural ureter. (Courtesy of Dr. A. A. Z. Hanna.)

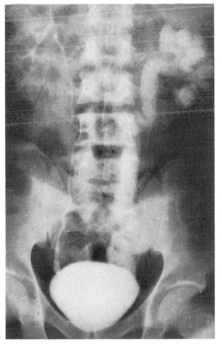

Figure 7-129. Urinary bilharziasis. *Excretory urogram.* Marked dilatation and tortuosity of whole left ureter secondary to stricture in intramural ureter and resulting in left hydronephrosis and nephrolithiasis. (Courtesy of Dr. A. A. Z. Hanna.)

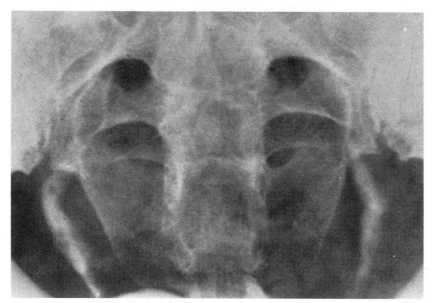

Figure 7–130.   **Bilharziasis.** *Excretory urogram.* Negative shadows caused by bilharzial papillomatosis of both ureters. (Courtesy of Prof. J. Bitschai.)

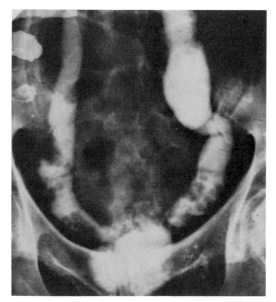

Figure 7–131.   **Urinary bilharziasis.** *Excretory urogram.* Multiple filling defects in lower third of both ureters resulting from bilharzial ureteritis cystica with marked dilatation and tortuosity of proximal parts of ureters. (Courtesy of Dr. A. A. Z. Hanna.)

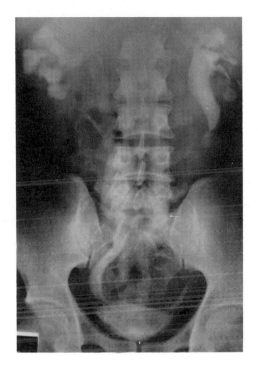

Figure 7–132. Urinary bilharziasis. *Excretory urogram.*
General features of urinary bilharziasis in addition to
calculi and calcification of bladder wall seen in plain
film.(1) Right ureterovesical stricture. (2) Left ureteral
stricture at level of L-3 (Makar's stricture). (Courtesy of
Dr. F. Shehadeh.)

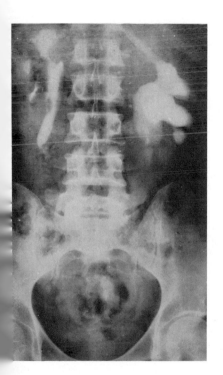

Figure 7–133. Urinary bilharziasis. *Excretory urogram.*
Bilateral ureteral stricture at level of third lumbar vertebra
(**Makar's stricture**) with resulting left hydronephrosis. (Courtesy
of Dr. A. A. Z. Hanna.)

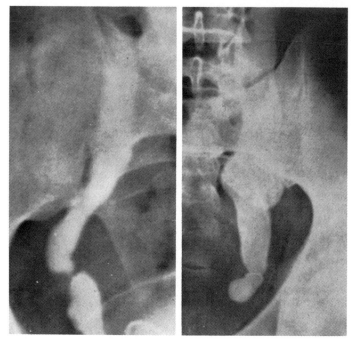

Fig. 7–134   **Fig. 7–135**

Figure 7–134. **Bilharziasis.** *Right retrograde pyelogram.* Typical annular type stricture in lower third of ureter with dilatation above and below. (Courtesy of Prof. J. Bitschai.)

Figure 7–135. **Bilharziasis.** *Plain film.* Giant "primary" ureteral calculus formed in situ in left ureter, which is markedly dilated because of bilharziasis. Stricture in terminal portion of ureter. (Courtesy of Prof. J. Bitschai.)

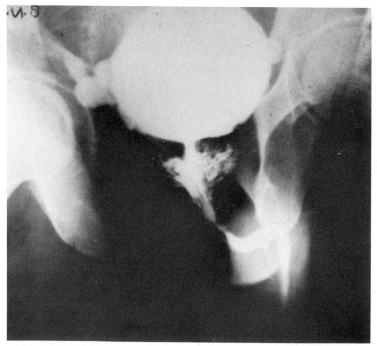

Figure 7–136. **Urinary bilharziasis.** *Voiding cystogram.* Constriction of vesical neck with dilatation and sacculation of prostatic urethra and extravasation of contrast medium in prostatic ducts. Note cellules and diverticula in bladder. (Courtesy of Dr. A. A. Z. Hanna.)

REFERENCES

Pyelonephritis

Beeson, P. B.: Urinary Tract Infection and Pyelonephritis. In Black, D. A. K.: Renal Disease. Ed. 2, Philadelphia, F. A. Davis Company, 1967, pp. 382-403.

Beeson, P. B., Rocha, H., and Guze, L. B.: Experimental Pyelonephritis: Influence of Localized Injury in Different Parts of the Kidney on Susceptibility to Hematogenous Infection. Tr. A. Am. Physicians 70:120-126, 1957.

Braasch, W. F.: Clinical Data Concerning Chronic Pyelonephritis. J. Urol. 39:1-25 (Jan.) 1938.

de Navasquez, S.: Experimental Pyelonephritis in the Rabbit Produced by Staphylococcal Infection. J. Path. & Bact. 62:429-436 (July) 1950.

de Navasquez, S.: Further Studies in Experimental Pyelonephritis Produced by Various Bacteria, With Special Reference to Renal Scarring as a Factor in Pathogenesis. J. Path. & Bact. 71:27-32 (Jan.) 1956.

Emmett, J. L., Alvarez-Ierena, J. J., and McDonald, J. R.: Atrophic Pyelonephritis Versus Congenital Renal Hypoplasia. J.A.M.A. 148:1470-1477 (Apr. 26) 1952.

Guze, L. B., and Beeson, P. B.: Observations on the Reliability and Safety of Bladder Catheterization for Bacteriologic Study of the Urine. New England J. Med. 255:474-475 (Sept 6) 1956.

Gwinn, J. L., and Barnes, G. R., Jr.: Striated Ureters and Renal Pelves. Am. J. Roentgenol. 91:666-668 (Mar.) 1964.

Heptinstall, R. H.: Limitations of Diagnosis in Chronic Pyelonephritis. In Black, D. A. K.: Renal Disease. Ed. 2, Philadelphia, F. A. Davis Company, 1967, pp. 350-381.

Hinman, F., Jr., and Hutch, J. A.: Atrophic Pyelonephritis From Ureteral Reflux Without Obstructive Signs ("Reflux Pyelonephritis"). J. Urol. 87:230-242 (Mar.) 1962.

Hodson, C. J.: The Radiological Diagnosis of Pyelonephritis: Acute Pyelonephritis. Proc. Roy. Soc. Med. 52:669-672 (Aug.) 1959.

Hodson, C. J.: Radiology of the Kidney. In Black, D. A. K.: Renal Disease. Ed. 2, Philadelphia, F. A. Davis Company, 1967a, pp. 136-169.

Hodson, C. J.: The Radiological Contribution Toward the Diagnosis of Chronic Pyelonephritis. Radiology 88:857-871 (May) 1967b.

Hodson, C. J., and Craven, J. D.: The Radiology of Obstructive Atrophy of the Kidney. Clin. Radiol. 17:305-320 (Oct.) 1966.

Hodson, C. J., and Edwards, D.: Chronic Pyelonephritis and Vesico-ureteric Reflux. Clin. Radiol. 11:219-231 (Oct.) 1960.

Hutch, J. A., Hinman, F., Jr., and Miller, E. R.: Reflux as a Cause of Hydronephrosis and Chronic Pyelonephritis. J. Urol. 88:169-175 (Aug.) 1962.

Hutch, J. A., Miller, E. R., and Hinman, F., Jr.: Perpetuation of Infection in Unobstructed Urinary Tracts by Vesicoureteral Reflux. J. Urol. 90:88-91 (July) 1963.

Kass, E. H.: Asymptomatic Infections of the Urinary Tract. Tr. A. Am. Physicians 69:56-64, 1956.

Kass, E. H.: Bacteriuria and the Diagnosis of Infections of the Urinary Tract: With Observations on the Use of Methionine as a Urinary Antiseptic. A.M.A. Arch. Int. Med. 100:709-714 (Nov.) 1957.

Kimmelstiel, P., Kim, O. J., Beres, J. A., and Wellman, K.: Chronic Pyelonephritis. Am. J. Med. 30:589-607 (Apr.) 1961.

King, M. C., Friedenberg, R. M., and Tena, L. B.: Normal Renal Parenchyma Simulating Tumor. Radiology 91:217-222 (Aug.) 1968.

Monzon, O. T., Ory, E. M., Dobson, H. L., Carter, E., and Yow, E. M.: A Comparison of Bacterial Counts of the Urine Obtained by Needle Aspiration of the Bladder: Catheterization and Midstream-Voided Methods. New England J. Med. 259:764-767 (Oct. 16) 1958.

Prather, G. C., and Sears, B. R.: Pyelonephritis: In Defense of the Urethral Catheter. J.A.M.A. 170:1030-1035 (June 27) 1959.

Rosenheim, M. L.: Problems of Chronic Pyelonephritis. Brit. M. J. 1:1433-1440 (June) 1963.

Sanford, J. P., Favour, C. B., Mao, F. H., and Harrison, J. H.: Evaluation of the "Positive" Urine Culture: An Approach to the Differentiation of Significant Bacteria From Contaminants. Am. J. Med. 20:88-93 (Jan.) 1956.

Shopfner, C. E.: Urinary Tract Pathology With Sepsis. Am. J. Roentgenol. 108:632-640 (Mar.) 1970.

Renal Fibrolipomatosis

Faegenburg, D., Bosniak, M., and Evans, J. A.: Renal Sinus Lipomatosis: Its Demonstration by Nephrotomography. Radiology 83:987-998 (Dec.) 1964.

Hamm, F. C., and DeVeer, J. A.: Fatty Replacement Following Renal Atrophy or Destruction. J. Urol. 41:850-866 (June) 1939.

Kutzmann, A. A.: Replacement Lipomatosis of the Kidney. Surg., Gynec. & Obst. 52:690-701 (Mar.) 1931.

McDonald, D. F.: Renal Fibrolipomatosis. J. Urol. 94:43-47 (July) 1965.

Olsson, O., and Weiland, P.: Renal Fibrolipomatosis. Acta radiol. 1:1061-1070 (Sept.) 1963.

Tumefactive Xanthogranulomatous Pyelonephritis

Avnet, N. L., Roberts, T. W., and Goldberg, H. R.: Tumefactive Xanthogranulomatous Pyelonephritis. Am. J. Roentgenol. 90:89-96 (July) 1963.

Clark, R. L., McAllister, H. A., and Harrell, J. E.: An Exercise in Radiologic-Pathologic Correlation. Radiology 92:597-603 (Mar.) 1969.

Friedenberg, M. J., and Spjut, H. J.: Xanthogranulomatous Pyelonephritis. Am. J. Roentgenol. 90:97-108 (July) 1963.

Ghosh, H. H.: Chronic Pyelonephritis With Xanthogranulomatous Change: Report of 3 Cases. Am. J. Clin. Path. 25:1043-1049 (Sept.) 1955.

Kawaichi, G. K., and Reingold, I. M.: Xanthogranulomatous Pyelonephritis in the Paraplegic. J. Urol. 97:58-61 (Jan.) 1967.

Mitchell, R. E., Jr., Dodson, A. I., and Kay, S.: Xanthogranulomatous Pyelonephritis. Am. Pract. & Digest Treat. *10*:2150-2155 (Dec.) 1959.

Parker, J. M.: Xanthogranulomatous Pyelonephritis. J. Urol. *96*:290-292 (Sept.) 1966.

Selzer, D. W., Dahlin, D. C., and DeWeerd, J. H.: Tumefactive Xanthogranulomatous Pyelonephritis. Surgery *42*:874-883 (Nov.) 1957.

Vinik, M., Freed, T. A., Smellie, W. A. B., and Weidner, W.: Xanthogranulomatous Pyelonephritis: Angiographic Considerations. Radiology *92*:537-540 (Mar.) 1969.

Pyeloureterectasis and Pyelonephritis of Pregnancy

Crabtree, E. G., Prather, G. C., and Prien, E. L.: End-Results of Urinary Tract Infections Associated With Pregnancy. Am. J. Obst. & Gynec. *34*:405-417, 1937.

Dure-Smith, P.: Ureteric Dilatation: Its Anatomical Basis and Relation to Sex and Pregnancy. In Grady, F. O., and Brumfitt, W.: Urinary Tract Infection. London, Oxford University Press, 1968, pp. 172-175.

Fry, I. K., and Spiro, F. I.: Upper Urinary Tract Dilatation in Non-pregnant Women. In Grady, F. O., and Brumfitt, W.: Urinary Tract Infection. London, Oxford University Press, 1968, pp. 175-178.

Harrow, B. R., Sloane, J. A., and Salhanick, L.: Etiology of the Hydronephrosis of Pregnancy. Surg., Gynec. & Obst. *119*:1042-1048 (Nov.) 1964.

Heidrick, W. P., Mattingly, R. F., and Amberg, J. R.: Vesicoureteral Reflux in Pregnancy. Obst. & Gynec. *29*:571-578 (Apr.) 1967.

Hodson, C. J.: Radiologic Changes in the Urinary Tract Associated With Pregnancy in Relation to the Pathogenesis of Pyelonephritis. In Grady, F. O., and Brumfitt, W.: Urinary Tract Infection. London, Oxford University Press, 1968, pp. 172-175.

Hutch, J. A., Ayres, R. D., and Noll, L. E.: Vesicoureteral Reflux as Cause of Pyelonephritis of Pregnancy. Am. J. Obst. & Gynec. *87*:478-485 (Oct.) 1963.

Kincaid-Smith, Priscilla: Bacteriuria and Urinary Infection in Pregnancy. Clin. Obst. & Gynec. *11*:533-549 (June) 1968.

Kincaid-Smith, Priscilla, and Bullen, Margaret: Bacteriuria in Pregnancy. Lancet *1*:395-399 (Feb.) 1965.

Kretschmer, H. L., Heaney, H. S., and Ockuly, E. A.: Dilatation of the Kidney Pelvis and Ureter During Pregnancy and the Puerperium: A Pyelographic Study in Normal Women. J.A.M.A. *101*:2025-2028 (Dec. 23) 1933.

Marshall, S., Lyon, R. P., and Minkler, D.: Ureteral Dilatation Following Use of Oral Contraceptives. J.A.M.A. *198*:782-783 (Nov.) 1966.

Ureteritis and Ureteral Stricture

Mininberg, D. T., Andronaco, J., Nesbit, R. M., and Nagamatsu, G. R.: Nonspecific Regional Ureteritis. J. Urol. *98*:664-668 (Dec.) 1968.

Schofield, P. F., Staff, W. G., and Moore, T.: Ureteral Involvement in Regional Ileitis (Crohn's Disease). J. Urol. *99*:412-416 (Apr.) 1968.

Shopfner, C. E.: Nonobstructive Hydronephrosis and Hydroureter. Am. J. Roentgenol. *98*:172-180 (Sept.) 1966.

Cystitis Cystica; Pyelitis and Ureteritis Cystica; Chronic Proliferative Lesions of the Urinary Tract: Cystitis Glandularis, Cystitis Follicularis, Malacoplakia, etc.

Albarran, J.: Les tumeurs de la vessie. Paris, G. Steinheil, 1892, pp. 78-79.

Bothe, A. E., and Cristol, D. S.: Cystic Disease of the Upper Urinary Tract: Pyelitis Cystica and Ureteritis Cystica. Am. J. Roentgenol. *48*:787-793 (Dec.) 1942.

Broders, A. C.: Squamous-Cell Epithelioma of the Skin: A Study of 256 Cases. Ann. Surg. *73*:141-160 (Feb.) 1921.

Brown, R. C., and Smith, B. H.: Malacoplakia of the Testis. Am. J. Clin. Path. *47*:135-147 (Feb.) 1967.

Cederqvist, L. L.: Malacoplakia of the Urinary Tract. Arch. Path. *80*:495-499 (Nov.) 1965.

Emmett, J. L., and McDonald, J. R.: Proliferation of Glands of the Urinary Bladder Simulating Malignant Neoplasm. J. Urol. *48*:257-265 (Sept.) 1942.

Gibson, T. E., Bareta, J., and Lake, G. C.: Malacoplakia: Report of a Case Involving the Bladder and One Kidney and Ureter. Urol. internat. *1*:5-14, 1955.

Goldman, R. L.: A Case of Malacoplakia With Involvement of the Prostate Gland. J. Urol. *93*:407-410 (Mar.) 1965.

Hand, J. R., and Sullivan, A. W.: Malakoplakia of the Urinary Tract: Report of a Case. Portland Clin. Bull. *12*:1-10 (June) 1958.

Haukohl, R. S., and Chinchinian, H.: Malacoplakia of the Testicle: Report of a Case. Am. J. Clin. Path. *29*:473-478 (May) 1958.

Hinman, F., and Cordonnier, J.: Cystitis Follicularis. J. Urol. *34*:302-308 (Oct.) 1935.

Hoffmann, E., and Garrido, M.: Malakoplakia of the Prostate: Report of a Case. J. Urol. *92*:311-313 (Oct.) 1964.

Józsa, L.: Beiträge zur Pathogenese der Malakoplakie. Ztschr. Urol. *54*:465-470, 1961.

Kettle, E. H.: On Polymorphism of the Malignant Epithelial Cell. Proc. Roy. Soc. Med. (Section of Pathology) *12*:1-32, 1919.

Kolodny, G. M.: Ureteral Dilatation With Pyuria. J.A.M.A. *197*:577-578 (Aug. 15) 1966.

Lewis, J. A., Vieralves, G., Landes, R. R., and Powell, L. W.: Malakoplakia of the Renal Pelvis, Calyces and Upper Ureter: Case Report. J. Urol. *85*:243-245 (Mar.) 1961.

Loitman, B. S., and Chiat, H.: Ureteritis Cystica and Pyelitis Cystica: A Review of Cases and Roentgenologic Criteria. Radiology *68*:345-351 (Mar.) 1957.

McNulty, M.: Pyelo-ureteritis Cystica. Brit. J. Radiol. *30*:648-652 (Dec.) 1957.

Melicow, M. M.: Malacoplakia: Report of Case, Review of Literature. J. Urol. *78*:33-40 (July) 1957.

Michaelis, L., and Gutmann, C.: Ueber Einschlüssee in Blasentumoren. Ztschr. klin. Med. *47*:208-215, 1902.

Morse, H. D.: The Etiology and Pathology of Pyelitis Cystica, Ureteritis Cystica and Cystitis Cystica. Am. J. Path. *4*:33-50 (Jan.) 1928.

Patch, F. S., and Rhea, L. J.: The Genesis and Development of Brunn's Nests and Their Relation to Cystitis Cystica, Cystitis Glandularis and Primary Adeno-carcinoma of the Bladder. Canad. M. A. J. *33*:597-606 (Dec.) 1935.

Schneiderman, C., and Simon, M. A.: Malacoplakia of the Urinary Tract. J. Urol. *100*:694-698 (Nov.) 1968.

Scott, E. V. Z., and Scott, W. F., Jr.: A Fatal Case of Malakoplakia of the Urinary Tract. J. Urol. 79: 52-56 (Jan.) 1958.

Sözer, I. T.: A Rare Localization of Malakoplakia: Renal Pelvis. J. Urol. *95*:746-748 (June) 1966.

Stirling, C., and Ash, J. E.: Chronic Proliferative Lesions of the Urinary Tract. J. Urol. *45*:342-360 (Mar.) 1941.

von Brunn, A.: Ueber drüsenähnliche Bildungen in der Schleimhaut des Nierenbeckens des Ureters und der Harnblase beim Menschen. Arch. f. mikr. Anat. *41*:294-302, 1893.

von Hansemann, D.: Über Malakoplakie der Harnblase. Arch. path. Anat. *173*:302-308, 1903.

Gas Producing Infections

Boijsen, E., and Lewis-Jonsson, J.: Emphysematous Cystitis. Acta radiol. *41*:269-276 (Mar.) 1954.

Burger, R. H., Ward, J. N., and Draper, J. W.: Perinephric Abscess With Gas Formation. Am. Surgeon *30*:302-305 (May) 1964.

Faingold, J. E., Hansen, C. O., and Rigler, L. G.: Cystitis Emphysematosa: Review of the Literature and Report of Four Cases Diagnosed by Roentgen Examination. Radiology *61*:346-354 (Sept.) 1953.

Ganem, E. J., Calitri, J., and Glidden, H. S.: The Roentgenographic Diagnosis of Cystitis Emphysematosa. J. Urol. *78*:245-251 (Sept.) 1957.

Gillies, C. L., and Flocks, R.: Spontaneous Renal and Perirenal Emphysema: Report of a Case in a Diabetic From Escherichia coli Infection. Am. J. Roentgenol. *45*:173-174 (Aug.) 1941.

Kent, H. P.: Gas in the Urinary Tract. J. Faculty Radiol. *7*:57-65, 1955.

Klein, D. E., Mahoney, S. A., Youngen, R., and Schneider, D. H.: Renal Emphysema. J. Urol. *95*:625-629 (May) 1966.

Milner, W. A., Garlick, W. B., and Mamonas, C.: Cystitis Emphysematosa: Case Report With Clinical Diagnosis and Review of the Literature. New England J. Med. *246*:902-905 (June) 1952.

Stokes, J. B., Jr.: Emphysematous Pyelonephritis. J. Urol. *96*:6-11 (July) 1966.

Teasley, G. H.: Cystitis Emphysematosa: Case Report With a Review of Literature. J. Urol. *62*:48-51 (July) 1949.

Renal Parenchymal (Cortical) Infection—Cortical Abscess; Renal "Carbuncle"; Perinephritis; Perinephric Abscess; Pyonephrosis

Becker, J. A., Fleming, R., Kanter, I., and Melicow, M.: Misleading Appearances in Renal Angiography. Radiology *88*:691-700 (Apr.) 1967.

Beer, E.: Roentgenographic Evidence of Perinephritic Abscess. Am. J. Surg. n.s. *4*:446-447 (Apr.) 1928; J.A.M.A. *90*:1375-1376 (Apr. 28) 1928.

Cabot, H.: Perinephritic Abscess—Ureteral Stone—Kidney Stone. Interstate Postgrad. M. A. North America, 1930, pp. 1-5.

Cabot, H.: Blood Stream Infections of the Kidney. Brit. J. Urol. *8*:233-256, 1936.

Cabot, H., and Montgomery, T. R.: The Diagnosis and Management of Subacute Blood Stream Infections of the Kidney. New York State J. Med. *39*:818-828 (Apr. 15) 1939.

Doolittle, K. H., and Taylor, J. N.: Renal Abscess in the Differential Diagnosis of Mass in Kidney. J. Urol. *89*:649-651 (May) 1963.

Mathé, C. P.: A New Sign for the Diagnosis of Perinephritic Abscess, Perinephritis, Renal Carbuncle and Cortical Abscess of the Kidney. Urol. & Cutan. Rev. *38*:639-642 (Sept.) 1934.

Menville, J. G.: The Lateral Pyelogram as a Diagnostic Aid in Perinephric Abscess. J.A.M.A. *111*: 231-233 (July 16) 1938.

Parks, R. E.: The Radiographic Diagnosis of Perinephric Abscess. J. Urol. *64*:555-563 (Oct.) 1950.

Prehn, D. T.: A Pyelographic Sign in the Diagnosis of Perinephric Abscess. J. Urol. *55*:8-17 (Jan.) 1946.

Salvatierra, O., Jr., Bucklew, W. B., and Morrow, J. W.: Perinephric Abscess: A Report of 71 Cases. J. Urol. *98*:296-302 (Sept.) 1967.

Shane, J. H., and Harris, M.: Roentgenologic Diagnosis of Perinephritic Abscess. J. Urol. *32*:19-26 (July) 1934.

Cystitis

Adams, P., and Kraus, J. E.: Eosinophilic Granuloma: An Unusual Case With Involvement of the Skin, Lungs and Kidneys. Arch. Dermat. *61*:957-970 (June) 1950.

Brown, E. W.: Eosinophilic Granuloma of the Bladder. J. Urol. *83*:665-668 (May) 1960.

Champion, R. H., and Ackles, R. C.: Eosinophilic Cystitis. J. Urol. *96*:729-732 (Nov.) 1966.

Cristol, D. S., Greene, L. F., and Thompson, G. J.: Interstitial Cystitis of Men: A Review of Seventy-eight Cases. J.A.M.A. *126*:825-828 (Nov.) 1944.

Farber, S., and Vawter, G. F.: Clinical Pathological Conference. J. Pediat. *62*:282-287 (Feb.) 1963.

Hand, J. R.: Interstitial Cystitis: Report of 223 Cases (204 Women and 19 Men). J. Urol. *61*:291-310 (Feb.) 1949.

Higgins, C. C.: Hunner Ulcer of the Bladder (Review of 100 Cases). Ann. Int. Med. *15*:708-715 (Oct.) 1941.

Hunner, G. L.: A Rare Type of Bladder Ulcer: Further Notes, With a Report of Eighteen Cases. J.A.M.A. *70*:203-212 (Jan.) 1918.

Kopp, J. H.: Pyelitis, Ureteritis and Cystitis Cystica. J. Urol. *56*:28-34 (July) 1946.

Palubinskas, A. J.: Eosinophilic Cystitis: Case Report of Eosinophilic Infiltration of the Urinary Bladder. Radiology *75*:589-591 (Oct.) 1960.

Warrick, W. D.: Cystitis Cystica: Bacteriological Studies in a Series of 28 Cases. J. Urol. *45*:835-843 (June) 1941.

Wenzl, J. E., Greene, L. F., and Harris, L. E.: Eosinophilic Cystitis. J. Pediat. *64*:746-749 (May) 1964.

Brucellosis of the Urinary Tract

Abernathy, R. S., Price, W. E., and Spink, W. W.: Chronic Brucellar Pyelonephritis Simulating

Tuberculosis. J.A.M.A. *159*:1534-1537 (Dec. 17) 1955.

Boyd, M. L.: Human Prostatic Infection With Brucella abortus (Alcaligenes abortus). J. Urol. *39*: 717-721 (May) 1938.

Buckley, T. I.: Brucellosis of the Male Genitalia. California & West. Med. *48*:175-177 (Mar.) 1938.

Clark, A. L.: Urinary Tract Infections Accompanying Brucellosis. J. Urol. *42*:249-256 (Aug.) 1939.

Forbes, K. A., Lowry, E. C., Gibson, T. E., and Soanes, W. A.: Brucellosis of the Genito-urinary Tract: Review of the Literature and Report of a Case in a Child. Urol. Survey *4*:391-412, 1954.

Greene, L. F., and Albers, D. D.: Brucellosis of the Urinary Tract. Proc. Staff Meet., Mayo Clin. *25*: 638-640 (Nov. 8) 1950.

Greene, L. F., Weed, L. A., and Albers, D. D.: Brucellosis of the Urinary Tract. J. Urol. *67*:765-772 (May) 1952.

Hardy, A. V., Jordan, C. F., and Borts, I. H.: Undulant Fever: Further Epidemiologic and Clinical Observations in Iowa. J.A.M.A. *107*:559-563 (Aug. 22) 1936.

Hardy, A. V., Jordan, C. F., Borts, I. H., and Hardy, G. C.: Undulant Fever: With Special Reference to a Study of Brucella Infection in Iowa. Nat. Inst. Health Bull. *158*:75 (Dec.) 1930.

Harris, H. J.: Brucellosis (Undulant Fever): Clinical and Subclinical. New York, Paul B. Hoeber, Inc., 1941.

Herrell, W. E., and Barber, T. E.: The Combined Use of Aureomycin and Dihydrostreptomycin in the Treatment of Brucellosis. Proc. Staff Meet., Mayo Clin. *24*:138-145 (Mar. 16) 1949.

Honey, R. M., Gelfand, M., and Myers, N. H.: Chronic Brucellar Pyelonephritis With Calcification: Short Review of the Literature and Report of a Case. Central African J. Med. *3*:465-468 (Nov.) 1957.

Isaac, A. G.: Orchitis and Epididymitis Due to Undulant Fever. J. Urol. *40*:201-207 (July) 1938.

Kelalis, P. P., Greene, L. F., and Weed, L. A.: Brucellosis of the Urogenital Tract: A Mimic of Tuberculosis. J. Urol. *88*:347-353 (Sept.) 1962.

Martin, W. J., Nichols, D. R., and Beahrs, O. H.: Chronic Localized Brucellosis: With Recurrent Constitutional Manifestations. Arch. Int. Med. *107*:75-80 (Jan.) 1961.

Fungal Infections of the Kidney

Abbott, D. P.: Primary Actinomycosis of the Kidney. J.A.M.A. *82*:1414-1415 (May) 1924.

Albers, D. D.: Monilial Infection of the Kidney: Case Reports. J. Urol. *69*:32-38 (Jan.) 1953.

Baron, E., and Arduino, L. T.: Primary Renal Actinomycosis. J. Urol. *62*:410-416 (Oct.) 1949.

Cowan, D. E., Dillon, J. R., Jr., Talbot, B. S., and Bridge, R. A. C.: Renal Moniliasis: A Case Report and Discussion. J. Urol. *88*:594-596 (Nov.) 1962.

Hunt, V. C., and Mayo, C. W.: Actinomycosis of the Kidney. Ann. Surg. *93*:501-505 (Feb.) 1932.

Granulomatous Prostatitis

Kelalis, P. P., and Greene, L. F.: Carcinoma of the Prostate — or Granulomatous Prostatitis? GP *32*: 86-89, 1965.

Kelalis, P. P., Greene, L. F., and Harrison, E. G., Jr.: Granulomatous Prostatitis: A Mimic of Carcinoma of the Prostate. J.A.M.A. *191*:287-289 (Jan. 25) 1965.

Kelalis, P. P., Harrison, E. G., Jr., and Greene, L. F.: Allergic Granulomas of the Prostate in Asthmatics. J.A.M.A. *188*:963-967 (June 15) 1964.

Kelalis, P. P., Harrison, E. G., Jr., and Utz, D. C.: Allergic Granulomas of the Prostate: Treatment With Steroids. J. Urol. *96*:573-577 (Oct.) 1966.

Melicow, M. M.: Allergic Granulomas of the Prostate Gland. J. Urol. *65*:288-296 (Feb.) 1951.

Tanner, F. H., and McDonald, J. R.: Granulomatous Prostatitis: A Histologic Study of a Group of Granulomatous Lesions Collected From Prostate Glands. Arch. Path. *36*:358-370 (Sept.) 1943.

Thompson, G. J., and Albers, D. D.: Granulomatous Prostatitis: A Condition Which Clinically May Be Confused With Carcinoma of Prostate. J. Urol. *69*:530-538 (Apr.) 1953.

Yalowitz, P. A., Greene, L. F., Sheps, S. G., and Carlin, M. R.: Wegener's Granulomatosis Involving the Prostate Gland: Report of a Case. J. Urol. *96*: 801-804 (Nov.) 1966.

Urinary Bilharziasis

Afifi, M. A.: Roentgenographic Manifestations of Urinary Bilharziasis and Calculous Formations in Egypt, and Intravenous Pyelography. Am. J. Roentgenol. *31*:208-223 (Feb.) 1934.

Atala, A., and Zaher, M. F.: Bilharzial Calcification of the Renal Capsule: A Case Report. J. Urol. *101*:125-126 (Feb.) 1969.

Atala, A., Zaher, M. F., and Ragy, I.: Bilharzial Bladder Outlet Obstruction. J. Urol. *101*:183-185 (Feb.) 1969.

El-Badawi, A. A.: Bilharzial Polypi of the Urinary Bladder. Brit. J. Urol. *38*:24-35 (Feb.) 1966.

Faust, E. C., and Russell, P. F.: Craig and Faust's Clinical Parasitology. Ed. 7, Philadelphia, Lea & Febiger, 1964, pp. 553-564.

Maged, A., and Soliman, L. A. M.: Bilharzial Pseudocalculus of the Ureter. J. Urol. *99*:30-34 (Jan.) 1968.

Makar, N.: Urological Aspects of Bilharziasis in Egypt. Cairo, Société Orientale de Publicite, 1955.

Manson-Bahr, P. H.: Manson's Tropical Diseases: A Manual of the Diseases of Warm Climates. Ed. 14, Baltimore, The Williams & Wilkins Company, 1954, pp. 702-719.

Ragheb, M.: The Radiological Manifestation in Bilharziasis. Brit. J. Radiol. *12*:21-27 (Jan.) 1939.

Vermooten, V.: Bilharziasis of the Ureter and Its Pathognomonic Roentgenographic Appearance. J. Urol. *38*:430-441 (Nov.) 1937.

Wolstenholme, G. E. W., and O'Connor, M.: Ciba Foundation Symposium — Bilharziasis. Boston, Little, Brown and Company, 1962, 433 pp.

CHAPTER 8

Tuberculosis of the Genitourinary Tract

By HARRY W. ten CATE

GENERAL CONSIDERATIONS

Pathogenesis

Tuberculosis of the genitourinary tract is generally considered to be a metastatic infection resulting from hematogenous dissemination of tubercle bacteria. The primary lesion usually is tuberculosis of the lungs or occasionally of bones and joints (Medlar, 1926; 1948; Medlar, Spain, and Holliday). In almost all cases of renal tuberculosis a healed or still active pulmonary lesion is present. Renal tuberculosis essentially is a bilateral disease. Consequent to its hematogenous origin, multiple tiny miliary tubercles can be found on serial sections in both kidneys. Most of these small lesions tend to heal either spontaneously or as the result of chemotherapy instituted for the primary pulmonary disease. In relatively rare cases tuberculosis spreads rapidly within both kidneys, involving the ureters, bladder, and genital tract in a short time. If miliary foci do not heal, they usually behave as silent lesions, sometimes for years, before they eventually become manifest;

often the primary pulmonary process has by that time healed completely. Sometimes only a small scar is found on roentgen examination of the chest, and the primary lesion may have been completely forgotten by the patient or may never have been detected. It is not unusual for a latent period of 10, 15, or even 20 years to elapse between the pulmonary infection and the first clinical manifestations of the disease in the genitourinary tract. One might argue that in such cases the renal disease must be due to a new tuberculous infection. On the other hand, it is quite reasonable to conclude that the primary pulmonary infection acquired some 10 to 20 years previously had not been treated adequately or timely enough to heal its metastatic lesions elsewhere in the body.

Tuberculosis rarely involves the external genitalia primarily. Contiguous spread of tuberculous lesions of the lumbar spine to the kidney or ureter is equally rare. Coincidental tuberculous lesions of the spine, joints, intestines, and genital organs are not uncommon, and in some cases urinary tuberculosis may be a tertiary manifestation due to hematogenous spread from such lesions. In renal tuberculosis

855

careful attention should be given to possible coincidental involvement of these organs (Fig. 8–1). Tuberculosis of the ureter and bladder is almost always secondary to renal tuberculosis consequent to bacteriuria, as is probably true of tuberculous prostatitis and tuberculosis of the seminal vesicles and epididymis. Medlar expressed the view that tubercle bacteria in the urine bathing the prostate enter the prostatic ducts to infect the prostate gland; bacteria also enter the ejaculatory ducts to infect the seminal vesicles, vasa deferentia, and epididymides. Genital tuberculosis, however, is occasionally manifest in males in whom a tuberculous infection of the kidneys cannot be demonstrated (Cooper; Ross, Gow, and St. Hill). In such cases a direct hematogenous infection of the genital organs from a primary source in the lungs should be considered a possibility. Even then, at a later time renal tuberculosis may become manifest.

The first renal tuberculous emboli are found in the glomerular and cortical arterioles, causing small tubercles. Healing depends on the number and virulence of the contained bacteria, on the local and general resistance of the host, and on the sensitivity of the strain of bacteria to the chemotherapy used. If healing does not occur, a necrotizing lesion develops and bacteria pass down the tubules and may be detected in the urine with or without pyuria. New tubercles form at the narrow portion of the loop of Henle in the medulla, necrotize, and coalesce, involving the calyceal wall usually at the tip of the papilla. This small, irregular, ulcerating cavitation represents the first lesion that can be detected urographically. The ulcerocavernous papillitis may be a solitary lesion in one kidney or may be multiple in one or both kidneys. With progression of the infection the lesion enlarges, causing a cavernous process of the entire pyramid. Further calyceal deformity develops as an enlargement of the calyx with disappearance of the calyceal tips or

as one or more separate cavities connected by fistulous tracts with one or more calyces. The disease spreads by secondary infection of the mucous membrane of the other calyces and the renal pelvis, ureter, and bladder. Multiple granulomatous lesions, usually ulcerating, cause edema, round cell infiltration, cavitation, and fibrosis. At the areas of physiologic narrowing in the urinary tract, such as calyceal infundibula, ureteropelvic junction, the ureter overlying the sacro-iliac joint, and the vesicoureteral junction, such lesions cause hydrocalyx, hydronephrosis, or hydroureter, with consequent further destruction of the renal parenchyma. Rapid healing with an adequate chemotherapeutic regimen may enhance fibrosis and stricture formation in the same areas. Thus all or part of the kidney may become "silent" on excretory urography, a condition known as autoamputation of a calyx or as partial or complete autonephrectomy. Such "autonephrectomized" kidneys may be asymptomatic for many years, the complete obstruction preventing further contamination.

The healing of extensive tuberculous lesions in the urinary tract is characterized by calcification, fibrosis, and stricture formation. Calcium deposits may be found in the linings of tuberculous cavities owing partially to the healing process and partially to sedimentation of urinary calcium salts on necrotic surfaces. Stricture and scarring consequent to the healing process are particularly important in the areas of physiologic narrowing. The number, extent, and progress of such strictures can be followed closely by roentgenographic methods so that careful consideration of reconstructive surgical possibilities at the optimal moment may prevent further destruction of the functioning renal tissue secondary to obstruction. Rapid stricture formation is well known as a complicating consequence of chemotherapy in tuberculosis of the urinary tract. The bladder may contract down to the size of an egg or a walnut, causing incontinence of urine, stricture of the ureteral orifices, and incompetence of the vesicoureteral junction resulting in vesicoureteral reflux. Thus stricture or reflux at the ureteral orifice in tuberculosis of the bladder with unilateral renal disease may seriously threaten function of the contralateral, clinically healthy kidney, even with an adequate chemotherapeutic regimen.

Diagnosis

As the therapeutic attitude toward genitourinary tuberculosis has changed completely through the years, so has the nature of the diagnostic problem. First, renal tuberculosis was regarded as a unilateral disease, and immediate nephrectomy of the diseased kidney was the only hope of cure. It was at that time of paramount importance to demonstrate beyond doubt and as early as possible which kidney was diseased. Excretory urography was only of relatively poor diagnostic quality and retrograde studies were usually necessary bilaterally for both roentgenographic and bacteriologic diagnosis. In 1926 Medlar demonstrated that renal tuberculosis is essentially a bilateral disease from the outset. Nephrectomy still was considered the only way of effective treatment but its immediate indication gradually changed into a more careful consideration of the time element, depending on the general condition of the patient, the degree of involvement of each kidney, and the assessment of renal function of both kidneys together and each kidney separately. The concept of immediate nephrectomy changed into that of nephrectomy when the patient's condition was considered at its best. After the period 1947 to 1952, when powerful therapeutic agents became available in the battle against *Mycobacterium tuberculosis* and diagnostic methods became more elaborate and refined, surgical therapy was first combined with chemotherapy and finally was completely

or almost completely replaced by a conservative regimen. At present this conservative attitude employing treatment with multiple drugs for at least 2 years has yielded such good results that surgical intervention is now rarely considered indicated in genitourinary tuberculosis.

Available diagnostic methods are used to (1) establish the tuberculous nature of the disease, (2) estimate the extent of the lesion in each kidney, (3) estimate the remaining amount of functioning renal tissue, (4) follow the progress of healing, and (5) detect complications of the healing process.

Tuberculosis of the genitourinary tract can be diagnosed only by demonstrating the presence of *M. tuberculosis* in urine or tissue specimens. Only a positive culture or a positive guinea pig inoculation test may be considered as conclusive evidence of tuberculosis, unless of course a histologic diagnosis is made beyond doubt from removed tissue. Demonstration of acid-fast bacteria in the urine sediment (Ziehl-Neelsen stain) is not sufficiently positive proof of urinary tract tuberculosis but should be categorized as "suggestive." False-positive results with this test are well known and no therapeutic regimen should be instituted on such evidence alone. In recent years some atypical mycobacterial strains that are clinically, histologically, and radiographically indistinguishable from those of human tuberculosis have been demonstrated to cause granulomatous disease in man. So far, renal disease has not been associated with these atypical mycobacteria, in contrast to disease of other organs such as the lungs. Recently Gould warned that the appearance of such atypical strains may be expected also in the urinary tract in the near future.

If symptoms and signs in a patient with pyelonephritis or cystitis do not respond readily to adequate treatment of nonspecific infection, tuberculosis should be suspected and ruled out by repeated cultures and inoculation of guinea pigs with early morning specimens of urine. This is particularly true if pyuria exists yet the gram stain of the urinary sediment fails to show bacteria. A positive gram stain does not, however, exclude tuberculosis, since secondary infection by nonspecific organisms is possible in urinary tract tuberculosis; moreover, tubercle bacteria may be present in the urine even though few or no leukocytes are present. Gross and microscopic hematuria not readily explained by other disease should always lead one to suspect tuberculosis. Chronic prostatitis and vesiculitis and chronic epididymitis may also be caused by tuberculosis. A fistula situated in the lateral or posterior part of the scrotum and leading to the epididymis is highly suspect. Tuberculous prostatitis on rectal palpation may closely resemble carcinoma of the prostate gland or nonspecific granulomatous prostatitis. The history may give an important clue that tuberculosis is the cause of the underlying disease; previously known or even slightly suspected tuberculous infection elsewhere in the body that could have acted as a source for hematogenous dissemination is as good a reason as any for performing urine culture and guinea pig inoculation.

A woman physician aged 39 years was admitted in 1964 because of attacks of renal colic on the left. This was the first and only sign or symptom of urinary tract disease that she had ever had. From 1943 through 1945 she had passed through several German concentration camps and had miraculously escaped the gas chamber and death. In 1944 she had had "nonspecific pleuritis" that had cleared up without medication. Otherwise she had always been healthy, apart from physical and mental distressing experiences in the camps. On excretory urography no function was evident in the left kidney. The right kidney was normal. Urine cultures were positive for tuberculosis. Left nephroureterectomy was performed because of persistent pain and pyuria. Extensive destruction of the kidney with several large cavities containing caseous material and with active tuberculous ureteritis was found (Fig. 8–2). The renal tuberculosis was thought to be secondary to tuberculous pleuritis and to have been silently destroying the kidney for almost 20 years.

Place of Roentgenography in Diagnosis

The early diagnosis of genitourinary tuberculosis requires the physician to be aware at all times of this possibility and to search carefully for *M. tuberculosis* in the urine, to do skin tests for tuberculosis, and to perform excretory urography. Renal tuberculosis does not produce pyelographic changes that are pathognomonic. Even a normal pyelogram does not exclude renal tuberculosis. On the other hand, tuberculosis often does produce significant, highly suggestive, or even characteristic pyelographic alterations. However, renal tuberculosis after all is only another chronic inflammatory disease almost all of whose roentgenographic manifestations can be mimicked by nontuberculous pyelonephritis. Such diseases as medullary sponge kidney, nonspecific papillary necrosis, and renal neoplasm are sometimes confusing in differential diagnosis and rarely may be present coincidentally with tuberculosis. Therefore urograms that suggest lesions other than tuberculosis should never prevent the physician from doing urine cultures and inoculation tests if tuberculosis has already been suspected for other reasons; on the other hand, such tests should be performed as the appropriate result of suspicious urograms made for other reasons in patients not suspected of having tuberculosis. Finally, in all films suggestive of urinary tract tuberculosis careful attention should be given to possible tuberculous lesions of the spine, sacro-iliac joints, and bony pelvis, and anteroposterior and lateral chest films should be made.

Once genitourinary tuberculosis has been diagnosed additional roentgenographic means other than routine excretory urography may help establish the extent of the lesions in each kidney separately and the amount of remaining functioning tissue. Retrograde pyelograms are sometimes necessary to outline renal cavities that do not show up on excretory films; a definite disadvantage is eventual introduction of secondary infection by nonspecific organisms or even tubercle bacteria in a previously uncontaminated kidney. It is therefore important that retrograde pyelography, if indicated, be carried out under the prophylactic protection of streptomycin in all cases in which tuberculosis is suspected.

Often retrograde pyelography can be dispensed with if newer methods are utilized such as the infusion type of excretory urography using high doses of contrast medium and combined with nephrotomography. Aortography and renal arteriography are advocated by some authors as helpful in advanced cases of renal tuberculosis in which either large parts of the kidney or the entire kidney does not visualize with more conventional methods. Retrograde cystography and micturition cystourethrography may be employed to visualize irregularities or defects in the bladder outline, vesicoureteral reflux, and cavitation in the prostatic urethra. Seminal vesiculography may help establish the extent of tuberculous vesiculitis. Other diagnostic methods that are occasionally helpful are isotope renography and renal scanning.

Of much importance are well-coordinated roentgenographic follow-up studies in all cases of established urinary tract tuberculosis. They are necessary to observe healing and to detect eventual complications of the healing process due to stricture formation.

ROENTGENOGRAPHIC ASPECTS OF GENITOURINARY TUBERCULOSIS

The Plain Film
(Figs. 8–2 through 8–25)

Roentgenographic diagnosis in genitourinary tuberculosis begins with careful examination of the plain film. Deposition of calcium by the body in an attempt to heal tuberculous lesions often provides a diagnostic clue in the roentgenogram. Among the more important findings are: (1) irregularity or enlargement or both of the soft-tissue shadows of the involved kidney—sometimes a large mass of caseous material in a tuberculous cavitation may cause pressure on the renal capsule with consequent bulging outside the normal contour; (2) calcific shadows overlying the kidneys, ureters, bladder, seminal vesicles, vasa deferentia, and prostate gland, and (3) associated tuberculous lesions in the bony structure (Fig. 8–1; see also Figs. 3–133 and 3–162 through 3–166). Calcific shadows must not be regarded too seriously until they are identified by means of urograms, as they may be produced by stones or calcification elsewhere than in the genitourinary organs. Certain characteristics of these shadows, however, may suggest genitourinary calcification caused by tuberculosis. Calcified lymph glands, often seen on the plain film of the abdomen, could be confused with renal calcification, but are not, ipso facto, suggestive of a tuberculous etiology.

RENAL CALCIFICATION

Calcific shadows produced by tuberculosis in the kidney tend to be indefinite and irregular in outline and are not as a rule so dense and well-defined as renal calculi. Often they are indistinct and involve a fairly large portion of the kidney. Such shadows tend to lie in the cortex of the kidney, whereas calculi are more commonly seen in the vicinity of the pelvis and calyces. However, it may be difficult at times, even by means of urography, to distinguish tuberculous calcification from renal calculi in the tips of the calyces or from nephrocalcinosis. In a study of this subject Apperson, Wechsler, and Lattimer found either calcification or calculi in 18% of 161 cases of renal tuberculosis. Although at times they were not entirely sure that they could distinguish between calcification and calculi, from their roentgenographic study they estimated that the two conditions occurred approximately equally. Also of interest in their study was the finding of a nontuberculous (secondary) infection in addition to the tuberculous infection in approximately a third of the cases in which either calcification or calculi were present. This was in contrast to an incidence of associated nontuberculous infection in 10% of the cases of renal tuberculosis generally.

The most poorly defined shadows of poor density seen in cases of renal tuberculosis are those produced by caseation with a limited amount of calcification (Figs. 8-3, 8-4, and 8-5). Such faint shadows may be recognized only after exceedingly careful examination of the plain film, as they may be only slightly more dense than normal renal tissue. Although most tuberculous calcification is minimally or moderately dense, variations of density are encountered until the other extreme is reached, in which shadows are so dense as to simulate stone. The size of the area involved with calcification may also vary greatly from a few minute areas to a cast of the entire kidney and ureter like that seen in advanced cases in which so-called autonephrectomy has occurred.

Although calcification occurs commonly in tuberculosis and suggests strongly the presence of tuberculosis, it is by no means pathognomonic. It must be remembered that the process of calcification simply represents the power of the body to localize and heal an inflammatory lesion, and although it occurs with much greater frequency in tuberculosis than in other inflammatory lesions, still it may be found as the end result in almost any nontuberculous infection. Gow (1965) has expressed the belief that tuberculous calcification of the renal parenchyma is an unfavorable prognostic sign when nonsurgical therapy is used: it would point to a smaller chance of stable urinary conversion and to more progressive deterioration of renal function than in renal

tuberculosis without calcification (Figs. 8-6 through 8-14; see also Fig. 3-47).

CALCIFICATION OF URETER AND BLADDER

Tuberculous calcification of the ureter is not as common as renal calcification. Calcification of the bladder is relatively rare. Calcification of the ureter usually is not difficult to recognize, because of its position and contour. At times it is difficult to distinguish calcification of the ureteral wall from ureteral calculi (Figs. 8-15A and B through 8-19). Tuberculous calcifications may be seen as mottled and irregular areas in various segments, or more homogeneous for a greater length. According to Friedenberg, Ney, and Stachenfeld, tuberculous calcification of the ureteral wall should be differentiated from calcification due to schistosomiasis (bilharziasis); in such cases the ureter is dilated and the calcification is limited to the lower ureteral segment. (See discussion, Chapter 7, page 839.) Calcification of the wall of the bladder, although uncommon, is easily recognized (Figs. 8-20 and 8-21).

CALCIFICATION OF SEMINAL TRACT (PROSTATE, SEMINAL VESICLES, VASA DEFERENTIA, AND AMPULLAE)

Tuberculous calcification of the prostate gland may be impossible to distinguish from nontuberculous calculous prostatitis without additional clinical data (Fig. 8-22; see also Fig. 1-63). In differential diagnosis it should be remembered that prostatic calculi occur much more commonly than does tuberculous calcification of the prostate. Demonstration of tubercle bacteria in the urine would of course lend weight to the diagnosis of tuberculous calcification, although renal tuberculosis and prostatic calculi of nonspecific origin may occur together (Fig. 8-23A and B). Calcification of the seminal vesicles may occur in tuberculosis (Fig. 8-24) but it is ot common. Calcification of the vasa eferentia is more commonly encount- red. Diabetes, however, is often found an etiologic factor in calcification of the

vasa, and certainly more often than is tuberculosis (Fig. 8–25; see also Figs. 8–22 and 3–105 through 3–111 and Table 3–1).

(Text continued on page 871.)

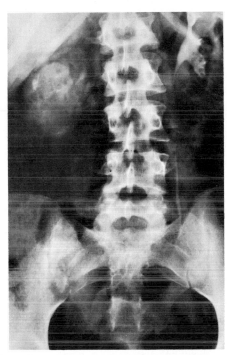

Figure 8–1. Right renal tuberculosis. Patient admitted to hospital with serious tuberculosis of right acro-iliac joint. On plain film (not shown) coincidentally a grossly calcified asymptomatic right kidney as seen (**autonephrectomy**). *Excretory urogram.* Left kidney normal. Note irregular areas of decalcification f right sacro-iliac joint. Right nephroureterectomy. Ureter was normal and no pathologic relationship was oted between ureter and sacro-iliac joint.

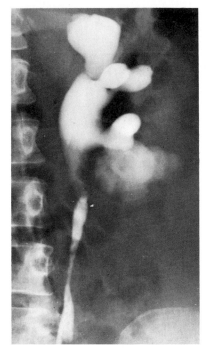
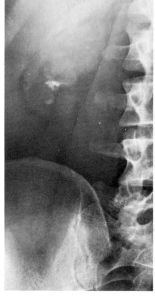

Fig. 8-2   Fig. 8-3

Figure 8-2. *Retrograde pyelogram.* **Left renal tuberculosis.** Note large cavity in lower pole, grade 2 hydronephrosis, and irregular upper ureter. Left nephrectomy was done. (There was no function evident on excretory urogram [see text].)

Figure 8-3. *Plain film.* **Diffuse tuberculous calcification** of right kidney in case of **autonephrectomy,** with no function remaining, as demonstrated by excretory urogram (not shown here).

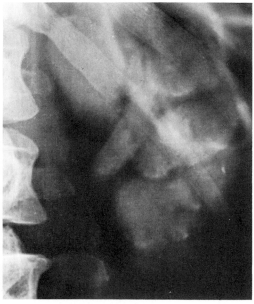
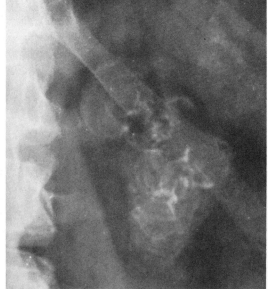

Fig. 8-4   Fig. 8-5

Figure 8-4. *Plain film.* **Extensive caseation and necrosis** caused by tuberculous left kidney. Minimal degree of calcification but sufficient to outline pelvis and upper portion of ureter.

Figure 8-5. *Plain film.* Note calcification in midureter. **Extensive calcification of nonfunctioning left kidney (autonephrectomy).**

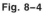

862

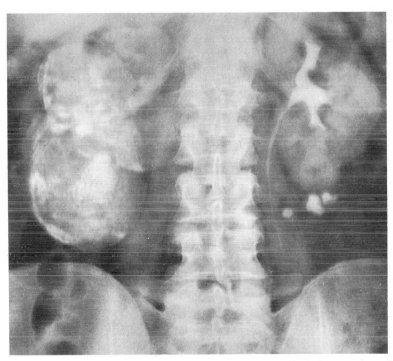

Figure 8–6.   *Excretory urogram.* **Autonephrectomy of tuberculous right kidney** with marked calcification of calyceal walls and calcium deposits in contents of collecting system. Marked stricture of ureteropelvic junction. Urine specimens negative for tuberculosis. Nephrectomy done. There was no parenchyma remaining; kidney contained yellow sterile fluid contents. Microscopy and bacteriologic examination of tissue and fluid contents failed to show tubercle bacteria, but there was little doubt that destruction must have been of tuberculous origin.

Fig. 8–7   Fig. 8–8

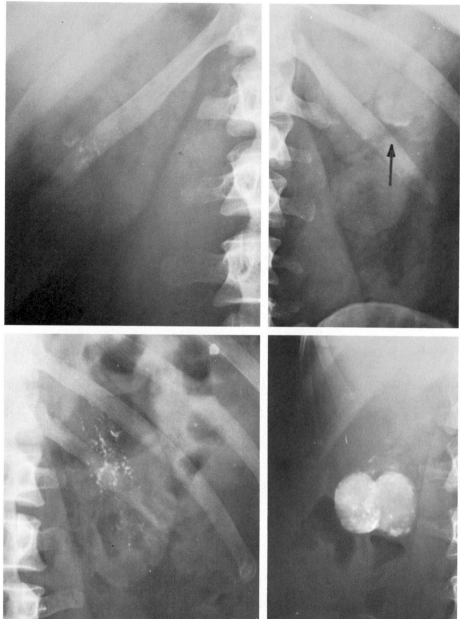

Fig. 8–9   Fig. 8–10

Figure 8–7. *Plain film.* **Tuberculous calcification of right kidney.** Shadows are indefinite and irregular in outline. Distribution of shadows would suggest tuberculous calcification.

Figure 8–8. *Plain film.* **Tuberculous calcification of left kidney.** Irregularity of calcific area and its position near lateral margin of kidney suggest tuberculosis rather than stone.

Figure 8–9. *Plain film.* **Tuberculous calcification of left kidney.** Calcific areas are indefinite and irregular in outline and seem to overlie pelvis and calyces. Differs from nephrocalcinosis in that renal pyramids do not seem to be outlined. Filigree appearance suggests tuberculosis rather than calculi. Brucellosis with calcification must also be considered in differential diagnosis.

Figure 8–10. *Plain film.* **Tuberculous calcification of right kidney,** of unusual density, which might be confused with renal stone.

Fig. 8–11

Fig. 8–12

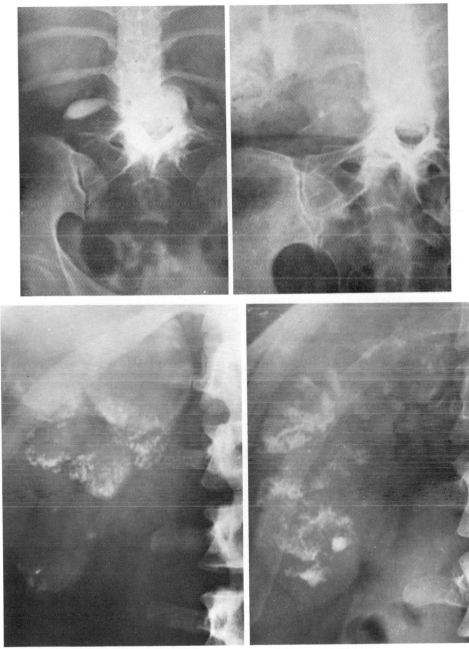

Fig. 8–13

Fig. 8–14

Figure 8–11. *Plain film.* Calcification of psoas abscess secondary to tuberculosis of lumbosacral vertebrae (Pott's disease). Right kidney was also involved by tuberculosis and showed no function in excretory urogram. Right nephrectomy was done. Films made 1 year after operation showed no change in calcific shadow.

Figure 8–12. *Excretory urogram.* Same case as in Figure 8–11 but 17 years later. Most of calcium has been absorbed; only small amount remains. Left kidney is grossly normal.

Figure 8–13. *Plain film.* Diffuse tuberculous calcification of right kidney in case of autonephrectomy, with no function remaining.

Figure 8–14. *Plain film.* Extensive tuberculous calcification of nonfunctioning right kidney (autonephrectomy), which might be confused with advanced stage of nephrocalcinosis.

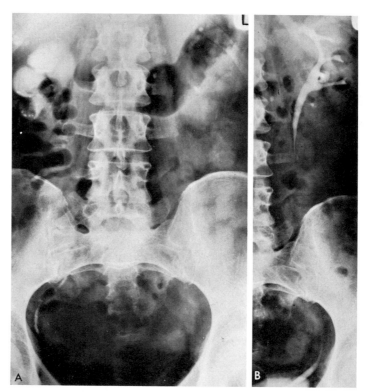

Figure 8–15.   Bilateral renal tuberculosis with calcification of kidney and ureter. **A,** *Plain film.* Calcifie nonfunctioning right kidney (**autonephrectomy**). Note calcified pelvic portion of right ureter, and calciu deposit in lower pole of left kidney. Urine negative for tubercle bacteria. **B,** *Excretory urogram.* Deforme left kidney with autoamputation of lower pole.

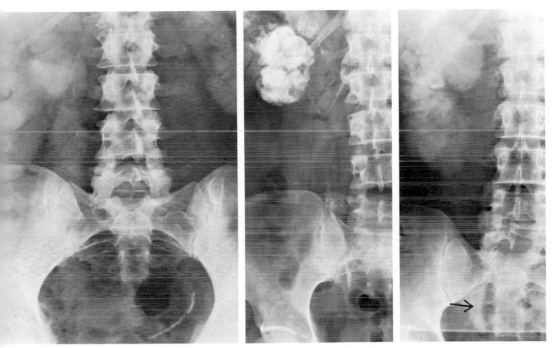

Fig. 8-16   Fig. 8-17   Fig. 8-18

Figure 8-16. *Excretory urogram.* Bilateral renal tuberculosis in woman, 57 years of age, with 30-year history of tuberculosis. Nonfunctioning left kidney with calcification (autonephrectomy) and calcification of lower part of left ureter. Stricture of terminal part of right ureter produced hydronephrosis. Cutaneous ureterostomy performed on right.

Figure 8-17. *Excretory urogram.* Long-standing right renal tuberculosis in man, 38 years of age, with draining psoas abscess. Nonfunctioning calcified right kidney (autonephrectomy) with calcified psoas abscess and calcification of ureter. Left kidney was normal.

Figure 8-18. *Plain film.* Autonephrectomy of right kidney, from tuberculosis. Diffuse caseation with calcification of right kidney and calcification of ureter (*arrow*).

Fig. 8–19

Fig. 8–20

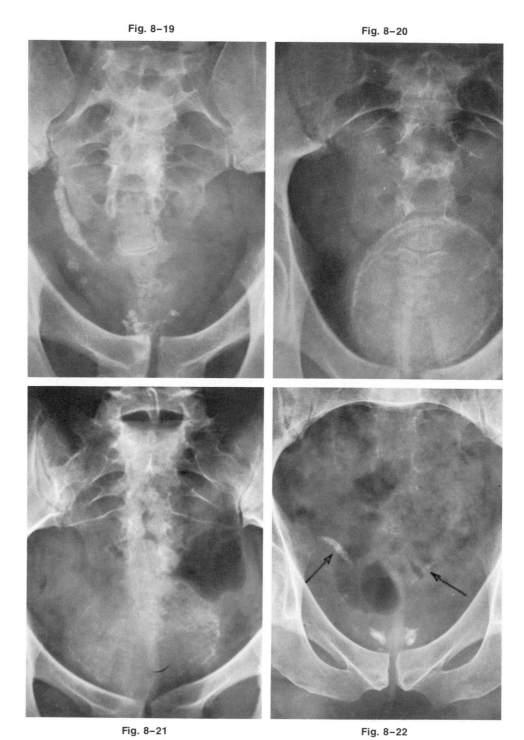

Fig. 8–21

Fig. 8–22

Figure 8–19. *Plain film.* Tuberculous calcification of lower part of right ureter and also of prostate gland

Figures 8–20 and 8–21. *Plain film.* Tuberculous calcification of wall of urinary bladder.

Figure 8–22. *Plain film.* Tuberculous calcification of vasa (*arrows*) and prostate gland.

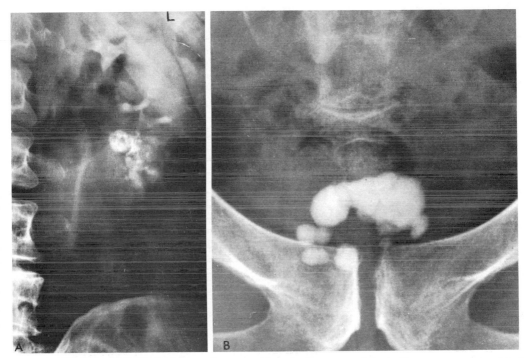

Figure 8–23. Left renal tuberculosis and nonspecific calculous prostatitis. A, *Excretory urogram.* Marked destruction and calcification of left lower pole. B, *Plain film.* Marked calculous prostatitis. Transurethral prostatic resection was performed and prostatic calculi removed. No tuberculosis could be demonstrated in tissue.

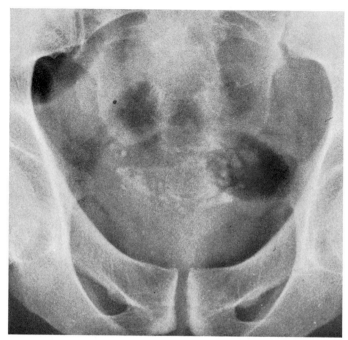

Figure 8–24.   *Plain film.* Tuberculous calcifications of both ampullae and seminal vesicles.

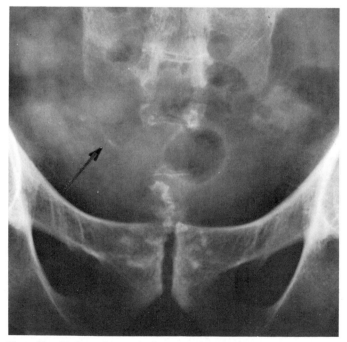

Figure 8–25.   *Plain film.* Tuberculous calcification of ampulla of vas (*arrow*) and prostate gland.

The Urogram in Tuberculosis of the Urinary Tract
(Figs. 8–26 through 8–81)

Tuberculosis of the kidney is essentially a disease of the renal parenchyma. It can be diagnosed with certainty only if the lesion has ulcerated into a calyx or the renal pelvis, causing bacteriuria, pyuria, and roentgenographically detectable deformities of the collecting system. Excretory urography is a roentgenographic method primarily used to outline the renal collecting system, but does not give visible information of localized lesions confined to the parenchyma. The diagnostic quality of the excretory urogram is an expression of the excretory and concentrating powers of the diseased kidney. Most clinicians feel that the density of contrast medium in the collecting system during intravenous pyelography reflects more or less acceptably the function of that kidney. In renal tuberculosis the excretory urogram does not give reliable information on the functional capacity of the kidney. It is well known that a good contrast density in the collecting system may be found if only a fairly small portion of the kidney has good function; on the other hand, poor visualization of contrast medium or absence of contrast density in the excretory urogram by no means necessarily represents complete destruction of the kidney, as Olsson (1943; 1946) pointed out. In addition, an excretory urogram alone may give an impression of renal status at that particular moment, but certainly has no prognostic value in tuberculosis. A tuberculous kidney not visualized on excretory urography may benefit from prolonged adequate therapy to such extent that its collecting system is surprisingly well visualized after some months of treatment (Figs. 8–26 and 8–27A and B). Also, according to Fritjofsson and co-workers, the results of para-aminohippurate clearance tests compared with the impression gained from excretory urography in renal tuberculosis show that intravenous pyelography is a poor renal function test. If a tuberculous kidney does not seem to function on excretory urography, it should not be removed for that reason alone, certainly not promptly and generally not before it has had ample opportunity to show its healing tendency after several months of chemotherapy.

The modern triiodinated contrast media are excreted mainly by the glomeruli whereas the biiodinated drugs previously used were excreted mainly by the tubules. Even though the first tuberculous lesion in the kidney is the small tubercle located in the glomerulus or cortical arterioles, the more important and extensive tuberculous lesion in the renal parenchyma is essentially a tubular one. This causes impaired tubular reabsorption and decreased concentration of contrast medium as it is excreted into the collecting system. In early tuberculosis, this impaired function is not represented by poor visualization of the corresponding calyx. The remaining parenchyma usually excretes well-concentrated contrast medium into the collecting system, and the calyx corresponding to the diseased area is usually well filled in a retrograde manner. As long as the calyceal lining is intact, the calyx shows up clearly and well defined and thus camouflages the corresponding diseased parenchymal area.

Patients with tuberculosis of the lungs, bones, or other organs may have roentgenologically detectable renal disease that is not necessarily tuberculous. Coincidental renal deformities such as those due to nontuberculous chronic pyelonephritis, papillary necrosis secondary to diabetes or misuse of acetophenetidin, medullary sponge kidney, calyceal diverticulum, or hypernephroma may simulate renal tuberculosis and lead to an erroneous diagnosis. Renal tuberculosis should never simply be diagnosed on the basis of such "typical" lesions seen on excretory urograms. The demonstration of tubercle bacteria in the urine is an absolute pre-requisite for the diagnosis.

In discussion of the pathogenesis of renal tuberculosis the medullary lesion eroding through the renal papilla and producing a cavity communicating with a calyx was described as the first urographically demonstrable lesion. Such a lesion is the classic erosion, that is, the "moth-eaten" or "feathery" irregularity of a calyx considered characteristic of renal tuberculosis. In 1938 Emmett and Braasch determined the frequency of the various changes in the excretory urograms as observed in 100 consecutive cases of proved renal tuberculosis when the patient was first seen. In descending order of frequency the changes were as follows: (1) absence of visualization, (2) delayed and impaired visualization, (3) calycectasis, (4) evidence of parenchymal necrosis as shown by "fuzzy," irregular, or "moth-eaten" outline of the calyces, (5) cicatricial deformity of the calyces with pinching off of the tips of minor calyces and obliteration of the calyces, (6) deformity or dilatation of the ureter, and (7) pyelectasis.

Calycectasis is demonstrated more commonly than erosion or destruction of the renal papilla. The inflammatory changes in the calcyes and renal pelvis may be readily demonstrable, while the cortical abscess from which such changes originate may not be as readily visualized. Severe nontuberculous pyelonephritis may produce almost exactly the same urographic changes, so that roentgenologic distinction between tuberculous and non-tuberculous pyelonephritis may be difficult or impossible.

Chemotherapy for tuberculosis apparently has not decreased the *incidence* of genitourinary tuberculosis. Siegel and Lattimer stated in 1964 that the overall incidence of advanced lesions had not changed during the previous 17 years as observed in their material, but that the incidence of far-advanced lesions had dropped significantly* (see classification of renal tuberculosis given in Tables 8–1 and 8–2). They felt that this might be the first indication of a decline in severity if not in incidence of renal tuberculosis. This would mean that at present such first findings as absence of function or poor visualization on excretory urograms in renal tuberculosis would no longer head the list of urographic findings as it did in Emmett and Braasch's survey in 1938; on the other hand, stricture formation with consequent hydronephrosis and loss of renal function is one of the sacrifices to be partly attributed to chemotherapy. Therefore, poor visualization or even nonfunctioning kidneys, if not the first urographic finding, will still be encountered in the course of the therapeutic regimen of this disease on follow-up studies.

UROGRAPHIC CHANGES IN RENAL CALYCES AND PELVIS

It is quite natural that the earliest and most frequent urographic changes should occur in the calyces, as the renal pyramid is the site of the key lesion of the kidney (Lieberthal). As mentioned previously calycectasis is one of the earliest and most frequent findings.

Minimal calyceal dilatation may be the first telltale sign of the tuberculous process. In other cases, minimal erosion of a tip of one calyx (indicating involvement of the tip of a pyramid) may be the earliest urographic finding. Such minimal calyceal irregularity may be difficult or impossible to distinguish from pyelosinous backflow or a variation of the normal (see Figs. 4-108 through 4-132). In many cases, final decision must rest on clinical and labor-

---

*In a recent (October 1969) personal communication Frimann-Dahl (Professor of Radiology, Ulleval Hospital, Oslo, Norway) stated "kidney tuberculosis is nearly eradicated with us now; we only occasionally see a case." J.L.E.

atory rather than on urographic data (Figs. 8–28 through 8–33). As the infection proceeds, greater changes in the calyces occur. Increased calycectasis associated with irregularity in contour indicates erosion of the pyramids and cortical necrosis. These changes have been described by such terms as "fuzzy," "feathery," and "moth-eaten." Depending on the amount of necrosis and whether the cavity contains caseous or liquid material, deposits of contrast medium in varying densities may be seen outside the calyx. Sometimes such collections are connected by a short or long tiny fistulous tract with the calyx or the renal pelvis. Cicatrization of calyces is seen not uncommonly. Stricture of the infundibula may incompletely isolate parts of the collecting system, which then has the image of a butterfly; or parts of a calyx may be isolated so that it appears in the urogram as a pinched-off dilated cyst-like structure (Figs. 8–34 through 8–42). Indeed, it is sometimes impossible to decide whether such a cavity partially filled with contrast medium represents a diseased and dilated calyx or whether it is a primary cavity ruptured into the collecting system (Fig. 8–43). If the connection between cavity and collecting system has a fine but irregular outline, probably caseation is present and incomplete filling of the cavity has occurred. Crimann-Dahl (1955) emphasized the diagnostic importance of the "lipping" type of cavity which resembles the rupture of a normal calyx as seen in so-called pyelosinous transflow (Fig. 8–31; see Figs. 4–112, 4–113, and 4–117). If such a cavity projects in the medial direction, he considers it pathognomonic of tuberculosis. It should be remembered that a calyceal diverticulum or a composite calyx with broad papillae may be mistaken for a tuberculous cavity (see Figs. 4–75, 4–76, 4–46, and 5–47). The tuberculous cavity and the "pinched-off" calyx usually have an irregular outline but they may become

smooth-walled during healing under antibiotic treatment. Also, nontuberculous pyelonephritis may cause similar deformities. Total occlusion of a calyceal infundibulum by tuberculous cicatrization may be recognized as an abrupt or sharp-tipped ending of the neck of the calyx with the calyceal tips missing where they would be expected.

It is evident that with such a severe infectious process almost any bizarre dilatation or cicatricial deformity of the calyces might occur. When the process becomes more advanced, a whole group of calyces may become entirely obliterated or destroyed, owing to cicatrization or destruction and caseation of large portions of the kidney (Figs. 8–44 through 8–47).

As the pathologic changes are occurring in the calyces the renal pelvis and ureter are being bathed with urine containing tubercle bacteria and they may also become the site of severe disease which may produce pathologic deformity. Marked dilatation of the renal pelvis often is due to an inflammatory stricture at the ureteropelvic junction or almost anywhere in the ureter, and therefore is a relatively late phenomenon in the course of the disease. Again, nontuberculous pyelonephritis or other nontuberculous obstruction at the ureteropelvic junction, in the ureter, or at the vesicoureteral orifice may produce almost identical roentgenographic findings. Discrete tuberculous changes can be easily missed or interpreted as nontuberculous. If one waits for urographic evidence of pyramidal erosion and cortical necrosis, many early lesions will be missed (Figs. 8–48 through 8–54). A careful search for acid-fast bacteria in the urine sediment, particularly if the gram stain is negative in the presence of pyuria, and in addition repeated culture and guinea pig inoculation of early morning urine specimens may occasionally be rewarding and should certainly not be omitted if there is any doubt at all.

(Text continued on page 888.)

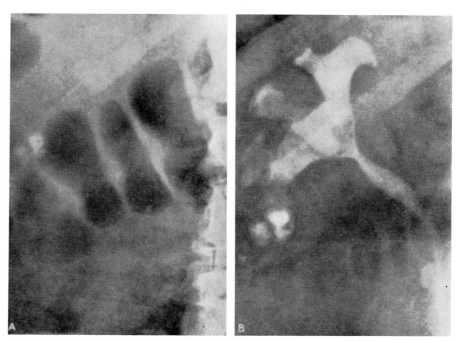

Figure 8–26. Results of chemotherapy in renal tuberculosis. Right renal tuberculosis with no function on excretory urography. Small calcification is noted in one of lower calyces. **A,** *Excretory urogram* before treatment was begun. **B,** *Excretory urogram* after 4½ months of triple-drug therapy. Kidney has resumed function. Calcification is contained in deformed lower calyceal group. (Courtesy of Dr. P. G. Hoorweg, Amsterdam.)

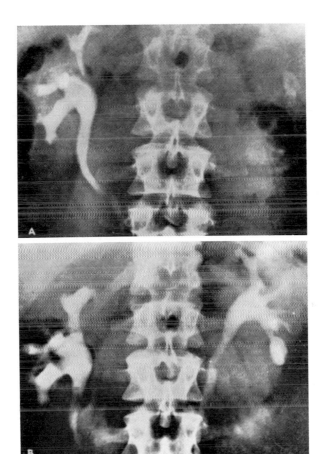

Figure 8–27.   Results of chemotherapy in renal tuberculosis. Bilateral renal tuberculosis with no function of left kidney evidenced in excretory urography. **A,** *Excretory urogram.* Nonfunctioning left kidney with calcification in lower pole. Tuberculous changes in upper and middle calyceal groups of right kidney with pinching off of right upper calyceal infundibulum. **B,** *Excretory urogram* after 5 months of triple-drug therapy. Left kidney resumed function after 3 months of treatment. Right kidney also improved. Five years later, urograms were exactly the same as in **B.** Stable urinary conversion. (Courtesy of Dr. P. G. Hoorweg, Amsterdam.)

Fig. 8–28

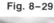

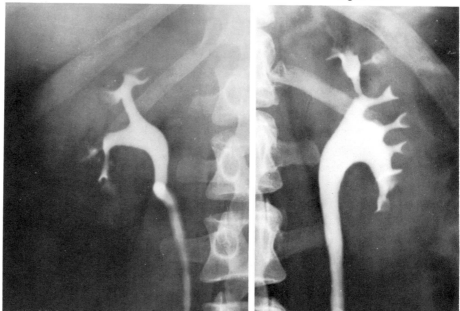

Fig. 8–30

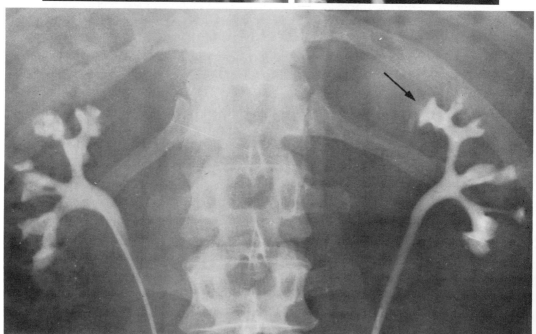

Figure 8–28. *Right retrograde pyelogram.* **Early tuberculous involvement of lower calyces.** Small area of cortical necrosis beyond tip of lower calyx, which could easily be mistaken for pyelosinous backflow.

Figure 8–29. *Left retrograde pyelogram.* **Early tuberculous involvement of upper calyces.** Small area of cortical necrosis beyond tip of upper calyx, which could be mistaken for pyelosinous backflow.

Figure 8–30. **Right renal tuberculosis.** *Bilateral retrograde pyelogram.* Minimal amount of erosion of lateral branch of upper calyx of right kidney, which might easily be confused with atypical calyx with some extravasation. Pyelotubular backflow from upper calyx of left kidney (*arrow*).

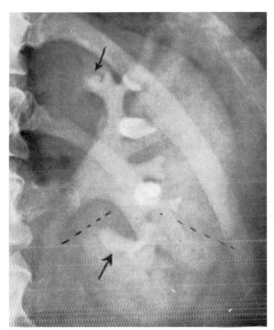

Figure 8–31. Renal tuberculosis. "Lipping-type" cavity of lower calyx which projects medially could be mistaken for "pyelosinous transflow." Also there is small pyelogenic cyst of upper calyx. (From Frimann-Dahl, 1955.)

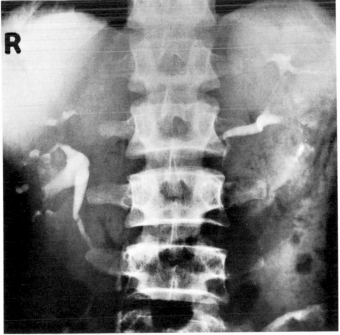

Figure 8–32. Bilateral renal tuberculosis; *excretory urogram* of man aged 22 years who presented with scrotal fistula from right tuberculous epididymitis.

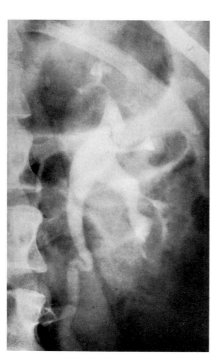

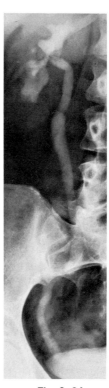

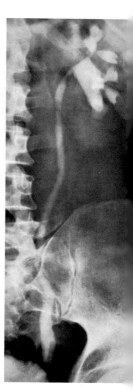

Fig. 8–33   Fig. 8–34   Fig. 8–35

Figure 8–33. Tuberculosis of upper pole of left kidney. Kink in upper ureter over psoas line is not pathologic. Six years previously, right nonfunctioning tuberculous kidney was removed. Left kidney was normal then.

Figure 8–34. *Excretory urogram.* Right renal tuberculosis, with butterfly type of calyceal pattern due to moderate strictures of calyceal infundibula and ureteropelvic junction. Note **ureteral strictures** opposite third lumbar vertebra and at ureterovesical junction.

Figure 8–35. *Excretory urogram.* Left renal tuberculosis. Butterfly type of calyceal pattern in upper pole; ureteral stricture of intramural portion. (Right kidney was normal.)

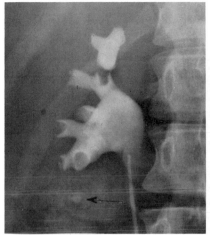

Fig. 8–36

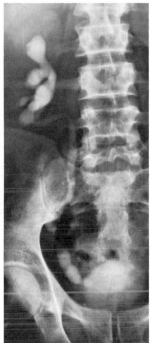

Fig. 8–37

Figure 8–36. *Right retrograde pyelogram.* **Right renal tuberculosis.** Minimal atypical irregularity of middle calyx. "Pinched-off" tip of lower calyx; some contrast medium seen in lower pole of kidney (*arrow*) with no apparent connection with lower calyces.

Figure 8–37. *Excretory urogram.* Solitary right kidney. **Mild dilatation of calyces,** which are smooth in outline and do not especially suggest tuberculous process. Pelvis normal. Ureter dilated throughout and lower third is markedly involved in tuberculous process, which has caused irregular areas of dilatation and constriction. **Early tuberculous stricture at ureterovesical juncture.**

Figure 8–38. *Excretory urogram.* Right renal tuberculosis; multiple confluent small cavities ulcerating in most of calyces.

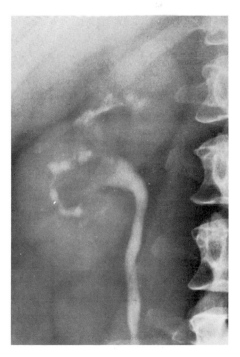

Fig. 8–39

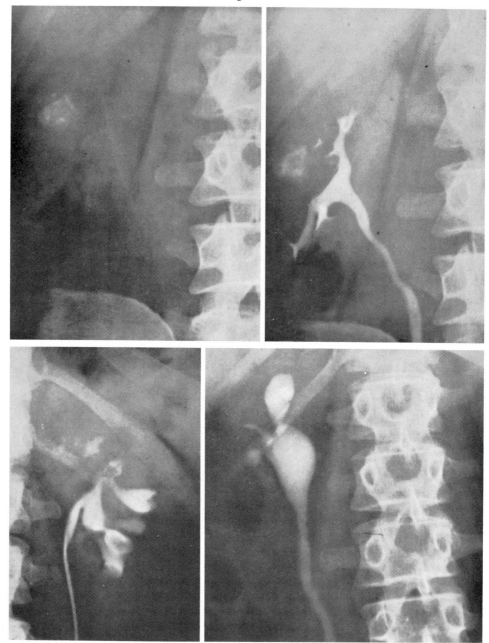

Fig. 8–40   Fig. 8–41

Figure 8–39.   **Right renal tuberculosis with calcification. A,** *Plain film.* Tuberculous calcification of right kidney. **B,** *Right retrograde pyelogram.* Tuberculous lesion involves middle portion of kidney, apparently completely destroying middle calyx. Pelvis and upper and lower calyces are almost normal urographically.

Figure 8–40.   *Left retrograde pyelogram.* **Advanced left renal tuberculosis.** Almost complete obliteration of upper calyces, with pyelocaliectasis of lower.

Figure 8–41.   *Right retrograde pyelogram.* **Right renal tuberculosis.** Partial obliteration of middle and lower calyces, with moderate dilatation of upper calyx and pelvis. Mild ureterectasis suggests involvement of ureter in tuberculous process.

Fig. 8–42

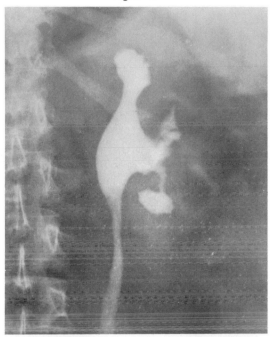

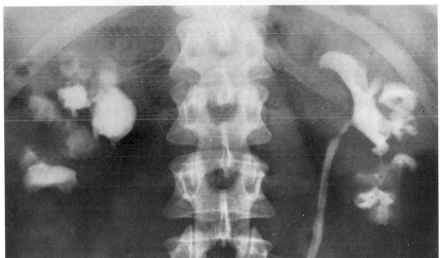

Fig. 8–43

Figure 8–42. *Left retrograde pyelogram.* **Advanced renal tuberculosis.** Destruction of middle calyces. 'Pinched-off" lower calyx, which is irregularly dilated, indicating cortical necrosis. Minimal dilatation of upper calyx, pelvis, and ureter.

Figure 8–43. *Bilateral retrograde pyelogram.* **Advanced bilateral renal tuberculosis** with extensive cortical necrosis.

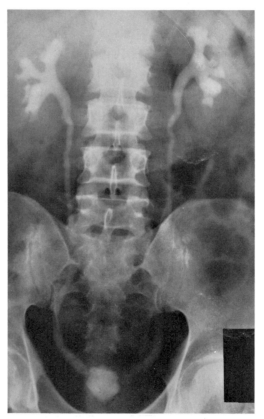

Figure 8–44.   *Excretory urogram.* Bilateral renal tuberculosis (acute). Moderate calycectasis and ureterectasis. Marked contracture of bladder from acute tuberculous cystitis.

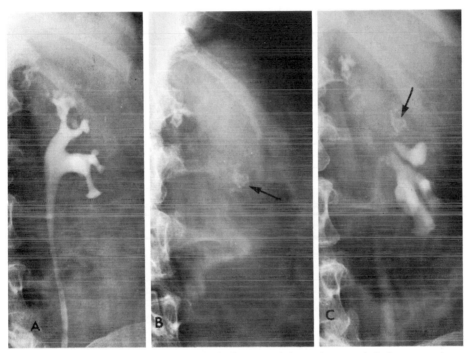

Figure 8–45.   Progression of renal tuberculosis before era of chemotherapy. **A,** *Left retrograde pyelogram.* Minimal dilatation and erosion of upper calyx of left kidney, associated with calcification. Remainder of pelvis, calyces, and ureter within normal limits. Pott's disease of thoracolumbar portion of spinal column. **B,** and **C,** Five years later. **B,** *Plain film.* Calcification persists and has increased in size and degree of density over upper pole of left kidney. Pott's disease of thoracolumbar portion of spinal column easily seen in film. **C,** *Excretory urogram.* Complete destruction of upper calyx of kidney, apparently without function. Moderate involvement of middle and lower calyces, which are now dilated grade 2.

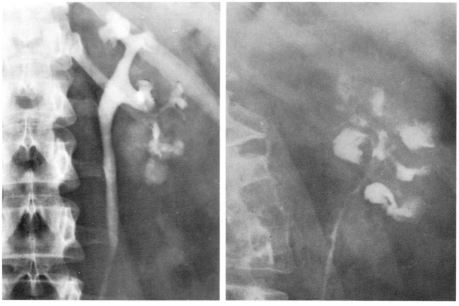

Fig. 8–46   Fig. 8–47

Figure 8–46. *Left retrograde pyelogram.* **Advanced tuberculosis involving chiefly lower pole of left kidney,** with marked irregularity of lower group of calyces, suggesting cortical necrosis.

Figure 8–47. *Left retrograde pyelogram.* **Advanced tuberculosis of left kidney,** with marked irregularity of all calyces, suggesting advanced cortical necrosis. Scoliosis of thoracolumbar portion of spinal column (old Pott's disease). Left nephrectomy for tuberculosis.

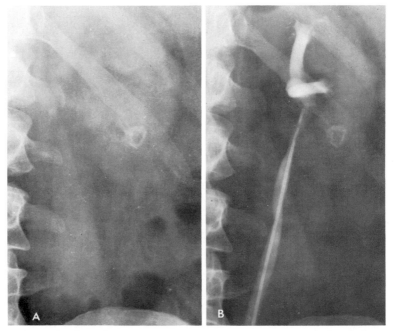

Figure 8–48. **Left renal tuberculosis with calcification.** **A,** *Plain film.* Calcific shadow over lower pole of left kidney. **B,** *Left retrograde pyelogram.* Marked cicatrization, erosion, and deformity of pelviocalyceal system. Lower calyx almost obliterated. Calcification in lower calyx. **Tuberculous ureteritis.**

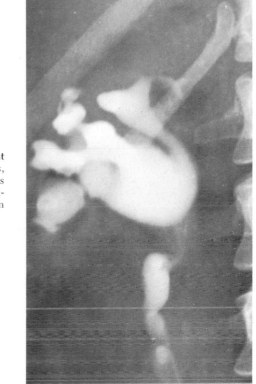

Figure 8–49. *Right retrograde pyelogram.* **Right renal tuberculosis.** Dilatation of pelvis and calyces, with minimal evidence of cortical necrosis in this film. Marked involvement of ureter, which is visualized in upper third as irregular areas of dilatation and constriction.

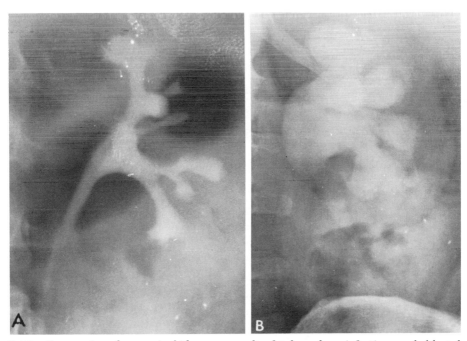

Figure 8–50. **Progressive changes in kidney as result of tuberculous infection,** probable **tuberculous** stricture of intramural portion **of ureter,** and obstruction from small, **contracted bladder. A,** *Left retrograde pyelogram* of "good" kidney (right kidney shown in previous films to be greatly destroyed with tuberculosis). Urine from left kidney showed pus grade 1 (20 cells per high-power field), acid-fast stains negative, but results of inoculation of guinea pigs were positive. Right nephrectomy performed. **B,** *Excretory urogram* 4 years later. Marked pyelocaliectasis of solitary left kidney. No doubt combination of tuberculous infection, obstruction of intramural portion of ureter, and obstruction from contracted, irritable bladder. Cystoscopy not done. Cutaneous ureterostomy advised but refused.

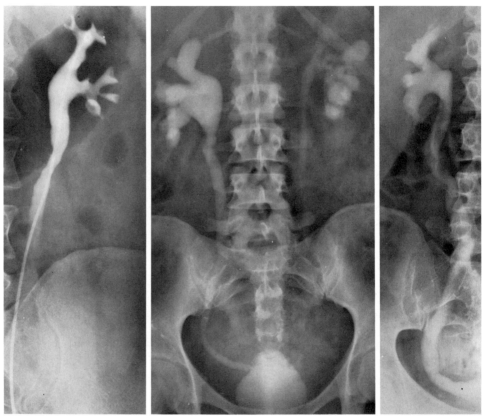

Fig. 8–51　　　　　　　　　　Fig. 8–52　　　　　　　　　　Fig. 8–53

Figure 8–51. **Left renal tuberculosis.** *Left retrograde pyelogram.* No definite urographic changes in upper and middle calyces—questionable lower calyx. Pelvis and upper part of ureter are moderately dilated and irregular from tuberculous process. At nephrectomy caseous tuberculosis was found.

Figure 8–52. *Excretory urogram.* **Bilateral renal tuberculosis, with extensive involvement of left kidney.** Dilatation of all calyces. Marked pyeloureterectasis on right. Some of this dilatation might be explained on obstructive basis from contracted, irritable bladder. However, positive results of inoculation of guinea pigs were reported from urine obtained from right kidney.

Figure 8–53. *Excretory urogram.* **Tuberculous solitary right kidney** (left nephrectomy previously for tuberculosis). Only mild pyelocaliectasis but marked ureterectasis, caused by both **tuberculous involvement of ureter** and obstruction from small, **contracted tuberculous bladder.**

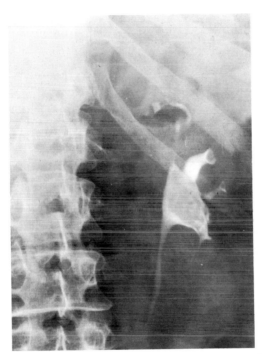

Figure 8–54. *Left retrograde pyelogram.* **Left renal tuberculosis.** Unusual filling defect of left renal pelvis, apparently caused by caseation. Could be confused with filling defect from nonopaque stone or epithelial tumor in renal pelvis. Irregular deformity of upper calyx suggests marked involvement of upper pole of kidney.

UROGRAPHIC CHANGES IN THE URETER

Tuberculous changes in the ureter are almost always secondary to renal tuberculosis, the kidney manifesting roentgenographic changes also. Primary tuberculosis of the ureter is rare. Infection and ulceration of the ureteral mucosa are caused by tuberculous bacteriuria.

Early urographic changes are ureteral dilatation and a slightly irregular outline that often extends from the renal pelvis to the bladder. The dilatation is caused by inflammatory changes with edema and infiltration in the narrow intramural portion, whereas the slight irregularities are due to multiple small ulcerations. As ureteral involvement increases, the wall of the ureter may become thickened so that the ureter loses its normal elasticity and peristalsis. Areas of fibrosis, cicatrization, and constriction may alternate with areas of dilatation. Stricture formation may occur in any portion of the ureter, but most often in the terminal portion. Strictures may be short, single, or multiple, or they may be long. Usually the ureter is dilated above and below the stricture, the distal dilatation being secondary to severe inflammatory involvement or to another stricture more distally. Sometimes areas of stricture and dilatation seem to alternate, giving the characteristic image of a string of pearls ("beaded" ureter) and finally resulting in a tortuous course due to confluent strictures and ulcerations. Such an extremely irregular outline of the ureter ("corkscrew" ureter) strongly suggests tuberculosis. In advanced cases another variety of ureteral involvement is represented by the thick-walled shortened ureter with a narrow lumen. This "pipestem" ureter runs a course almost as straight as a pencil toward the bladder. It has no peristalsis and is not dilated. In Figure 8–55 a schematic presentation is given of these ureteral changes. Particularly, multiple strictures and the "beaded," the "corkscrew," and the "pipestem" ureter are to be considered almost characteristic of tuberculous ureteritis (Figs. 8–56 through 8–63). A single short stricture caused by tuberculosis is not common, but does occur. It will be seen in all films of the same series of the pyelogram, in contrast to the "kink" (Fig. 8–55A) in a normal ureter, often seen where it passes over the psoas line just distal to the renal pelvis. The "kink" represents a peristaltic wave and is not continuously reproduced in all films of the pyelographic series. Incomplete filling, also due to normal peristalsis of the ureter, and spastic contraction sometimes simulate a stricture, but neither is reproducible in all films.

Stricture and fibrosis of the intramural ureter of the contralateral healthy kidney may be secondary to tuberculosis of the bladder. Thus the remaining nontuberculous kidney and ureter may be severely damaged from fibrotic obstruction. In such cases it may be extremely difficult to decide whether one is dealing with bilateral renal tuberculosis or with unilateral renal disease and bladder involvement. This type of obstruction may be so severe that a ureteral catheter cannot be passed to verify the diagnosis by examination of separate ureteral samples. A therapeutic dilemma is, then, whether ureteroneocystostomy or urinary diversion should be undertaken. The degree of bladder involvement is usually judged from the cystogram and from cystoscopic examination. Thus the best judgment in such cases depends on the degree of bladder involvement. Vesical contracture may be treated by cystoplasty and the healthy ureter may be reimplanted in the bowel segment used for enlargement of the bladder. Even a temporary cutaneous ileoureterostomy can later eventually be converted into a ureteroileocystoplasty (Moonen). Vesicoureteral reflux into a nontuberculous ureter and kidney may also be due to vesical tuberculosis with unilateral renal disease. Here, the contracted bladder with fibrosis of the vesical wall has caused a rigid, wide-open, golf-hole type of ureteral orifice. This is seen particularly in those cases in which vesical neck contracture exists in addition to the small-capacity contracted bladder, and may be a consequence of rapid healing under the influence of chemotherapy.

A complete work-up including micturition cystourethrography and cystoscopy, if possible, is indicated before sound judgment can be passed on the surgical management of bilateral (pyelo-) ureterectasis in cases of unilateral or bilateral renal tuberculosis. A careful follow-up is equally essential both in cases in which the results of chemotherapy are watched and in those in which reconstructive surgery has been combined with chemotherapy.

ADVANCED RENAL TUBERCULOSIS; RENOCOLIC FISTULA AND AUTONEPHRECTOMY; SILENT TUBERCULOUS KIDNEY

When the disease is advanced and destruction of the renal parenchyma is marked, the resulting urogram may show such great deformity that all semblance to the original anatomic form is lost. In such cases irregular areas of contrast medium may be seen in any part of the renal region. These represent sinuses and pockets dispersed throughout the masses of necrotic caseation. The pelvis and calyces may be damaged so much that they cannot be recognized. Erosion of the tuberculous process into the bowel (Bhisitkul and Burros) with resultant nephrocolic fistula is not uncommonly seen (see Chapter 15). Fistulae and sinuses draining through the flank or abdominal wall were not uncommon in the past.

One of the end results of such neglected, advanced disease is the condition known as "autonephrectomy." In this type of case, renal function is completely lost because of complete destruction of the renal parenchyma, and the drainage system of the kidney becomes completely obstructed or obliterated so that it no longer communicates with the bladder. The end result may be a quiescent, caseous, fibrotic kidney with or without calcification (Figs. 8–64 through 8–69; see also Figs. 8–6 and 8–15).

The silent tuberculous kidney may present a problem both in correct diagnosis and in treatment. Not all silent tuberculous kidneys are "autonephrectomized," and certainly not all are lost for future function (see Figs. 8–26 and 8–27). If the affected kidney is not visualized on the excretory urogram, retrograde pyelography is indicated. If the ureter can be catheterized, usually the diagnosis is made easily by roentgenographic and and bacteriologic studies. Such kidneys should not be removed promptly; instead, even if the destructive lesions seem extensive, conservative treatment should be tried for at least some months. The remaining portion of potentially functioning renal parenchyma may be estimated by additional diagnostic means such as nephrotomography, renal scanning, or renal arteriography.

If the ureter is completely obstructed and the bladder is normal, urine cultures may well be negative for tuberculosis even though a tuberculous autonephrectomized kidney is present. In such cases of unilateral autonephrectomy and a normal remaining contralateral kidney, calcification in the parenchyma or in the wall of the calyces may be the only lead to the correct diagnosis. In such kidneys the tuberculous process may be completely extinguished, and after nephrectomy it may be impossible to recognize microscopically or bacteriologically the tuberculous origin of the disease. In most of these autonephrectomized kidneys it is impossible to know whether its contents are still infectious. Prompt removal is therefore not advisable. Some clinicians feel that such kidneys have been present over many years, and that there is no reason to remove them. Others feel that they should be removed, because they may endanger the patient in the future. At any rate, if nephrectomy seems to represent the best judgment, at least some weeks or months of prophylactic chemotherapy should be instituted before operation is undertaken.

(Text continued on page 896.)

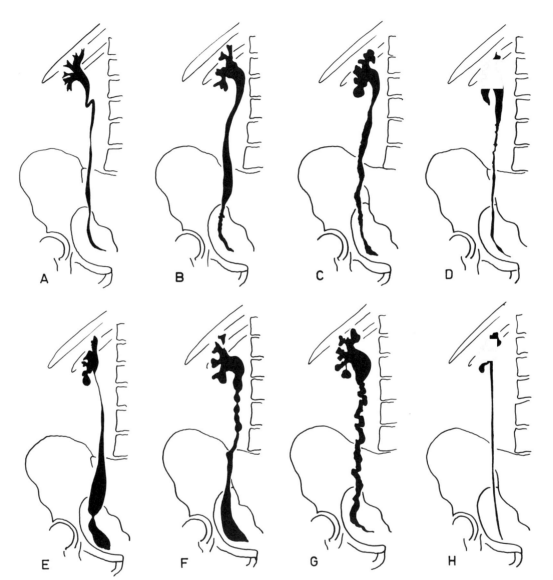

Figure 8–55.   Tuberculous urographic changes of ureter. *Schematic drawing.* **A,** Normal ureter; kink in ureter overlying psoas line and different caliber of ureteral outline are due to normal peristalsis; they are not exactly reproducible in all films of same series of urograms. **B,** Irregular outline of pelvic ureter due to tuberculous ulcerations. **C,** Moderately dilated ureter with multiple marginal irregularities representing tuberculous ulcerations. **D,** Long ureteral stricture. **E,** Multiple (two) ureteral strictures in pelvic ureter. **F,** "Beaded" ureter representing alternating strictures and dilatations (see text). **G,** "Corkscrew" ureter (see text). **H,** "Pipestem" ureter (see text).

Fig. 8–56   Fig. 8–57

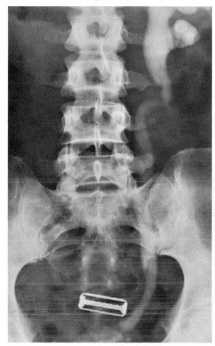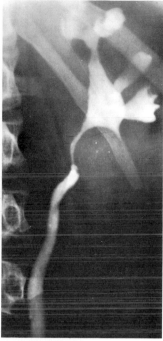

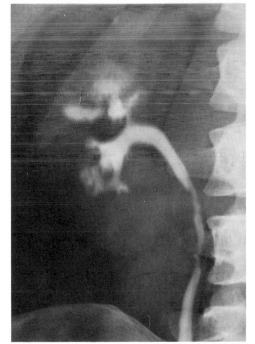

Fig. 8–58

Figure 8–56. *Excretory urogram.* **Solitary left tuberculous kidney.** (Right kidney removed previously for tuberculosis.) Pyeloureterectasis resulting from obstruction from **contracted tuberculous bladder. Tuberculous stricture of intramural portion of ureter** and tuberculous infection of kidney and ureter.

Figure 8–57. *Left retrograde pyelogram.* **Left renal tuberculosis.** Destruction and obliteration of lower calyx. **Stricture of ureter** adjacent to pelvis, with irregular dilatation below.

Figure 8–58. *Right retrograde pyelogram.* **Right renal tuberculosis.** Marked irregularity of calyces from cortical destruction and caseation. Tuberculous **stricture of upper third of ureter.**

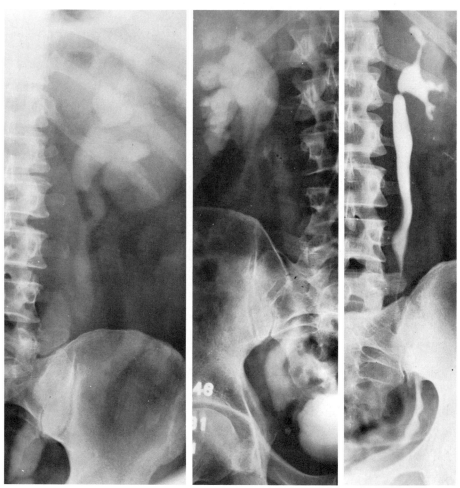

Fig. 8–59   Fig. 8–60   Fig. 8–61

Figure 8–59. *Excretory urogram.* **Solitary tuberculous left kidney.** (Previous right nephrectomy for tuberculosis.) Moderate pyeloureterectasis caused by tuberculous infection and obstruction of lower part of ureter from **contracted tuberculous bladder.**

Figure 8–60. *Excretory urogram.* **Right renal tuberculosis.** Pyelocaliectasis grade 2, with dilatation of entire ureter. Abrupt ending of terminal portion of ureter caused by marked granulomatous reaction in right half of bladder in region of right ureteral orifice, apparently also involving intramural portion of ureter.

Figure 8–61. *Left retrograde pyelogram.* **Left renal tuberculosis.** Apparent obliteration of lateral branch of upper calyx. Moderate **tuberculous involvement of ureter,** with beginning stricture at ureteropelvic juncture and at level of fifth transverse process and sacrum.

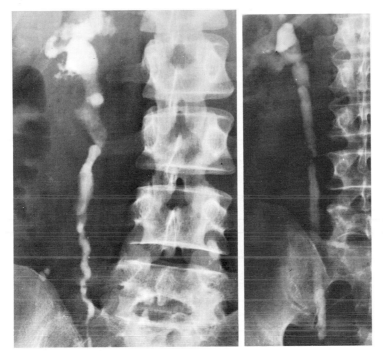

Fig. 8-62   Fig. 8-63

Figure 8-62. *Retrograde pyelogram.* **Advanced tuberculosis.** "Pipestem" **ureter.** Marked cortical destruction of kidney.

Figure 8-63. *Retrograde pyelogram.* Urinary tuberculosis. "Pipestem" **ureter** and marked destruction of kidney. Wall of ureter is thickened, fixed, and contains alternate areas of dilatation and narrowing.

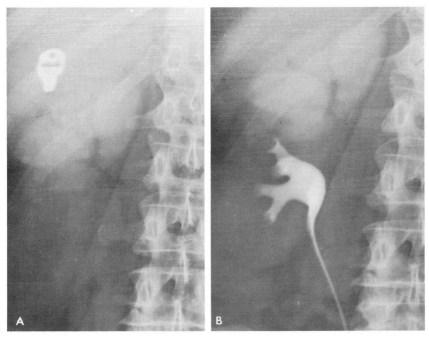

Figure 8-64. Duplicated kidney with **autonephrectomy** of upper segment from old **tuberculosis.** Caseation f upper segment casts dense shadow. **A,** *Plain film.* **B,** *Retrograde pyelogram.* (Courtesy of Dr. R. B. Carson.)

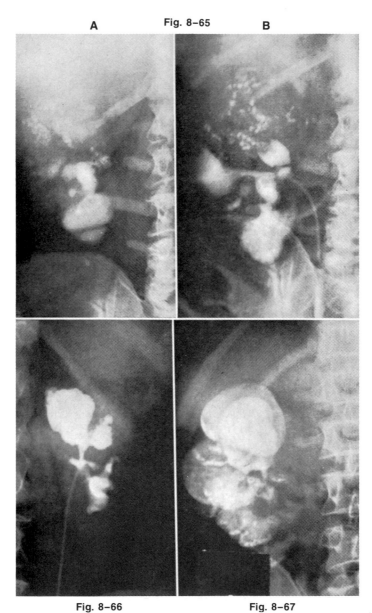

Fig. 8–65

Figure 8–65. A, *Plain film.* Extensive tuberculous calcification of right kidney, which is greatly enlarge and deformed. B, *Right retrograde pyelogram.* Only middle and lower groups of calyces outlined, whic show marked dilatation and erosion from cortical necrosis.

Figure 8–66. *Left retrograde pyelogram.* Advanced left renal tuberculosis. Extensive cortical necrosi leaving large pockets of contrast medium throughout renal substance.

Figure 8–67. *Plain film.* Extensive tuberculous calcification of nonfunctioning right kidney (auton phrectomy).

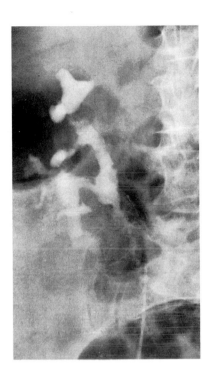

Figure 8–68. *Retrograde pyelogram.* **Far-advanced right renal tuberculosis;** nonfunctioning right kidney. Marked cortical necrosis. Note bizarre outline of collecting system and irregularity of renal pelvis and ureter.

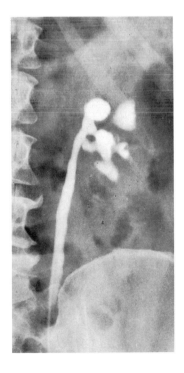

Figure 8–69. Left renal tuberculosis; *retrograde pyelogram* of **nonfunctioning kidney** presenting with gross hematuria and left flank pain. On retrograde pyelogram, upper pole does not visualize, suggesting possibility of expanding lesion. Collections of medium are partially in calyces, partially perhaps in non-calyceal cavities. Nephrectomy done. Removed specimen contained **large caseous abscess in upper pole of kidney.** Ureter markedly infiltrated and thickened.

RENAL TUBERCULOSIS SIMULATING OTHER LESIONS; COINCIDENTAL HYPERNEPHROMA AND CYST

Unusual deformities in renal tuberculosis may simulate other conditions and cause confusion. At times one encounters lesions of the renal parenchyma which simulate expanding lesions such as solitary abscess, renal carbuncle, hamartoma, or hypernephroma (Figs. 8–70, 8–71, and 8–72). (Renal brucellosis simulating tuberculosis has been discussed in Chapter 7, page 825, Figs. 7–104, 7–105, and 7–106.)

Coincidental disease in the tuberculous kidney occurs only rarely. Coincidental lesions are most often hypernephroma and cyst (Figs. 8–73 and 8–74). At least 36 cases have been reported (Steyn and Logie), including 19 cases reviewed in 1948 by Neibling and Walters, who added 7 cases from the Mayo Clinic. If hypernephroma is suspected of being present in a tuberculous kidney, renal angiography is warranted to verify the diagnosis and facilitate the decision regarding nephrectomy.

TUBERCULOSIS OF THE BLADDER

The unusual finding of calcification of the wall of the bladder was illustrated in Figures 8–20 and 8–21. The most common urographic finding is a contracted, spastic bladder of small capacity. At times, however, one encounters cystograms of unusual contour which usually represent a tuberculous lesion that has been confined to one portion of the bladder (usually the side of the involved kidney and ureter) and has caused localized deformity from spasticity, cicatrization, and fibrosis. Filling defects simulating tumor, soft stone, or diverticulum may be caused by marked cicatrization with deformity of one portion of the bladder or by a hyperplastic, granular-appearing inflammatory lesion that has the gross appearance of tumor. In some cases advanced inflammation of a ureteral orifice produces a rosette of inflammatory reaction and edema sufficient to cause a negative filling defect in the cystogram (Figs. 8–75, 8–76, and 8–77; see also Fig. 8–44). Vesical involvement may cause stricture or incompetence of a ureteral orifice, even if the upper tract on that side has no tuberculous changes. Particularly fibrosis and contracture of the bladder occurring during the healing process may lead to "death of the remaining kidney."

TUBERCULOUS PERINEPHRIC ABSCESS AND PSOAS ABSCESS

Tuberculous perinephric abscess associated with advanced renal tuberculosis, although rare, must be kept in mind. Tuberculous psoas (cold) abscess arising from tuberculosis of the lower thoracic and lumbar portions of the vertebral column may also become so large as to displace the kidneys and ureter. A careful examination of the films for evidence of Pott's disease will occasionally clarify the diagnosis in difficult and unusual cases (Figs. 8–78, 8–79, and 8–80; see also Figs. 8–1, 8–11, and 8–12 and Figs. 3–162 through 3–166). Scheinin and Kontturi found in their material on 232 patients with various manifestations of bone and joint tuberculosis that 23 patients (9.9% had renal tuberculosis, in 3 of whom both kidneys were affected. On the other hand not all urographic renal changes in patients with skeletal tuberculosis are due to tuberculous infection of the kidney. Here again, urine cultures and guinea pig inoculation tests are prerequisite to correc diagnosis.

ROENTGENOGRAPHIC CLASSIFICATION OF RENAL TUBERCULOSIS

Several investigators have tried t classify tuberculous lesions of the kidne

Table 8–1 **Classification of Renal Tuberculosis***

GROUP	DESCRIPTION
1	Unilateral renal tuberculosis: minor lesions without cystitis
2	Unilateral renal tuberculosis: major lesion necessitating nephrectomy; cystitis
3	Bilateral renal tuberculosis: nephrectomy for more-advanced lesion
4	Tuberculosis occurring in remaining kidney subsequent to nephrectomy for unilateral disease
5	(a) Major bilateral tuberculous lesions
	(b) Minor bilateral tuberculous lesions

*After Jacobs, A., and Borthwick, W. M. (1950).

on the basis of roentgenographic changes. In previous years, when nephrectomy or partial resection of the kidney still formed an important part of the therapeutic program, such classifications were useful to compare results of treatment for different grades of involvement. Not all urologists have abandoned surgical therapy, however, and apart from surgical indications it is still of interest to compare results of medical treatment. For this reason some of the most widely used systems of classifications are here included. It should be remembered that all methods to classify the seriousness of renal tuberculous lesions in grades of involvement are necessarily based on roentgenographically visible changes. As stated above, not all lesions can be demonstrated by urographic means equally well, and some not at all. In 1950 Jacobs and Borthwick presented a classification (Table 8–1), which was accepted in 1953 by the British Medical Research Council and which had primarily to do with indications for surgical intervention.

As can be seen from Table 8–1, a division is made only between cases suitable for nephrectomy and cases suitable for conservative medical treatment. Partial nephrectomy or cavernotomy is not represented in the classification. Since 1950 the therapeutic attitude toward renal tuberculosis has grown so much more conservative that a classification into nephrectomy and non-nephrectomy cases has become outdated.

Lattimer introduced in 1953 his classification in grades 0 through 4 based only on roentgenographic changes and not primarily with the intention of separating surgical from nonsurgical cases (Table 8–2).

In grades 1 and 2, only one cavity may be present; grades 2, 3, and 4 may be termed "advanced lesions," of which

Table 8–2 **Classification of Renal Tuberculosis***

GRADE	DESCRIPTION	SIZE OF LESIONS
0	No roentgen abnormality visible but ureteral urine positive for tubercle bacilli	Small
1	Definite slight roentgen abnormality, but not diagnostic for tuberculosis; includes doubtful calyceal distortions and slight but definite irregularities of pelvis and upper ureter; ureteral urine positive for tubercle bacilli	Medium
2	One calyx only, with definite roentgen changes characteristic of tuberculosis; culture of ureteral or voided urine positive	Medium
3	Two calyces showing distortions of tuberculosis; culture of ureteral or voided urine positive	Large
4	Three or more calyces obviously tuberculous by x-ray; culture of ureteral or voided urine positive; massive putty-type lesions in this category	Large

After Lattimer, J. K. (1953).

grade 4 lesions are "far-advanced" ones (massive lesions involving three or more calyces, including "putty kidney" with positive urine cultures). In 1964 Siegel and Lattimer stated that, according to this classification, the incidence of grade 4 (far-advanced) lesions had dropped from 70% in 1957 to 0% in 1962, whereas the overall incidence of advanced lesions (grades 2, 3, and 4 together), amounting to 80%, had not changed in 17 years. From 1957 on, no nephrectomies had been done for renal tuberculosis.

Still another classification, again directed more toward surgical intervention, particularly partial nephrectomy, was given by Semb (1955) (Fig. 8–81). In his classification six groups are recognized; one black point means destruction of one calyx (one segment), three black points mean destruction of the upper division, and two black points mean destruction of the intermediate or the lower division. Semb's classification according to the extent of destructive changes and the relation to the pyramids, the calyces, and the three divisions of the kidney was adopted by the "European Symposium on Urogenital Tuberculosis" in 1953. Group 1 represents no destructive changes and includes the "parenchymatous" type of renal tuberculosis. Group 2 comprises the least destruction with one single focus within one pyramid (one segment) in connection with one calyx or one pair of calyces. Group 3 covers destruction of one division of the kidney. This may vary from destruction of two pyramids (segments) or calyces to destruction of up to a total of all pyramids (segments) within this division. This distribution represents approximately one third of the kidney substance. Group 4 represents destruction of one division and one pyramid (one segment) of another division— roughly speaking, one and one-half divisions or approximately half the total kidney volume. Group 5 comprises destruction of two divisions, that is, two groups of pyramids or calyces, involving approximately two-thirds the kidney substance. Group 6 represents destruction in all three divisions, or the "total destructive" type.

On the basis of this classification Semb propagated selective partial nephrectomy for renal tuberculosis. This procedure is only rarely performed any more, since prolonged chemotherapy has proved to be preferable.

(Text continued on page 904.)

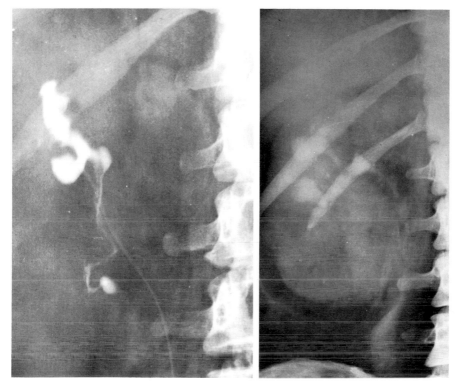

Fig. 8-70   Fig. 8-71

Figure 8-70. *Right retrograde pyelogram.* Advanced renal tuberculosis with marked destruction, producing bizarre deformity which simulates hypernephroma.

Figure 8-71. *Excretory urogram.* Advanced tuberculosis of right kidney, which forms extensive lesion of lower pole that displaces right ureter medially. Could be mistaken for either cortical abscess or hypernephroma. Left kidney normal.

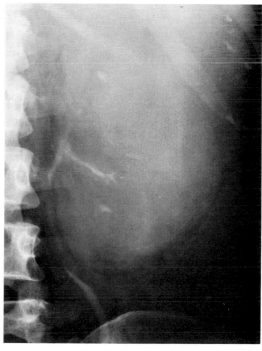

Figure 8-72. *Excretory urogram.* Left renal tuberculosis simulating tumor. At operation extensive caseous tuberculosis with cavitation. Right kidney normal.

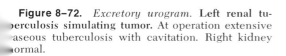

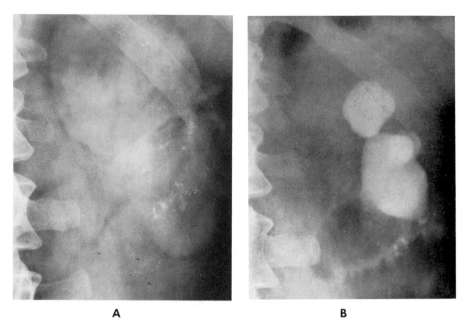

A   B

Figure 8–73. Adenocarcinoma associated with tuberculosis with calcification. **A,** *Plain film.* Enlargement of upper pole of left kidney. Irregular areas of calcification over lower pole. **B,** *Excretory urogram.* Obliteration of lower calyces from tuberculosis with calcification. Irregular dilatation of upper calyces found to be due to adenocarcinoma (hypernephroma) of upper pole. (Courtesy of Dr. T. D. Moore.)

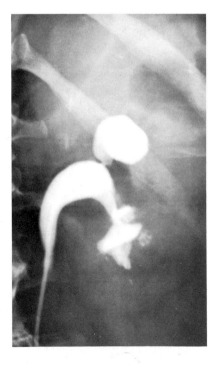

Figure 8–74. Renal cyst and tuberculosis. *Left retrograde pyelogram.* Destructive lesion from renal tuberculosis involving lower pole of kidney. Deformity of upper calyx found on surgical exploration to be caused by simple cyst. (Courtesy of Dr. E. W. Campbell.)

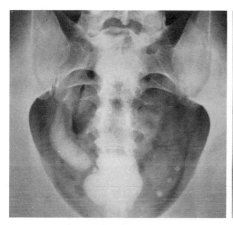
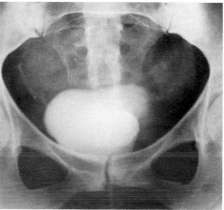

Fig. 8–75   Fig. 8–76

Figure 8–75. *Excretory cystogram.* Marked deformity of vesical outline from tuberculous cystitis. Calcareous lesion in region of right ureteral orifice which causes filling defect of bladder and apparent abrupt termination of right ureter, which is dilated grade 3.

Figure 8–76. *Excretory urogram.* Left renal tuberculosis with tuberculous involvement of left half of bladder, causing marked deformity.

Figure 8–77. *Excretory urogram.* Left renal tuberculosis and marked tuberculous changes of bladder. Normal right kidney. Opacifications over lumbar spine from contrast studies of vertebral canal. Patient presented with low back pain and recurrent cystitis.

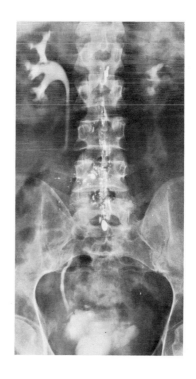

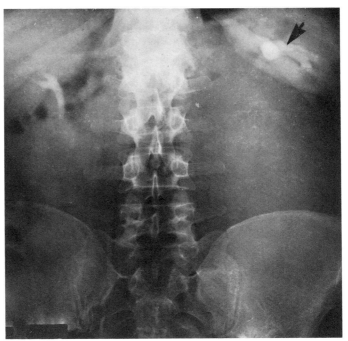

Figure 8–78. *Excretory urogram.* **Pott's disease with bilateral tuberculous psoas abscesses.** Tuberculos of lower dorsal and upper lumbar spine. Outline of psoas muscles obliterated. Abscesses displace both kic neys laterally and upward.

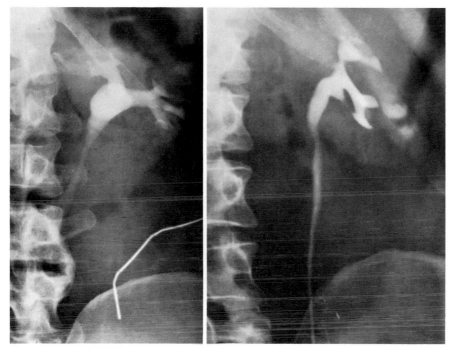

Fig. 8–79   Fig. 8–80

Figure 8–79. *Excretory urogram.* **Tuberculous psoas abscess** displacing left kidney.
Figure 8–80. *Left retrograde pyelogram.* **Tuberculous perinephric abscess from advanced tuberculosis of kidney,** with much destruction of calyces and renal parenchyma. Lower pole of kidney displaced laterally and upward from abscess.

CLASSIFICATION OF PATHOLOGY IN RENAL TUBERCULOSIS

GROUP	DESTROYED TISSUE	UPPER PART	LOWER PART	INTERMED. PT.	UPP.+ LOW. PT.	CLASSIFICATION ~
1	NO DESTR.	(img)				PARENCHYMATOUS TUBERCULOSIS 12%
2	ONE SEGM.	(img)	(img)	(img)		LOCAL DESTRUCTIVE TUBERCULOSIS 54%
3	ONE DIV.	(img)	(img)	(img)		
4	ONE DIV.+ ONE SEGM.	(img)	(img)		(img)	
5	TWO DIV.	(img)	(img)		(img)	
6	THREE DIV.	(img)				TOTAL DESTRUCTIVE TUBERCULOSIS 34%

Figure 8–81. Classification of renal tuberculosis according to Semb. (From Semb, C., 1955.)

Additional Diagnostic Methods

RETROGRADE PYELOGRAPHY

In many cases of renal tuberculosis the excretory urogram, even after careful preparation of the patient, is not of sufficient quality to permit accurate interpretation. This may be due to insufficient function of the diseased kidney or to incomplete filling of the collecting system or of pathologic cavities. Sometimes a part of the collecting system is missing (see Fig. 8–15). Retrograde pyelography is often carried out in such cases to delineate more sharply the areas involved; only in a relatively small percentage of cases, however, does retrograde pyelography result in films of better diagnostic quality than excretory urography. Sometimes a cavity or dilated calyx faintly shown on the excretory urogram cannot be visualized at all on retrograde pyelography. This negative result may of course be used as an argument for the diagnosis of a tuberculous cavity or diseased calyx, but still is a negative result. Frimann-Dahl (1955), commenting on the value of retrograde pyelography, stated that of 91 patients with renal tuberculosis in whom retrograde pyelography was performed it was superior to excretory urography in only 11 patients. In only four patients was a decisive accurate diagnosis based on retrograde studies. In 69 patients results were equal to those of excretory urography and in 11 patients poor results were obtained. Significant pyelolymphatic, pyelosinous, or pyelovenous backflow occurred in six patients, and in two patients unsatisfactory results were obtained. He stated that the main value of retrograde studies is to confirm the diagnosis based on excretory urograms, and that these may be valuable in many cases when it is important to demonstrate the degree and localization of destruction. An advantage is that one can obtain oblique projections without being dependent on compression. If retrograde pyelography is performed in patients with proven or suspected renal tuberculosis, prophylatic antibiotic therapy should be given, and if bilateral studies are necessary, one side should be examined at a time, the second side being examined after an interval of 4 to 6 days. Particularly the risk of renal reflux caused by back pressure with spread of bacteria into the renal tissues, the lymphatic system, or the bloodstream should be considered. Such studies should be made preferably under fluoroscopic control with accurate positioning of the catheter tip and with low pressure-piston injection of a carefully measured amount of contrast material, in order to avoid backflow. Backflow may occasionally even lead to incorrect interpretation or diagnosis with regard to the amount of destroyed renal tissue.

Retrograde pyelography is seldom necessary in patients with a solitary kidney suspected of having a tuberculous infection. Usually the remaining kidney shows up well on excretory urography.

INFUSION PYELOGRAPHY; NEPHROTOMOGRAPHY*

Retrograde pyelography can in many cases be dispensed with by using higher doses of contrast medium, eventually combined with tomography (Schencker Marcure, and Moody). In 1966 Ludvik Pecherstorfer, and Opl commented on the diagnostic results obtained with infusion pyelography in 43 patients with renal tuberculosis, using 80 ml of undiluted 76% meglumine diatrizoate (Urographin administered by intravenous drip in 5 to 10 minutes as an out-clinic procedure In 41 patients the results were so good that previously planned retrograde pyelography could be circumvented. Optimal pictures were obtained in moderately

---

*See discussion of technique, Chapter 1, pages 5 and 55.

diseased kidneys after an average of 40 minutes, and in poorly functioning kidneys after up to 6 hours. The nephrographic effects were better than with routine excretory urography; the intensity of the contrast material in the collecting system is comparable to that obtained with retrograde pyelography, and one has ample time to make tomograms or shift and oblique exposures. Nephrotomography is of no diagnostic value in early tuberculous lesions confined to calyceal irregularity. It does demonstrate areas of absent or poor vascularization in advanced cases that may be interpreted as hydronephrosis or as collections of caseous material in relation to areas of normal or near-normal vascularization. Becker, Weiss, and Lattimer, using 150 ml of 90% sodium diatrizoate (Hypaque) with 150 ml of 5% dextrose in water by intravenous drip, found that nephrotomography performed in 27 patients was of value only in demonstrating hydronephrosis or areas of retained caseous material in advanced renal tuberculosis. In such cases the nephrotomograms documented the nature of the remaining renal substance even better than did the arteriogram.

ARTERIOGRAPHY*

Renal angiography has only limited value in the diagnosis of tuberculosis. No significant changes on the arteriogram are seen in early tuberculosis with small calyceal deformities. Although it has been suggested that changes in the small ramifications of the arterial pattern (De Nunno) and obliteration of small vessels (Frimann-Dahl, 1966; Olsson, 1967) are sometimes seen as early changes, most authorities in this field agree that such changes are insignificant, and that early renal tuberculosis can be better diagnosed by excretory urography than by renal angiography. In advanced cases, renal arteriography may help particularly to study vascularization of renal segments that do not show up on excretory urography or retrograde pyelography. Angiography will then permit one to recognize avascular areas where, in the arterial phase, the renal vessels stretch around dilated calyces or granulomatous abscesses. In the nephrographic phase the areas are seen as filling defects, and the amount of well-vascularized or reasonably well-vascularized renal parenchyma may be judged. The angiographic phase usually is confirmative, but only rarely gives important additional information. It should be remembered that the urogram delineates primarily the collecting system, whereas the angiogram reflects essentially the renal parenchyma. In this respect, renal angiography has been advocated in advanced cases of tuberculosis to permit a forecast of possible healing with medication; only if the vascularization of diseased segments of the kidney is intact or fair are chemotherapeutic agents able to reach the diseased parenchyma. Fritjofsson and co-workers found that the urogram often shows more pathologic change than the angiogram does, and in their experience the angiogram never showed more extensive pathologic changes than did the urogram. Fritjofsson and Edsman noted that the angiogram occasionally helps in accurate localization of advanced lesions and its extensions with respect to conservative surgical treatment (partial nephrectomy). Becker, Weiss, and Lattimer stated that in their experience renal arteriography only confirmed the findings of nephrotomography in advanced cases, but did not yield any additional information; neither method influenced the therapy of any of their patients with renal tuberculosis. At the present writing it seems correct to say, in summary, that renal arteriography is not advised as a routine method of examination in suspected renal tuberculosis, that it is of no help in detecting early

---

See discussion of technique, Chapter 2.

lesions, that it only confirms the findings of nephrotomograms in advanced cases, and that it occasionally may be indicated in the patient with silent kidney of obscure etiology or with suspected renal hypertension associated with tuberculosis.

ISOTOPE RENOGRAPHY; ISOTOPE RENAL SCAN*

In the diagnosis of renal diseases the use of radioactive substances has gained a definite place in recent years. For renal tuberculosis the isotope renogram and renal scan are of only limited diagnostic value. Kirsch and Hennig discussed its applications in tuberculosis of the urinary tract. They stressed that this type of examination may be used for screening in follow-up studies during the course of chemotherapy. Its advantages are that it represents a split-function test of the renal parenchyma and carries little risk of overexposure to the patient who otherwise would be subjected to repeated x-ray studies. If progressive deterioration of renal function or ureteral obstruction is found with renography or renal scan, it should be followed by more accurate diagnostic tests such as excretory urography or retrograde studies. In this respect it could find a place in sanatoria for renal tuberculosis, where routinely a large volume of urographic follow-up studies might be replaced by isotope examinations. Occasionally it may be used in silent kidney in order to determine the loss of functioning parenchymal tissue versus ureteral obstruction due to stricture or coincidental calculous disease. For the diagnosis of tuberculosis, ipso facto, it has no value. In the future it could probably be used also to determine and follow up the extent of vesicoureteral reflux generally and the extent in cases of vesical tuberculosis

---

*See discussion of technique, Chapter 20.

particularly, although at present these studies cannot compete in accuracy with more conventional methods such as cystography, micturition cystourethrography, and cystoscopy.

The Urogram in Genital Tuberculosis
(Figs. 8–82 through 8–87)

It is still a matter of discussion whether genital tuberculosis can occur without infection of the kidneys. There is no question that in most cases of genital tuberculosis, bacteriuria secondary to renal tuberculosis is evident. As discussed previously, the generally accepted route of infection in the male is the posterior urethra, being bathed in urine containing mycobacteria that enter the prostatic and ejaculatory ducts and from there infect the prostate, seminal tract, and epididymis. It is probable that in some cases the genital tract in the male is infected by hematogenous dissemination from a primary focus in lungs or bones, whereas in the female this route represents the usual method of infection. Occasionally the genital organs may be infected by the lymphogenic route. It is of interest to note, then, that tuberculous epididymitis, vesiculitis, or prostatitis can occur without renal tuberculosis or bacteriuria. Palmlöv described a patient who died of miliary tuberculosis and tuberculous meningitis secondary to tuberculous prostatovesiculitis. There were no bacteriuria or urographic changes. At autopsy the kidneys contained only small miliary foci. On the other hand genital tuberculosis may be present but difficult to detect in renal tuberculosis. It is important therefore in all cases of urinary tuberculosis to search for lesions in the genital tract both in male and female patients.

Generally speaking, the diagnosis of genital tuberculosis is more a clinical than a roentgenographic problem; occasionally roentgenographic changes are helpful in diagnosis.

IN THE MALE

The organs affected by tuberculosis in the male are the prostate gland, the seminal vesicles, and the epididymis. A primary focus in the testis is rare, but the testis may be affected by direct spread from the epididymis.

A scrotal fistula from tuberculous epididymitis is not an unusual first sign of urogenital tuberculosis. It is often located posteriorly or on the lateral border of the scrotum, in contrast to a syphilitic fistula of the testis that presents anteriorly but has become extremely rare.

Calcifications of the spermatic tract and prostate are visible on a plain film but occur relatively rarely in tuberculosis and are by no means characteristic. Prostatic calculi are often seen and are usually due to nonspecific chronic low-grade inflammation. They even may occur coincidentally in the presence of renal tuberculosis without tuberculous prostatitis (Figs. 8–82 and 8–83; see also Figs. 8–22, 8–23, and 8–25). Calcification of the vasa and ampullae is associated more often with diabetes than with tuberculosis (see Figs. 8–22, 8–24, and 8–25 and also Figs. 3–105 through 3–111 and Table 3–1).

Tuberculous seminal vesiculitis is rare as an isolated disease; it almost always is associated with tuberculous prostatitis. In suspected cases seminal vesiculography may be carried out by injection of contrast medium in the ductus deferens through a small scrotal incision (see Figs. 1–62, 1–63, and 1–64). A tuberculous abscess of a seminal vesicle that became sufficiently large to encroach on and distort the urinary bladder is shown in Figure 8–84.

Tuberculous prostatitis is an important disease and occurs more often than one would think from studying the literature. It is more resistant to treatment than renal tuberculosis, may cause considerable destruction, and is sometimes difficult to detect owing to lack of characteristic symptoms. Retrograde urethrography and micturition cystourethrography are important methods for accurate diagnosis (Figs. 8–85 and 8–86). May and co-workers reported on roentgenographic diagnosis and course of the disease in 91 cases. They found definite evidence of prostatic involvement in 22 patients in whom no suspicion was aroused by rectal digital palpation. In 38 patients urethrography confirmed the rectal findings, and in 31 patients with positive rectal palpatory changes in the prostate gland no communication of prostatic cavities with the urethra could be demonstrated by urethrography. They stressed that in the presence of urethrographically demonstrable prostatourethral fistulae, healing may be hastened by performing transurethral prostatic resection in combination with chemotherapy (Fig. 8–87). They advocated routine urethrography in patients with suspected or proven renal tuberculosis. On digital rectal examination prostatic tuberculosis may be difficult to differentiate from prostatic carcinoma when the prostate gland is hard and nodular and urinary specimens are negative for tubercle bacteria. In such cases, transrectal or perineal biopsy may be done under protection of a prophylactic chemotherapeutic regimen. The biopsy specimen should be examined both microscopically and by culture. Granulomatous prostatitis of nonspecific origin may also mimic carcinoma of the prostate gland on rectal palpation (see discussion, Chapter 7, pages 832 and 833), whereas it is microscopically difficult sometimes to distinguish from tuberculous prostatitis because of the presence of granulomatous lesions with giant cell formation.

IN THE FEMALE

Genital tuberculosis in the female should be searched for if urinary tuberculosis is present. Only rarely does roentgenographic examination yield results in these instances. Genital tuberculosis may produce pelvic inflammatory masses large enough to displace and distort the lower third of the ureters and the bladder (Sutherland). Fistulous communications involving the lower parts of the ureters, bladder, and intestine have been reported (see Fistulas and Sinuses, Chapter 15). Menstrual blood samples should be cultured for tuberculosis if possible in all cases of urinary tuberculosis in the female. Overbeck and Keller reported that use of this method disclosed that 9.7% of 187 female patients with renal tuberculosis had positive cultures for otherwise unsuspected genital tuberculosis.

(Text continued on page 911.)

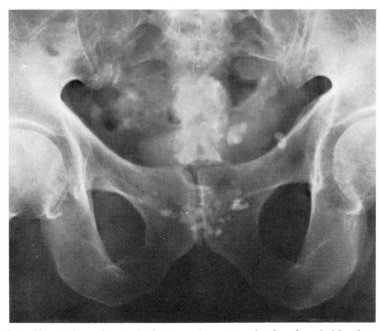

Figure 8–82. *Plain film.* **Tuberculous calcification of prostate gland** and probably also of right ampulla.

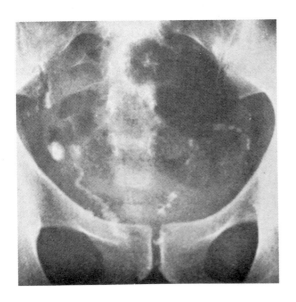

Figure 8–83. *Plain film.* **Tuberculous calcification of vasa and seminal vesicle.** (Courtesy of Dr T. Leon Howard.)

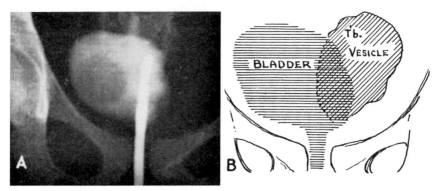

Figure 8–84. **Tuberculosis of seminal vesicle.** A, *Cystogram* showing vesical displacement to right and flattening of left bladder wall by enlarged tuberculous left seminal vesicle. B, Schema of condition present. (Courtesy of Bellevue Hospital; from Campbell's Urology, vol. 2, p. 1576.)

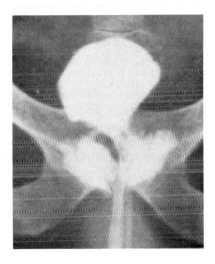

Figure 8–85. *Cystourethrogram.* Tuberculous abscesses of prostate which have sloughed and evacuated leaving large irregular cavities. (Courtesy of Dr. J. K. Lattimer.)

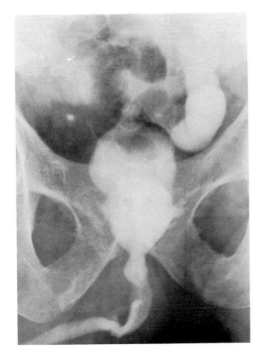

Figure 8–86. *Retrograde cystourethrogram.* Almost complete **sloughing of prostate from extensive tuberculous abscesses.** Vesicoureteral obstruction with reflux which increased in severity during chemotherapy.

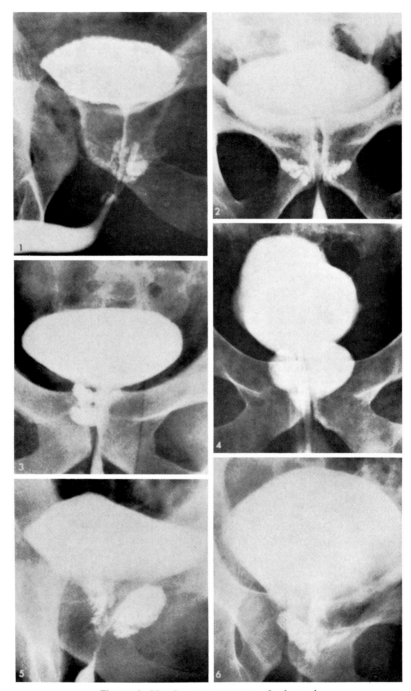

Figure 8–87 *See opposite page for legend.*

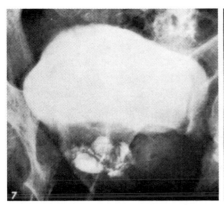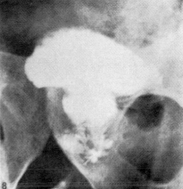

Fig. 8–87. *(Continued)*

Figure 8–87. Tuberculous prostatitis. *Retrograde urethrograms.* 1, Bilateral periurethral cavities and beginning tuberculous contracture of bladder. 2, Symmetrical extravasation of contrast medium in prostatic urethra. 3, Large prostatic cavity on right; small cavities on left. 4, Complete destruction of prostatic parenchyma. Formation of so-called anterior bladder. 5, Extensive cavernous prostatitis bilaterally. 6, Same patient as in 5 after transurethral prostatic resection. 7, Extensive cavernous prostatitis bilaterally. 8, Same patient as in 7 after 2 years. Complete liquefaction of prostatic parenchyma, marked "anterior bladder." (From May, P., Hohenfellner, R., König, E., and König, K.)

MODERN CHEMOTHERAPY OF GENITOURINARY TUBERCULOSIS
(Figs. 8–88 through 8–108)

One of the greatest triumphs of modern medicine since World War II has been the chemotherapeutic treatment of tuberculosis. The effectiveness of prolonged multiple drug therapy has been reflected in the fact that most of the tuberculosis sanatoria in North America and Western Europe have been closed. Ample evidence of the magnificent results of chemotherapy can be found in the extensive literature on this subject. Contrary to prewar opinion, tuberculosis of the urinary tract is no longer considered primarily a surgical disease. Surgical intervention for renal tuberculosis, whether it be nephrectomy, partial nephrectomy, or cavernotomy, is therefore now only rarely undertaken (Fig. 8–88), and then only in carefully selected patients who show little progress in spite of prolonged therapy, onset of renal hypertension, or coincidental renal disease which requires surgical treatment (Kaufman and Goodwin; Lattimer and co-workers). Even so, some authorities still prefer to reserve resection as a possible alternative or as part of a combined medical and surgical therapeutic regimen (Beck and Marshall; Gow, 1966; Malament, Auerbach, and Harris; Puigvert and Gittes; Strauss).

When chemotherapy was first instituted, it was thought that only the relatively small lesions could be expected to heal, larger lesions requiring surgical extirpation. As time passed, however, it was astounding to see that even large lesions were being controlled in a high percentage of cases. At present, almost all lesions are first subjected to chemotherapy. Hanley stated in 1960 that regardless of how much of a kidney has been destroyed, "it is unwise to express an opinion regarding ultimate prognosis on an initial pyelogram"; he advised waiting until the end of 2 months of intensive treatment. Lattimer alone (1955b) and with his associates (1954; 1956; 1965) now advises a minimum of 2 years of triple-drug treatment in renal tuberculosis. Nonfunctioning tuberculous kidneys as evidenced on the excretory urogram may resume function within a few months of intensive treatment. Examples of healing in renal tuberculosis and comparisons of treated and untreated patients are shown in Figures 8–89 through 8–95. All workers interested in this subject indicate that the disease may be only arrested and quiescent even though the urine has become sterile. Periodic urograms and urine cultures are necessary for many years. A combination of streptomycin, para-aminosalicylic acid (PAS), and isoniazid is commonly used for 2 or more years in treatment. PAS is preferably administered in the form of sodium-PAS, which causes less gastrointestinal disturbances than does the acid form. Isoniazid given over long periods may cause peripheral or optical neuritis. For this reason it should be combined with administration of vitamin B_6 (pyridoxine) in doses of 50 mg twice daily. Lattimer and co-workers reported that cycloserine may effectively replace streptomycin, thus doing away with the inconvenience and discomfort of intramuscular injections of streptomycin. Ethionamide is another drug effective against *M. tuberculosis*. It is given orally, and may replace streptomycin. Occasionally it causes jaundice, and monthly liver-function tests are advocated if ethionamide is used over a prolonged period (Lattimer and colleagues).

Follow-up Studies

In all patients treated for tuberculosis of the genitourinary tract, careful follow-up roentgen examinations at regular intervals are mandatory both for evaluation of therapeutic results and for early detection of complications during the healing process. From the outset it should be explained to all patients that such studies are an essential part of the therapeutic program and that conservative or reconstructive surgical treatment is occasionally necessary as adjunctive treatment. Gow (1963) advised that urine cultures and inoculation tests together with intravenous pyelography be performed on admission, then after 3, 6, 9, and 15 months, and subsequently once yearly for 10 years, unless complications should call for earlier examinations. In such a program the exposure to x-rays, particularly in children, should be guarded; it may be reduced by limitation of the number of films in each series and, as mentioned above, by screening tests with isotope compounds.

Complications During Healing Process

The particular need of follow-up studies stems from the tendency of tissues affected by tuberculosis to contract from fibrosis in healing. Healing of superficial ulcerations affecting only the mucous membrane produces a small scar that does not cause stricture. Deeper destruction produces considerable fibrosis on healing. Areas of predilection for stricture formation with important consequences are the ureter and more particularly its terminal and intramural portions, the ureteropelvic junction, and the calyceal infundibulum.

Stricture of a Calyx

Contracture of the outlet of a calyx causes retention of urine or caseous material or both, resulting in hydrocalycosis and occasionally a large caseous abscess. Caseous material often is so thick and viscous that it will not drain sufficiently through a narrowed calyceal infundibulum even though urine still passes. It may be difficult sometimes to decide whether retention in a dilated calyx is due to accumulation of caseous material with moderate stricture of the calyceal neck or to retention of urine trapped behind a tight stricture. Hanley (1961) suggested that if the cavity fills partially with contrast medium on excretory urography but none enters it during retrograde pyelography, stricture is likely. If, on the other hand, the cavity is outlined only during retrograde filling and even then only faintly, it is probably just filled with caseous material which has not evacuated. Hanley suggested that multiple examinations over a fairly long period may be necessary before the diagnosis can be established, as often a calyx considered to be blocked may open up a few months later, evacuate the caseous material, and again communicate with the pelvis (Figs. 8-96 through 8-101; see also Figs. 8-26, 8-27, 8-94, and 8-95). The decision to undertake partial nephrectomy or cavernotomy should thus clearly be postponed until more definite proof of irreparable damage is evident. Even then the necessity of surgical intervention is questionable. Hanley stated that a large closed abscess cavity containing caseous material will not heal. If on repeated urographic examinations such a cavity remains obliterated, evacuation of its contents by cavernotomy should be seriously considered. He warned that one should be as certain as possible that the cavity is completely closed. Otherwise troublesome urinary fistulae may result. In his opinion, cavernotomy is preferable to partial nephrectomy in the majority of such cases (Figs. 8-88, 8-102, and 8-103). At present, cavernotomy and partial nephrectomy are only rarely considered necessary or advisable.

Strictures of Ureter; Contracted Bladder; Vesicoureteral Reflux

Progressive stricture of the ureteropelvic junction in the course of treatment is seen occasionally. As an isolated lesion it is rare in tuberculosis because other tuberculous changes are usually found in calyces and the ureter. Because of the resulting hydronephrosis, the diagnosis is easily made on excretory urography. The length of the stricture can be determined by retrograde ureterography (bulb catheter), and its functional importance can be judged from delayed retrograde pyelograms made with the patient upright. Plastic repair may be considered necessary if the stricture proves to be progressive on follow-up pyelograms after 6 to 12 weeks or if renal function deteriorates from back pressure. Depending on the condition and pliability of the pelvic and ureteral wall (induration, thickness, succulence) and the length of the stricture, pyeloplasty (Culp-DeWeerd) or intubated ureterotomy (Davis) is performed. In Hanley's experience the latter procedure is preferred for tuberculous strictures.

Stricture of the lower part of the ureter, especially the intramural portion, is a relatively common finding in the natural course as well as in the chemotherapy of tuberculosis. It may be due to ureteral disease in this area, but also may result from contracture of the tuberculous bladder. Unilateral or bilateral vesicoureteral reflux may also be a sequela of the contracted tuberculous bladder. It is not always easy to decide whether ureterectasis is due to contracture of the bladder, to vesicoureteral reflux, or to tuberculous stricture of the ureter. Establishing the cause may require many attempts at ureteral catheterization, dilatation, and cystography. If renal function becomes threatened, the obstruction or reflux must be relieved by ureteroneocystostomy or urinary diversion (Figs. 8-104 through 8-108; see also Figs. 8-56 through 8-61).

Contracture of the bladder caused by a slowly progressive fibrosis should be differentiated from an acute spastic condition. The small-capacity bladder, shrunken and contracted, is another end product of urinary tuberculosis that may require reconstructive surgical treatment. Cystoplasty with use of a bowel segment and eventual ureteral reimplantation in the isolated loop of bowel employed for reconstruction has become accepted as a beneficial procedure for the small contracted tuberculous bladder.

Transurethral resection of the vesical neck is another procedure occasionally indicated for relief of tuberculous contracture in this region. Large caseous abscesses may be drained into the prostatic urethra by transurethral procedures, if spontaneous drainage is insufficient. Healing may be hastened by evacuation of caseous material from prostatic cavities (see Figs. 8–85, 8–86, and 8–87). In the indication of all these types of reconstructive or conservative surgical treatment for genitourinary tuberculosis, periodic roentgenographic examinations play a dominant role.

In conclusion, tuberculosis of the genitourinary tract is at present less frequently encountered than previously and this holds true especially for far-advanced disease. Yet it is not as rare as one might expect from the glorious triumph of tuberculostatic medication. As urologists deal with an increasing number of disease entities, tuberculosis could become a forgotten disease in the future. It should not be forgotten, and a warning may be sounded that in all not readily explained pathology of the genitourinary tract the possibility of tuberculosis should be thought of and appropriately be proven or excluded. In the present era, when travel has become so easy and foreign labor, perhaps from countries where tuberculosis is still endemic, enters our production process, tuberculosis should still be seriously looked for, as this is the type of disease that continues to take both patients and doctors by surprise.

(References begin on page 928.)

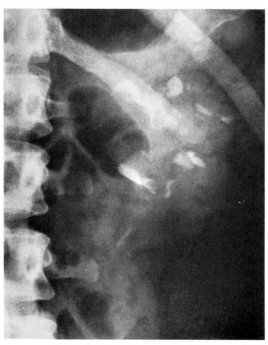

Figure 8–88. *Excretory urogram.* **Healed tuberculosis of left kidney treated by partial nephrectomy of lower pole and multiple-drug administration.** Stable urinary conversion for 5 years. Remaining portion of kidney functions well. Bizarre pattern due to tuberculous deformities and previous operation.

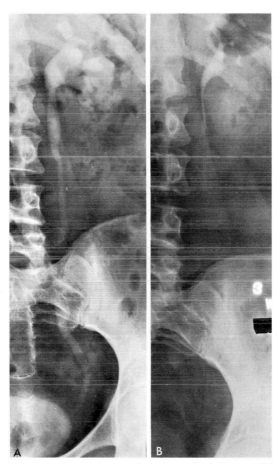

Figure 8–89. Left renal tuberculosis. **Healing with antimicrobial therapy.** Woman, 36 years of age. *Excretory urograms.* **A,** Before antimicrobial therapy was begun. Moderate dilatation of calyces, pelvis, and ureter. **B,** After 1 year of antimicrobial therapy. Lower calyx still shows evidence of dilatation and cavitation, but remainder of calyces, pelvis, and ureter have returned to normal.

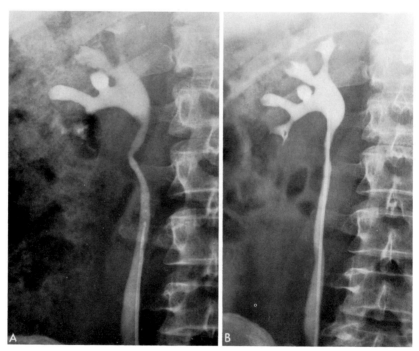

Figure 8–90. Results of antimicrobial therapy. Right renal tuberculosis in woman, 50 years of age. *Retrograde pyelograms.* **A,** Before therapy. Destructive tuberculous lesion involving lower calyx. Lesser changes in upper calyces. Left kidney was not involved. **B,** After 9 months of antimicrobial therapy. Almost normal appearance.

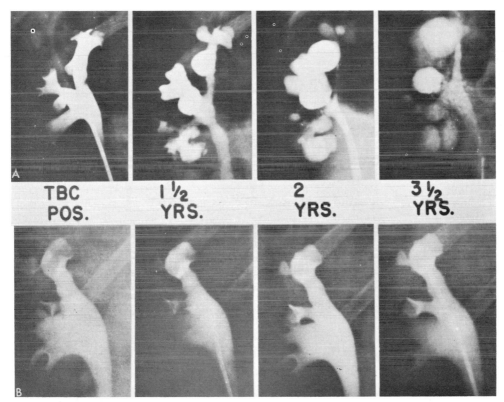

Figure 8–91. Value of chemotherapy in renal tuberculosis. **A,** Untreated "control" kidney of man, 30 years of age, with right renal tuberculosis. *Initial pyelogram* (far left) shows no urographic deformity, but *Mycobacterium tuberculosis* was demonstrated in urine. Subsequent films show course of disease during 3½ years (last film far right). **B,** Similar condition subjected to chemotherapy. No progression of disease. (From Lattimer, J. K., and Kohen, R. J.)

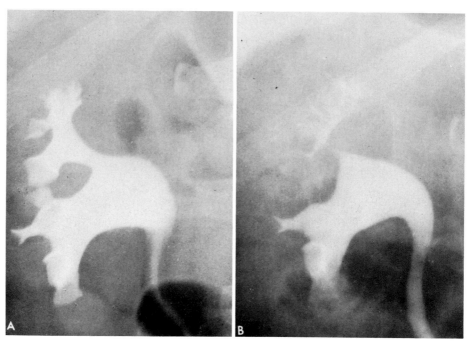

Figure 8–92. Example of progression of renal tuberculosis before era of chemotherapy. Man, 54 years of age. *Retrograde pyelograms.* **A,** Minimal erosion of upper calyx. **B,** Three years later. Marked destruction of upper calyces. Nephrectomy. Extensive involvement of upper pole with tuberculosis.

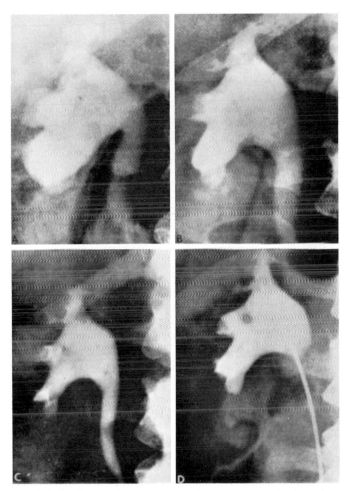

Figure 8–93. Results of chemotherapy in renal tuberculosis. Right renal tuberculosis; follow-up excretory urograms during chemotherapy. **A,** On admission; delayed function with grade 2 hydronephrosis and dilated ureter. **B,** Definite improvement of function and deformity after 9 months of multiple-drug therapy. **C,** Almost normal urogram and normal function after 2 years of treatment. **D,** *Retrograde pyelogram* does not give additional information on "hazy" outline of upper calyceal group. (Courtesy of Dr. P. G. Hoorweg, Amsterdam.)

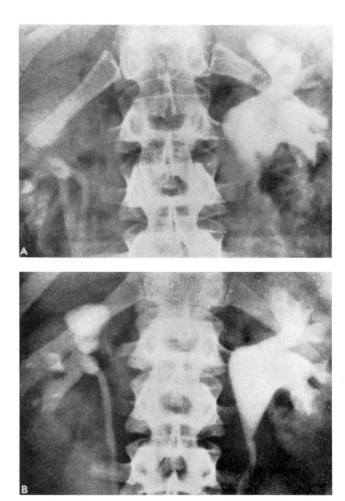

Figure 8–94. Results of chemotherapy in renal tuberculosis. Bilateral renal tuberculosis; follow-up urograms during prolonged chemotherapy. **A,** *Excretory urogram* before treatment. Poor function of right kidney; calycectasis in upper pole, irregular outline of middle and lower calyces. Moderate hydronephrosis of left kidney with irregular outline of all calyces. **B,** *Excretory urogram* after 7 months of chemotherapy. Marked improvement in function of both kidneys. Reduction of hydrocalycosis in right upper pole and of hydronephrosis of left kidney. Calyceal details are now sharply outlined. (Courtesy of Dr. P. G. Hoorweg, Amsterdam.)

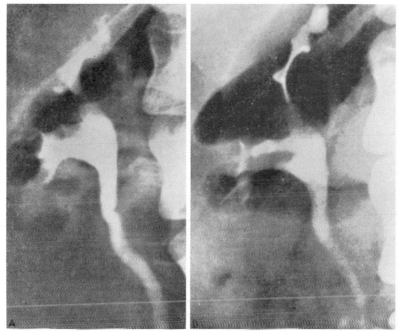

Figure 8–95. Results of chemotherapy in renal tuberculosis. Right renal tuberculosis. A, *Excretory urogram* before treatment. Irregular and "fuzzy" appearance of all calyces. B, *Excretory urogram* after 10 weeks of treatment. Details of calyces are sharply defined; urine cultures have become negative. (Courtesy of Dr. P. G. Hoorweg, Amsterdam.)

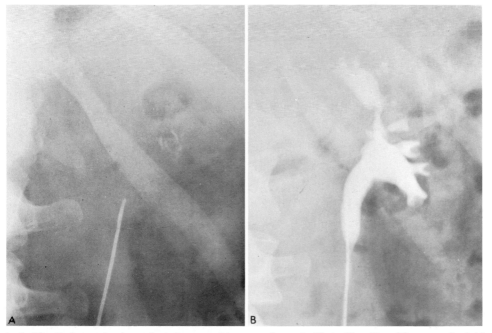

Figure 8–96. Left renal tuberculosis in man, 34 years of age. A, *Plain film.* Ring-like area of calcification over middle of left renal area suggests calcified aneurysm of renal artery. Two months' history. Had had no treatment. B, *Left pyelogram.* Tuberculous stricture of infundibulum of upper calyx, with calycectasis above. Calcification overlies area of stricture and apparently involves calyx which is projected in anteroposterior dimension.

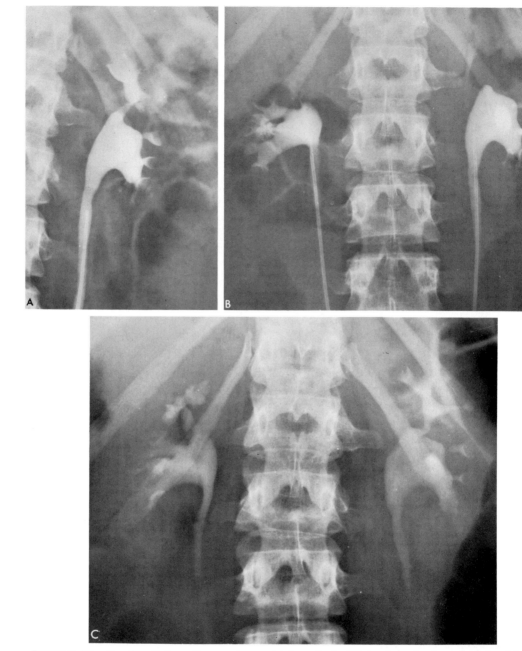

Figure 8–97.   Results of chemotherapy in renal tuberculosis. Bilateral renal tuberculosis in girl, 17 year
of age. **A**, *Left retrograde pyelogram.* Tuberculous erosion of upper and lower calyces. Narrowing (stricture)
of infundibulum. Right pyelogram (not shown here) revealed similar involvement principally of upper calyces. **B**, *Bilateral retrograde pyelograms* a few days after **A**. Incomplete obstruction of infundibulum of upper
calyces prevents contrast medium from entering upper calyces readily. **C**, *Excretory urogram* after 1 year of
chemotherapy. Great improvement; left kidney almost normal; right still shows mild stricture of infundibulum
of upper calyx at juncture with minor calyx.

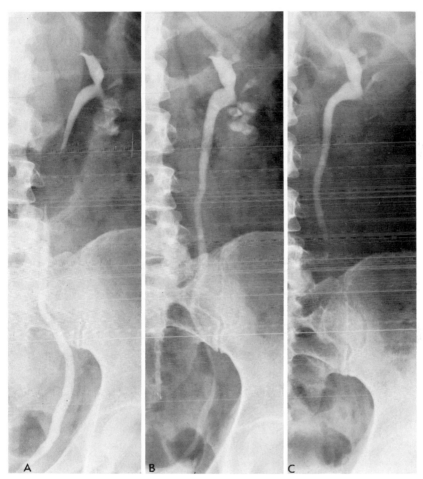

Figure 8-98.   Renal tuberculosis; healing with chemotherapy. **A,** *Retrograde pyelogram* before treatment. Gross involvement of lower calyces and ureter (ureterectasis). Plain film showed some irregular calcification in region of lower calyx. **B,** *Excretory urogram* after 2 months of chemotherapy. Narrowing (beginning stricture) of infundibulum of lower calyx. **C,** *Excretory urogram* after 14 months of chemotherapy. **Stricture of infundibulum** has progressed with almost complete occlusion of calyx. There is no contrast medium in lower calyx. Irregular shadows are areas of calcification.

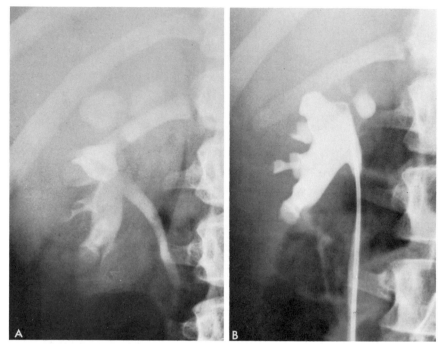

Figure 8–99.   Results of chemotherapy for renal tuberculosis in boy, 13 years of age. **A,** *Excretory urogram* of right kidney. Tuberculosis most marked in upper pole. Left kidney was normal. **B,** *Retrograde pyelogram* of right kidney after 2 years of chemotherapy. Stricture of upper calyx. Some visualization of dilated upper calyces was demonstrated with excretory urogram. Patient clinically well, with sterile urine and no symptoms.

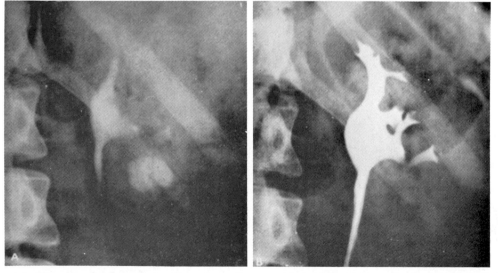

Figure 8–100.   Renal tuberculosis. Caseous cavity associated with stricture of calyceal infundibulum. **A,** *Excretory urogram.* Cavity associated with lower calyceal group. **B,** *Retrograde pyelogram.* Cavity does not fill, indicating **stricture of infundibulum.** (From Hanley, H. G., 1961.)

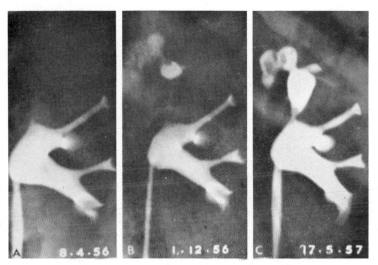

Figure 8-101. Renal tuberculosis. Caseous cavity without evidence of stricture of infundibulum. *Retrograde pyelograms* made during treatment. **A,** Upper calyces not filled; suggests either stricture of neck of calyx or complete filling of cavity by caseous material. **B,** Six months after **A. C,** Eleven months after **A.** Caseous material has been evacuated from cavities in upper calyces. Film made 2 years after **C** showed no change in appearance of upper calyces. Urine is sterile. (From Hanley, H. G., 1961.)

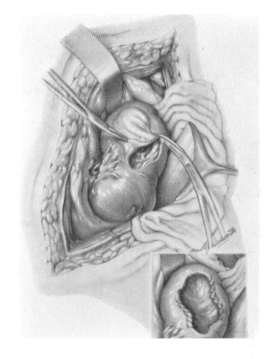

Figure 8-102. Renal cavernotomy for caseated tuberculous abscess. Abscess has been aspirated through wide-bore needle. As roof collapses limits of cavity are clearly defined. Center of roof, which is relatively avascular, is resected, care being taken to preserve overhanging edge which can be oversewn for hemostatic purposes when necessary (*inset*). Remaining caseous material is gently removed with dry gauze swabs. Undue roughness at this stage will result in troublesome oozing of blood from granulating walls. (From Hanley, H. G., 1961.)

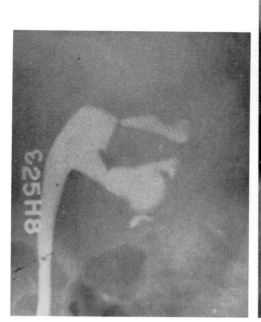

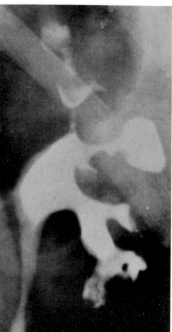

Fig. 8–103   **Fig. 8–104**

Figure 8–103. Renal tuberculosis. *Retrograde pyelogram.* Space-filling lesion due to large closed abscess cavity in upper pole of kidney. **Cavernotomy** done and 40 ml of thick pus was evacuated. (From Hanley, H. G., 1961.)

Figure 8–104. Renal tuberculosis. **Complications resulting from chemotherapy.** Strictures of both ureter and calyces developed during healing process. (Courtesy of Dr. J. K. Lattimer and Dr. Jerome Siegel.)

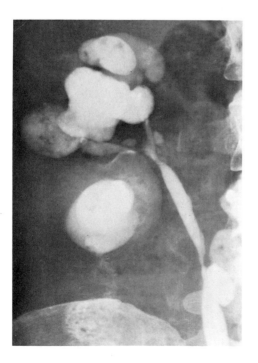

Figure 8–105. Renal tuberculosis. Complication resulting from chemotherapy. Strictures of both ureter and calyces developed during healing process. (Courtesy of Dr. J. K. Lattimer and Dr. Jerome Siegel.)

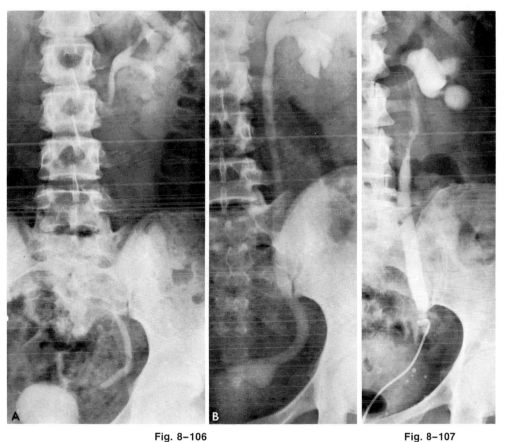

Fig. 8–106   Fig. 8–107

Figure 8–106.   Urinary tuberculosis. **Complications resulting from chemotherapy.** Bilateral renal tuberculosis in girl, 13 years of age. Complete destruction of right kidney, for which nephrectomy was performed. *A, Excretory urogram.* Solitary left kidney. Normal condition aside from mild dilatation of lower third of ureter and small contracted tuberculous bladder. **Chemotherapy begun. B,** *Excretory urogram* following 20 months of chemotherapy. Marked scarring of bladder apparently result of healing. Pyeloureterectasis seems to be result of contracted bladder and reflux rather than of ureteral stricture. Localized area of dilatation is main cavity of deformed bladder rather than deformity of ureter. Permanent left nephrostomy done.

Figure 8–107.   *Retrograde pyelogram.* **Tuberculous stricture, left ureter** (lower one third), in woman, aged 59. Marked destruction of kidney (which did not visualize on excretory urogram).

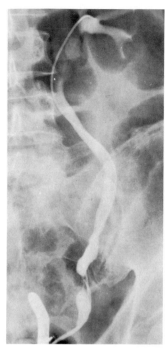

Figure 8–108. *Retrograde pyelogram.* **Tuberculous stricture of lower third of left ureter simulating primary carcinoma** in man, 68 years of age. Erroneous preoperative diagnosis made of primary carcinoma of ureter. True diagnosis discovered at operation.

REFERENCES

Anderson, F. E., Duca, C. J., and Scudi, J. V.: Some Heterocyclic Thiosemicarbazones. J. Am. Chem. Soc. 73:4967-4968 (Oct.) 1951.

Apperson, J. W., Wechsler, H., and Lattimer, J. K.: The Frequent Occurrence of Both Renal Calculi and Renal Calcifications in Tuberculous Kidneys. J. Urol. 87:643-646 (May) 1962.

Barrie, H. J., Kerr, W. K., and Gale, G. L.: The Incidence and Pathogenesis of Tuberculous Strictures of the Renal Pyelus. J. Urol. 98:584-589 (Nov.) 1967.

Beck, A. D., and Marshall, V. F.: Is Nephrectomy Obsolete for Unilateral Renal Tuberculosis? J. Urol. 98:65-70 (July) 1967.

Becker, J. A.: The Nonvisualized Kidney: The Value of Nephrotomography. Radiology 89:676-681 (Oct.) 1967.

Becker, J. A., Weiss, R. M., and Lattimer, J. K.: Renal Tuberculosis: The Role of Nephrotomography and Angiography. J. Urol. 100:415-419 (Oct.) 1968.

Bhisitkul, I., and Burros, H. M.: Tuberculous Renocolic Fistula: A Report of Two Cases. J. Urol. 85:716-719 (May) 1961.

Bruce, A. W., Awad, S. A., and Challis, T. W.: The Recognition and Treatment of Tuberculous Pyocalyx of the Kidney. J. Urol. 101:127-131 (Feb.) 1969.

Campbell, M.: Urology. Philadelphia, W. B. Saunders Company, 1954, vol. 1, pp. 656, 657; vol. 2, p. 1576.

Carr, D. T.: Current Status of Antimicrobial Therapy in Tuberculosis. J.A.M.A. 150:1170-1172 (Nov. 22) 1952.

Carr, D. T., Hinshaw, H. C., Pfuetze, K. H., and Brown, H. A.: The Use of Dihydrostreptomycin in the Treatment of Tuberculosis. Dis. Chest 16:801-815 (Dec.) 1949.

Carr, D. T., and Karlson, A. G.: Optimal Regimens of Antituberculous Drugs. Am. Rev. Resp. Dis. 84: 90-92 (July) 1961.

Cooper, H. G.: Treatment of Genitourinary Tuberculosis: Report After 14 Years. J. Urol. 86:719-72 (Dec.) 1961.

De Nunno, R.: Selective Instrumental Arteriographic Study in the Diagnosis of Renal Tuberculosis. J. Internat. Coll. Surgeons 32:523-529 (Nov.) 1959.

Emmett, J. L., and Braasch, W. F.: Has Excretory Urography Replaced Retrograde Pyelography in the Diagnosis of Renal Tuberculosis? J. Urol. 40:15-23 (July) 1938.

Emmett, J. L., and Kibler, J. M.: Renal Tuberculosis

Prognosis Following Nephrectomy; Based on Pre-operative Observations in the "Good" Kidney. J.A.M.A. 111:2351-2355 (Dec. 24) 1938.

Faulkner, J. W., Carr, D. T., and Emmett, J. L.: Collective Review: Current Status of Antimicrobial Therapy in Genitourinary Tuberculosis. Internat. Abstr. Surg., Surg., Gynec. & Obst. 98:417-426 (May) 1954.

Friedenberg, R. M., Ney, C., and Stachenfeld, R. A.: Roentgenographic Manifestations of Tuberculosis of Ureter. J. Urol. 99:25-29 (Jan.) 1968.

Frimann-Dahl, J.: Radiological Investigations of Urogenital Tuberculosis. Urol. internat. 1:396-426, 1955.

Frimann-Dahl, J.: Selective Angiography in Renal Tuberculosis. Acta radiol. 49:31-41, 1958.

Frimann-Dahl, J.: Angiography in Renal Inflammatory Diseases. In Kincaid, O. W.: Renal Angiography. Chicago, Year Book Medical Publishers, Inc., 1966, pp. 230-252.

Fritjofsson, Å., and Edsman, G.: Angiography in Renal Tuberculosis. Acta chir. Scandinav. 118:60-71, 1959.

Fritjofsson, Å., Helander, C.-G., Lindell, S.-E., and Obrant, K. O.: Roentgenological Findings and Clearance Functions in Cases of Renal Tuberculosis. Urol. internat. 17:106-114, 1964.

Gould, R. S.: Current Concepts of Renal Tuberculosis. J. Urol. 100:124-127 (Aug.) 1968.

Gow, J. G.: Genito-urinary Tuberculosis: A Study of 700 Cases. Lancet 11:261-265 (Aug. 10) 1963.

Gow, J. G.: Renal Calcification in Genito-urinary Tuberculosis. Brit. J. Surg. 52:283-288 (Apr.) 1965.

Gow, J. G.: The Surgery of Genito-urinary Tuberculosis. Brit. J. Surg. 53:210-216 (Mar.) 1966.

Grunberg, E., and Schnitzer, R. J.: Studies on Activity of Hydrazine Derivatives of Isonicotinic Acid in Experimental Tuberculosis of Mice. Quart. Bull. Sea View Hosp. 13:3-11 (Jan.) 1952.

Hanley, H. G.: The Scope of Surgery in Renal Tuberculosis. In Riches, E.: Modern Trends in Urology. New York, Paul B. Hoeber, Inc., 1960, pp. 131-146.

Hanley, H. G.: Conservative Surgery in Renal Tuberculosis Including Renal Cavernotomy. Brit. J. Surg. 48:415-420 (Jan.) 1961.

Hanley, H. G.: Treatment of Renal Tuberculosis. Brit. Med. J. 2:1611-1612 (Dec. 28) 1963.

Hinshaw, H. C., Feldman, W. H., Carr, D. T., and Brown, H. A.: The Clinical Administration of Dihydrostreptomycin in Tuberculosis: A Preliminary Report. Am. Rev. Tuberc. 58:525-530 (Nov.) 1948.

Hinshaw, H. C., and Herrell, W. E.: The Clinical Administration of Streptomycin. M. Clin. North America July 1966, pp. 855-861.

Jacobs, A., and Borthwick, W. M.: Streptomycin in Urinary Tuberculosis. Brit. J. Urol. 22:238-243, 1950.

Kaufman, J. J., and Goodwin, W. E.: Renal Hypertension Secondary to Renal Tuberculosis: Report of Cure in Four Patients Treated by Nephrectomy. Am. J. Med. 38:337-344 (Mar.) 1965.

Kerr, W. K., Gale, G. L., and Peterson, K. S. S.: Reconstructive Surgery for Genitourinary Tuberculosis. J. Urol. 101:254-266 (Mar.) 1969.

Kirsch, E., and Hennig, K.: Neue Gesichtspunkte zur Diagnostik und Therapie der Urotuberkulose unter Anwendung der Isotopen-Nephrographie und Szintigraphie. Ztschr. Urol. 58:769-785 (Oct.-Nov.) 1965.

Lattimer, J. K.: Caution Necessary in Treatment of Renal Tuberculosis With Isoniazid. J.A.M.A. 150:981-983 (Nov. 8) 1952.

Lattimer, J. K.: A Roentgenographic Classification of Tuberculosis: Lesions of the Kidney. Am. Rev. Tuberc. 67:604-612 (May) 1953.

Lattimer, J. K.: Partial Resection of Kidney for Tuberculosis. J. Urol. 73:455-459 (Mar.) 1955a.

Lattimer, J. K.: The Treatment of Tuberculous Infections of the Genitourinary Tract. J. Urol. 74:291-300 (Sept.) 1955b.

Lattimer, J. K., and Kohen, R. J.: Renal Tuberculosis. Am. J. Med. 17:533-539 (Oct.) 1954.

Lattimer, J. K., Reilly, R. J., Segawa, A., Wechsler, H., Siegel, J., Girgis, A., and Cleason, D.: Injections Are No Longer Necessary in the Treatment of Renal Tuberculosis. J. Urol. 93:735-738 (June) 1965.

Lattimer, J. K., and Spirito, A. L.: The Current Status of the Chemotherapy of Renal Tuberculosis. J. Urol. 75:375-379 (Mar.) 1956.

Lattimer, J. K., and Vasquez, G.: Renal Tuberculosis in Children. Postgrad. Med. 28:336-342 (Oct.) 1960.

Lattimer, J. K., Vasquez, G., and Wechsler, H.: New Drugs for Treatment of Genitourinary Tuberculosis: A Comparison of Efficacy. J. Urol. 83:493-497 (Apr.) 1960.

Lehmann, J.: Para-aminosalicylic Acid in the Treatment of Tuberculosis. Lancet 1:15-16 (Jan. 5) 1946.

Lehmann, J.: Kemoterapi av tuberkulos: p-Aminosalicylsyra (PAS) och närstående derivats bakteriostatiska effekt på tuberkelbacillen jämte djurexperimentella och kliniska försök med PAS. Nord. med. 33:140-145 (Jan. 10) 1947.

Lieberthal, F.: Renal Tuberculosis: The Development of the Renal Lesion. Surg., Gynec. & Obst. 67:26-37 (July) 1938.

Ludvik, W., Pecherstorfer, M., and Opl, G.: Infusionspyelographie und Tuberkulose. Ztschr. Urol. 59:561-573 (Aug.) 1966.

Malament, M., Auerbach, O., and Harris, J. T.: Limitation of Chemotherapy in Advanced Cavitary Tuberculosis of the Kidney. J. Urol. 99:700-706 (June) 1968.

May, P., Hohenfellner, R., König, E., and König, K.: Diagnostik und Therapie der Prostatatuberkulose. Urol. internat. 21:329-337, 1966.

Medlar, E. M.: Cases of Renal Infection in Pulmonary Tuberculosis: Evidence of Healed Tuberculosis Lesions. Am. J. Path. 2:401-413 (Sept.) 1926.

Medlar, E. M.: The Pathogenesis of Minimal Pulmonary Tuberculosis: A Study of 1,225 Necropsies in Cases of Sudden and Unexpected Death. Am. Rev. Tuberc. 58:583-611 (Dec.) 1948.

Medlar, E. M., Spain, D. M., and Holliday, R. W.: Post-mortem Compared With Clinical Diagnosis of Genito-urinary Tuberculosis in Adult Males. J. Urol. *61*:1078-1088 (June) 1949.

Miyake, K., Smith, M. J. V., and Lattimer, J. K.: Drug Resistance of Acid Fast Bacilli in the Urine. J. Urol. *98*:263-266 (Aug.) 1967.

Moonen, W. A.: Stricture of the Ureter and Contracture of the Bladder and Bladder Neck Due to Tuberculosis: Their Diagnosis and Treatment. J. Urol. *80*:218-228 (Oct.) 1958.

Neibling, H. A., and Walters, W.: Adenocarcinoma and Tuberculosis of the Same Kidney: Review of the Literature and Report of Seven Cases. J. Urol. *59*:1022-1035 (June) 1948.

Olsson, O.: Die Urographie bei der Nierentuberkulose. Acta radiol., Suppl. 47, 1943, pp. 7-162.

Olsson, O.: Urography in Renal Tuberculosis: Roentgen Diagnostic Investigations. (Abstr.) Radiology *47*:428-429 (Oct.) 1946.

Olsson, O.: Die Kontrastmittel im klinischen Gebrauch. In Encyclopedia of Medical Radiology. III. Roentgen Diagnostic Procedures. Berlin, Springer-Verlag, 1967, pp. 583-599.

Olsson, O., and Jönsson, G.: Roentgen Examination of the Kidney and the Ureter. In Encyclopedia of Urology. V/1. Diagnostic Radiology. Berlin, Springer-Verlag, 1962, pp. 1-365.

Overbeck, L., and Keller, L.: Über den Wert der Menstrualblutuntersuchung bei Frauen mit Nieren-tuberkulose. Zentralbl. Gynak. *88*:1105-1116, 1966.

Palmlöv, A.: Tuberculous Prostatovesiculitis Complicated by Miliary Tuberculosis: Report of One Case of Diagnostic Difficulty. Acta chir. scandinav. *123*:490-493 (May-June) 1962.

Puigvert, A., and Gittes, R. F.: Partial Nephrectomy in the Solitary Kidney. II. Experience With 20 Cases of Renal Tuberculosis. J. Urol. *100*:243-250 (Sept.) 1968.

Reinhard, J. F., Kimura, E. T., and Schachter, R. J.: Some Pharmacologic Characteristics of Isonicotinyl Hydrazide (Pyricidin): A New Anti-tuberculosis Drug. Science *116*:166-167 (Aug. 15) 1952.

Robitzek, E. H., Selikoff, I. J., and Ornstein, G. G.: Chemotherapy of Human Tuberculosis With Hydrazine Derivatives of Isonicotinic Acid (Preliminary Report of Representative Cases). Quart. Bull. Sea View Hosp. *13*:27-51 (Jan.) 1952.

Ross, J. C., Gow, J. G., and St. Hill, C. A.: Tuberculous Epididymitis: A Review of 170 Patients. Brit. J. Surg. *48*:663-666 (May) 1961.

Schatz, A., Bugie, E., and Waksman, S. A.: Streptomycin, a Substance Exhibiting Antibiotic Activity Against Gram-Positive and Gram-Negative Bacteria. Proc. Soc. Exper. Biol. & Med. *55*:66-69 (Jan.) 1944.

Scheinin, T. M., and Kontturi, M.: Incidence and Fate of Renal Tuberculosis in Patients With Bone and Joint Tuberculosis. Ann. chir. et gynaec. Finniae *55*:36-39, 1966.

Schencker, B., Marcure, R. W., and Moody, D. L.: Simplified Nephrotomography: The Drip Infusion Technique. Am. J. Roentgenol. *95*:283-290 (Oct.) 1965.

Scher, S.: Complications Following the Use of Streptomycin and Para-amino-salicylic Acid in Advanced Renal Tuberculosis. Brit. J. Urol. *25*:103-108 (June) 1953.

Semb, C.: Partial Resection of the Tuberculous Kidney. J. Oslo City Hosp. *3*:45-114, 1953.

Semb, C.: The Selective Principle in the Treatment of Urogenital Tuberculosis: Partial Resection of the Kidney and of the Ureter. Urol. internat. *1*:359-395, 1955.

Siegel, J., and Lattimer, J. K.: Renal Tuberculosis Has the Incidence of Advanced Lesions Decreased in the Past Two Decades? J. Urol. *91*:330-33 (Apr.) 1964.

Steyn, J. H., and Logie, N. J.: Coincident Tuberculous Perinephric Abscess and Carcinoma of the Kidney. Brit. J. Urol. *38*:7-8 (Feb.) 1966.

Strauss, Ingrid: Klinische und pathologisch-anatomische Beobachtungen über Verlaufsformen der Nierentuberkulose. Urologe *4*:29-42 (Jan.) 1965

Sutherland, A. M.: Genital Tuberculosis in Women. Am. J. Obst. & Gynec. *79*:486-497 (Mar.) 1960.

Wechsler, H., Westfall, M., and Lattimer, J. K.: The Earliest Signs and Symptoms in 127 Male Patients With Genitourinary Tuberculosis. J. Urol. *83*:80-803 (June) 1960.

Youmans, G. P., and McCarter, J. C.: Streptomycin in Experimental Tuberculosis: Its Effect on Tuberculous Infections in Mice Produced by M. Tuberculosis var Hominis. Am. Rev. Tuberc. *5* 432-439 (Nov.) 1945.

CHAPTER 9

Renal Cysts

CLASSIFICATION

Detailed evaluation of renal serous cysts an result in a large and extensive classfication. For instance, in 1950 Abeshouse numerated 16 varieties of renal cysts, and n 1967 Wahlqvist enumerated 29 variees, many of which had several subvarietes. For practical purposes, however, most enal cysts can be included in the following simple classification which is based argely on the classification of Spence, aird, and Ware.

I. Simple cyst
   A. Single or multiple
   B. Unilateral or bilateral
   C. Serous or hemorrhagic
II. Peripelvic cyst
III. Calyceal cyst (hydrocalyx, hydrocalycosis, calyceal diverticulum, pyelogenic cyst) (Considered in Chapter 5.)
IV. Cyst associated with neoplastic disease
   A. Cystic degeneration of parenchymal carcinoma
   B. Malignant change occurring in wall of simple cyst
   C. Cystadenoma
V. Cyst secondary to nonneoplastic renal pathology
   A. Inflammatory (tuberculosis, calculus formation, pyelonephritis)
   B. Echinococcus cyst
VI. Congenital renal cystic disease
   A. Polycystic disease
      1. In newborn babies, infants, and children
      2. In adults
   B. Multilocular cyst
   C. Unilateral multicystic disease
   D. Cystic disease associated with obstruction of the lower urinary tract
   E. Medullary sponge kidney
VII. Perinephric cyst

The lesions to be discussed in this chapter are simple cyst, peripelvic cyst, congenital cystic disease, echinococcus cyst, and perinephric pseudocyst (urinoma). The remaining cysts and cyst-like lesions are discussed elsewhere in this volume in the chapters dealing with their underlying pathology.

SIMPLE CYSTS

The simple solitary cyst arises from the renal parenchyma, usually near the periphery, and tends to grow away from the kidney. Except in rare instances of spontaneous rupture, it does not communicate with the pelviocalyceal system. It may not encroach on the pelviocalyceal system so that roentgenographically it is seen only as a circular soft-tissue shadow overlying the renal margin or projecting from it, or both. If the cyst tends to remain intrarenal and enlarges substantially, the calyces may be distorted. Cysts vary greatly in size from those less than a centimeter in diameter to those containing several liters of fluid (Hepler). The term *solitary cyst* is really a misnomer, because necropsy studies (Robertson) have demonstrated that simple cysts rarely occur singly. In most cases one large cyst may be seen in the renal tissues, but if a careful search is made, at least one or more comparatively small cysts may be found in addition to the large one. Simple cysts are primarily unilateral but may involve both kidneys.

Multiple, large, simple cysts are frequently found at operation, and these have been confused with congenital cystic disease of the kidney. Simple cysts are discrete and separated by normal renal tissue in contrast to the generalized involvement of the so-called congenital polycystic disease. Simple cysts usually involve only one kidney; therefore, if the deformity is unilateral, polycystic disease is unlikely.

Histopathogenesis of Simple Cysts in General

The cyst wall is composed of fibrous tissue and lined with a simple layer of flat endothelium. Most cysts are filled with a simple serous fluid. About 10% to 15% contain hemorrhagic fluid (Hepler).

Hepler's concept of the origin of cysts is generally accepted. His experimental work in 1930 showed that tubular obstruction plus vascular block and ischemia in the obstructed area causes the rapid development of a cyst. The facts that most cysts are encountered in adult life and that diseases of late adult life can cause the necessary tubular and vascular obstruction lend support to the thesis that most cysts are acquired. That congenital factors may sometimes result in cysts is supported by the occasional involvement of infants (Travers).

Incidence of Tumor Associated With Simple Cysts

The most difficult diagnostic problems posed by cysts arise from (1) the fear that a malignant tumor may be associated with (or lie within) the cyst and (2) the danger of making an erroneous diagnosis of cyst when the lesion is actually a solid tumor. The advent of nephrotomography and renal arteriography has greatly reduced the chance of confusing a cyst and a tumor, but the fear that a tumor may be associated with (or lie within) the cyst continues.

Various estimates of the incidence of malignant tumor within or associated with cysts can be found in the literature. Many loose statements have been made, so that estimates are not reliable. The most common estimate given is 7% (Gibson; Walsh). If the content of the cyst is hemorrhagic, the incidence of tumor is said to increase upward to as high as 25% or 30%. It has been our opinion at the Mayo Clinic that these estimates are too high. In fact, we have thought for some time that the incidence of tumor within the wall of a cyst is rare and we have been in agreement with Ainsworth and Vest that many of the reported cases of cysts associated with tumor would not stand critical evaluation. The article by Rehm, Taylor, and Taylor reporting three cases of malignant tumor within the wall of a cyst seen during years at the Department of Urology of the Ohio State University College of Medicine, has caused us concern. In 1963 we (Emmett, Levine, and Woolner) reevaluated 1,000 consecutive cases of renal exploration for expanding renal masses in order to determine the incidence of tumor occurring with cysts. Our findings suggested that tumor and cyst occur together in less than 1% of cases.

If a tumor is located within the cyst, it is nearly always found in the part of the cyst wall that is attached to the solid renal parenchyma. Gibson postulated the s quence of events in such a situation as follows: (1) the tumor develops in the renal parenchyma, (2) the tumor causes both tubular and vascular obstruction with ischemia, and (3) the obstruction and ischemia provide Hepler's ideal situation for the production of a cyst distal to the point of obstruction. Thus, the tumor is always in the portion of the cyst wall that is contiguous (attached) to the renal parenchyma. Rehm, Taylor, and Taylor's case 1 is an excellent example of Gibson's postulate (Fig. 9–1). The most disconcerting factor, however, is illustrated by their case 3 in which sheets of malignant tumor cells were found within the cyst wall although the wall appeared to be normal on gross examination.

Nephrogenic Polycythemia

Within the past few years the association of polycythemia and renal lesions, especially cysts and tumors, has been observed (Forssel; Jacobson and associates, 1957). A selective review of the literature by Nixon and co-workers in 1960 showed reports of polycythemia in association with 30 cases of hypernephroma, 4 cases of polycystic disease, 1 case of bilateral unilocular cysts, 1 case of adenoma, and cases of hydronephrosis (Gardner and Freymann). To this group these workers (Nixon and co-workers) added three cases (one of solitary simple cyst and two of multiple cysts). They estimated that 1% to 2% of patients with polycythemia have an underlying renal carcinoma. Although fewer cases of renal cystic disease have been reported in the literature, they are inclined to believe that the incidence of polycythemia in renal cystic disease is equal to that of hypernephroma. Jacobson and associates (1957; 1959) postulated that the kidneys secrete a substance generally referred to as erythropoietin and are the principal organs, not the only organs, which elaborate a factor necessary to the maintenance of erythropoietic equilibrium. Rosse, Wald-

mann, and Cohen reported nine cases of polycythemia associated with renal cysts. In six of these, definite erythropoietin activity was found in fluid aspirated from the cysts. High concentrations of erythropoietin have been found in the walls of renal cysts, and excision of cysts has resulted in remission of polycythemia. Remission has followed nephrectomy for renal tumor (Conley, Kowal, and D'Antonio; Cooper and Tuttle; DeWeerd and Hagedorn; Frey; Lawrence and Donald), only to recur with the onset of metastasis (Damon and associates; Omland).

Urographic Diagnosis of Simple Cysts

The Plain Film

Diagnosis of simple cyst may be suggested by the plain film, if one recognizes the soft-tissue outline of an expanding lesion adjacent to, or overlying, the kidney. The plain film may show the round dense shadow of the cyst which apparently overlies, or partly overlies, the renal outline (usually the upper or lower pole). The outline is smooth and round and in sharp contrast to the irregular contour likely to be produced by solid tumors (Fig. 9–2). In an occasional case the wall of the cyst may be calcified and may appear in the plain film as a thin curved line of calcification (Figs. 9–3, 9–4, and 9–5). Mottled calcification, although occasionally seen in cysts (Figs. 9–6, 9–7, and 9–8), is more commonly seen in renal tumors. A note of caution: A number of authors (Cannon, Zanon, and Karras; Lalli, 1966) have reported cases in which curvilinear calcifications typical of those seen in the walls of simple cysts have been found in renal carcinomas. We have encountered similar lesions and believe that the presence of a thin curvilinear calcification in the wall of a mass does not distinguish cyst from tumor (Fig. 9–9).

The Urogram

Urographic deformity depends on the situation of the cyst. When it is located in the periphery and grows away from the kidney, the renal pelvis and calyces may not be deformed (Fig. 9–10). The mass may go undetected unless tomograms are made as a routine part of the excretory urogram (Fig. 9–11). When it lies deeper within the renal parenchyma, the calyces and pelvis may be considerably distorted. One would expect that the urographic deformity would simulate that of any expanding lesion, such as a solitary abscess or neoplasm, and to a large extent this is true. The differential factor, which is sometimes helpful, is that with most cysts the normal terminal irregularities of the minor calyces involved are retained even though the renal pelvis or calyces, or both, are extensively deformed; whereas, in the presence of renal tumors, the normal terminal irregularities of the involved calyces may be lost. Urographic changes caused by renal cysts which may be noted in the calyces are crescentic outline, flattening with "splaying," abbreviation, dilatation, displacement, elongation, and even complete obliteration. Flattening or crescentic deformity of the medial border of the pelvis is also a common finding (Figs. 9–12 through 9–21).

Not only are calyces distorted, but when cysts are of moderate or large size the entire kidney may be rotated or twisted on its perpendicular, anteroposterior, or transverse axis, resulting in most peculiar types of malrotation and distortion (Fig. 9–22). After surgical excision of the cyst, the pyelogram usually shows a return to normal (Figs. 9–23, 9–24, and 9–25). Occasionally, a simple cyst will disappear spontaneously (Fig. 9–26). Generally speaking, it is not roentgenographically possible to distinguish between a simple solitary cyst and a *multilocular cyst* (Fig. 9–27). Although obstruction of the pelvis or calyces or both is relatively common in cases of peripelvic cyst, it is rather un-common in association with simple parenchymal cysts although it does occur occasionally. Secondary calculi may form in a dilated calyx as a result of the obstruction and stasis (Fig. 9–28).

Multiple Renal Cysts. *Multiple renal cysts* may be grouped together in one part of the kidney so that urographically they may appear as a simple solitary cyst (Fig. 9–29), or they may be distributed throughout the kidney causing a change in contour of several or all the calyces (Figs. 9–30 and 9–31). When the cysts are of moderate or large size, their presence is easily detected and the benign nature of the lesion can be suspected from the typical deformity of the calyces (Figs. 9–32, 9–33, and 9–34). Smaller cysts, however, may be difficult or impossible to diagnose without the use of tomography. As a matter of fact, it is now becoming apparent that many of the pyelograms which we formerly described as "variations of normal" were in reality exhibiting minimal deformities caused by multiple cysts (see "Nephrotomography" later in this chapter).

Differential Diagnosis: Cyst Versus Tumor.[*] As intimated previously, the great diagnostic problem has always been the differentiation of cyst from malignant tumor. The reason is obvious: If the lesion is a cyst, surgical removal usually is not indicated because it rarely (unless unusually large) causes symptoms. On the other hand, a malignant tumor demands nephrectomy. Before the era of arteriography and nephrotomography a positive diagnosis could not be made on the basis of the plain film and urogram; surgical exploration was required in almost all cases. Only too often cysts produced urograms that suggested tumor and vice versa. As a matter of fact, some of the most convincing and typical "cysts" turned out to be tumors at operation. **In other words, calyceal deformity was not sufficiently pathogn-**

---

[*]See also discussion in Chapter 10, pages 1087–108

monic to permit accurate diagnosis (Figs. 9–35 through 9–41). With the introduction of nephrotomography and arteriography this situation has radically changed (Evans; Evans, Dubilier, and Monteith; Watson, Fleming, and Evans).

(Text continued on page 957.)

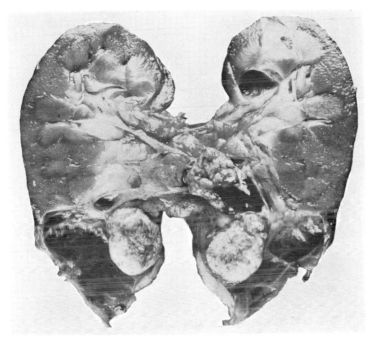

Figure 9–1.   Solitary cyst with tumor, 3 by 5 cm in diameter, in base adjacent to renal parenchyma. (Microscopic examination showed clear cell carcinoma.) (From Rehm, R. A., Taylor, W. N., and Taylor, J. N.)

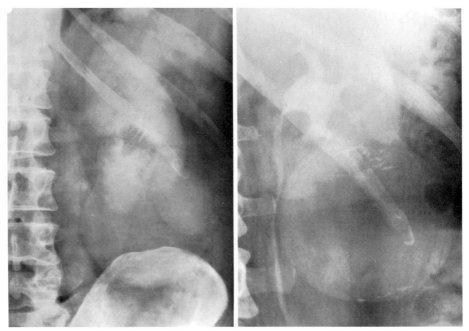

Fig. 9–2   Fig. 9–3

Figure 9–2. *Plain film.* Soft-tissue outline of moderate-sized **simple cyst** of lower pole of left kidne
Figure 9–3. *Excretory urogram.* **Simple (solitary) cyst** of lower pole of left kidney with typical **curv**
linear calcification of cyst wall.

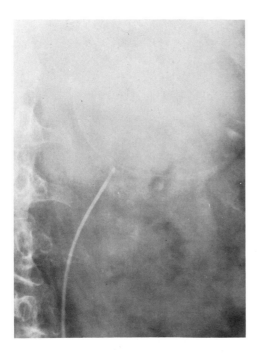

Figure 9–4. *Plain film.* Ureteral catheter in left uret.
Simple (solitary) cyst arising from upper pole of kidn
Curvilinear calcification of cyst wall.

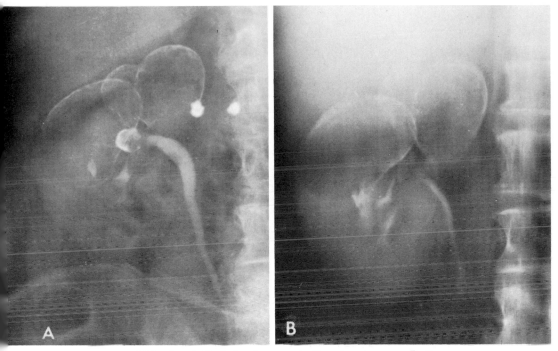

Figure 9–5. Multiple calcified simple cysts. A, *Excretory urogram.* B, *Tomogram.*

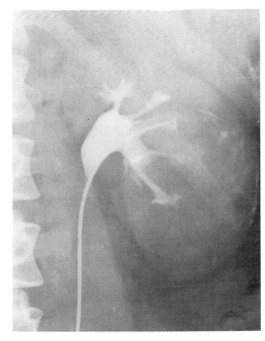

Figure 9–6. *Left retrograde pyelogram.* Simple (solitary) cyst arising from lower pole of kidney with both curvilinear and mottled calcification of cyst wall.

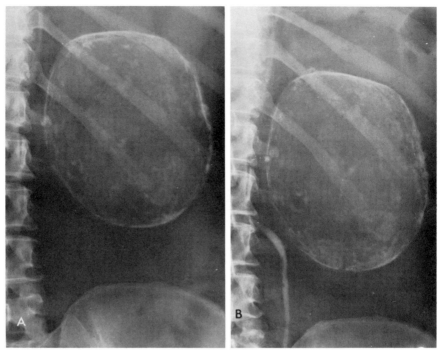

Figure 9–7. A, *Plain film.* Large simple cyst showing both curvilinear and mottled calcification in wall B, *Attempted left pyelogram.* Block is apparent at ureteropelvic juncture. (Nephrectomy. Pathologic diagnosis: large calcareous cyst which contains numerous cholesterol crystals.)

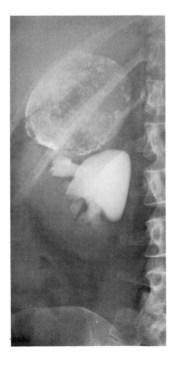

Figure 9–8. *Excretory urogram.* Mottled type of calcification in cyst (?) in upper pole of right kidney. (Lesion was thought clinically to be cyst, but no operation was performed.)

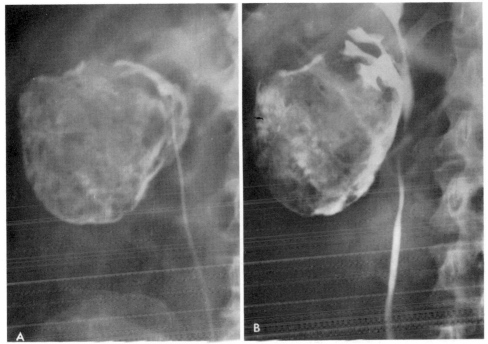

Figure 9–9. Calcified multilocular cyst with areas of hypernephroma. A, *Plain film* with lead catheter in right ureter. Large calcified lesion overlying lower pole of right kidney. B, *Right retrograde pyelogram.* Pelvis and calyces seem to be "displaced rather than involved" by calcific process (Surgical exploration and nephrectomy. Lobulated lesion was found, 8 cm in diamter, filled with numerous cysts varying from 1 to 2.5 cm in diameter. Several small yellowish nodes throughout lesion showed hypernephroma on microscopic examination.) (Courtesy of Dr J A. Taylor.)

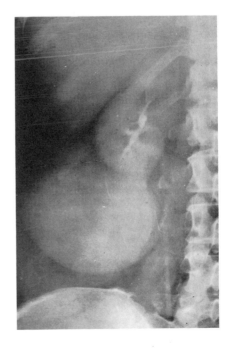

Figure 9–10. *Excretory urogram.* Large, circular soft-tissue shadow of **simple cyst** arising from lower pole of right kidney. Cyst is growing away from kidney and not encroaching on pelviocalyceal system.

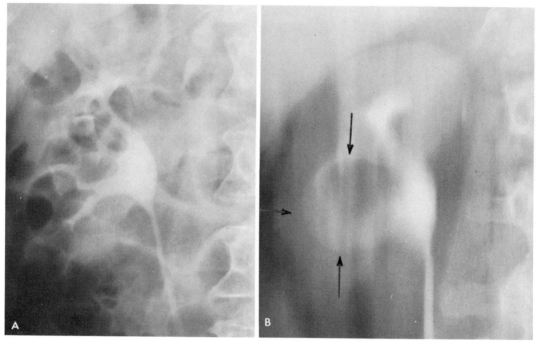

Figure 9–11.   Simple cyst. A, *Excretory urogram.* No evidence suggesting presence of renal mass is seen (Gas in bowel partially obscures kidney.) **B,** *Tomogram* made routinely as part of excretory urogram. Four-centimeter mass (*arrows*) on posterior aspect of kidney (later this proved to be cyst).

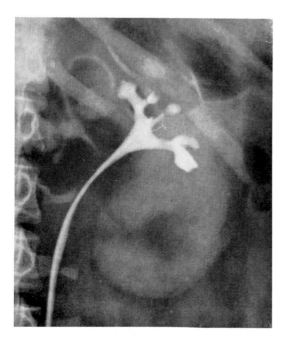

Figure 9–12. *Left retrograde pyelogram.* Well defined circular soft-tissue outline of **large simple cyst** of lower pole of left kidney, which is causing some flattening and splaying of lower calyx with slight upward and lateral displacement.

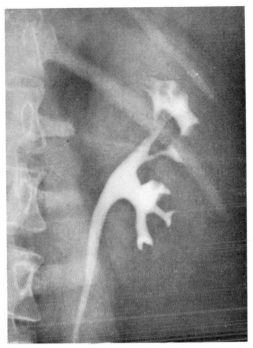

Figure 9–13. *Left retrograde pyelogram.* Small simple cyst of upper pole of kidney compressing medial branch of composite T-shaped upper calyx, producing typical crescentic deformity.

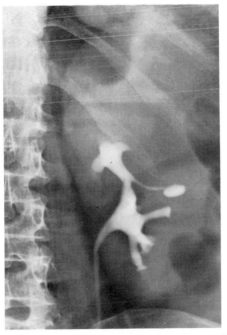

Figure 9–14. *Left retrograde pyelogram.* **Large simple (solitary) cyst** of upper pole of kidney growing away from kidney and encroaching on upper calyx, producing typical crescentic deformity.

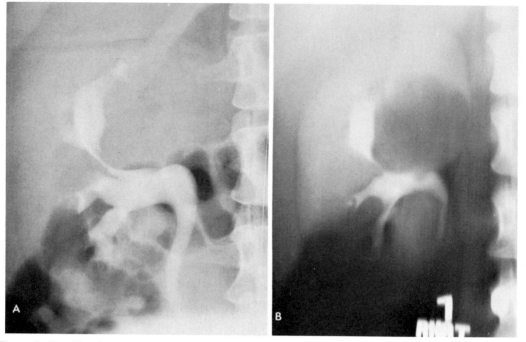

Figure 9–15. **Simple cyst. A,** *Excretory urogram.* Cyst producing crescentic deformity of renal pelvis and upper calyx. **B,** *Tomogram* shows relationship between radiolucent cyst and pelvis and calyces.

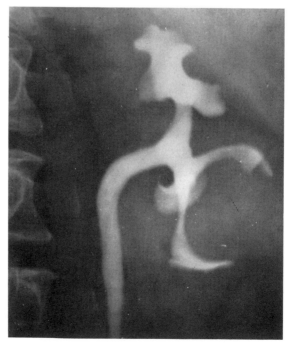

Figure 9–16. *Left retrograde pyelogram.* **Simple cyst** of lower pole of left kidney, causing crescentic deformity of lower calyx.

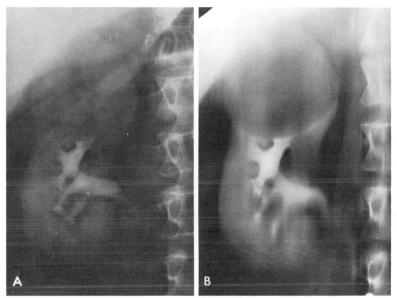

Figure 9–17.   **Simple cyst,** upper pole of right kidney. **A,** *Excretory urogram.* Mass in upper pole of right kidney producing only minimal flattening of upper-pole calyx. **B,** *Tomogram* demonstrates sharp demarcation between cyst and renal parenchyma.

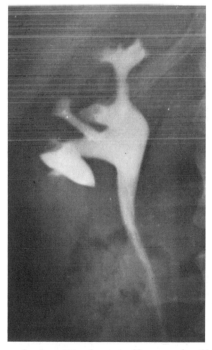

Figure 9–18.   *Right retrograde pyelogram.* **Simple cyst** of lower pole of kidney. Flattening and splaying of ⊃wer calyx with some upward and medial displacement.

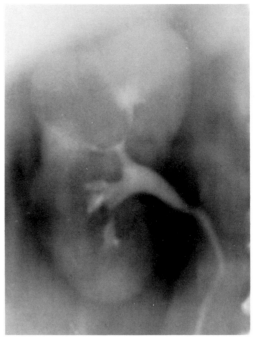

Figure 9–19. *Excretory urogram with tomogram.* Solitary **simple cyst** producing radiolucent defect in cortex of upper lateral portion of right kidney and slight spreading of upper calyces.

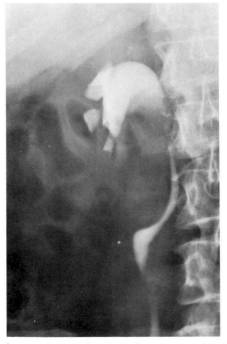

Figure 9–20. *Retrograde pyelogram.* **Large simple (solitary) cyst** of kidney displacing proximal ureter medially.

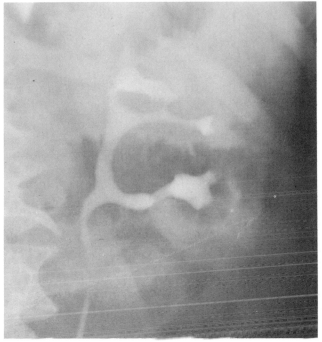

Figure 9–21. *Excretory urogram.* Solitary **peripelvic cyst** producing crescentic deformity of medial aspect of left renal pelvis.

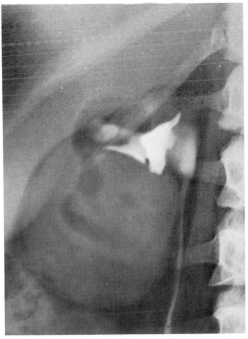

Figure 9–22. *Right retrograde pyelogram.* **Simple (solitary) cyst** of lower pole of right kidney, causing rotation around anteroposterior axis. Some of calyces are projected in anteroposterior plane. Middle calyx compressed by cyst, with typical crescentic deformity.

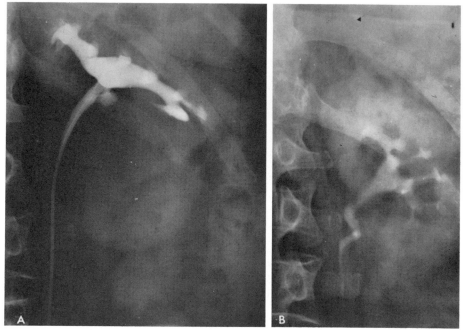

Figure 9–23. Simple cyst. *Retrograde pyelograms.* **A,** Solitary cyst of lower pole causing rotation around both anteroposterior and perpendicular axes. **B,** After surgical excision of cyst.

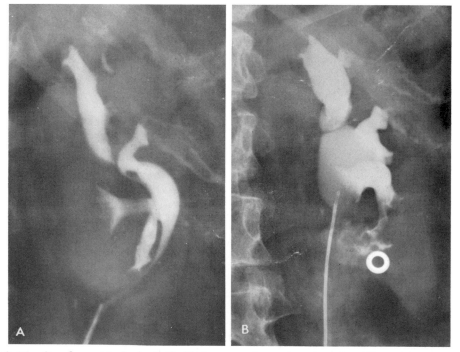

Figure 9–24. Simple cyst in lower half of kidney, causing malrotation of middle and lower calyces and displacement and deformity of pelvis. **A,** *Left retrograde pyelogram, preoperative,* suggests possible duplication. Difficult to tell whether malrotation is due to cyst or is of congenital origin. **B,** *Left retrograde pyelogram after surgical removal of cyst.* Pelvis and calyces have returned to normal, indicating that cyst was responsible for malrotation. No duplication present.

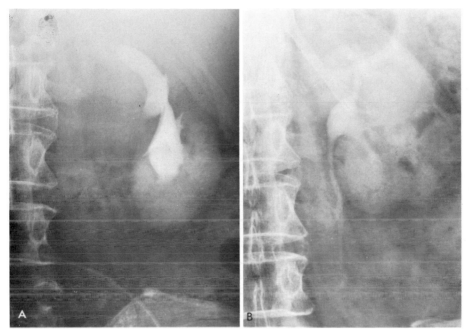

Figure 9–25. Simple (solitary) cyst of left kidney. *Excretory urograms.* **A,** Marked malrotation of kidney on its perpendicular axis. **B,** Cyst has been excised and kidney has returned to normal position.

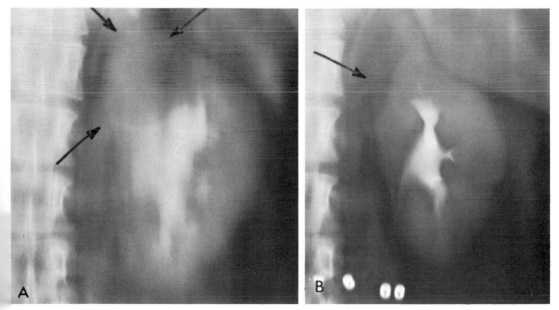

Figure 9–26. Spontaneous regression of simple cyst. **A,** *Excretory urogram with tomogram.* Simple cyst *(arrows)* of upper pole. **B,** *Excretory urogram with tomogram* (2 years later). Cyst has disappeared and only minimal scarring of cortex remains *(arrow).* (No operation performed.)

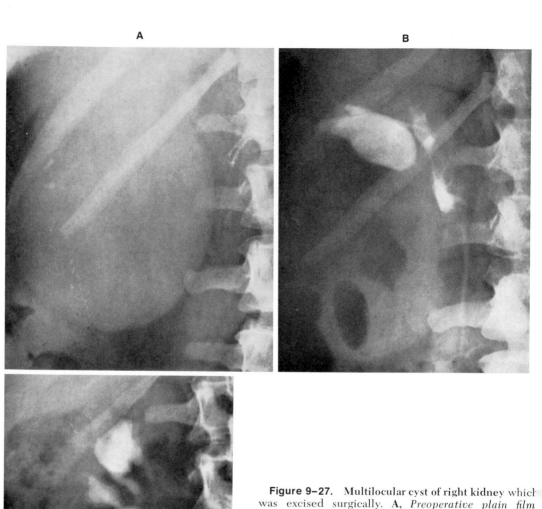

Figure 9–27. Multilocular cyst of right kidney which was excised surgically. **A,** *Preoperative plain film.* Soft-tissue outline suggests simple (solitary) cyst. **B,** *Preoperative excretory urogram.* Marked deformity of pelvis and calyces of right kidney from cyst. **C,** *Postoperative excretory urogram* (approximately 4 years after surgical removal of cyst). Position of calyces has returned to normal, although some pyelocaliectasis still persists.

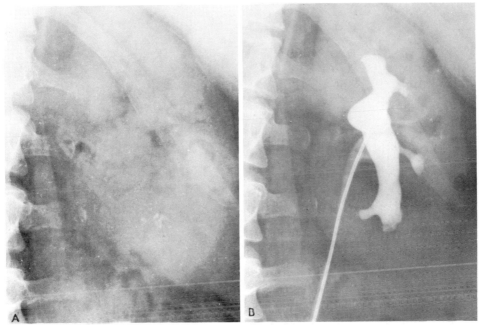

Figure 9-28.   Simple (solitary) cyst of lower pole of left kidney causing malrotation and obstruction of calyces resulting in secondary calculi in lower calyx. Surgical exploration and excision of cyst. A, *Plain film.* Multiple calculi can be seen in lower pole. B, *Retrograde pyelogram.*

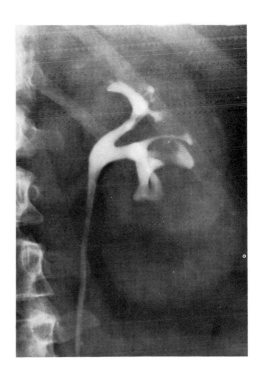

Figure 9-29.   *Left retrograde pyelogram.* Multiple simple cysts. Pyelogram suggests large simple (solitary) cyst.

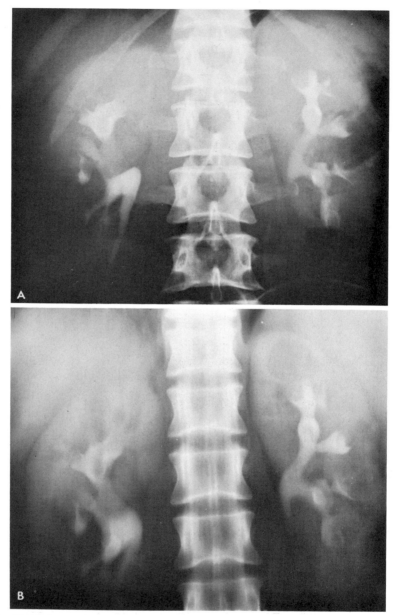

Figure 9–30.   **Multiple simple cysts. A,** *Excretory urogram.* Large kidneys with somewhat distorted calyces which show spreading and flattening especially on right. **B,** *Excretory urogram with tomogram.* Multiple simple cysts scattered in both kidneys.

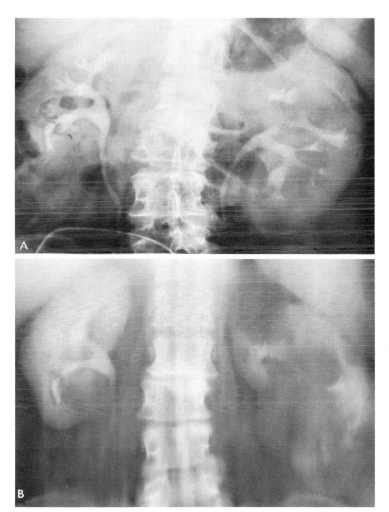

Figure 9–31.   Bilateral multiple simple cysts. **A,** *Excretory urogram.* Bilateral calyceal deformity with slightly enlarged left kidney. **B,** *Excretory urogram with tomogram.* Single cyst, lower medial aspect of right kidney, and multiple cysts of various sizes on left.

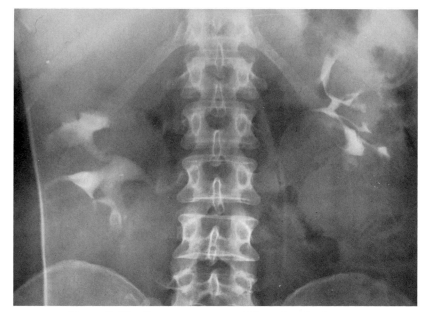

Figure 9–32. *Excretory urogram.* Bilateral multiple cysts.

Fig. 9–33

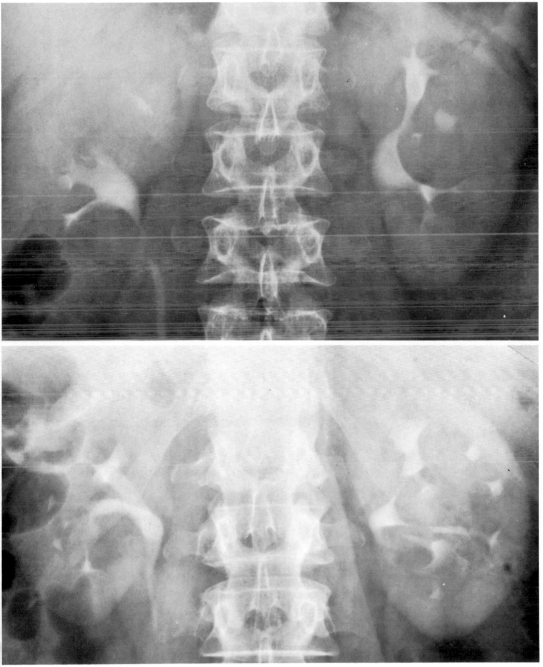

Fig. 9–34

Figures 9–33 and 9–34. *Excretory urograms.* Bilateral multiple renal cysts.

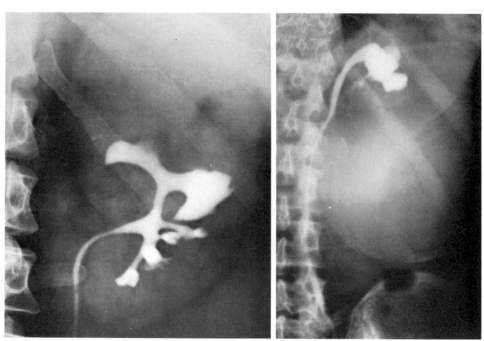

Fig. 9–35   Fig. 9–36

Figure 9–35. *Left retrograde pyelogram.* Large simple (solitary) cyst of upper pole of left kidney, causing irregular deformity of upper calyx. Cyst would be **difficult to distinguish from renal tumor without exploration.**

Figure 9–36. *Left retrograde pyelogram.* Large simple (solitary) cyst of lower pole of left kidney, causing irregular deformity of lower calyces. Cyst would be **difficult to distinguish from renal tumor without exploration.**

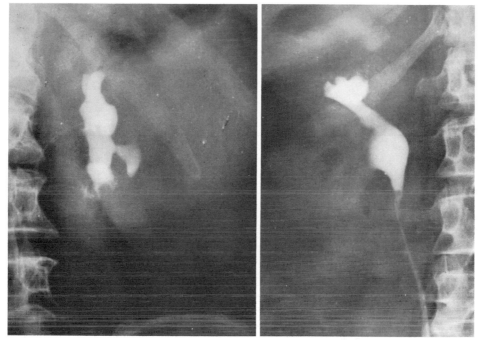

Fig. 9–37	Fig. 9–38

Figure 9–37. *Left retrograde pyelogram.* Large simple (solitary) cyst of left kidney, causing malrotation with flattening, broadening, and splaying of calyces. Cyst would be **impossible to distinguish from renal tumor** without further study.

Figure 9–38. *Right retrograde pyelogram.* Large simple (solitary) cyst of middle portion and lower pole of right kidney, producing so much pressure on middle and lower calyces that they will not fill. This pyelogram cannot be distinguished from that of renal tumor or cortical abscess of kidney. Further study would be necessary for accurate diagnosis.

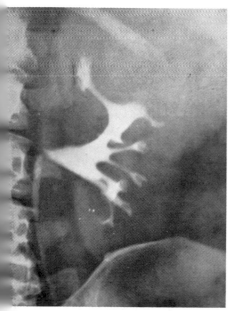
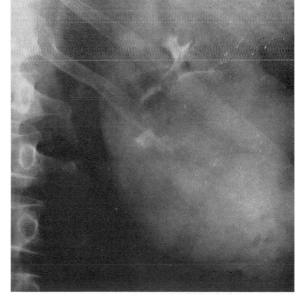

Fig. 9–39	Fig. 9–40

Figure 9–39. *Left retrograde pyelogram.* Renal cyst. Complete obliteration of one of upper calyces simulates destruction or "amputation" of calyx by tumor.

Figure 9–40. *Excretory urogram.* Multiple simple cysts involving left kidney, producing marked irregular deformity of pelviocalyceal system. They suggest tumor rather than cyst.

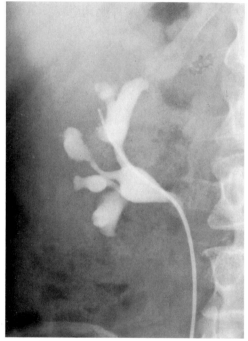

Figure 9–41. *Right retrograde pyelogram.* Case of **tumor simulating cyst.** Deformity of upper calyx compatible with either tumor or cyst. Patient brought excretory urograms which had been made 3 years earlier, and there was no change in contour of calyces. For this reason, lesion was considered cyst. There were no symptoms. One year later patient died; necropsy showed hypernephroma with metastasis.

The Nephrotomogram and Arteriogram

Simple cysts arising from the parenchyma of the kidney are avascular thin-walled lesions which produce sharply circumscribed radiolucent defects in the opacified parenchyma on both the **nephrotomogram** and the **renal arteriogram.** In the arterial phase of the nephrotomogram the renal arteries approach the cyst but do not enter it (Fig. 9–42). Since the cyst is avascular and filled with fluid, it retains a homogeneous radiolucent appearance throughout the examination. Intense opacification of the renal parenchyma is seen during the nephrographic phase of the nephrotomogram. During this phase, the radiolucent cyst contrasts sharply with the opaque parenchyma and the cyst wall is more clearly demonstrated than on films made during the preceding arterial phase. The wall of the cyst is smooth in outline and clearly defined. If it protrudes outside the surface of the kidney it is identified as a thin radiopaque line which rarely exceeds 1 mm in thickness. At the point of protrusion of the cyst from the renal parenchyma, a crescentic or beak-like deformity of the renal cortex may be seen. This feature is characteristic of simple cyst and is an important sign differentiating cyst from tumor (Figs. 9–43 through 9–53).

Chynn and Evans have reported their accuracy in differentiating cyst from tumor at 95% with nephrotomography. Southwood and Marshall have concurred with this evaluation. Our own experience, based on more than 4,000 intravenous nephrotomograms made at the Mayo Clinic, would tend to agree that nephrotomography is an accurate diagnostic aid. It is our feeling that, when *strict diagnostic criteria* are observed in differentiating cyst from tumor, that is, when diagnosis is based only on the classical signs, the accuracy is very high and falls within the range reported by Chynn and Evans. We

have found, however, that approximately 20% of our studies do not show the classical signs which clearly distinguish cyst from tumor. In these cases we think further evaluation by means of **renal arteriography** or **percutaneous puncture** of the mass is required for diagnosis or that the patient be explored for diagnosis and appropriate therapy. *It is axiomatic that a roentgenographic diagnosis of simple cyst can be made and accepted only when the classical roentgenographic signs are present.*

The arteriographic characteristics of renal cysts (Figs. 9–54 through 9–57) are essentially the same as the nephrotomographic characteristics. In almost all instances, however, the renal arteries are demonstrated more clearly by arteriography than by nephrotomography, and abnormalities of the renal vasculature which suggest tumor are more easily recognized. (See Chapter 10.) Typically, on the early films of either a midstream or selective renal arteriogram, the arteries in the vicinity of a cyst are displaced by the mass and are seen to course over its surface without penetration into its substance. In contrast to the findings in cases of carcinoma, arterial branching is normal and "tumor vessels" are not observed. Late in the filming sequence of the arteriogram (nephrographic phase), the renal parenchyma is densely opacified and contrasts sharply with the unopacified cyst. The walls of the cyst are well delineated and smooth *but often this feature as well as the thin wall of the cyst is not as well demonstrated by arteriography as by nephrotomography.*

Some cysts, because of their locations on the anterior or posterior surfaces of the kidney, their small sizes, the thickness of their walls, or their relationships to the renal parenchyma, do not exhibit the classical features described. In these cases differential diagnosis between cyst and tumor becomes more difficult and less reliable (Fig. 9–58).

(Text continued on page 970.)

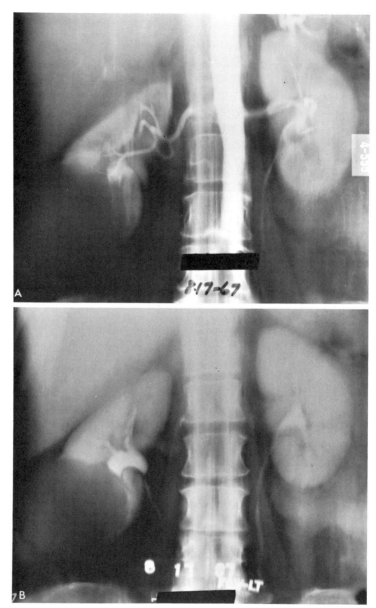

Figure 9–42. Simple cyst of right kidney. *Nephrotomograms.* **A,** *Arterial phase.* Cyst is avascular. No "tumor type" vessels or "tumor stain" is visible. **B,** *Nephrographic phase.* Cyst does not opacify and is of homogeneous density throughout. Wall is paper-thin and sharply demarcated from adjacent renal parenchyma.

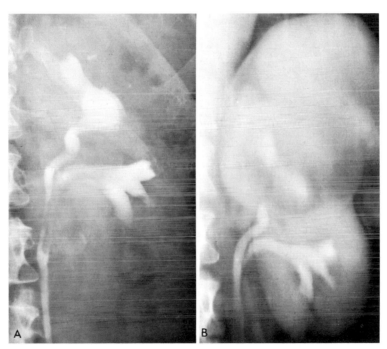

Figure 9–43.   Simple cyst upper pole of duplex kidney. **A**, *Excretory urogram.* Broadening, flattening, and splaying of calyces serving upper segment. **B**, *Nephrotomogram.* Circular radiolucent shadow of cyst with thin walls with typical acute crescentic angle visible laterally at junction of cyst wall with cortex.

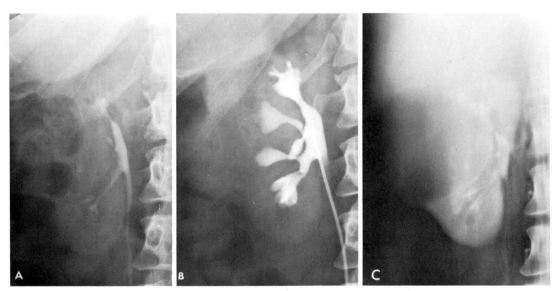

Figure 9–44. **Simple cyst. A,** *Excretory urogram.* **B,** *Retrograde pyelogram.* Both show expanding lesion in right kidney compressing middle calyces. **Cyst or tumor (?).** **C,** *Nephrotomogram.* Circular radiolucent avascular shadow proved to be **simple cyst.** In vascular phase (not shown here) blood vessels skirted cyst.

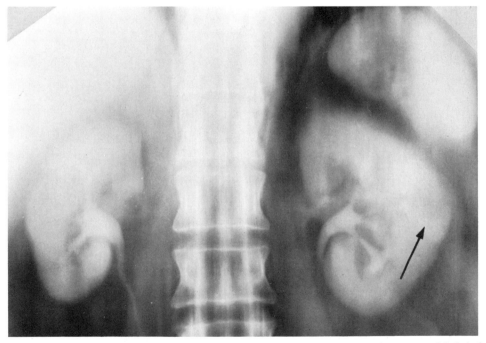

Figure 9–45. *Nephrotomogram.* Small circular radiolucent shadow at lateral margin of left kidney is **simple cyst** (*arrow*). Normal right kidney.

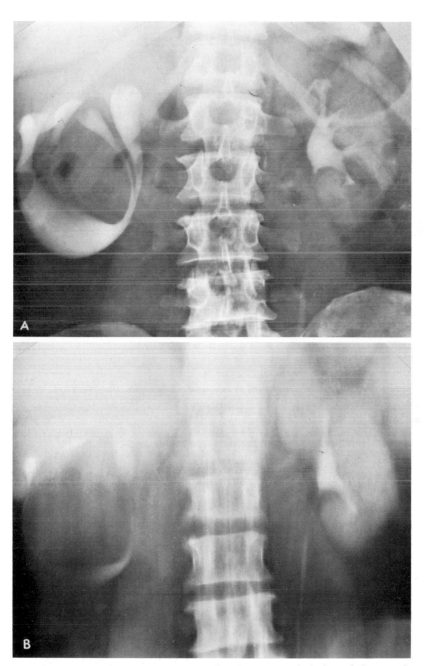

Figure 9–46. A, *Excretory urogram.* Peculiar expanding lesion in right kidney deforms pelvis and calyces. B, *Nephrotomogram.* Large circular radiolucent shadow shows lesion to be **simple cyst.** (Lesion incompletely demonstrated on single tomographic section shown here.)

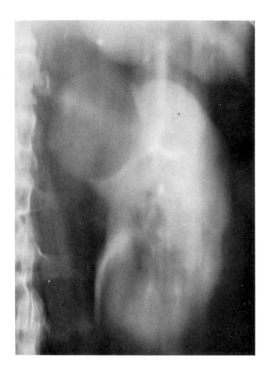

Figure 9–47. *Nephrotomogram.* Large **solitary simple cyst** of left kidney.

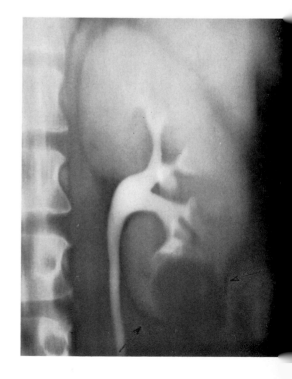

Figure 9–48. *Nephrotomogram, nephrographic phase.* Small **simple cyst** of lower pole of left kidney produces sharply circumscribed lucent filling defect in opacified renal parenchyma. Acute crescentic angles (*arrows*) are formed by protrusion of cyst outside kidney.

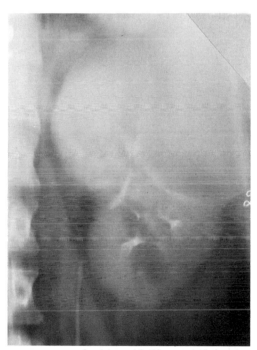

Figure 9–49.   *Nephrotomogram.* **Multiple cysts.** Two in upper pole are very large.

Fig. 9–50

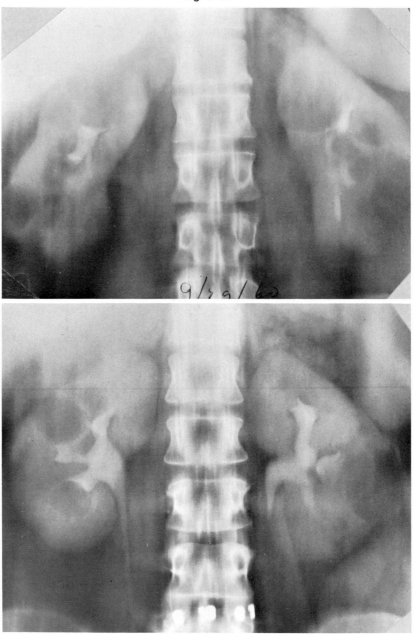

Fig. 9–51

Figure 9–50. *Nephrotomogram.* **Bilateral multiple renal cysts.** Multiple circular radiolucent shadows are well delineated.

Figure 9–51. *Nephrotomogram.* Multiple circular radiolucent shadows in both kidneys, indicating bilateral multiple renal cysts.

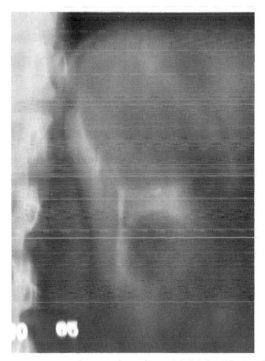

Figure 9–52. *Nephrotomogram, nephrographic phase.* **Multiple (2) simple cysts** of left kidney.

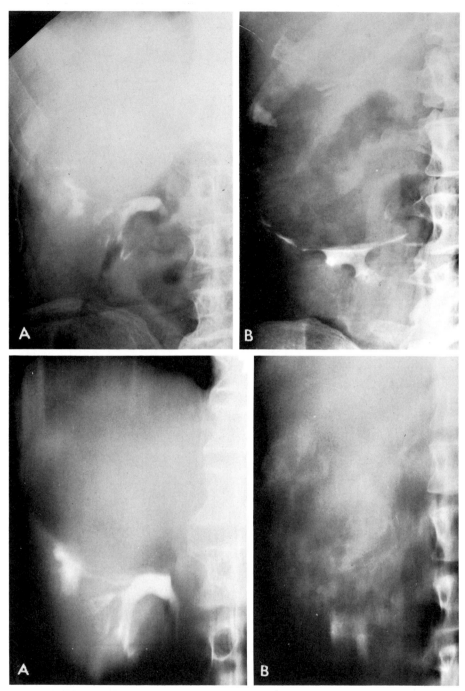

Figure 9–53. Problem of differential diagnosis (cyst versus tumor) in two cases in which excretory uro grams were similar. **A,** *Excretory urogram.* Lesion in upper pole of right kidney suggests **either cyst or tumo** **A′,** *Nephrotomogram* in same case as **A.** Radiolucent shadow without vascularization **shows that lesion** cyst. **B,** *Excretory urogram* in another case. Similar in appearance to **A. B′,** *Nephrotomogram.* **Increase** density with mottling of pathologic vascularization, "puddling," and "tumor staining" **shows lesion to b** **tumor.**

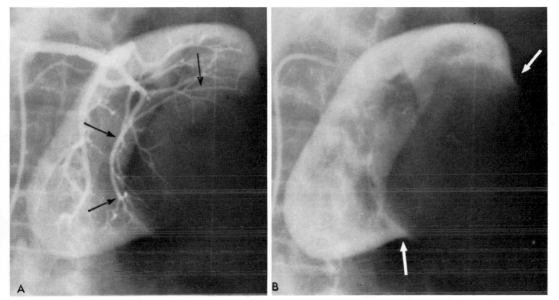

Figure 9–54.   Simple cyst. *Selective renal arteriograms.* **A,** *Arterial phase.* Renal arteries are displaced and stretched around cyst (*arrows*). No arteries enter mass. **B,** *Nephrographic phase.* Mass remains lucent and wall is sharply defined. Typical acute crescentic angles (*arrows*) are formed by renal cortex at junctions with cyst wall.

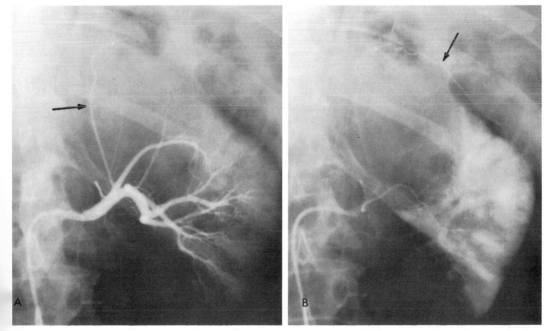

Figure 9–55.   Simple cyst, upper pole of left kidney. *Selective renal arteriograms.* **A,** *Arterial phase.* Arteries are stretched over and around cyst. No "tumor type" vessels are seen. Lower pole is supplied by accessory artery and is therefore unopacified in this selective arteriogram. **B,** *Nephrographic phase.* Cyst in upper pole is avascular and sharply demarcated from renal parenchyma. Prominent capsular artery (*arrow*) stretched over cyst.

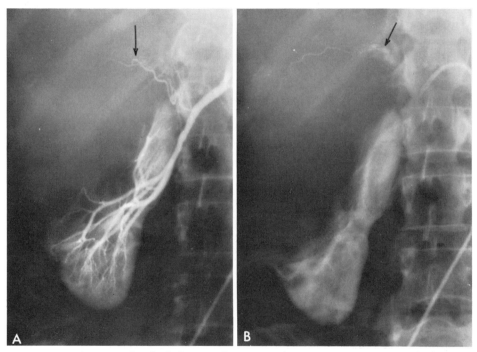

Figure 9–56. **Simple cyst** of right kidney. *Selective renal arteriograms.* **A,** *Arterial phase.* Intrarenal arteries and renal parenchyma are displaced by large avascular renal cyst. Capsular artery (*arrow*) courses over surface of cyst. **B,** *Nephrographic phase.* Cyst does not opacify, signifying its avascular character. Wall of cyst is not well seen after it protrudes through wall of kidney. Right adrenal gland is opacified (*arrow*).

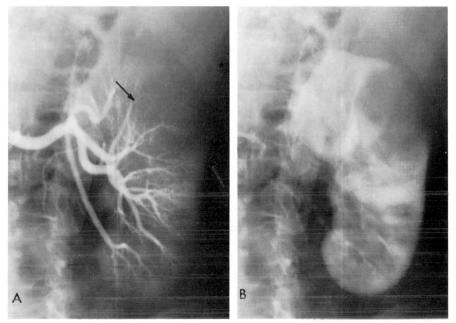

Figure 9–57.   **Simple cyst** of left kidney. *Selective renal arteriograms.* **A,** *Arterial phase.* Because of peripheral location of cyst (*arrows*), little displacement of renal arteries is present and lesion is difficult to identify in early arterial phase. **B,** *Nephrographic phase.* Radiolucent cyst is easily identified because of its sharp contrast with surrounding densely opacified renal parenchyma.

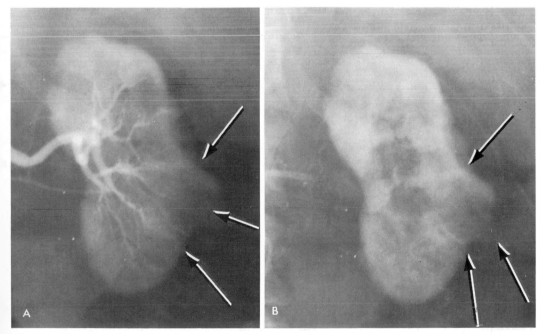

Figure 9–58.   Cyst simulating hypovascular hypernephroma. *Selective renal arteriograms.* **A,** *Arterial phase.* **B,** *Nephrographic phase.* Small cyst (*arrows*) is almost completely surrounded by normal renal parenchyma and appears to opacify. No "tumor type" vessels are seen, but appearance of mass simulates poorly vascularized hypernephroma.

Percutaneous Aspiration and Injection of Contrast Medium: The Renal Cystogram

Percutaneous needle aspiration of a renal cyst through the lumbar area (Dean) and injection of contrast medium into the cyst (DeWeerd; Lindblom, 1946; 1952) have been advocated in differential diagnosis. Aspiration of 15 ml or more of clear fluid plus the x-ray demonstration of a contrast-filled smooth-walled cavity without intracystic filling defects (Figs. 9–59 through 9–62) suggests cyst (DeWeerd). Findings which cause one to suspect tumor include the aspiration of turbid, cloudy, or hemorrhagic fluid, tissue, or debris and a plain film suggesting an irregular cavity with filling defects or no cavity at all. Although there has been considerable criticism of this procedure, much of it does not appear to be valid. Use of Papanicolaou's stain for the aspirated fluid is, of course, a routine procedure.

Recently we have begun evaluating expanding lesions of the kidney in selected cases by percutaneous aspiration in a manner similar to that recommended by Lalli (1967) (Figs. 9–63, 9–64, and 9–65). We do this under local anesthesia, on an outpatient basis, using image-intensification techniques. Although our experience as yet is quite limited, we think this approach to the problem of cyst versus tumor holds promise. We have not used it as a routine procedure, but we have found it to be of definite value in evaluation of the elderly patient who has a renal mass which is not clearly a cyst or a tumor by nephrotomography and whose physical condition makes him a significant surgical risk.

The Problem of Management

The clinical decision of when to explore and when not to explore a presumed renal "cyst" is not as simple as it appears to be. The dogmatic statement that every case must be explored may represent oversimplification of the problem. For instance, in clinical practice this problem is especially troublesome in aged patients, usually 65 years or older, who are being examined for problems totally unrelated to the kidney. Many of these patients are obese and have many physical and mental problems associated with degenerative disease. Surgical exploration of such patients carries not only a definite risk but also a definite morbidity, and it introduces socioeconomic problems that may strain the resources of their families. One must ask if it is sound medical practice to submit 300 or 500 such patients to operation to find one tumor; also, if this one tumor is found, is nephrectomy a sufficiently "curative procedure" to justify exploration of so many patients who do not have tumors. At times the effort toward diagnostic perfection may be pushed to ridiculous and unrewarding heights.

(Text continued on page 976.)

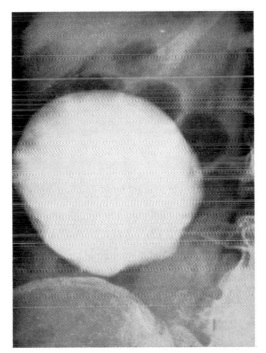

Figure 9–59. *Percutaneous renal cystogram.* **Simple cyst.** (From Ainsworth, W. L., and Vest, S. A.)

Fig. 9–60

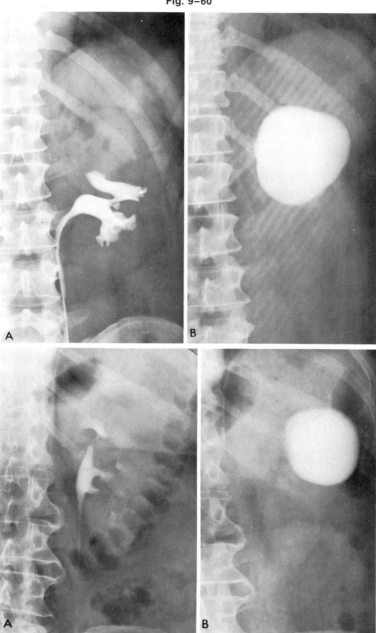

Fig. 9–61

Figure 9–60.   Simple cyst. **A,** *Retrograde pyelogram* suggests either cyst or tumor of upper pole of kidney. **B,** *Percutaneous renal cystogram* (contrast medium injected through needle introduced in lumbar area) shows smooth-walled cyst. (From DeWeerd, J. H.)

Figure 9–61.   Simple cyst. **A,** *Excretory urogram.* Expanding lesion of right kidney, cyst or tumor (?) **B,** *Percutaneous renal cystogram.* Clear fluid aspirated plus smooth walls confirms diagnosis of **simple cyst.** (From DeWeerd, J. H.)

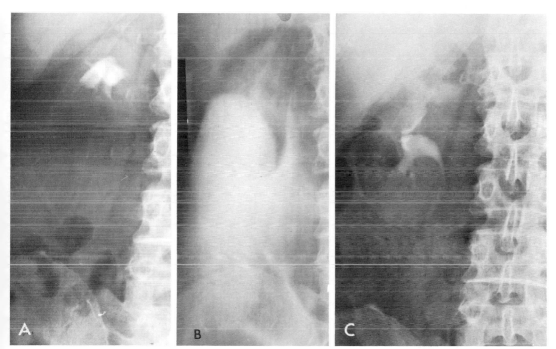

Figure 9–62. Large simple cyst which "disappeared" following percutaneous renal cystogram. **A,** *Excretory urogram* show large circular soft-tissue shadow compressing calyces of right kidney. **B,** *Percutaneous renal cystogram*. Film shows extravasation of medium outside cyst. **C,** *Excretory urogram* several weeks after aspiration. Cyst has disappeared and pyelogram shows return to normal. (From DeWeerd, J. H.)

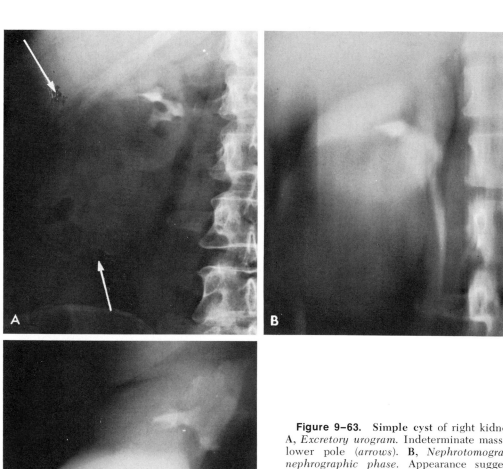

Figure 9–63. Simple cyst of right kidney.
A, *Excretory urogram.* Indeterminate mass at
lower pole (*arrows*). **B,** *Nephrotomogram,*
nephrographic phase. Appearance suggests
cyst, but necrotic carcinoma is not excluded.
C, *Percutaneous renal cystogram.* Cyst was
filled with straw-colored fluid, and wall has
smooth outline.

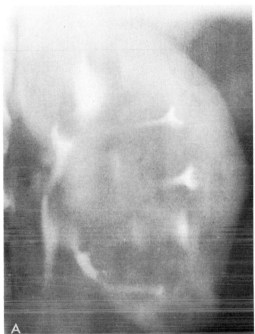

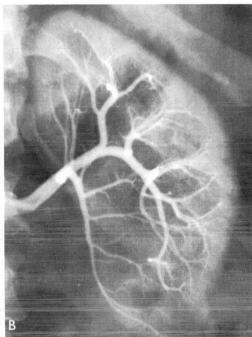

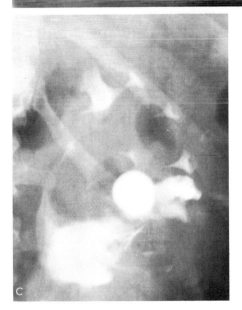

Figure 9–64.   Multiple simple cysts of left kidney. **A,** *Nephrotomogram* and **B,** *selective left renal arteriogram* demonstrate avascular aspect of mass. **C,** *Percutaneous renal cystogram.* Several cysts are outlined. There is some leakage of contrast medium around cysts. (From Lalli, A. F.)

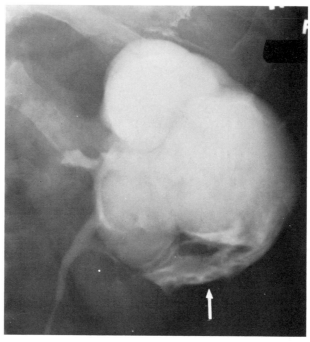

Figure 9–65. *Percutaneous renal cystogram.* **Cyst with multiple septa.** Small amount of medium has extravasated from cyst puncture site into perirenal tissues (*arrow*).

PERIPELVIC CYSTS

Peripelvic cyst is a loosely used clinical term to describe cysts which arise in the region of the hilus of the kidney. Because of the restricted confines of the area, their expansion is limited and they rarely become larger than 5 cm in diameter. They tend to insinuate themselves so deeply into the sinus renalis that at operation they may not be apparent until all of the connective tissue has been carefully cleaned away from the renal pelvis and calyces.

There are several theories of pathogenesis. Most peripelvic cysts are no doubt simple cysts arising from the renal parenchyma in the region of the sinus renalis. The others are more difficult to explain. Henthorne postulated a lymphatic origin. His reasons were that they seemed to be inseparable from the renal pelvis, were insinuated deeply into the sinus renalis, and coursed along the major blood vessels in a fashion suggestive of lymphatic trunks. The histologic composition of the cyst wall has been described as concentric layers of fibrocytes similar in appearance to the wall of a lymphatic cyst. Thompson more recently concluded that there is insufficient evidence that lymphatic ectasia is responsible. Scholl suggested the possibility that some may arise from remnants of the wolffian body.

Growth of the cyst is usually at the expense of the renal pelvis, the encroachment producing unusual types of pelvic distortion as well as occasional obstruction (pyelectasis or calycectasis or both) (Jordan; Lieberthal). Obviously a wide variety of pelvic and calyceal deformity results in rather bizarre types of urograms. These urographic changes are difficult to describe but when once seen are usually not difficult to recognize if the possibility of peripelvic cyst is kept in mind (Figs. 9–66 through 9–75; see also Fig. 5–41).

(Text continued on page 981.)

Fig. 9–66 Fig. 9–67

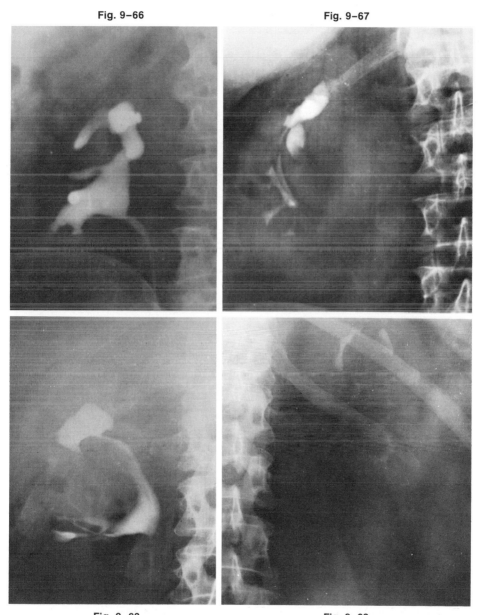

Fig. 9–68 Fig. 9–69

Figures 9–66, 9–67, 9–68, and 9–69. *Retrograde pyelograms.* Examples of peripelvic cysts.

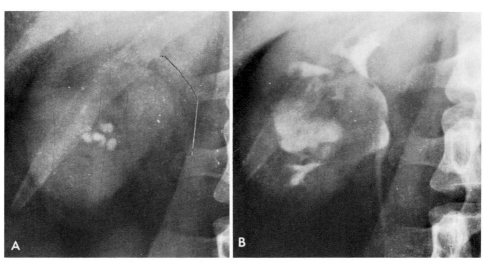

Figure 9–70. Peripelvic cyst obstructing middle calyx resulted in formation of secondary calculi. **A,** *Plain film.* Multiple calculi overlying lower pole of right kidney. **B,** *Excretory urogram.* Peripelvic cyst, which has obstructed one of middle calyces resulting in calycectasis and secondary calculi. (Diagnosis proved surgically.)

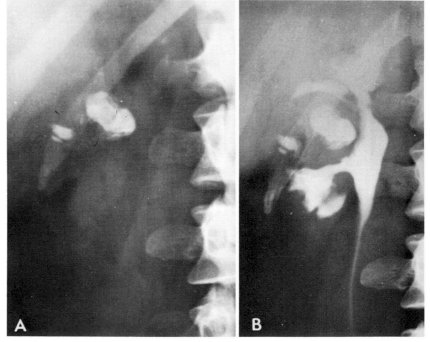

Figure 9–71. Peripelvic cyst causing calyceal obstruction and nephrolithiasis. **A,** *Plain film.* Calcific shadows overlying right renal area. **B,** *Right retrograde pyelogram.* Deformity of lateral margin of pelvis and apparent obliteration of middle calyces which seem to include calculi. (Surgical exploration showed stone in middle calyx, marked cortical infection, and many cysts of various sizes arising from renal pelvis.)

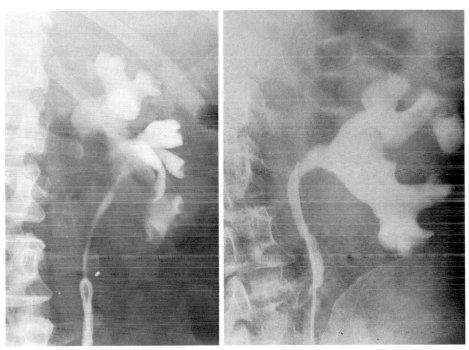

Fig. 9–72   Fig. 9–73

Figure 9–72. *Retrograde pyelogram.* **Peripelvic cyst.** Note ureteral catheter looped back on itself.

Figure 9–73. *Retrograde pyelogram.* **Multiple peripelvic cysts** (largest was 4 cm in diameter) causing calycectasis in man, 76 years of age. (Diagnosis proved surgically. Nephrectomy done because surgeon could not be sure tumor was not present.)

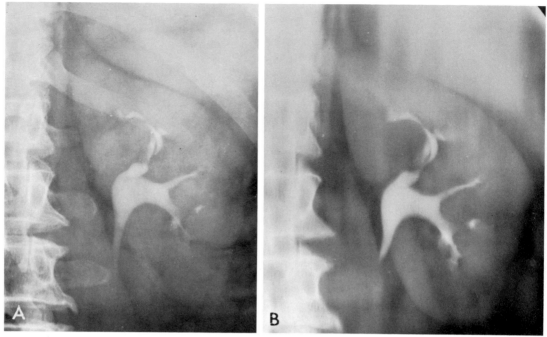

Figure 9–74. Peripelvic cyst in man, 52 years of age. **A,** *Retrograde pyelogram.* Crescentic deformity of upper calyces of left kidney. **B,** *Nephrotomogram.* Small circular radiolucent shadow of cyst situated medial to infundibulum of upper calyx. Difficult to decide whether this should be classified as simple cyst or peripelvic cyst.

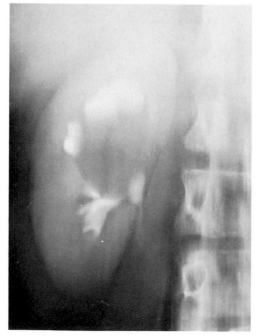

Figure 9–75. *Nephrotomogram.* Rather large **peripelvic cyst.** Circular radiolucent shadow encroaches on pelvis and obstructs middle and upper calyces.

CONGENITAL RENAL CYSTIC DISEASE

by

Charles C. Rife

and

David M. Witten

Classification and Pathogenesis

Classification of congenital renal cystic disease is confused and controversial. Uniform terminology has been slow in developing, and the confusion surrounding these lesions is made worse by the multiplicity of names which have been given to various pathologic entities as well as by attempts to classify lesions which are in all likelihood distinct separate entities as of one type. In the final analysis, however, the basic difficulty is our incomplete knowledge of the pathogenesis and natural history of renal cystic disease.

Most authors recognize a number of types of congenital cysts, including such clinical entities as multilocular cyst, unilateral multicystic disease, medullary sponge kidney, and the various forms of congenital polycystic disease. A number of other lesions such as calyceal "cysts" or diverticula, parapelvic cysts, and even simple serous cysts have been considered congenital by some authors; but the evidence to support this view is inconclusive.

The greatest uncertainty and confusion surround *congenital polycystic disease.* Traditionally, two major types, adult and infantile, have been recognized; but most authorities (Arey; Gwinn and Landing; Morehead; Osathanondh and Potter; Spence, Baird, and Ware; Wahlqvist) now agree that the term *congenital polycystic disease,* as commonly used, includes a number of clinically distinct and pathologically unrelated cystic malformations of the kidney.

Microdissection Studies of Osathanondh and Potter

In 1964, Osathanondh and Potter published the results of a series of excellent microdissection studies of kidneys from patients with "polycystic" disease, which have provided new insight into the pathogenesis, histopathology, and anatomic interrelationships of the various forms of congenital cystic disease. These studies revealed a number of previously unrecognized anatomic differences between types of polycystic disease which had been regarded as clinically similar by most investigators and at the same time demonstrated that lesions such as multilocular cyst, unilateral multicystic kidney, and medullary sponge kidney may be localized or limited forms of these same processes. From their dissections, Osathanondh and Potter have reclassified the congenital cystic diseases on the basis of pathogenesis. They recognize four types.

CLASSIFICATION OF OSATHANONDH AND POTTER

Type I. Type I cystic disease is *thought to develop from hyperplasia of the interstitial* portions of the collecting tubules *developing from the ureteral bud.* This lesion is found only in newborn infants and is apparently incompatible with prolonged life. Associated cystic changes are always found in the liver. The disease is probably hereditary with transmission as a non-sex-linked (autosomal) recessive trait. It includes the classical form of "infantile polycystic disease" and has been described at times by the terms *polycystic disease of the newborn, hamartomatous polycystic kidney,* and *sponge kidney.*

Type II. Type II cystic disease *results from inhibition of developmental activity in the ampullary portions* of the develop-

---

° According to Osathanondh and Potter, the youngest branches of the ureteral bud consist of two parts: the *ampulla,* which is the zone of growth at the end of the tubule, and the *interstitial portion,* which is the part formed and left behind as the ampulla advances.

ing renal tubules, which interferes with division of tubules and induction of nephrons. As a result, few branches of collecting tubules and few nephrons are formed. In this condition, cysts are limited to the terminal or ampullary portions of the collecting tubules and no normal renal tissue is found in involved regions. Associated ureteral abnormalities are commonly seen, such as ureteral agenesis, atresia, and irregular dilatations of the ureter. The lesion may involve only a portion of a kidney, the entire kidney, or in rare instances both kidneys. It is commonly known as *multilocular cystic disease* when only a portion of one kidney is involved and as *unilateral multicystic disease* when an entire kidney is involved. It has also been described in the literature as *hypoplastic, aplastic, dysgenetic,* and *dysplastic cystic kidney.* If localized, the lesion is compatible with a normal life, but the rare bilateral form seen in newborn infants is not compatible with life. In contrast to types I and III, this lesion is apparently not familial and does not occur in association with cystic abnormalities of the liver, pancreas, or lung.

Type III. Type III is the common form of "adult type" polycystic disease and is the form most frequently encountered in clinical practice. It is almost always bilateral and is found in children as well as in adults. The renal malformation is much less uniform than in types I and II, and normal and abnormal areas are intermixed. It appears to *result from multiple abnormalities of development which include abnormalities of both the interstitial* (see preceding footnote) *and ampullary portions of the collecting tubule as well as abnormalities of branching of ampullae and induction of nephrons.* Any part of the nephron or collecting tubule may become enlarged and cystic. The lesion is often seen with a definite familial predisposition and may be transmitted as an autosomal dominant trait. Associated cysts of the liver are found in about one third of the cases.

Type IV. In this type, the abnormalities in the kidneys are *associated with urethral obstruction in early fetal life.* The cysts are usually small and located mainly beneath the renal capsule. They result from dilatation of Bowman's space and may be associated with diffuse mild dilatation of collecting tubules resulting from increased intralobular pressure. Cystic changes in the liver are not found in association with this type and no familial tendency is present.

While the classification proposed by Osathanondh and Potter just outlined has been of great help in clarifying the pathogenesis and structural relationships of the various types of congenital cystic disease, it is often difficult to correlate these concepts with the clinical problems of diagnosis, treatment, and prognosis. For this reason we have chosen to retain the more conventional clinical nomenclature and classification, as follows:

CLINICAL CLASSIFICATION OF CONGENITAL RENAL CYSTIC DISEASE

   I. Congenital polycystic disease
     A. In newborn babies, infants, and children
     B. In adults
  II. Multilocular cyst
 III. Unilateral multicystic kidney
 IV. Cystic disease associated with obstruction of the lower urinary tract
  V. Medullary sponge kidney

Congenital Polycystic Disease

Polycystic Disease of Infants and Children

Polycystic malformations of the kidney found in newborn babies, infants, and children have been grouped together by most authors under the term *infantile type polycystic disease.* Until recently, the

ajority have considered these lesions
be one disease or one disease with sev-
ral subvarieties. Recent evidence sug-
ests that this is a greatly oversimplified
iew and that a number of distinct types
an be identified which differ in their
inical and pathologic pictures, genetic
ansmission, and roentgenographic char-
cteristics. (See preceding discussion
ncerning classification and pathogene-
s of congenital renal cystic diseases.)

Infantile Polycystic Disease. Infantile
ype of polycystic disease, also referred
as *polycystic disease of the new-*
orn, hamartomatous polycystic disease,
ponge kidney, and more recently by
Osathanondh and Potter as *congenital*
enal cystic disease, type I, is found only
the newborn infant, is invariably bi-
ateral, and is incompatible with pro-
nged survival. Siblings may be affected
nd the disease is hereditary with non-
ex-linked (autosomal) recessive inher-
ance (Dalgaard; Lundin and Olow). The
asic abnormality, according to Osatha-
ondh and Potter, is hyperplasia of the
nterstitial portions of the collecting tu-
ules which develop from the ureteral
uds. *Grossly,* the kidneys are symme-
rically enlarged with the cortical surface
tudded with small cysts. The *cut surface*
as the appearance of a sponge, with gross
ystic dilatation of tubules radiating
hrough the entire thickness of the kid-
ey (Fig. 9–76). Cystic proliferation of the
ile ducts is always present, prompting
Gwinn and Landing to suggest the name
nfantile polycystic disease of the kidney
nd liver for this syndrome. Pancreatic
r pulmonary cysts have been reported,
ut there is doubt that they in fact are
ound in this disease. *Clinically,* these
atients have large palpable kidneys and
re subject to respiratory and cardiac dif-
iculties as newborn infants. In those who
urvive the newborn period, hypertension
nd increasing renal insufficiency develop.
ccording to Gwinn and Landing, the
oentgenographic findings are striking.
hey describe the characteristic appear-
nce as follows:

. . . the massively enlarged kidneys can be seen
on the plain films of the abdomen as soft tissue
masses [Fig. 9–77]. In the excretory urogram,
there is often a delay of several minutes to
hours before there is visualization of contrast
medium in the kidneys. Usually, a nephrogram
effect is first seen, with the contrast medium
visible throughout the kidneys. The image has
a streaky pattern, from the medulla to the surface of the cortex, with a suggestion of alternating radiodense and radiolucent radially aligned
areas [Figs. 9–78 and 9–79]. There is typically
an insufficient concentration to visualize the
collecting structures and ureters, even though
contrast medium is seen in the bladder.

**"Adult Type" Polycystic Disease Found
in Children.** This disease also has been
referred to as *microcystic disease* and by
Osathanondh and Potter as *congenital
renal cystic disease, type III.* Although
this is the common form of polycystic disease found in adult patients, many authors
have recognized that it also may occur in
infancy and childhood. However, Osathanondh and Potter have pointed out that
when seen in pediatric patients it has been
confused with other types of polycystic
disease and that it is probably more common in infancy and childhood than had
been suspected previously. Their dissections revealed that the disease in infants
and adults is identical except for differences directly due to age.

Familial Bilateral Cystic Dysplasia.
Despite the facts that Osathanondh and
Potter have classified all renal cysts which
resemble those seen in adult polycystic
disease into type III and that this has been
accepted by many authors (Anderson;
Kissane and Smith), Gwinn and Landing
contend that another form of cystic disease
is seen in infants and children which does
not fit into either the infantile type I or
the adult type III groups. They have designated this lesion *familial bilateral cystic
dysplasia* and described it as bilateral with
kidneys which are large but of normal
shape and contour. "Cysts are located in
both cortex and medulla and are of varying size, but do not reach the size seen in
adult polycystic disease." Dysplastic features are prominent, and they think that

both the renal lesion and an associated lesion of the liver differ grossly and microscopically from corresponding lesions of infantile polycystic disease (type I). The condition may be found in siblings and appears to be a genetically determined disorder with autosomal recessive transmission which clearly would distinguish it from the adult type polycystic disease (type III). Clinically, this form is present in infancy, but it is much more likely to be recognized in early childhood. Roentgenographically, according to Gwinn and Landing, both kidneys are large and smooth in outline. The excretory urogram shows that

. . . the renal collecting structures are visualized, and contrast medium can be seen in the renal pyramids, presumably in the ectatic collecting ducts [Fig. 9–80]. It is not, as a rule, seen to the periphery of the kidney, as occurs in "infantile polycystic disease."

They also mentioned that the calyces are wide and blunted, with short wide infundibula but without the splayed appearance seen in adult type polycystic disease (Fig. 9–81).

(*Text continued on page 987.*)

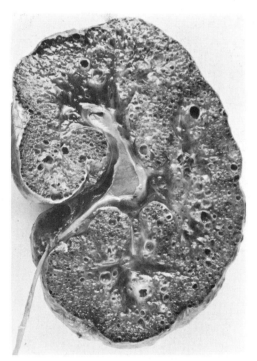

Figure 9–76.   Infantile type polycystic kidney. Cut section. Note uniformity of size of cysts.

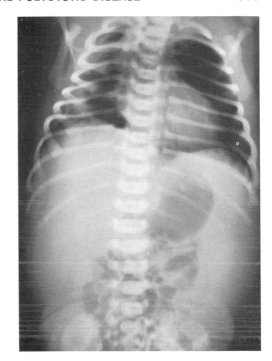

Figure 9–77. *Plain film.* Infantile polycystic disease. Massively enlarged kidneys displace gas-containing bowel to midline. (From Gwinn, J. L., and Landing, B. H.)

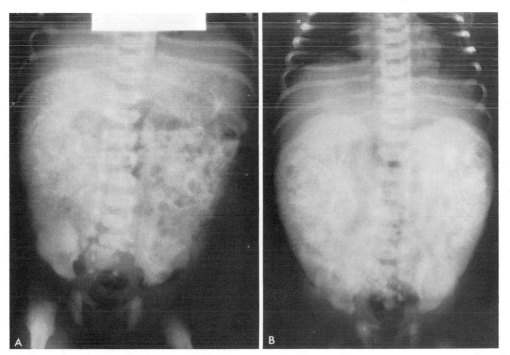

Figure 9–78. Infantile polycystic disease. **A,** *Five-hour* and **B,** *18-hour excretory urograms* of newborn infant. Nephrogram effect of huge kidneys is apparent, as is radially aligned pattern of streaky opacification of renal parenchyma. Pelviocalyceal structures are not visualized. (From Gwinn, J. L., and Landing, B. H.)

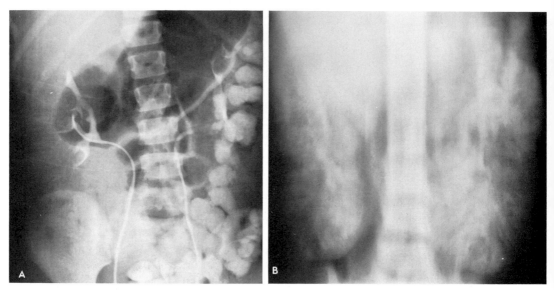

Figure 9–79. Congenital polycystic disease in 8-year-old girl. **A,** *Bilateral retrograde pyelogram.* Kidneys are enlarged and pelviocalyceal system is distorted. Opaque material in bowel obscures left kidney. **B,** *Excretory urogram with tomogram.* Markedly enlarged kidneys with streaky opacification of renal parenchyma, typical of infantile polycystic disease. (Courtesy of Dr. R. Nesbit.)

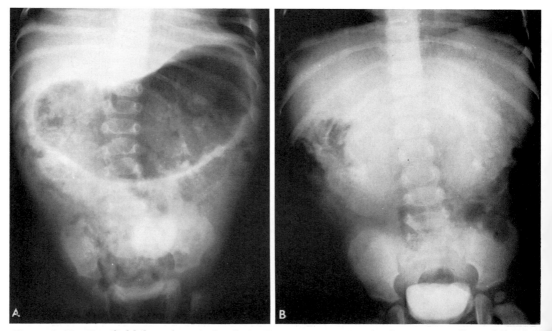

Figure 9–80. Familial bilateral cystic dysplasia. *Excretory urograms.* **A,** *Thirty-minute film* and **B,** *2-hour film.* Large kidneys, contrast medium in collecting ducts, and visualization of collecting structures. (From Gwinn, J. L., and Landing, B. H.)

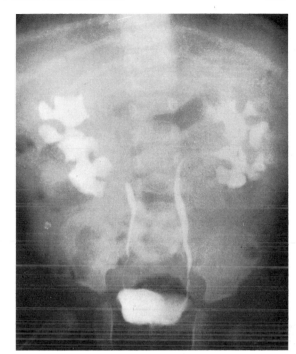

Figure 9–81. *Bilateral retrograde pyelogram.* **Familial bilateral cystic dysplasia.** Calyces are wide and blunted, and infundibula are short and wide (compare this with Fig. 9–79). (From Gwinn, J. L., and Landing, B. H.)

Polycystic Disease in Adults

"Adult type" polycystic disease is the most common form of polycystic disease encountered in clinical practice (Fig. 9–82). Bell has estimated its incidence at autopsy at 1:351. The malformation is considered by most authors to be bilateral and hereditary (Dalgaard) with transmission as an autosomal dominant trait. Many cases are seen, however, in which no family history suggestive of polycystic disease can be obtained. Associated cysts in the liver are found in about one third of the cases; in rare cases cysts are also encountered in the pancreas and lung. Osathanondh and Potter designate this lesion as *type III* in their classification and report that it results from multiple abnormalities of development of the renal tubules. They state that the lesion is generally but not always bilateral and that it is **characterized by an irregular intermixture of normal and abnormal tubules and nephrons.** Cysts of various sizes may be found arising from any part of the nephron, but most commonly they involve Bowman's space, the angle of the loop of Henle, or the proximal convoluted tubule. **Continuity of the cyst with the remainder of the nephron is maintained in all instances.** The onset of symptoms, Osathanondh and Potter think, varies in relation to the proportion of normal and abnormal structures present. If the abnormal structures predominate in the kidney, the disease may be evident at birth. This form often has been confused with other types of "infantile" polycystic disease in the past, where it usually has been called *microcystic disease* because of the small size of the cysts in patients at this age.

In most instances, normal structures predominate and diagnosis is usually not made until the fourth or fifth decade of life, after the cysts have slowly enlarged to the point where symptoms appear. At this stage, the kidneys are large and may be palpable, hypertension is often present, and pain and gross hematuria are common. Azotemia and progressive renal failure are evidence of far-advanced disease.

Preclinical polycystic disease of the "adult type" is rarely recognized, but careful examination of "suspected" patients (usually children of patients with proved polycystic disease) with tomography and large doses of urographic medium will often reveal early asymptomatic disease. We have, in a few instances, demonstrated its presence in asymptomatic children from 10 years to 15 years of age who were studied because of polycystic disease in the family. In these cases, the size of the kidneys may be normal or only slightly increased. The cysts are small, though numerous and variable in size.

Roentgenographic Diagnosis. The plain film usually demonstrates large irregular renal outlines. The psoas muscle shadows may be obscured, and the bowel may be displaced by the enlarged kidneys. Renal size varies widely; thus the kidneys may be only slightly enlarged in some instances, while in others they may be so large that they appear to fill the entire abdomen. Plaques of calcium may be seen scattered about in the walls of the cysts.

On the **urogram** the disease is characterized by elongation, irregular enlargement, and bizarre distortion of the calyces (Figs. 9–83 through 9–87). In some patients, one kidney is considerably larger than the other because of larger or more numerous cysts. Occasionally, the difference in size is so great that the disease appears to be unilateral. Bulbous enlargement or splaying of the ends of the calyces is often observed in contrast to the narrowing or tapering of the calyx seen frequently with neoplasm, but occasionally only one or two calyces appear involved and differentiation from simple cyst or carcinoma may be difficult. Often the ends of the calyces have a crescentic outline due to the presence of an adjacent cyst. The outline of the pelvis itself may not be greatly altered, in contradistinction to the deformity often observed in the pelvic outline in cases of neoplasm or of large or multiple simple cysts. In some in-

stances, depression of renal function or deformity of the renal pelvis and calyces by cysts may result in such poor filling of the collecting system that a **retrograde pyelogram** must be employed for diagnosis.

The *renal parenchyma* is thickened and irregular. When adequate renal function and normal renal tissue remain to provide good opacification of the kidney, the nephrogram, in a typical case, has a distinctive mottled (nonhomogeneous) "honeycomb," "Swiss-cheese," or "sponge-like" appearance due to the presence of innumerable radiolucent cysts of various sizes throughout the kidney (Figs. 9–88 and 9–89). This feature may be seen on films of good quality made early in the filming sequence of the excretory urogram (30 seconds to 5 minutes) (Halpern, Dalrymple, and Young), but in our experience it is best seen on tomograms made 3 to 5 minutes after injection of a large volume (100 to 150 ml) of urographic contrast medium either by the drip infusion technique or by nephrotomography (Figs. 9–90, 9–91, and 9–92).

Arteriography may offer considerable help in the study of polycystic kidneys (Billing; Ettinger, Kahn, and Wise; Meaney and Corvalan). Intrarenal arterial branches are stretched, elongated, and displaced by the myriad of cysts (Figs. 9–93 and 9–94), and an abnormally large amount of renal substance peripheral to termination of arterial branches is noted usually. An absence of "tumor vessels" or "tumor stain" helps exclude renal neoplasm. During the late or nephrographic phase of the arteriogram (Figs. 9–95 and 9–96) the kidneys appear abnormally large and the distinctive mottled or Swiss-cheese appearance just described is seen in the majority of cases (seven of nine cases reported by Cornell).

The distinctive roentgenographic abnormality seen on the nephrogram has been recognized only in recent years, as the result of improvements in roentgenographic technique, and its recognition has facilitated the detection of polycystic disease, especially in patients who have not yet developed symptoms. Despite this, atypical or less-advanced cases are often encountered, in which it is difficult or impossible to distinguish polycystic disease from multiple bilateral simple cysts by excretory urography, nephrotomography, or angiography (Figs. 9–97 and 9–98). In such cases, one must rely on clinical data and the family history. Even with this information, however, borderline cases with minimal involvement are encountered, in which it may be difficult even for a pathologist to make an unequivocal distinction.

Cystic Disease (Dysplasia) Associated With Obstruction of Lower Urinary Tract

Cystic disease associated with urethral or other lower urinary tract obstruction which Osathanondh and Potter have designated type IV is rarely recognized as a clinical entity but appears to be a rather common finding on pathologic examination of the kidneys from patients with obstruction of the lower urinary tract in fetal life, especially in boys with congenital urethral valves. Apparently the renal abnormalities develop during the early fetal period, when renal collecting tubules are relatively short and straight. The obstruction to the flow of urine at the proximal part of the urethra transmits a back pressure to the bladder, ureters, renal pelvis, and nephron with resultant dilatation and thickening of the more proximal transport system along with formation of numerous tiny cysts throughout the renal cortex. The degree and severity of involvement depend on the degree of obstruction and the fetal age at which urinary obstruction occurs. Apparently lesser degrees of involvement are compatible with a normal life-span. Hydronephrosis, which accompanies this abnormality, obscures roentgenographic evidence of the cystic changes in the kidney so that the condition is rarely if ever suspected on the basis of urography.

(Text continued on page 1007.)

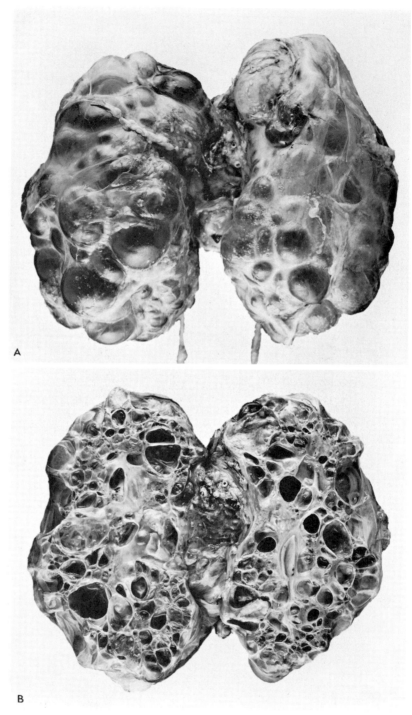

Figure 9–82.   Adult type polycystic kidney. **A,** *Uncut surfaces.* Note renal contour is retained. **B,** *Cu section.* There is no uniformity in size of cysts.

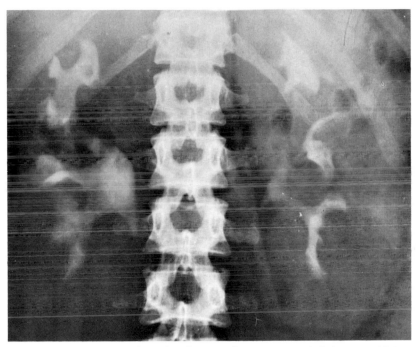

Figure 9–83. *Excretory urogram.* **Bilateral polycystic disease.** Typical deformity of bilateral polycystic disease. Note large size of both kidneys, which can be seen best on left.

Fig. 9–84

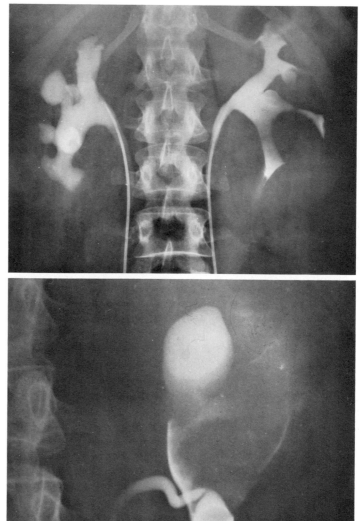

Fig. 9–85

Figure 9–84. *Bilateral retrograde pyelogram.* Deformity of left kidney suggests large simple cyst of lowe pole of left kidney. However, large kidney on right, with broad flaring calyces, suggests possible polycysti disease. (Surgical exploration of left kidney revealed typical **polycystic disease**.)

Figure 9–85. *Left retrograde pyelogram.* **Polycystic disease associated with hydronephrosis.** (Surgica exploration showed multiple cysts projected against pelvis and producing marked hydronephrosis. Lef nephrectomy. Polycystic disease, corroborated on pathologic examination.)

Fig. 9–86

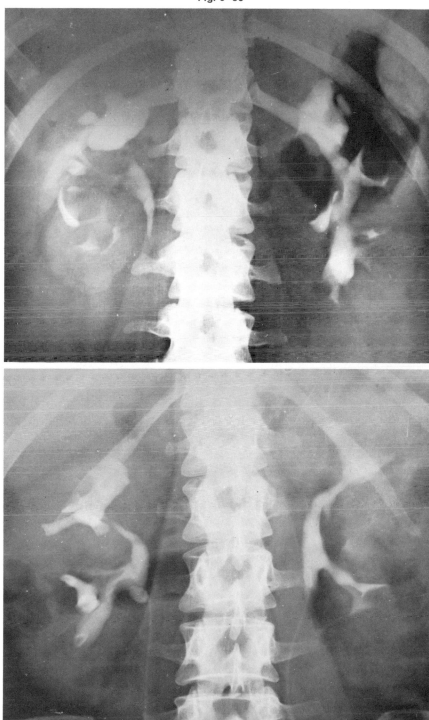

Fig. 9–87

Figure 9–86. *Excretory urogram.* Typical urographic deformity of **bilateral polycystic disease.**
Figure 9–87. *Bilateral retrograde pyelogram.* Urographic deformity of **bilateral polycystic disease.**

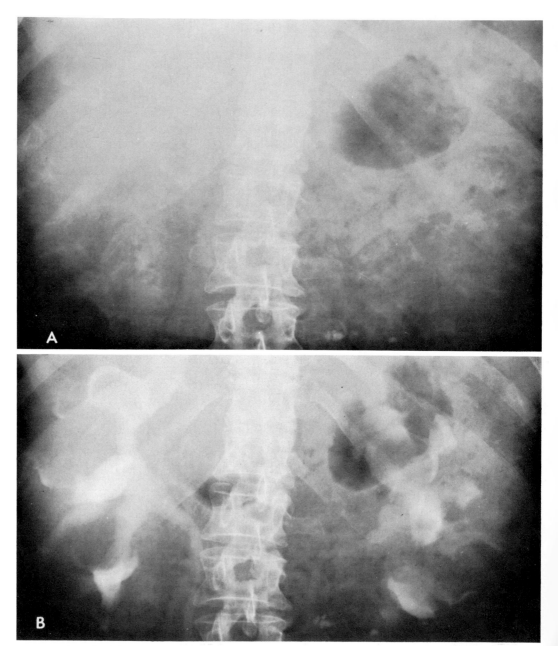

Figure 9–88. "Adult type" polycystic disease. *Excretory urograms.* **A,** *Ten-minute film.* Large kidney with mottled opacification of parenchyma due to presence of innumerable cysts. Mottling is disordered contrasted to "streaky" pattern of infantile polycystic disease. **B,** *Forty-five-minute film.* Typical distortio of calyces due to cystic abnormality.

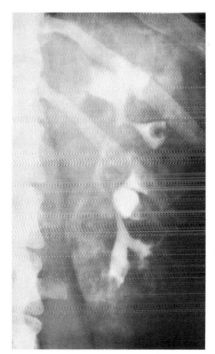

Figure 9–89. *Excretory urogram.* **"Adult type" polycystic disease.** Mottled opacification of renal paren-
hyma due to presence of innumerable lucent cysts. Typical spreading and deformity of calyces are present.

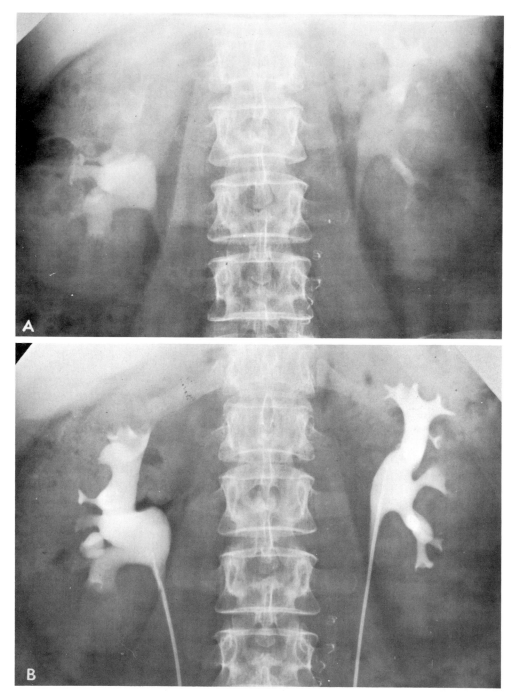

Figure 9–90. *See legend on facing page.*

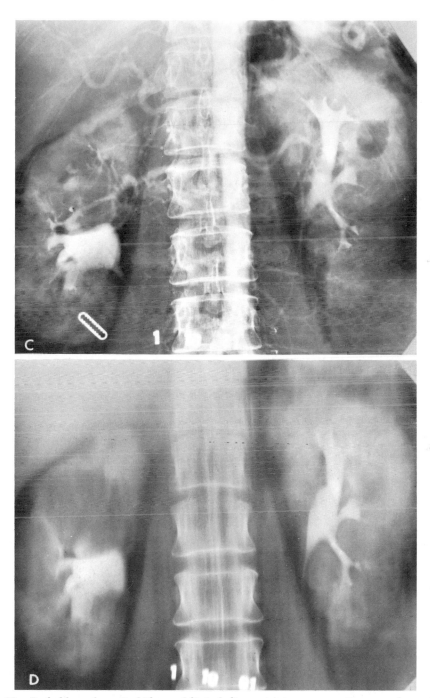

Figure 9–90. Probable polycystic kidneys (clinical diagnosis) in woman, 49 years of age. No familial story could be elicited and patient had no hypertension as yet. **A** (*see facing page*), *Excretory urogram.* (*see facing page*), *Bilateral retrograde pyelograms.* Peculiar broad calyces could be considered either riation of normal or pathologic. **C,** *Nephrogram* (not tomogram), *arterial phase.* **D,** *Nephrotomogram,* *phrographic phase.* Multiple cysts of various sizes (radiolucent areas), produce mottled or honeycombed pearance in the opacified renal parenchyma.

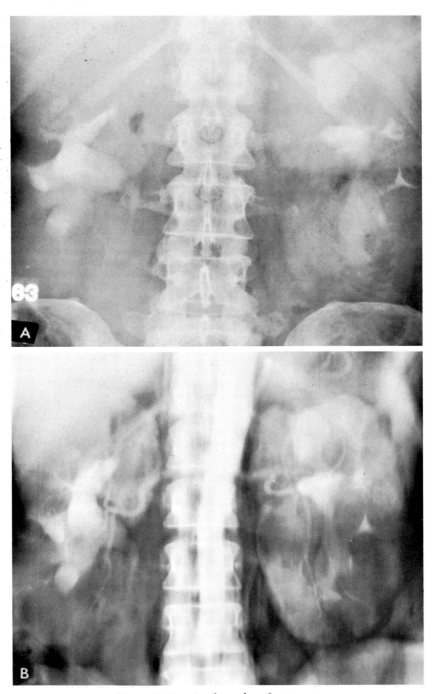

Figure 9–91   *See legend on facing page.*

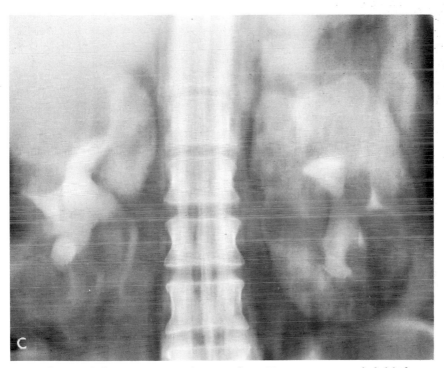

Figure 9–91.   Polycystic kidneys in woman, 53 years of age. Ten years previously left kidney was explored urgically because of pain and about 50 cysts varying in size from that of baseball to 0.5 cm in diameter were xcised or punctured. **A** (*see facing page*), *Excretory urogram.* **B** (*see facing page*), *Nephrotomogram* (vascular hase). **C**, *Nephrotomogram (nephrographic phase).* Note "honeycomb" or "Swiss-cheese" appearance of arenchyma from innumerable cysts. No areas of parenchyma free of cysts can be identified.

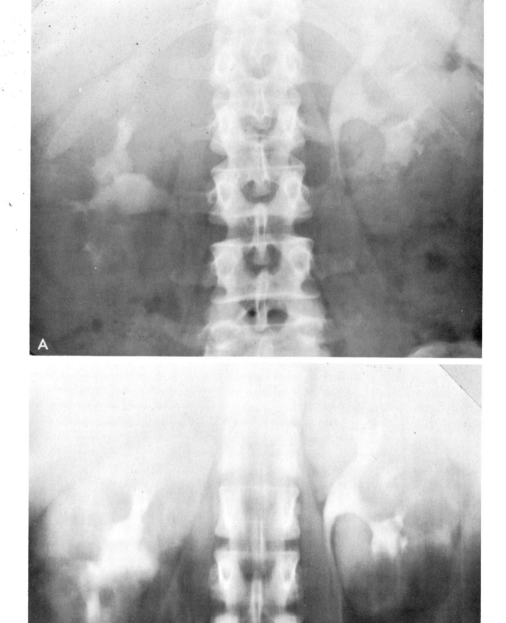

Figure 9–92. Polycystic kidneys in woman, 38 years of age. **A,** *Excretory urogram.* **B,** *Nephrotomogram.*
Both kidneys are filled with radiolucent shadows from innumerable cysts of greatly varying sizes.

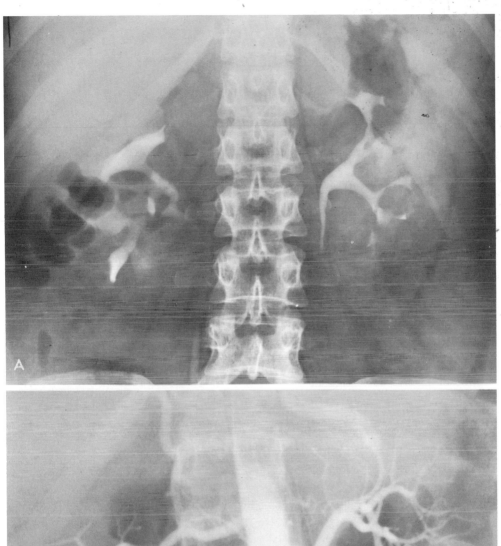

Figure 9–93. "Adult type" polycystic disease. **A,** *Excretory urogram.* Enlarged kidneys with typical alyceal deformity. **B,** *Arteriogram.* Renal arteries within kidneys are stretched, elongated, and displaced y cystic malformation.

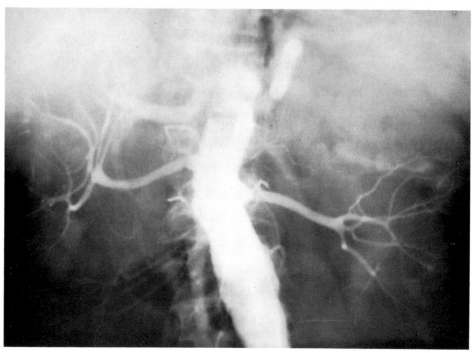

Figure 9–94. *Transfemoral aortogram* of 67-year-old man. Midstream injection. "**Adult type**" polycystic **disease.** Kidneys are enlarged. Renal artery branches within kidneys are stretched and displaced by myriad of cysts.

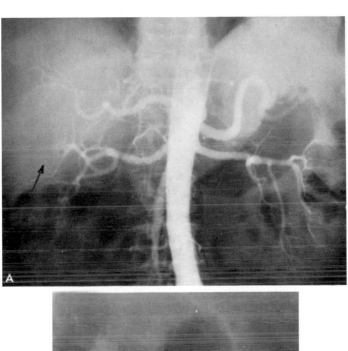

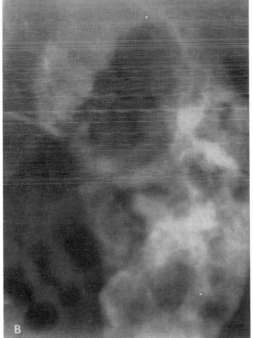

Figure 9–95. "Adult type" polycystic disease. **A,** *Transfemoral aortogram* of 68-year-old man. Displacement and stretching of intrarenal branches with changes more advanced on right (*arrow*) than on left. **B,** *Selective left renal arteriogram, nephrographic phase.* Distinctive "mottled" or "honeycomb" appearance produced by innumerable radiolucent cysts throughout kidney.

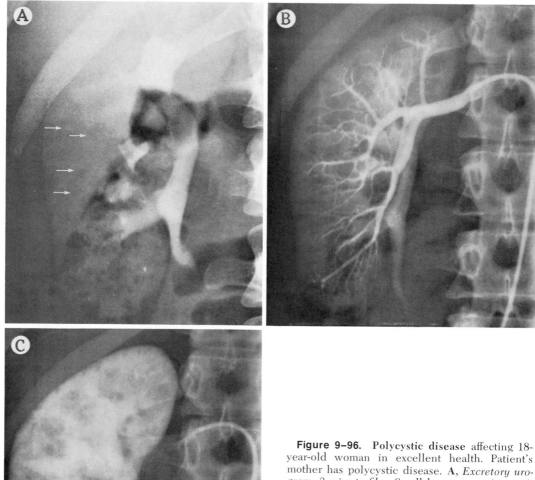

Figure 9–96. Polycystic disease affecting 18-year-old woman in excellent health. Patient's mother has polycystic disease. **A,** *Excretory urogram, 3-minute film.* Small lucent cysts (*arrows*). **B** and **C,** *Selective renal arteriograms.* Minimal displacement of intrarenal arteries on early film (**B**) and mottled (nonhomogeneous) density of parenchyma on nephrogram (**C**). (From Halpern, M., Dalrymple, G., and Young, J.)

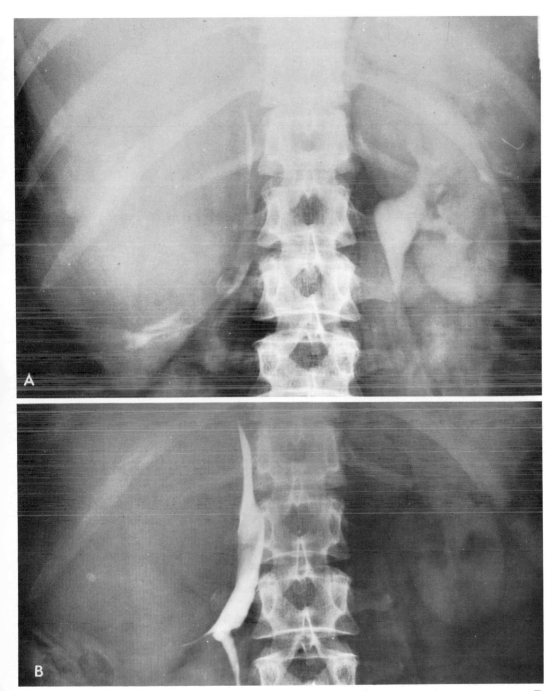

Figure 9–97. Unilateral polycystic kidneys versus multiple simple cysts. **A,** *Excretory urogram.* Deformity from what appears to be large simple cyst or tumor of right kidney. Left kidney of normal size, although calyces are poorly outlined and pelvis is dilated grade 1. **B,** *Right retrograde pyelogram.* Deformity similar to that seen in excretory urogram; suggests large solitary cyst. (*Right nephrectomy.* Pathologic examination showed "polycystic kidney" with 90% destruction. Questions arise whether this was unilateral polycystic disease, with minimal lesions in opposite side which are not urographically apparent, or multiple cysts of right kidney.)

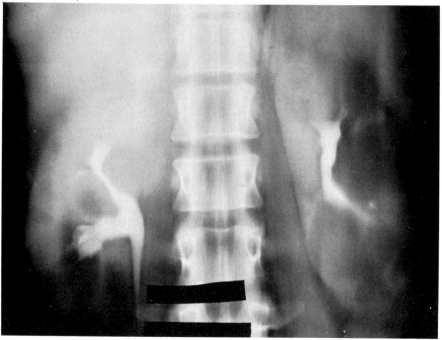

Figure 9–98. *Nephrotomogram.* **Polycystic disease?** Multiple large and small cysts of both kidneys with no family history, clinical signs, or symptoms suggestive of congenital polycystic disease. In cases such as this, differentiation of polycystic disease from multiple bilateral simple cysts is difficult or impossible.

Multilocular Cysts

In the past, multilocular cysts have been classified with simple unilocular cysts because of similarities in their gross appearance and clinical characteristics. However, differences in gross anatomic characteristics of these lesions and probable differences in their histopathogenesis suggest that these rare renal malformations should be differentiated from solitary and multiple simple cysts and classified among the congenital cystic diseases.

Multilocular cysts (Fig. 9–99) are unilateral and localized to one portion of the kidney. The uninvolved portions of the kidney remain normal. The lesion consists of one or more large cysts divided by septa into a number of separate smaller cystic cavities. The septa are complete and the loculi do not communicate with one another or with the renal pelvis.

Boggs and Kimmelstiel concluded that multilocular cysts do not represent "mere dilatation of tubules as a result of nonunion (Hildebrandt) or persistence of tubules which normally disintegrate (Kampmeier)," but rather new growth from residual elements of the metanephric blastema. They suggested that a better term than *multilocular cysts* for this condition would be *benign multilocular cystic nephroma*.

In support of this theory they called attention to the presence of embryonic mesenchyme with "frustrated formation of renal tubules and glomerular anlagen" in the walls of the cysts and the septa between them. They emphasized the difference between this condition and the ordinary types of polycystic disease. The *multilocular cyst* is sharply set apart from adjacent renal tissue and contains no mature functioning nephrons within its septa, whereas in the "adult form" of *polycystic disease* the cysts are scattered more or less densely throughout normal renal parenchyma. Boggs and Kimmelstiel furthermore viewed the presence of embryonic mesenchyme (anlagen of renal tubules and glomeruli) in the multilocular cyst as evidence of an undeniable relationship with Wilms' tumor.

More recently, Osathanondh and Potter, supported by evidence obtained through the use of microdissection techniques, have proposed that multilocular cyst should properly be considered as a form of congenital cystic disease. They classified this lesion as a localized form of their type II cystic disease and suggested that it is closely related to unilateral multicystic disease as well as to a form of bilateral polycystic disease seen in newborn infants, which is not compatible with life. (See prior discussion.) This lesion is not familial and is not associated with cysts of the liver.

Urographically, a multilocular cyst is difficult to differentiate from a solitary simple cyst and multiple closely associated simple cysts. On the plain film, there may be enlargement of one kidney or a definite mass may be seen. On the excretory urogram, the lesion distorts and displaces calyces and the renal pelvis in a manner indistinguishable from that of simple cyst (see Fig. 9–27). **Retrograde pyelography** may help to determine the presence of a mass in an occasional case but is of no value in differential diagnosis. **Arteriography** can be used effectively to differentiate this lesion from malignant tumor, as abnormal "tumor vessels" and "tumor stain" will not be present. In our experience, **nephrotomography** has been of relatively little assistance in differential diagnosis, since the presence of multiple cavities with relatively thick walls makes this lesion difficult to distinguish from a necrotic or cystic tumor.

Multicystic Disease (Unilateral Multicystic Disease)

Unilateral multicystic kidney is a term first used by Schwartz in 1936 to describe an unusual kidney which he had removed from a male infant, 4 months of age. The lesion is encountered most frequently in infants and children but has been reported in patients of all ages. In 1955, Spence collected 15 cases from the literature and presented 4 cases of his own. Of the 15 cases from the literature, 14 involved infants or children less than 2 years of age. Of his own cases, two involved infants, one a woman 21 years of age, and one a woman 70 years of age. Feinzaig, in a study of 29 cases at the Mayo Clinic, found 21 lesions (72%) in newborn infants or children under 3 years of age and 8 (28%) in patients more than 16 years of age. Gwinn and Landing said, "unilateral multicystic kidney. . .is the most common cystic disorder of the kidney in the first month of life."

The condition is considered to be a congenital fetal maldevelopment. It is *not familial, does not occur in conjunction with cystic abnormalities of the liver, pancreas, or lung,* and has no predilection for either sex. Its histopathogenesis is not fully understood, but as pointed out previously, the studies of Osathanondh and Potter suggest that unilateral multicystic disease and multilocular cyst are forms of the same basic developmental defect which they designate type II. (See prior discussion of multilocular cyst, page 1007.) In a few isolated cases, a kidney typical of unilateral multicystic disease has been found on one side and a kidney typical of congenital polycystic disease on the contralateral side (Charlton and Evans; Osathanondh and Potter). The embryologic significance of these cases is unknown but the two processes do not appear to be related.

The condition as seen clinically is *unilateral* with *a normal opposite kidney.* In most instances the ureter on the involved side is atretic or absent but in a few cases a microscopically patent ureter has been reported. Rarely a bilateral form is seen in newborn infants; it is not compatible with life. In many instances, the bilateral form is accompanied by other congenital anomalies.

Grossly, the kidney is described as having the appearance of a bunch of grapes with the entire kidney replaced by a lobulated mass of cysts which may vary from 0.5 to 8 cm in diameter (Figs. 9-100A and B and 9-101). The renal pedicle may be absent or reduced in size. In most cases no renal pelvis can be identified, but if it can be identified, it does not communicate with the cysts. *Histologically,* there is abundant fibrous connective tissue with complete loss of the normal renal architecture. Only an occasional nubbin of solid tissue can be found, which on section may show some infantile tubules or glomeruli. The cyst walls are composed of fibrous tissue and are lined by flattened or cuboidal epithelial cells.

Diagnosis in children is usually made by palpation of a flank or abdominal mass. In adults, most multicystic kidneys are asymptomatic and are found incidentally when a soft-tissue mass is noted, in the region of the diseased kidney, on the **plain film** or when an unexplained unilateral absence of renal function is noted on an **excretory urogram** done for unrelated urologic complaints. The involved kidney does not function and cannot be visualized by excretory urography (Fig. 9-102A). The opposite kidney is roentgenographically normal. If a ureteral orifice is present and patent, the blind ending or partially atretic ureter may be demonstrated by **retrograde pyelography** (Figs. 9-102B and 9-103). In many cases, however, a ureteral orifice cannot be found on the involved side at cystoscopy. Rarely, the walls of the cysts are calcified and can be seen on the plain film (Figs. 9-104 and 9-105).

(Text continued on page 1013.)

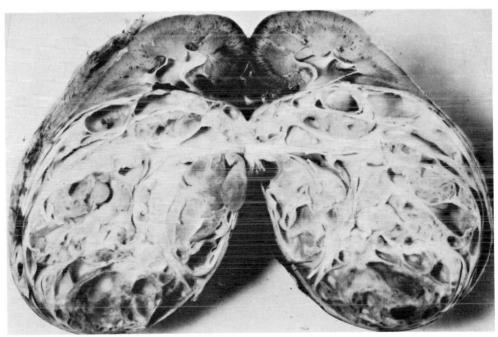

Figure 9–99. **Multilocular cyst.** Note gross resemblance to cystadenoma. Thick capsule separates cystic mass from normal upper pole of kidney. (From Frazier, T. H.)

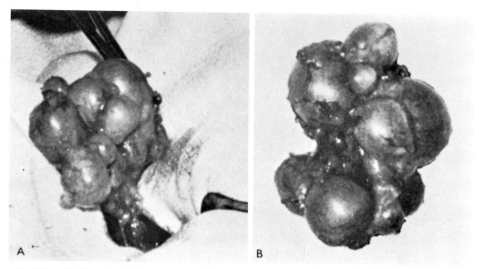

Figure 9–100. Multicystic kidney removed from girl, 4 years of age. **A**, Exposed during operation. **B**, Specimen after removal. (From Spence, H. M.)

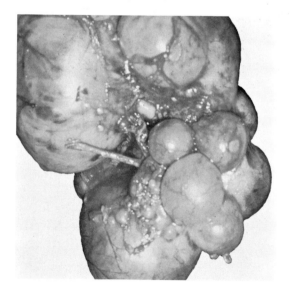

Figure 9–101. Multicystic kidney. Gross specimen.

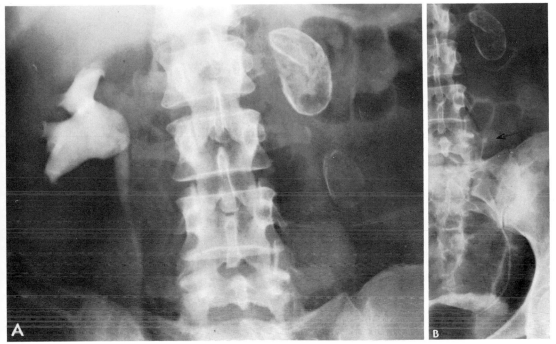

Figure 9–102. Multicystic kidney, left. **A,** *Excretory urogram.* Partially calcified mass in region of left kidney. No renal function is present on that side. Right kidney is normal. **B,** *Left retrograde ureterogram.* Left ureter is thin and terminates in small bulbous dilatation just above sacrum (*arrow*).

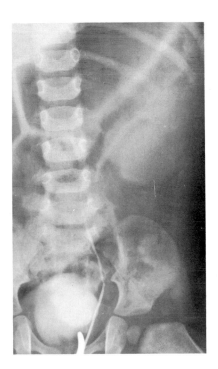

Figure 9–103. *Left retrograde ureterogram.* Multicystic kidney. Only lower half of ureter is delineated. Soft-tissue mass is seen in left upper quadrant of abdomen which corresponds to multicystic kidney.

Fig. 9–104

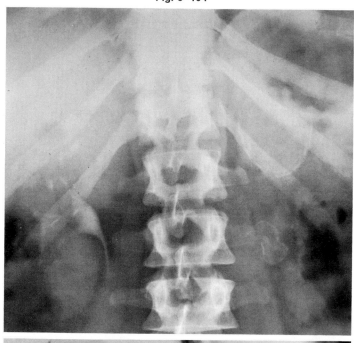

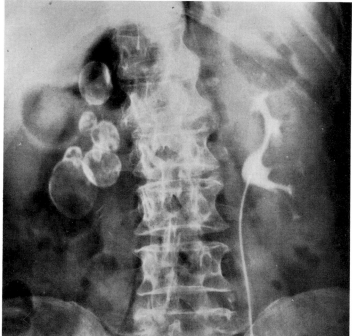

Fig. 9–105

Figure 9–104. *Excretory urogram.* **Unilateral multicystic left kidney with calcification** and no function. Right kidney normal. (At operation small left renal pedicle could be identified, but there were no pulsations. Ureter was identified but was not more than 2 mm in diameter.)

Figure 9–105. *Bilateral retrograde pyelogram.* **Unilateral multicystic right kidney with calcification of** cysts. No function on right. Right ureteral catheter stopped at brim of pelvis. Left retrograde pyelogram normal. (From Spence, H. M.)

Medullary Sponge Kidney
(Sponge Kidney; Cystic Disease of Renal Pyramids; Cystic Dilatation of Renal Pyramids; Congenital Cystic Dilatation of Renal Collecting Tubules; Renal Tubular Ectasia)

Medullary sponge kidney was first described by Lenarduzzi in 1939 but received little attention in the English literature until the past 15 years. It has been defined as a "developmental defect occurring in the medulla of the kidney, characterized by cystic dilatation of the collection tubules" (Miller). In most instances, both kidneys are involved, but lesions localized to one kidney or even a single calyx are frequently seen. Pathologically, the collecting tubules in the renal pyramids are dilated and numerous small cysts and cyst-like structures arise from the tubules. The amount of tubular dilatation varies widely from case to case and from pyramid to pyramid in the same individuals (Palubinskas, 1961; 1963). Cysts usually range from less than 1 mm to 6 mm or more in diameter; in rare instances larger cysts are observed. Grossly, on cut section, the surfaces of the pyramids appear porous or spongy. In advanced cases the pyramids are enlarged and irregularly flattened. Microscopically, the cysts are lined by cylindrical low-columnar of flattened-cuboidal epithelium (Abeshouse and Abeshouse; Mulvaney and Collins). Small calculi may be present in the cysts or dilated tubules, and it is often the calculi observed on roentgen examination that call attention to the condition.

The disease occurs in persons of all ages (Abeshouse and Abeshouse; Murphy, Palubinskas, and Smith; Smith and Graham) and is more frequent in males than in females, ratio 2.5 to 1 (Abeshouse and Abeshouse). It is rare in the general population, with an incidence of approximately 0.5% (29 cases) in 2,465 consecutive patients having urograms reported on by Palubinskas (1961).

Etiology and Pathogenesis

The cause of the disease is not definitely known. Among the theories which have been advanced may be mentioned (1) faulty ontogenetic development (Cacchi and Ricci), (2) hamartomatous changes, and (3) tubular obstruction (Vermooten, 1941; 1951). Calculi, found in the dilated collecting tubules in many cases, may result from stasis of urine in the dilated and cystic tubules (Vermooten, 1951). Currently most authors agree that medullary sponge kidney is a developmental defect affecting the formation of the collecting tubules (Palubinskas, 1961). Osathanondh and Potter point out that, in this disease, the principal abnormality is hyperplasia of the portions of the collecting tubules that lie within the medulla, but there is generally some involvement of the nephrons. On this basis they classify this lesion as a form of their type III ("adult type") polycystic disease. Support for this theory is lent by Vespignani who described a case in which sponge kidney involved the lower pole of one kidney; the upper pole and the entire opposite kidney were polycystic. We have observed a similar case in which medullary sponge kidney, with changes ranging from mild dilatations of the collecting tubules to gross cystic changes in the papillae, was found in association with cystic disease of both kidneys. The polycystic changes in this case differed somewhat from ordinary polycystic disease ("adult type"), however, in that fewer cysts were identified and some areas of uninvolved cortex appeared to be present. A heredofamilial tendency has been described and siblings with medullary sponge kidney have been recorded (Dell'Adami and Meneghini; Fleischner, Bellman, and Henken; Palubinskas, 1961), but the mode of transmission is not well-defined.

Symptoms and Findings

Sponge kidney is compatible with a normal life expectancy (Murphy, Palubinskas, and Smith), although cases are occasionally encountered in which the disease appears to be progressive, with gradual loss of renal function (Lindvall).

Symptoms only arise from complications of the disease, especially the passage of calculi, and associated urinary infection. Gross hematuria is the most common symptom, with backache and renal colic next. Urinary symptoms and pyuria may be present. As mentioned, in most cases renal function is not altered.

Diagnosis; Urographic Findings

In the absence of symptoms, recognition of the disease is usually more or less accidental, calculi being discovered on a routine plain film of the abdomen or lumbar vertebrae, the characteristic urographic deformity being observed in an excretory urogram made for other reasons. It is important to stress that excretory urography is essential to diagnosis, since the dilated collecting tubules and cysts are filled by this technique. Retrograde pyelography, on the other hand, is of little value in diagnosis, since the dilated tubules and cysts rarely fill when medium is introduced from below (Fig. 9–106).

Urographically the condition has been described as demonstrating grape-like clusters of dilated ducts and small cysts confined to the pyramids adjacent to and surrounding the terminal calyces. The urographic appearance depends on the type of tubular changes present (Di Sieno and Guareschi; Palubinskas, 1963) (Figs. 9–107, 9–108, and 9–109). They form a spectrum which ranges from mild dilatation of the renal collecting tubules (often referred to as renal tubular ectasia) producing fan-like opacification of the renal papilla through increasing severity of tubular dilatation and cystic change to gross deformities with multiple cyst and cyst-like cavities of various sizes with beaded or striated cavities extending through the pyramid from tip to base. The calyces in the full-blown case tend to be broad, shallow, distorted, and widely cupped. If calculi are present (Figs. 9–110 through 9–116), they tend to be arranged in groups around a calyx, which may at times suggest the diagnosis even on the basis of a plain film.

Differential Diagnosis. The following must be ruled out: calyceal diverticula and pyelogenic cysts, tuberculosis, necrotizing papillitis, pyelosinous backflow, and nephrocalcinosis. As pointed out by Lindvall, nephrocalcinosis is a broad term that includes several unrelated morbid conditions. In its conventional use there is no connotation of tubular dilatation associated with cystic cavities.

(Text continued on page 1022.)

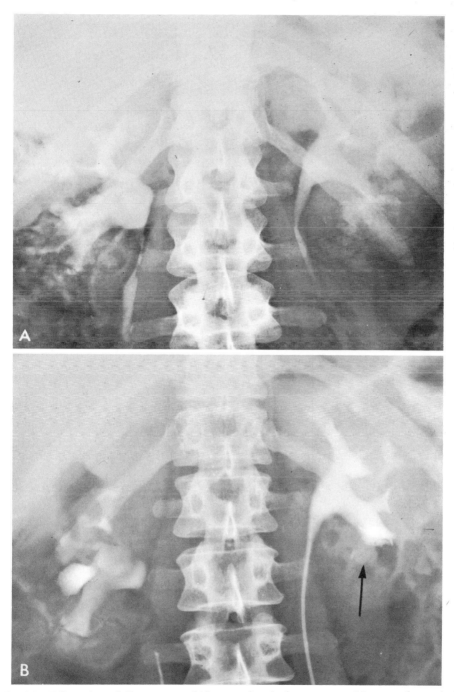

Figure 9–106. Bilateral medullary sponge kidney with calculi in woman, 31 years of age. **A,** *Excretory urogram.* Grape-like clusters of cystic cavities especially surrounding lower calyces, more marked in left kidney than right. One-centimeter calculus in left kidney was well shown in plain film (not shown). **B,** *Bilateral retrograde pyelogram.* Little evidence of cystic dilatation, as contrast medium has not entered collecting tubules except to small degree in left lower calyx, which is dilated and includes calculus (*arrow*).

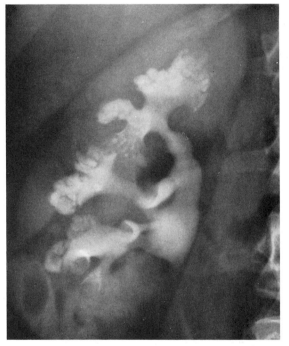

Figure 9–107.   *Excretory urogram.* **Medullary sponge kidney.** Wide variation in severity of cystic change is seen from pyramid to pyramid. Some pyramids are normal; others show mild dilatation of collecting tubules, while still others show marked cystic changes with gross deformity.

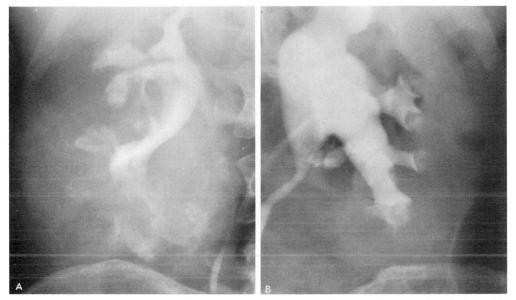

Figure 9–108. Medullary sponge kidneys. *Excretory urograms.* **A,** *Right kidney.* **B,** *Left kidney.* Marked variation in severity of involvement in kidneys of one patient. Advanced cystic changes in pyramids on right (**A**) are associated with multiple parenchymal cysts (polycystic disease?). Medullary sponge kidney proved at operation. Changes on left (**B**) are much less advanced.

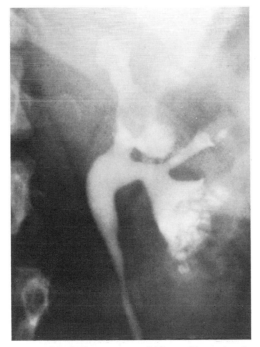

Figure 9–109. *Excretory urogram.* **Medullary sponge kidney.** Extensive involvement of pyramids in left lower pole. Calyx is broadened and shallow, and advanced cystic changes are present in collecting tubules. Remaining calyces are much less severely involved.

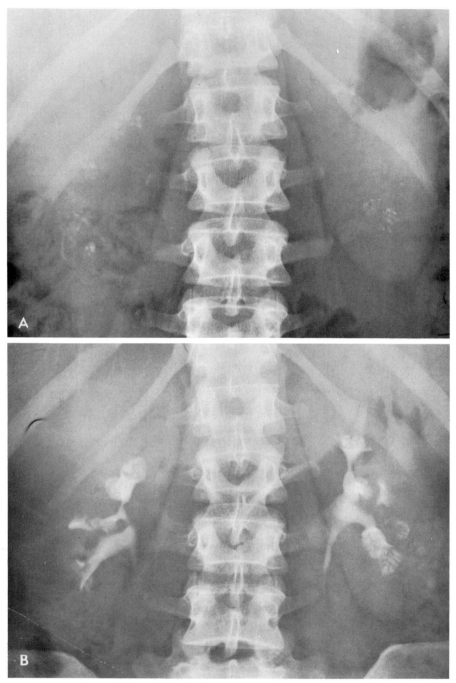

Figure 9–110. Bilateral medullary sponge kidney with associated calculi in man, 34 years of age. **A,** *Plain film.* **B,** *Excretory urogram.* Fan-like appearance of dilated tubules projecting from lower calyces of left kidney; grape-like cystic cavities adjacent to upper calyces of both kidneys.

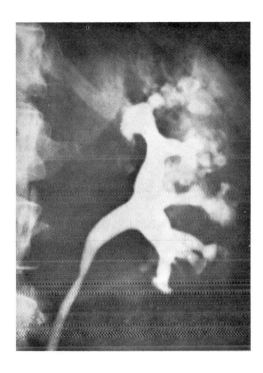

Figure 9–111. *Retrograde pyelogram.* **Medullary sponge kidney** in man, 38 years of age. Grape-like clusters of cystic cavities filled with contrast medium (this was also shown in previous excretory urogram). Right kidney appeared to be normal. (From Mulvaney, W. P., and Collins, W. T.)

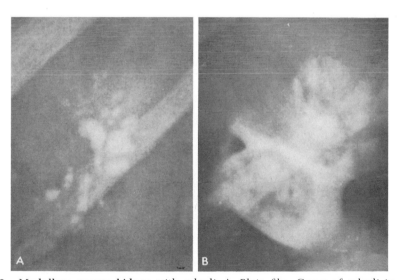

Figure 9–112. **Medullary sponge kidney** with calculi. **A,** *Plain film.* Group of calculi in upper pole of kidney. **B,** *Excretory urogram.* Calculi are situated in cavities filled with contrast medium adjacent to enlarged widely cupped calyces. (From Lindvall, N.)

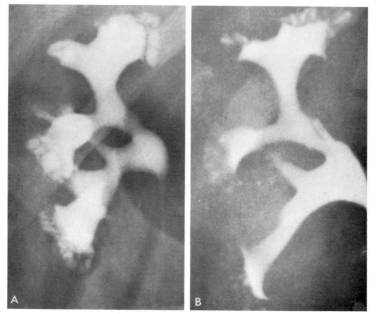

Figure 9–113.   Medullary sponge kidney with calculi. **A,** *Excretory urogram.* Grape-like clusters of contrast medium filled cystic cavities surrounding minor calyces. Many are filled with calculi. **B,** *Retrograde pyelogram.* Only few of cavities are filled. (From Lindvall, N.)

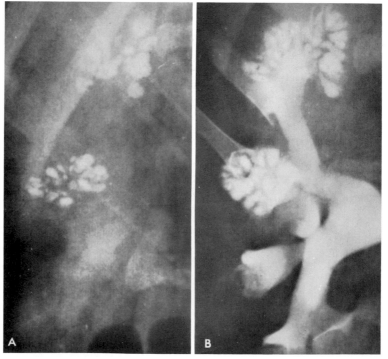

Figure 9–114.   Medullary sponge kidney with calculi. **A,** *Plain film.* Kidney appears to be enlarged. Grouped distribution of calculi suggests sponge kidney. **B,** *Excretory urogram.* Calculi appear to be in cystic cavities which surround minor calyces. (From Lindvall, N.)

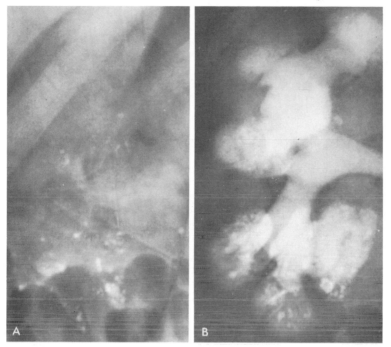

Figure 9–115. Medullary sponge kidney with calculi. **A,** *Plain film.* Small calculi diffusely distributed throughout medullary portion of kidney. **B,** *Excretory urogram.* Calculi appear to lie in cavities, some of which have appearance of dilated collecting tubules while others are cystic. (From Lindvall, N.)

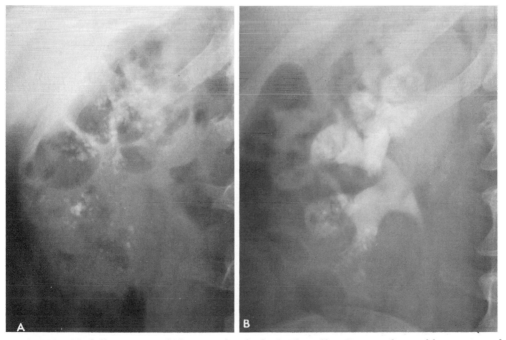

Figure 9–116. Medullary sponge kidney, with calculi. **A,** *Plain film.* Groups of smoothly marginated calculi in medullary portions of kidney. **B,** *Excretory urogram.* Fan-like opacification of collecting tubules with mild cystic changes. Calculi are contained within tubules and cysts.

ECHINOCOCCUS CYSTS
(RENAL HYDATIDOSIS)

by

Kamal A. Hanash

Hydatid disease results from human infestation by two species of the genus *Echinococcus: E. granulosus* and *E. multilocularis.* The disease is highly endemic in sheep- and cattle-raising countries. In the past, most of the cases of hydatidosis in the United States were discovered in immigrants; recent reports, however, indicate an increasing incidence among native-born residents. It is especially common among the Eskimo of Alaska where the disease is endemic in several areas (Faust and Russell).

Epidemiology

The adult tapeworm of *E. granulosus,* the most common species in human hydatidosis, is only 3 to 6 mm long; it inhabits the intestines of dogs and other canines which constitute the primary hosts in its life cycle. The eggs excreted in the dog's feces are ingested by the intermediate hosts such as man, sheep, cattle, and pigs. Dogs are infested by ingesting infected meat, usually mutton or beef, to complete the cycle.

When swallowed by a suitable intermediate host such as man, the egg hatches in the duodenum and the oncosphere migrates through the intestinal wall via the portal system to be lodged in any of several organs, mainly the liver and the lungs. The embryo then begins developing a cystic cavity which may reach a diameter of 1 cm by the fifth month. The covering of the cyst comprises three layers: (1) an outer non-nucleated laminated membrane (ectocyst), (2) an inner layer of germinal membrane (endocyst) which is responsible for the growth of the cyst and from which the brood capsules develop by budding, and

(3) an adventitia or pericyst which is contributed by the host (Fig. 9–117). Daughter cysts which form from the germinal layer of the mother cyst may remain attached to the endocyst and are encountered outside the cystic cavity only if the cyst ruptures.

Most hydatid cysts in man are acquired during childhood possibly because of the close contact of children with infected dogs.

Pathogenesis of Genitourinary Infestation

The genitourinary system may be involved *primarily* or *secondarily.* Renal hydatidosis comprises 2% to 3% of human cases; it usually is produced during *primary infestation* with the hydatid worms which reach the kidney via the arterial system.

As illustrated by Kirkland, *secondary infestation* of any part of the genitourinary tract may result from spread of a hydatid cyst located in an adjacent organ or tissue. For instance, the kidney or ureter may be involved by a direct spread from a hepatic, splenic, or retroperitoneal cyst. Rupture of an echinococcus cyst located in the abdomen may result in discharge and seeding of daughter cysts and scolices in the pelvis with involvement of the retrovesical tissue and organs, such as the prostate gland, vas deferens, and seminal vesicles; these provide new sites for the growth of mature cysts. Vesical irritability, probably the most common symptom of secondary infestation of the genitourinary tract, may be caused by compression of the bladder by a large pelvic cyst. In the kidney, the cyst always originates in the cortex and is invariably subcapsular.

A cyst is considered *closed* if all three layers are intact; when it is no longer protected by the third layer (adventitia or pericyst) or by the lining of the collecting system, it is considered to be an *exposed* cyst. If all three of the layers of the cyst have ruptured, resulting in free communication with the calyces and pelvis, it is described as an *open* or *communicating* cyst (Kirkland).

The renal cyst may grow rapidly, compressing and destroying the kidney, or slowly and insidiously over a period of many years, causing minimal clinical symptoms but eventually resulting in marked distortion of the kidney and loss of renal function. Leakage of the contents of a cyst through incompetent cystic membranes (or layers) or gross rupture of the cyst may produce serious anaphylactic reactions. Some cysts, however, never produce brood capsules, and sometimes the *Echinococcus* is killed by bacterial infection and fibrosis, which may result in calcification of the cyst.

Diagnosis

The diagnosis of hydatid disease may be suspected from a history of previous infestation. The passage of grape-like debris in the urine, intermittent dull flank pain, a renal mass with a hydatid thrill, and renal or ureteral colic produced by daughter cysts obstructing the ureter or ureteropelvic junction are suggestive. Eosinophilia and positive intradermal (Cassoni), precipitin, complement-fixation, and hemagglutination tests are confirmatory.

ROENTGENOGRAPHIC DIAGNOSIS

The Plain Film

The plain film may be of diagnostic help by revealing soft-tissue masses, either calcified or noncalcified, that could represent possible cysts. If calcification is present, daughter cysts may be evident because of a mottled appearance of the calcific distribution or by definite outlining of the various cysts (Figs. 9–118, 9–119, and 9–120A).

The Urogram

It is important to remember that echinococcus cysts may be located almost anywhere in the region of the abdomen. They commonly involve organs such as the kidneys, spleen, and liver, but they may occur in other intra-abdominal or retroperitoneal locations, including the pelvis where they may involve the bladder and genitalia secondarily (Figs. 9–121 and 9–122). In such cases, they may be difficult to distinguish from deep pelvic cysts (see Figs. 12–290, 12–291, and 12–292; 12–295 through 12–303).

Renal Cysts. Diagnosis is more easily made if the cyst is "open" because its communication with the collecting system then permits direct filling of the cyst with contrast medium (Fig. 9–123). When this is possible, the outlines of daughter cysts (which give the appearance of a cluster of grapes) are pathognomonic. A fluid level, indicating the presence of air, also may be seen occasionally. Surraco has emphasized the "goblet" and "crescent" signs which appear in "closed" or "exposed" cysts (Fig. 9–120B); they result from the smooth curvilinear compression of the renal pelvis and spreading and flattening of the calyces. In "exposed" cysts, however, the renal pelvis communicates with the pericystic space (not the cyst itself); thus, contrast medium escapes into the pericystic space, causing an irregular shadow around the cyst (Hanna and Sabry). Compression of a calyx by the cyst produces a crescentic shape that has been described as the sign of the claw (Figs. 9–124 and 9–125).

The urographic picture of renal hydatidosis may mimic a wide variety of other renal masses or mass-like lesions; and, if possible, they should be differentiated preoperatively because of the hazard of opening the cyst during operation. *Nephrotomography* and *selective renal arteriography* may be of value in making the correct differential diagnosis by demonstrating (1) a thick cyst wall, (2) nonhomogeneous radiolucency, as is seen in necrotic tumors, and (3) identification of cysts of extraurinary organs and structures which appear to involve the genitourinary system (Fig. 9–126).

Diagnostic Needle Puncture

Diagnostic needle puncture of the cyst with direct injection of contrast medium may provide extremely accurate diagnosis by graphically demonstrating the presence of daughter cysts (see Fig. 9–122). Such a procedure, however, carries a definite risk because as mentioned previously under the heading of pathogenesis the contents of the cyst apparently may be very toxic (Kirkland). If leakage occurs from either spontaneous or surgical rupture of the cyst wall, serious anaphylactic reactions may occur.

(Text continued on page 1033.)

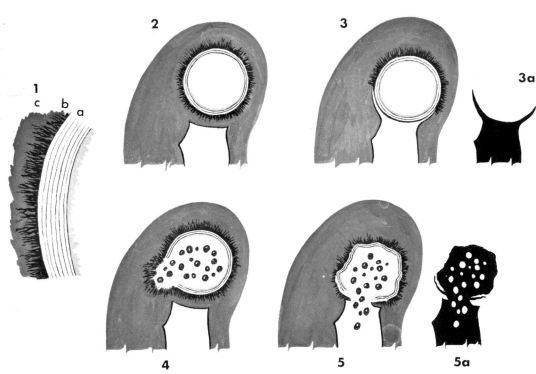

Figure 9–117. Three layers of renal hydatid cyst and its relationship to collecting system. 1, **Endocyst** (a), **ectocyst** (b), and **pericyst** (c) forming three layers. 2, "**Closed**" cyst with three membranes intact, overlying major calyx. 3, "**Exposed**" cyst with absence of adventitial layer or pericyst; cyst is in close contact with urine. 4 and 5, "**Open cysts**" resulting from rupture and discharge of daughter cysts. (From Kirkland, K.

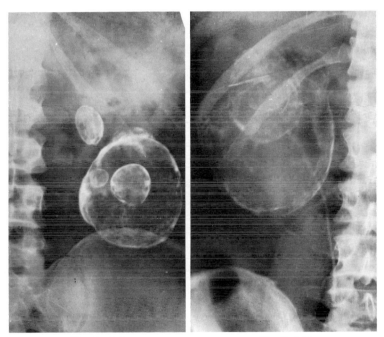

Fig. 9–118   Fig. 9–119

Figure 9–118. *Plain film.* Calcified **echinococcus cyst of left kidney**, showing daughter cysts.
   Figure 9–119. *Plain film* with lead catheter in right ureter. **Echinococcus cyst of right kidney** with calcification in walls. Multiple daughter cysts.

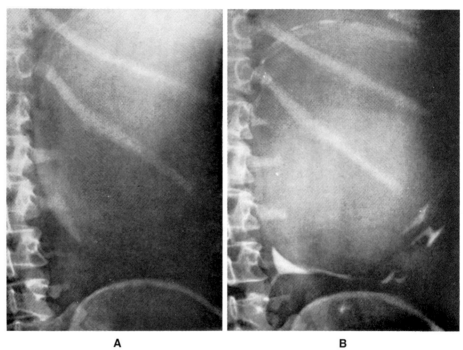

A   B

Figure 9–120.   **Echinococcus cyst of left kidney. A,** *Plain film.* Soft-tissue outline of large cyst with calcific deposits in wall. Some residual barium in transverse colon. **B,** *Excretory urogram.* Pelvis and calyces
outlined; they are pushed downward and laterally by large "exposed" cyst producing "goblet" or "crescent"
sign of Surraco.

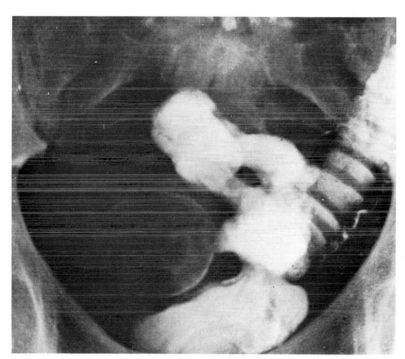

Figure 9–121. *Plain film.* **Genitourinary hydatidosis.** Secondary infestation of hydatid cyst in bony pelvis, involving vas deferens and lying in close relationship to rectum. (From Kirkland, K.)

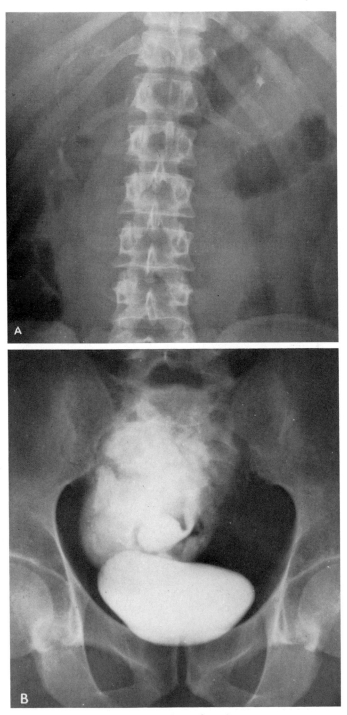

Figure 9–122. *See legend on facing page.*

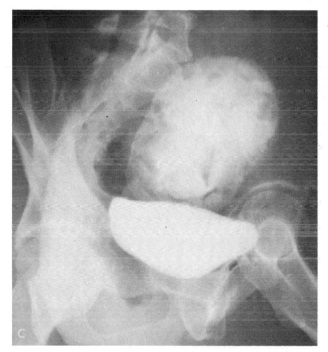

Figure 9–122. Echinococcus cyst of omentum, simulating urachal cyst, and echinococcus cyst of liver in ιan aged 36. Patient complained of large tender mass in lower midportion of abdomen. No residual urine. ., *Excretory urogram* demonstrated vaguely outlined ovoid mass extending from symphysis pubis to level ‹f lumbosacral joint (not included in this illustration) and calcified ring in region of liver, which was diagnosed s possible echinococcus cyst. (Needle-puncture aspiration yielded 300 ml clear colorless watery fluid. Micros-opy showed only epithelial cells.) **B** and **C,** *Renografin injection, anteroposterior* and *lateral views.* Iultiple daughter cysts are outlined. (At operation, freely movable ovoid cyst [12 by 8 cm] was found within mentum; it was attached to dome of bladder by adhesions. Cyst was removed. Pathology: typical cyst with ultiple daughter cysts. Microscopy showed typical scolices with hooklets.) (From Constantian, H. M., nd Bolduc, R. A.)

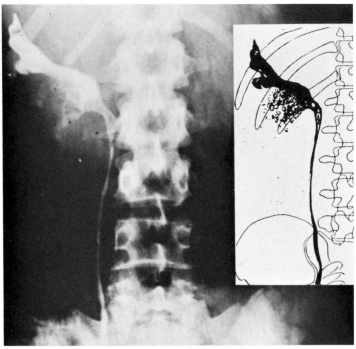

Figure 9–123. *Excretory urogram.* "**Open**" type renal hydatid cyst in 22-year-old female patient. Sile rupture of hydatid cyst in right kidney with discharge of daughter cysts, causing obstruction at ureteropelv junction. (From Kirkland, K.)

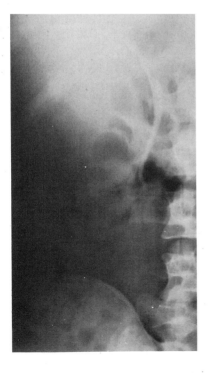

Figure 9–124. *Excretory urogram.* "**Exposed**" type rer hydatid cyst. Huge uncalcified echinococcus cyst in right kidn compressing pelvis and calyces. (Arteriography showed mass be avascular. Nephrectomy performed.) (Courtesy of Dr. Shehadeh.)

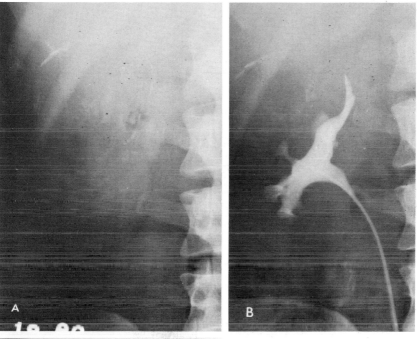

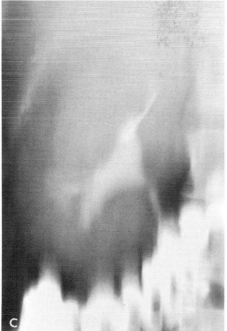

Figure 9–125. "Exposed" type renal hydatid cyst. A, *Plain roentgenogram.* Large partially calcified right renal mass. B, *Retrograde pyelogram.* Note impression on renal collecting system from cyst. C, *Nephrotomogram* confirms cystic characteristic of mass. (Hydatid cyst wall was incised, revealing numerous daughter cysts of various sizes, some of which were collapsed.) (From Henry, J. D., Utz, D. C., Hahn, R. G., Thompson, J. H., Jr., and Stilwell, G. G.)

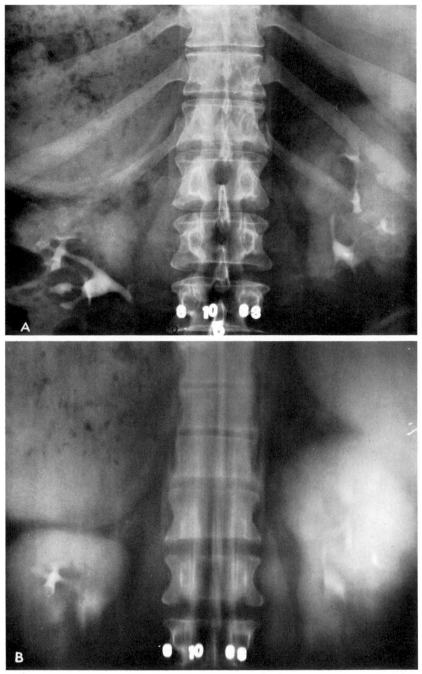

Figure 9–126. **Hydatid cyst of liver simulating cyst of kidney. A,** *Excretory urogram.* Large mass containing a myriad of lucent defects projects over and compresses upper pole of right kidney. This mass was thought to represent renal hydatid cyst. **B,** *Nephrotomogram.* Cyst is shown to be extrarenal arising from liver. Note increased density and relatively thick wall of hydatid cyst in contrast to simple serous cyst.

PARARENAL PSEUDOCYST (HYDROCELE RENALIS; URINOMA; PARARENAL PSEUDOHYDRONEPHROSIS; TRAUMATIC PERIRENAL OR PERINEPHRIC CYST)

Chronic urinary extravasation in the region of the kidney and upper part of the ureter (when the urine has no avenue for escape or drainage) may result in an encapsulated collection of urine. This condition has been given various names, such as *pararenal pseudocyst* (Sauls and Nesbit), *pseudohydronephrosis* (Crabtree), *hydrocele renalis* (Mulholland), *perirenal cyst* (Johnson and Smith), *perinephric cyst* (Spriggs), and *urinoma*. A pseudocyst may assume a myriad of shapes, sizes, and locations. On occasion, it may surround the kidney much as a hydrocele does a testis; this circumstance has given rise to the term *hydrocele renalis* (Figs. 9–127 through 9–130; see also Fig. 9–134E). The variety that lies alongside and only partially encompasses the kidney and upper part of the ureter, however, is the more common type.

Etiology

Most cases that have been reported in the literature have been the result of renal and ureteral trauma (automobile accidents, football injuries, and so on) (Gilliam; Hurwitz and Weisenthal; Sturdy and Magell; Veintraub and associates; Zufall). More recently, cases are being reported which have followed surgical operations on the kidney or ureter, or both, or diagnostic cystoscopic procedures with perforation of the ureter or renal pelvis (Fig. 9–131) (Arduino, Perlstein, and Glucksman; Hudson and Hundley; Pyrah and Smiddy; Sauls and Nesbit). For instance, in 1967 Hudson and Hundley reported two such surgical cases which they believed to be the sixth and seventh, respectively, reported in the literature.

There have been some cases reported in which a history of either trauma or previous operation could not be obtained; thus, they must be considered to be of idiopathic origin (Hyman). Such situations have been encountered in infants and children and may be associated with predisposing factors, such as congenital obstruction in the urinary tract (Pautler and Garvey). Spontaneous perforation of the urinary tract by a calculus has been described as the cause (Hyman). Predisposing factors, such as obstruction, pyelectasis, and ureterectasis, are not uncommonly encountered in the traumatic group.

Pathogenesis

The mechanism of pseudocyst formation is considered to be leakage of urine into the perirenal or periureteral tissues through a small opening in the calyces, pelvis, or ureter. The leakage may continue and become persistent; as already mentioned, it may be aided and abetted by obstruction below, such as at the ureteropelvic junction, or blockage of the ureter from a stone, blood clot, or external compression from a contiguous retroperitoneal hematoma.

Instead of the extravasated urine being absorbed by the tissues, it is thought to lyse fat cells and cause a fibroblastic reaction that may result eventually in complete enclosure of the collection of urine, simulating a cyst. It differs from a true cyst, however, in that the wall, although composed of fibrous tissue, has no epithelial lining. Razzaboni in 1922 showed experimentally in animals that such a fibrous sac wall could be formed within 12 to 40 days. The condition is slowly progressive; it may become clinically apparent within a few days or recognition may be delayed for weeks or months. The thickness of the cyst varies greatly and apparently bears direct relationship to the length of time the urinary leakage has been present. In Hurwitz and Weisenthal's case, when the pseudocyst was exposed surgically, the cyst wall was relatively thick. They said the lesion looked like Wilms' tumor (see Fig. 9–134E).

Clinical Signs and Symptoms

Presenting symptoms consist of a palpable flank mass associated with various degrees of pain. There is usually only slight tenderness to palpation and little if any increase in temperature. Urinalysis is usually normal.

Cases have been reported in the literature in which the pseudocyst produced renal hypertension which was promptly relieved by nephrectomy (Gilliam; Pautler and Garvey; Schroeder and Correa). Schroeder and Correa have postulated that the enveloping of the kidney (except for the hilar vessels) by the pseudocyst causes compression of the parenchyma with resulting ischemic hypertension as suggested by Page.

Roentgen Diagnosis

The lesion may be suspected from the plain film because of a large diffuse "soft-tissue mass" in one side of the abdomen. It is usually in one of the upper quadrants but may extend downward below the crest of the ilium. Diagnosis is usually suspected from an excretory urogram. The most common findings are (1) no excretion of contrast medium on the involved side or evidence of hydronephrosis with reduced renal function and (2) displacement of the kidney (usually upward and laterally) from the "soft-tissue mass" (pseudocyst) (Figs. 9–131 through 9–135). If there is a history of recent renal injury or operation, these findings should alert the physician to suspect the condition. If no contrast medium is excreted a retrograde pyelogram will be required; this may also demonstrate displacement of the ureter from the mass in addition to the pyelectasis above.

The point of leakage may be demonstrated by extravasation of the contrast medium: if renal function is good, this may be seen in the excretory urogram; if poor it may show in the retrograde pyelogram. In some cases the pseudocyst may be filled and outlined with contrast medium (Figs. 9–129, 9–130, 9–132, 9–134, and 9–135), but more often this is not possible. Surgical exploration may be required before a definite diagnosis can be made.

(References begin on page 1043.)

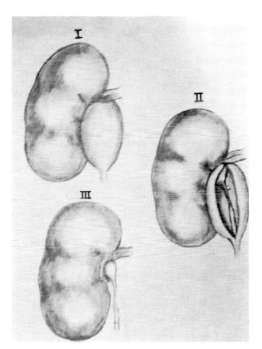

Figure 9–127. Drawing of **peripelvic pseudocyst surrounding pelvis and adjacent ureter** in woman aged 58. **I,** Condition as seen on exploration. **II,** Pseudocyst opened. **III,** Pseudocyst has been removed. Note stricture of ureter, which was contributing factor. Etiology uncertain. No history of trauma or previous operation. (From Hyman, J.)

Fig. 9-128

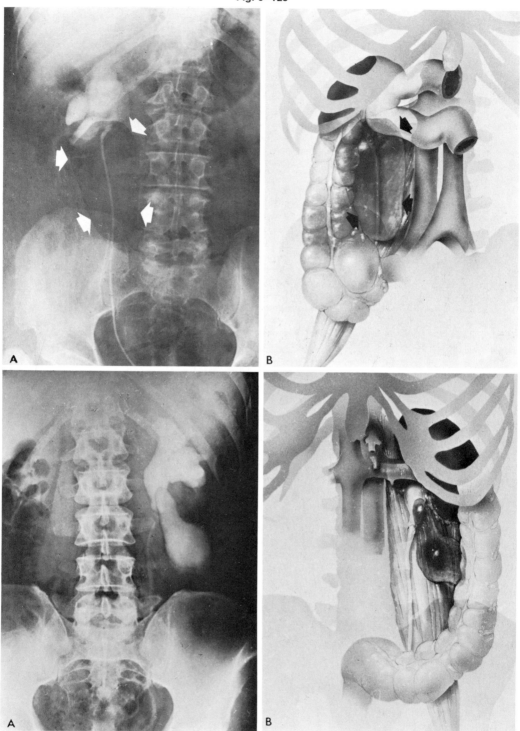

Fig. 9-129

Figure 9-128. Postoperative (pyelolithotomy) pararenal pseudocyst (right). **A,** *Retrograde pyelogram* Obstruction of kidney from pseudocyst which is also displacing upper part of ureter laterally. Lower pol of kidney appears to be moderately displaced upward and laterally. **B,** *Diagrammatic illustration of appea ance and position of pseudocyst* as found at operation. (From Sauls, C. L., and Nesbit, R. M.)

Figure 9-129. Postoperative (ureterolithotomy) pseudocyst (left) with psoas muscle forming posteri wall. **A,** *Excretory urogram.* Left pyelectasis, with efflux of contrast medium into juxta-ureteral space. *Drawing of findings at operation.* There is still communication between cyst and ureter. (From Sauls, C. L and Nesbit, R. M.)

1036

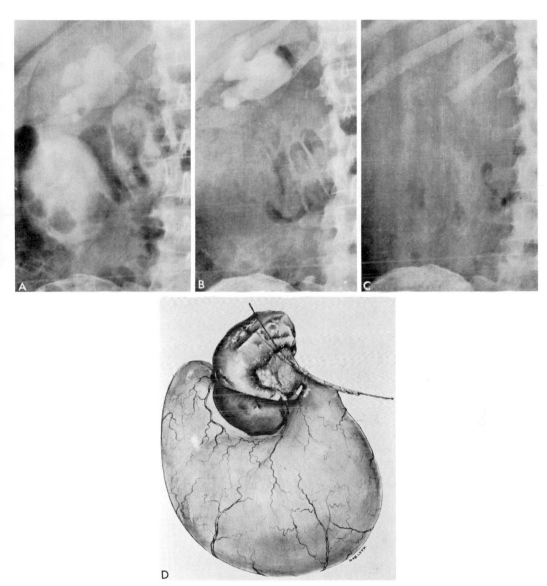

Figure 9–130. Postoperative pararenal pseudohydronephrosis (pseudocyst) associated with right kidney of obese woman with small intrarenal pelvis. **A,** *Excretory urogram* 3 weeks after difficult pelviolithotomy in which considerable trauma to pelvis necessitated extensive suturing. Hydronephrotic pelvis with kidney displaced upward and medially by mass below kidney, which fills with contrast medium, suggesting extravasation into mass. **B,** *Excretory urogram* 4 weeks after operation. Soft-tissue mass is larger, but no contrast medium enters it. This suggests that there is no longer any communication between pelvis and mass. **C,** *Excretory urogram* made almost 3 months after operation. Nonfunctioning right kidney with large soft-tissue shadow below filling right loin. **D,** *Composite drawing of surgical specimen after removal of right kidney.* Lower half of kidney invaginates upper portion of cyst. Cyst communicates by fairly wide opening with pelvis at pelvioureteral juncture. Renal pelvis, formerly intrarenal, is now extrarenal and shows early hydronephrosis. (From Pyrah, L. N., and Smiddy, F. G.)

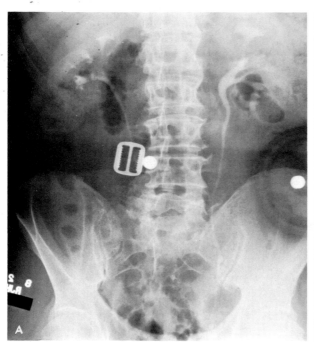

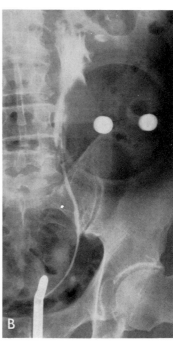

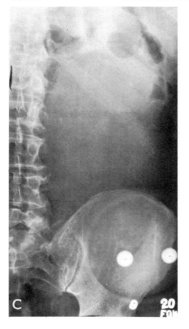

Figure 9–131. Pararenal pseudocyst secondary to perforation of upper left ureter during diagnostic cystoscopic examination. **A,** *Excretory urogram* before cystoscopic examination. Both kidneys normal. **B,** *Attempted left retrograde pyelogram.* Extravasation of contrast medium near ureteropelvic junction. **C,** *Excretory urogram,* 3 weeks later. Large soft-tissue mass in left side of abdomen which displaces kidney upward and extends downward below crest of ilium. (Colonic stoma obscures lower limits.) (At operation, mass was found to extend down to level of iliac arteries; 1,200 ml of urine was aspirated from fibrous-walled pseudocyst approximately 18 cm in diameter. Left nephrectomy. Pyelectasis grade 2.)

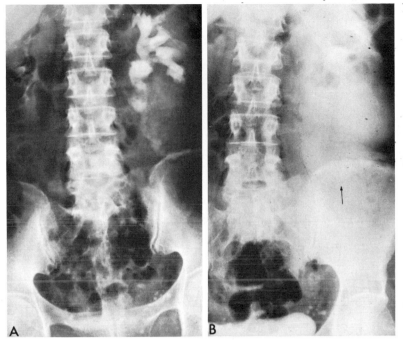

Figure 9–132. Postoperative pararenal pseudocyst (left) in woman, aged 53, after pelviolithotomy and excision of simple parenchymal cyst. **A,** *Excretory urogram* 11 days postoperatively. Extravasation of contrast medium outside left renal pelvis; moderate pyelectasis. **B,** *Excretory urogram* 5 weeks postoperatively. Large soft-tissue shadow in left flank extending slightly below iliac crest (*arrow*). Dilated upper calyces only faintly visible. (Treatment: Stab wound was made over bulging flank mass, yielding 400 ml of urine. Ureteral catheter was inserted in left ureter cystoscopically [remained indwelling for 11 days]. Drainage from flank wound ceased on 14th day. Follow-up excretory urogram 9 months postoperatively showed both kidneys normal.) (From Hudson, H. C., and Hundley, R. R.)

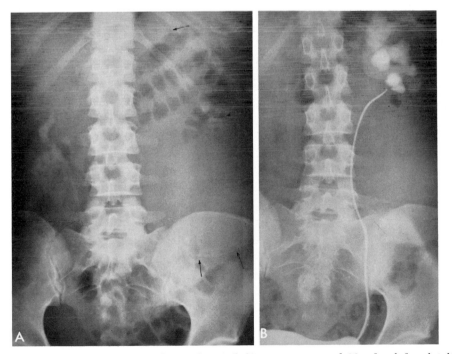

Figure 9–133. Postoperative pararenal pseudocyst (left) in woman, aged 30, after left pelviolithotomy. Films made approximately 5 weeks after operation. **A,** *Excretory urogram.* Large "soft-tissue" mass filling left side of abdomen and extending down over ilium (*vertical arrows*). Left kidney displaced upward and only dilated upper calyces visible (*horizontal arrows*). **B,** *Retrograde pyelogram.* Moderate pyelocaliectasis. Upper half of ureter is displaced medially by pseudocyst. (From Hudson, H. C., and Hundley, R. R.)

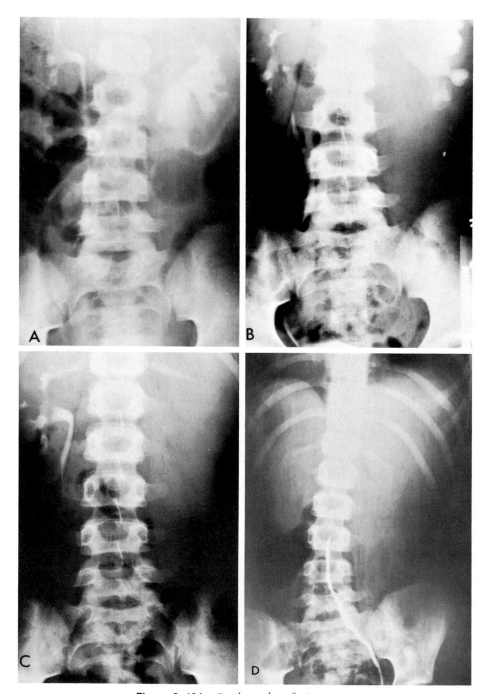

Figure 9–134. *See legend on facing page.*

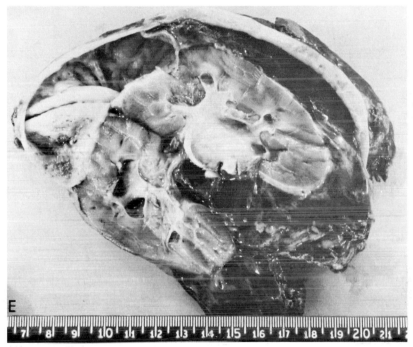

Figure 9–134. Post-traumatic pararenal pseudocyst in girl, aged 9, who had been struck by automobile. **A,** *Excretory urogram* 11 days after injury. Extravasation of contrast medium from region of ureteropelvic junction. **B,** *Excretory urogram* approximately 4 weeks after injury. Progressive hydronephrosis with upward and lateral displacement of kidney. **C,** *Excretory urogram* 3 months after injury. No function. Large "soft-tissue mass" in upper part of abdomen. **D,** *Retrograde pyelogram.* Ureter is displaced medially by mass and is obstructed at level of L3. (At operation, huge tense relatively indurated mass was found, which appeared to surround kidney and looked like Wilms' tumor. Mass and kidney removed.) **E,** *Gross specimen,* bisected. Kidney is surrounded by pseudocyst. Minute sinus tract between lower pole of kidney and pseudocyst could be demonstrated with fine probe. (From Hurwitz, S. P., and Weisenthal, C. L.)

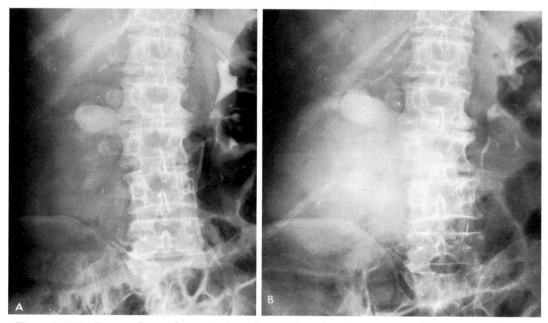

Figure 9–135. Pararenal pseudocyst (urinoma) on right side, of woman, aged 80 years, 30 days after anterior resection for carcinoma of sigmoid. (Uterus, tubes, and ovaries were removed at operation.) Lesion presented as large mass in right flank and upper quadrant of abdomen. *Excretory urograms.* **A,** *Ten-minute film.* Pyelocaliectasis with reduced function. Kidney is displaced medially by "soft-tissue mass." **B,** *Ninety-minute film.* Mass is now visualized with contrast medium from leakage through injured ureter. Lower margin of pseudocyst is seen easily below crest of ilium.

REFERENCES

General References

Abbe, R.: Paranephric Cysts. Tr. Am. S. A. 8:265-272, 1890.

Abeshouse, B. S.: Serous Cysts of the Kidney and Their Differentiation From Other Cystic Diseases of the Kidney. Urol. & Cutan. Rev. 54:582-602 (Oct.) 1950.

Abeshouse, B. S., and Abeshouse, G. A.: Sponge Kidney: A Review of the Literature and a Report of Five Cases. J. Urol. 84:252-267 (Aug.) 1960.

Ainsworth, W. L., and Vest, S. A.: The Differential Diagnosis Between Renal Tumors and Cysts. J. Urol. 66:740-749 (Dec.) 1951.

Anderson, W. A. D.: Pathology. Ed. 5, St. Louis, C. V. Mosby Company, 1966, vol. 1, pp. 646-647.

Arey, J. B.: Cystic Lesions of the Kidney in Infants and Children. J. Pediat. 54:429-445 (Apr.) 1959.

Begg, R. C.: Pyelography in Renal Hydatids. Brit. J. Surg. 24:691-702 (Apr.) 1937.

Bell, E. T.: Renal Diseases. Ed. 6, Philadelphia, Lea & Febiger, 1950, pp. 87-89.

Billing, L.: The Roentgen Diagnosis of Polycystic Kidneys. Acta radiol. 41:305-315 (Apr.) 1954.

Boggs, L. K., and Kimmelstiel, P.: Benign Multilocular Cystic Nephroma: Report of Two Cases of So-Called Multilocular Cyst of the Kidney. J. Urol. 76:530-541 (Nov.) 1956.

Cacchi, R., and Ricci, V.: Sur une rare maladie kystique multiple des pyramides rénales le "rein en éponge." J. Urol. 55:497-519, 1949.

Cannon, A. H., Zanon, B., Jr., and Karras, B. G.: Cystic Calcification in the Kidney: Its Occurrence in Malignant Renal Tumors. Am. J. Roentgenol. 84:837-848 (Nov.) 1960.

Charlton, C., and Evans, D. J.: Multicystic Kidney and Contralateral Polycystic Kidney in an Adult. Brit. J. Urol. 38:505-509 (Oct.) 1966.

Chynn, K. Y., and Evans, J. A.: Nephrotomography in the Differentiation of Renal Cyst From Neoplasm: A Review of 500 Cases. J. Urol. 83:21-24 (Jan.) 1960.

Conley, C. L., Kowal, J., and D'Antonio, J.: Polycythemia Associated With Renal Tumors. Bull. Johns Hopkins Hosp. 101:63-73 (Aug.) 1957.

Cooper, W. M., and Tuttle, W. B.: Polycythemia Associated With a Benign Kidney Lesion: Report of a Case of Erythrocytosis With Hydronephrosis, With Remission of Polycythemia Following Nephrectomy. Ann. Int. Med. 47:1008-1015 (Nov.) 1957.

Cornell, S. H.: Angiography in Polycystic Disease of the Kidneys. J. Urol. 103:24-26 (Jan.) 1970.

Dalgaard, O. Z.: Bilateral Polycystic Disease of the Kidneys: A Follow-up of Two Hundred and Eighty-four Patients and Their Families. Acta med. scandinav., Suppl. 328, 1957, pp. 13-255.

Damon, A., Holub, D. A., Melicow, M. M., and Uson, A. C.: Polycythemia and Renal Carcinoma: Report of Ten New Cases, Two With Long Hematologic Remission Following Nephrectomy. Am. J. Med. 25:182-197 (Aug.) 1958.

Dean, A. L.: Treatment of Solitary Cyst of the Kidney by Aspiration. Tr. Am. A Genito-Urinary Surgeons 32:91-95, 1939.

Dell'Adami, G., and Meneghini, C.: Il "rene a spugna": La prima osservazione in consanguinei. Arch. ital. urol. 27:81-89, 1954.

DeWeerd, J. H.: Percutaneous Aspiration of Selected Expanding Renal Lesions. J. Urol. 87:303-308 (Mar.) 1962.

DeWeerd, J. H., and Hagedorn, A. B.: Hypernephroma Associated With Polycythemia. J. Urol. 82:29-36 (July) 1959.

Di Sieno, A., and Guareschi, B.: Il quadro radiologico del rene a spugna midollare (R.S.M.): Revisione della letteratura e presentazione di due case. Radiol. clin. 25:80-103, 1956.

Ekström, T., Engfeldt, B., Lagergren, C., and Lindvall, N.: Medullary Sponge Kidney: A Roentgenologic, Clinical, Histopathologic and Biophysical Study. Stockholm, Almqvist & Wiksells, 1959, 73 pp.

Emmett, J. L., Levine, S. R., and Woolner, L. B.: Coexistence of Renal Cyst and Tumor: Incidence in 1007 Cases. Brit. J. Urol. 35:403-410 (Dec.) 1963.

Ettinger, Alice, Kahn, P. C., and Wise, H. M., Jr.: The Importance of Selective Renal Angiography in the Diagnosis of Polycystic Disease. J. Urol. 102:156-161 (Aug.) 1969.

Evans, J. A.: Nephrotomography in the Investigation of Renal Masses. Radiology 69:684-689 (Nov.) 1957.

Evans, J. A., Dubilier, W., Jr., and Monteith, J. C.: Nephrotomography: A Preliminary Report. Am. J. Roentgenol. 71:213-223 (Feb.) 1954.

Feinzaig, W.: Multicystic Dysplastic Kidney: A Clinical and Pathological Study of 29 Cases. Thesis, Mayo Graduate School of Medicine (University of Minnesota), Rochester, 1964.

Fleischner, F. G., Bellman, S., and Henken, E. M.: Papillary Opacification in Excretory Urography: The So-called Pyelotubular Reflux. Radiology 74:567-572 (Apr.) 1960.

Forssel, J.: Nephrogenous Polycythaemia. Acta med. scandinav. 161:169-179, 1958.

Frazier, T. H.: Multilocular Cysts of the Kidney. J. Urol. 65:351-363 (Mar.) 1951.

Frey, W. G., III: Polycythemia and Hypernephroma: Review and Report of a Case With Apparent Surgical Cure. New England J. Med. 258:842-844 (Apr. 24) 1958.

Gardner, F. H., and Freymann, J. G.: Erythrocythemia (Polycythemia) and Hydronephrosis: Report of a Case With Radio-iron Studies, With Recovery After Nephrectomy. New England J. Med. 259:323-327 (Aug. 14) 1958.

Gibson, T. E.: Interrelationship of Renal Cysts and Tumors: Report of Three Cases. J. Urol. 71:241-252 (Mar.) 1954.

Gwinn, J. L., and Landing, B. H.: Cystic Diseases of the Kidneys in Infants and Children. Radiol. Clin. North America 6:191-204 (Aug.) 1968.

Halpern, M., Dalrymple, G., and Young, J.: The Nephrogram in Polycystic Disease: An Important Radiographic Sign. J. Urol. 103:21-23 (Jan.) 1970.

Henthorne, J. C.: Peripelvic Lymphatic Cysts of the Kidney: A Review of the Literature on Perinephric Cysts. Am. J. Clin. Path. 8:28-38 (Jan.) 1938.

Hepler, A. B.: Solitary Cysts of the Kidney: A Report

of Seven Cases and Observations on the Pathogenesis of These Cysts. Surg., Gynec. & Obst. 50:668-687 (Apr.) 1930.

Hildebrandt: Quoted by Boggs, L. K., and Kimmelstiel, P.

Holm, H.: On Pyelogenic Renal Cysts. Acta radiol. 29:87-94, 1948.

Jacobson, L. O., Goldwasser, E., Fried, W., and Plzak, L.: Role of the Kidney in Erythropoiesis. Nature 179:633-634 (Mar. 23) 1957.

Jacobson, L. O., Goldwasser, E., Gurney, C. W., Fried, W., and Plzak, L.: Studies of Erythropoietin: The Hormone Regulating Red Cell Production. Ann. New York Acad. Sc. 77:551-573 (June 25) 1959.

Jordan, W. P., Jr.: Peripelvic Cysts of the Kidney. J. Urol. 87:97-101 (Feb.) 1962.

Kampmeier, O. F.: The Metanephros or So-Called Permanent Kidney in Part Provisional and Vestigial. Anat. Rec. 33:115-120 (June) 1926.

Kissane, J. M., and Smith, Margaret G.: Pathology of Infancy and Childhood. St. Louis, C. V. Mosby Company, 1967, pp. 526-541.

Lalli, A. F.: The Roentgen Diagnosis of Renal Cyst and Tumor. J. Canad. A. Radiol. 17:41-43 (Mar.) 1966.

Lalli, A. F.: Percutaneous Aspiration of Renal Masses. Am. J. Roentgenol. 101:700-704 (Nov.) 1967.

Lambert, P. P.: Polycystic Disease of the Kidney: A Review. Arch. Path. 44:34-58 (July) 1947.

Lawrence, J. H., and Donald, W. G., Jr.: Polycythemia and Hydronephrosis or Renal Tumors. Ann. Int. Med. 50:959-969 (Apr.) 1959.

Lenarduzzi: Reperto pielografico poco commune (dilatazione della vie urinarie intrarenali). Radiol. med. 26:346-347 (Apr.) 1939.

Lieberthal, F.: Multi-locular Solitary Cyst of the Renal Hilus. J. Urol. 42:321-325 (Sept.) 1939.

Lindblom, K.: Percutaneous Puncture of Renal Cysts and Tumors. Acta radiol. 27:66-72, 1946.

Lindblom, K.: Diagnostic Kidney Puncture of Cysts and Tumors. Am. J. Roentgenol. 68:209-215 (Aug.) 1952.

Lindvall, N.: Roentgenologic Diagnosis of Medullary Sponge Kidney. Acta radiol. 51:193-206 (Mar.) 1959.

Lundin, P. M., and Olow, I.: Polycystic Kidneys in Newborns, Infants and Children: A Clinical and Pathological Study. Acta pediat. 50:185-200 (Mar.) 1961.

Meaney, T. F., and Corvalan, J. G.: Angiographic Diagnosis of Polycystic Renal Disease. Cleveland Clin. Quart. 35:79-84 (Apr.) 1968.

Miller, F.: Sponge Kidney: Report of a Case in a 70-Year-Old Man. J. Urol. 87:770-773 (June) 1962.

Morehead, R. P.: Human Pathology. New York, McGraw-Hill Book Company, Inc., 1965, pp. 763-765.

Mulvaney, W. P., and Collins, W. T.: Cystic Disease of the Renal Pyramids. J. Urol. 75:776–779 (May) 1956.

Murphy, W. K., Palubinskas, A. J., and Smith, D. R.: Sponge Kidney: Report of Seven Cases. J. Urol. 85:866-874 (June) 1961.

Nixon, R. K., O'Rourke, W., Rupe, C. E., and Korst, D. R.: Nephrogenic Polycythemia. Arch. Int. Med. 106:797-802 (Dec.) 1960.

Omland, G.: Polycythemia in Renal Carcinoma. Acta med. scandinav. 164:451-454 (Aug.) 1959.

Osathanondh, V., and Potter, Edith L.: Pathogenesis of Polycystic Kidneys. Arch. Path. 77:459-512 (May) 1964.

Palubinskas, A. J.: Medullary Sponge Kidney. Radiology 76:911-918 (June) 1961.

Palubinskas, A. J.: Renal Pyramidal Structure Opacification in Excretory Urography and Its Relation to Medullary Sponge Kidney. Radiology 81:963-970 (Dec.) 1963.

Rehm, R. A., Taylor, W. N., and Taylor, J. N.: Renal Cyst Associated With Carcinoma. J. Urol. 86:307–309 (Sept.) 1961.

Robertson, H. E.: Personal communication to the author.

Rosse, W. F., Waldmann, T. A., and Cohen, P.: Renal Cysts, Erythropoietin and Polycythemia. Am. J. Med. 34:76-81 (Jan.) 1963.

Scholl, A. J.: Peripelvic Lymphatic Cysts of the Kidney. J.A.M.A. 136:4-7 (Jan. 3) 1948.

Schwartz, J.: An Unusual Unilateral Multicystic Kidney in an Infant. J. Urol. 35:259-263 (Mar.) 1936.

Smith, C. H., and Graham, J. B.: Congenital Medullary Cysts of the Kidneys With Severe Refractory Anemia. Am. J. Dis. Child. 69:369-377 (June) 1945.

Southwood, W. F. W., and Marshall, V. F.: A Clinical Evaluation of Nephrotomography. Brit. J. Urol. 30:127-141, 1958.

Spence, H. M.: Congenital Unilateral Multicystic Kidney: An Entity To Be Distinguished From Polycystic Kidney Disease and Other Cystic Disorder. J. Urol. 74:693-706 (Dec.) 1955.

Spence, H. M., Baird, S. S., and Ware, E. W., Jr.: Cystic Disorders of the Kidney—Classification, Diagnosis, Treatment. J.A.M.A. 163:1466-1472 (Apr. 20) 1957.

Surraco, L. A.: Renal Hydatidosis. Am. J. Surg. 44:581-586 (June) 1939.

Thompson, I. M.: Peripelvic Lymphatic Renal Cysts. J. Urol. 78:343-350 (Oct.) 1957.

Travers, E. H.: Solitary Cysts of the Kidney: Report of a Case in an Infant. J. Urol. 71:253-255 (Mar.) 1954.

Vermooten, V.: The Incidence and Significance of the Deposition of Calcium Plaques in the Renal Papilla as Observed in the Caucasian and Negro (Bantu) Population in South Africa. J. Urol. 46:193-200 (Aug.) 1941.

Vermooten, V.: Congenital Cystic Dilatation of the Renal Collecting Tubules. Yale J. Biol. & Med. 23:450-453 (June) 1951.

Vespignani, L.: Sull'associazione delle vaire forme della malattia cistica. Radiobiol. Radioter. Fis. Med. 5:483, 1951. (Quoted by Miller, F.)

Wahlqvist, L.: Cystic Disorders of the Kidney: Review of Pathogenesis and Classification. J. Urol. 97:1-6 (Jan.) 1967.

Walsh, A.: Solitary Cyst of the Kidney. Proc. Roy. Soc. Med. 44:437-441, 1951.

Watson, R. C., Fleming, R. J., and Evans, J. A.: Arteriography in the Diagnosis of Renal Carcinoma: Review of 100 Cases. Radiology 91:888-897 (Nov.) 1968.

Echinococcus Cysts

Begg, R. C.: Pyelography in Renal Hydatids. Brit. J. Surg. 24:691-702 (Apr.) 1937.

Constantian, H. M., and Bolduc, R. A.: Echinococcus Cyst Simulating Urachal Cyst. J. Urol. 99:755-758 (June) 1968.

Faust, E. G., and Russell, P. F.: Echinococcus granulosus. In: Craig and Faust's Clinical Parasitology. Ed. 7, Philadelphia, Lea & Febiger, 1964, pp. 678-688.

Hanna, A. A. Z., and Sabry, Y.: Personal communication to the author.

Henry, J. D., Utz, D. C., Hahn, R. G., Thompson, J. H., Jr., and Stilwell, G. G.: Echinococcal Disease of the Kidney: Report of Case. J. Urol. 96:431-435 (Oct.) 1966.

Kirkland, K.: Urological Aspects of Hydatid Disease. Brit. J. Urol. 38:241-254, 1966

Surraco, L. A.: Renal Hydatidosis. Am. J. Surg. 44: 581-586 (June) 1939.

Pararenal Pseudocyst

Arduino, L. J., Perlstein, G. B., Jr., and Glucksman, M. A.: Pararenal Pseudocyst. Am. J. Surg. 103: 758-760 (June) 1962.

Crabtree, E. G.: Pararenal Pseudo-hydronephrosis: With Report of Three Cases. Tr. Am. A. Genito-Urinary Surgeons 28:9-40 (June 6) 1935.

Gilliam, M. R.: Perirenal Cyst Associated With Hypertension: Report of a Case. J. Urol. 66:661-666 (Nov.) 1951

Hudson, H. C., and Hundley, R. R.: Pararenal Pseudocyst. J. Urol. 97:439-443 (Mar.) 1967.

Hurwitz, S. P., and Weisenthal, C. L.: Pararenal Pseudocyst. J. Urol. 97:8-15 (Jan.) 1967.

Hyman, J.: Peri-ureteropelvic Cyst. J. Urol. 70: 32-37 (July) 1953.

Johnson, C. M., and Smith, D. R.: Calcified Perirenal Pseudohydronephrosis: Hydronephrosis With Communicating Perirenal Cyst With Calcification. J. Urol. 45:152-164 (Feb.) 1941.

Mulholland, S. W.: A Cyst Involving the Entire Renal Capsule. J. Urol. 41:653-659 (May) 1939.

Page, I. H.: The Production of Persistent Arterial Hypertension by Cellophane Perinephritis. J.A.M.A. 113:2046-2048 (Dec. 2) 1939.

Pautler, E. E., Jr., and Garvey, F. K.: Perinephric Cyst: Report of Case Associated With Ureteropelvic Occlusion and Congenital Hydronephrosis. J. Urol. 70:840-845 (Dec.) 1953.

Pyrah, L. N., and Smiddy, F. G.: Pararenal Pseudohydronephrosis: A Report of Two Cases. Brit. J. Urol. 25:239-246, 1953.

Razzaboni, G.: Ricerche sperimentali sulla pseudo-idronefrosi. Arch. ital. chir. 6:365-372, 1922.

Sauls, C. L., and Nesbit, R. M.: Pararenal Pseudocysts: A Report of Four Cases. J. Urol. 87:288-206 (Mar.) 1962.

Schroeder, K. F., and Correa, R. J., Jr.: Hypertension Resulting From an Unusual Pararenal Pseudocyst. J. Urol. 96:119-121 (Aug.) 1966.

Spriggs, A. L.: Perinephric Cysts. J. Urol. 67:414-432 (Apr.) 1952.

Sturdy, D. E., and Magell, J.: Traumatic Perinephric Cyst ('Pseudohydronephrosis'). Brit. J. Surg. 48:315-318 (Nov.) 1960.

Weintraub, H. D., Rall, K. L., Thompson, I. M., and Ross, G., Jr.: Pararenal Pseudocysts: Report of 3 Cases. Am. J. Roentgen. 92:286-290 (Aug.) 1964.

Zufall, R.: Traumatic Avulsion of the Upper Ureter. J. Urol. 85:246-248 (Mar.) 1961.

CHAPTER 10

Tumors of the Genitourinary Tract

TUMORS OF THE KIDNEY, RENAL PELVIS, AND URETER

Classification

Tumors of the kidney are divided into two groups: (1) those arising from the cortex (parenchyma), called *cortical tumors*, and (2) those arising from the renal pelvis (and calyces). A simple but practical working classification follows.

I. Cortical (parenchymal) renal tumors
  A. Benign cortical tumors
    1. Epithelial tumors (renal cell tumors; tumors that arise from renal tubules)
      a. Adenoma
        (1) Papillary type (cystadenoma)
        (2) Alveolar type
        (3) Tubular type
    2. Mesenchymal tumors (connective tissue tumors; tumors that arise from connective tissue in either the renal cortex or capsule)
      a. Fibroma
      b. Myoma
      c. Lipoma
      d. Angioma
      e. Mixed mesenchymal tumors
        (1) Hamartoma (angiomyolipoma)
  B. Malignant cortical (parenchymal) tumors
    1. Epithelial tumors (renal cell tumors; tumors that arise from mature renal tubules)
      a. Adenocarcinoma (clear cell carcinoma; granular cell carcinoma; Grawitz's tumor; hypernephroma)
    2. Mesenchymal tumors (connective tissue tumors [arising from connective tissue of either the renal cortex or the capsule])
      a. Sarcoma
    3. Embryonal tumors (derived from embryonic renal blastema)
      a. Wilms' tumor (embryonal adenosarcoma; mesoblastic nephroma; malignant nephroma)
    4. Tumors that involve the cortex secondarily
II. Tumors of the renal pelvis and ureter
  A. Benign tumors (nonepithelial)

B. Malignant tumors
  1. Epithelial tumors (transitional cell epithelioma; transitional cell carcinoma; squamous cell epithelioma; squamous cell carcinoma; epidermoid carcinoma)
  2. Adenocarcinoma (mucinous adenocarcinoma)
  3. Secondary tumors
  4. Nonepithelial (mesenchymal) tumors (sarcoma)

Tumors of the renal cortex (parenchyma) may arise either from epithelial cells of the renal tubules or from mesenchymal (connective) tissue. Tumors which arise from epithelial cells are spoken of as *renal cell tumors.* Connective tissue tumors may arise from fibrous tissue located either in the renal parenchyma or in the renal capsule. Regardless of their site of origin, tumors may be either malignant or benign. Malignant tumors are the most common and of the greatest clinical importance.

Comparative Incidence of Various Types of Tumors of the Kidney and Renal Pelvis

The incidence of the various types of tumors, as reported in 1943 by McDonald and Priestley in 636 kidneys removed surgically for tumor at the Mayo Clinic from 1904 through 1940, in 1951 by Riches, Griffiths, and Thackray from

study of more than 2,000 cases of tumor of both the kidney and the ureter, and in 1957 by Lucké and Schlumberger, is given in Table 10–1.

Benign Tumors of the Renal Cortex (Parenchyma)

Incidence

Benign tumors of the renal parenchyma are of such minor clinical importance that most textbooks of pathology do little more than list their names. The overwhelming majority of these tumors are small (microscopic to 1 to 2 cm in diameter) and never reach sufficient size to be recognized clinically; they are usually found during routine autopsy. The incidence varies from 15 to 20% (Table 10–2). On the other hand, a few benign lesions become large enough to produce clinical signs and symptoms that permit their recognition during life. In a review of this subject, Foster found 135 reports of such tumors, which he listed as follows: 57 adenomas, 7 angiomas, 17 fibromas, 24 lipomas, 22 myomas, and 8 mixed tumors. He pointed out that occasionally these tumors reach enormous size and provide the largest tumors of the kidney that are encountered. He divided them into three groups: (1) intrarenal, (2) arising from the renal capsule, and (3) perinephric (retroperitoneal tumors). Foster's 43-lb fibroma in the kidney of an 8-

Table 10–1.   **Incidence of Renal Tumors by Type as Given by Various Authors**

| | PER CENT OF CASES | | |
TYPE OF TUMOR	McDonald and Priestley (636 kidneys)	Riches and associates (more than 2,000 cases)	Lucké and Schlumberger
Adenocarcinoma (hypernephroma)	80.0	75.0	83.4
Tumors of the renal pelves	11.9	12.5	7.7
Wilms' tumor	4.9	8.0	5.6
Sarcoma	3.1	—	3.3
Primary tumor of ureter	—	0.9	—
Miscellaneous	—	1.9	—

Table 10–2. **Incidence of Benign Tumors of the Renal Cortex**

TYPE OF TUMOR	NEWCOMB'S STUDY (1937) 1,172 NECROPSIES		APITZ' STUDY (1943) 4,309 NECROPSIES	
	Cases	Nodules	Cases	Nodules
Adenoma	84	147	305	725
Mesenchymal tumors	63	69	273	312
Adrenal nodules (rests*)	31	32	261	293
Total	178	248	839	1,330
Incidence, %	15.2	—	19.5	—

*Adrenal rests are not considered true tumors, but rather heteroplastic tissue which may occur anywhere within the kidney. Adrenal rests were formerly thought to result from active displacement of a bit of adrenal tissue in the metanephric blastema during embryogenesis. The opinion now is that the coelomic wall that normally forms the peripheral portions of the renal blastema also is able to form adrenal tissue (Gruenwald; Lucké and Schlumberger).

year old Negro boy appeared to be the largest intrarenal benign tumor on record. Demel's 63-lb lipoma appeared to be the largest tumor on record arising from the renal capsule. Perinephric tumors apparently reach even larger size. See section on "Retroperitoneal Tumors" in this chapter.)

EPITHELIAL TUMORS (ADENOMAS AND CYSTADENOMAS)
(Figs. 10–1 through 10–7)

Epithelial tumors are considered to arise from mature renal tubules and are called *adenomas*. Adenomas are usually small, varying in size from microscopic to to 2 cm in diameter; they are often multiple and usually occur in the peripheral portion of the cortex just under the renal capsule.

Pathologic Aspects

In the renal cortex adenomas are usually small, single or multiple grayish-white, yellow, or brown nodules. They are sharply circumscribed, but not encapsulated. They usually appear to be solid, although some appear cystic (cystadenomas). In rare instances an adenoma may become large enough to cause clinical symptoms. Gordon-Taylor reported one 3 inches in diameter that weighed 22 lb.

Histologically, adenomas of the renal cortex are of three types: (1) papillary (cystadenoma), (2) alveolar, and (3) tubular. The papillary variety, which is the most common, is composed of cystic spaces into which project numerous papillary branches composed of branching strands of connective tissue lined by cuboidal or cylindrical epithelium. The alveolar type is characterized by polyhedral cells arranged in alveolar fashion. The cells are cuboidal or cylindrical and usually large. They are often fatty. The tubular type, which is rare, is characterized by elongated irregular canals lined by small fat-free cells with prominent nuclei.

Roentgen Features

If an adenoma reaches substantial size it may distort the pelvis and calyces, as may any renal mass, but there is never any evidence of calyceal destruction. Basically it is an avascular tumor; the arteriogram shows no evidence of neovascularization, puddling, or tumor staining. Rabinowitz, Wolf, and Goldman found that in four of five cases the nephrotomogram revealed a relatively radiolucent mass with a smooth regular outline which suggested a simple cyst. The distinguishing factor, however, was the thick capsule in contradistinction to a thin capsule which is the rule with cysts. Also a simple cyst is often entirely intrarenal; an adenoma is never so. It should be remembered that occasionally a malignant hypernephroma with cystic degeneration may also appear translucent and have a thick capsule but in such cases the outline of the tumor is usually irregular as contrasted to the smooth regular outline of the benign adenoma.

MESENCHYMAL TUMORS (CONNECTIVE TISSUE TUMORS; FIBROMAS; ANGIOMAS; LIPOMAS)
(Figs. 10–8 through 10–12)

Nonepithelial tumors are thought to originate from connective tissue, adipose tissue, muscle, and vascular or lymphatic tissue of the kidney or renal capsule. Smooth muscle components are considered to originate either from smooth muscle fibers scattered in the inner layer of the renal capsule or from the walls of the stellate veins, which drain the superficial renal cortex. The commonest types of tumors are fibroma, myoma, lipoma, angioma, hemangioma, or various combinations, and mixed tumors. Combinations of more than one type of tissue such as fibromyoma are common. Fibrous tissue may undergo myxomatous change resulting in fibromyxoma. Renal lipomas were considered in detail by Robertson and Hand in 1941, Spillane, Singiser, and Prather in 1952, and Tahara and Hess in 1945.

Most benign mesenchymal tumors are small and are encountered only at necropsy. Fibromas, which are the most common, may be found either in the peripheral portion of the cortex or deeper in the medulla. Nearly all tiny tumors in the medulla are fibromas. Leiomyomas are probably the commonest mesenchymal tumors found in the peripheral portion of the cortex.

Roentgen and Clinical Data

Except possibly hemangioma, only tumors which attain considerable size be-come clinically apparent. *Hemangiomas,* however, cause gross hematuria in an appreciable percentage of cases regardless of size. A palpable mass, hematuria (in 50% of Foster's collected 135 cases), and occasional pain are the cardinal signs and symptoms of large benign tumors.

If the tumor becomes large enough to be recognized urographically it generally appears as a space-occupying lesion with few, if any, distinguishing characteristics.

Hamartoma (Angiomyolipoma; Mixed Tumors; Benign Mesenchymoma) (Figs. 10–13 through 10–22)

Although hamartoma is a mesenchymal tumor and belongs in the group discussed above, it is encountered sufficiently often and has such peculiar clinical and radiographic manifestations that it deserves individual consideration here.

Hamartoma is the name commonly employed in the literature for this group of tumors composed of blood vessels, smooth muscle, and adipose tissue. It is Albrecht's term for a tumor "due to over development of some tissue element which belongs normally at the site where it is found or to abnormal relationship of a normally situated tissue element." Boggs and Kimmelstiel defined hamartoma as "a tumorous structure composed of the tissue elements normally present in an adult organ but in abnormal proportions without evidence of active growth." This type of tumor accounts for most of the individual cases of unusual renal tumor reported in the literature.

Two types of hamartomas are recognized: (1) the small, multifocal medullary fibromas usually involving both kidneys and associated with tuberous sclerosis and (2) the single larger tumor of mixed mesenchymal origin which is *not* associated with tuberous sclerosis. Tumors of the latter type are found almost exclusively in women and in the sixth and seventh decades of life. From 50%

80% are of type 1 (associated with tuberous sclerosis) (Seabury, Ensor, and Wolfe). Grossly the tumor appears as a greasy, yellow, lobulated mass resembling fat, but is firmer and more friable than fatty tissue. Although the tumors may infiltrate into the perinephric tissues, it is doubtful whether they ever undergo malignant degeneration; distant metastasis has never been reported. Approximately 150 cases *without* tuberous sclerosis have been reported (Seabury, Ensor, and Wolfe).

One characteristic that sets hamartomas apart from other benign renal tumors is the tendency for spontaneous infarcts or hemorrhages to develop deep within the tumor and cause severe pain. Spontaneous rupture with massive retroperitoneal hemorrhage, severe pain, shock, and an accompanying mass in the flank has been reported (Keshin).

Radiographic Data. As in all benign tumors, the deformity of the collecting system in hamartoma is not diagnostic and cannot be distinguished from that of any other variety of renal tumor.

Because of the excessive amount of fat in the tumor, the low density of the fat decreases the opacity of the lesion so that it may be difficult to discern the contour and limits of the tumor. Radiolucent areas within the tumor are commonly seen and are thought to represent heavy concentrations of fat or infarcts and areas of hemorrhage. At times these areas suggest multiple cysts or even polycystic disease (if the disease is bilateral). A thick capsule may exclude the diagnosis of cysts (Adelman; Khilnani and Wolf) (Fig. 10–18). Infarction and hemorrhage with massive retroperitoneal hematoma may complicate diagnosis (Keshin) (Fig. 10–19).

Arteriography may also be misleading; even though this tumor is benign, often (because of its vascular nature) neovascularization with tumor vessels, puddling, and staining may be present and suggest a malignant lesion (Figs. 10–20, 10–21, and 10–22).

PATHOGENESIS OF BENIGN TUMORS

There are many theories concerning the origin of benign renal tumors. Foster has written an excellent summary of this subject as follows:

The multiplicity of theories purporting to explain the origin and nature of the benign renal tumors is an index of the complexity of the problem. There are two main schools of thought. The first favors the idea that these tumors are developmental or congenital in origin and the second that they are neoplastic in origin.

Colvin, an advocate of the developmental theory, listed the pathogenesis as follows: 1) from the wolffian body, 2) from renal blastema or nephrotome, 3) from a faulty segmentation of the nephrotome from the myotome and sclerotome, 4) from primordial segments or undifferentiated mesoderm included in the nephrogenic anlage, and 5) from endothelium. Fuchsman [and Angrist] states, "The basic linkage of these tumors is best seen in the mixed group. The adenomyomas, fibromyolipomas and the other permutations and combinations of epithelial and stromal tissues may properly be considered differentiated forms of Wilms's tumors. The diversified character of these neoplasms suggest [sic] that they are developmental tumors which, though differentiated, have a common embryonal origin . . . Some epithelial neoplasms and connective tissue tumors, and particularly the mixed forms, probably have a common origin, representing varying differentiation of original nephrogenic mesenchyme."

On the other hand advocates of the neoplastic theory, such as Bailey and Harrison and Herbut, believe that benign renal neoplasms may arise from any of the various elements of the kidney, originating from the tissues which they appear to represent or be derived from, as for example, lipoma from fat cells or their progenitors, fibroma from connective tissue cells or their progenitors, etc.

There is an additional theory regarding the origin of the adenomas and lipomas, i.e., that, in the case of the adenomas, they are a result of a reparative process and arise in association with arteriosclerotic and degenerative changes in the kidney, while in the case of lipomas they are the result of a degenerative process within the kidney resulting in fatty replacement.

Since benign renal tumors, especially the larger ones, are seldom "pure" but rather are composed of two or more types of tissue in various combinations, one author (Watson) advocated calling all benign renal tumors "mixed tumors," suggesting that this group of tumors constitutes a definite variety which probably arises in a manner not unlike mixed tumors in other locations. The present writer believes, however, that, although there is a great similarity among these tumors in gross appearances, clinical manifestations, symptoms, operative problems and prognosis, and from a practical standpoint they can be described together as a single group, yet (as Simon pointed out) these tumors fundamentally do not appear to have characteristics in common such as are possessed by the malignant types of mixed renal tumors but rather resemble the tumors of their predominant tissue. Their constituent tissues are practically always closely related and arise from one germinal layer only. Considerable confusion would be avoided if we continue to classify them according to the predominant tissue or tissues rather than to group them collectively as mixed tumors.

TUBEROUS SCLEROSIS (NEURILEMMOBLASTOSIS) (Figs. 10–23, 10–24, and 10–25)

The clinical syndrome of tuberous sclerosis was first described by Bourneville in 1880. The classic triad of the disease consists of mental retardation, epilepsy, and sebaceous adenomas of the face (butterfly distribution on the bridge of the nose and nasolabial folds). The disease has been referred to as one of the neurocutaneous syndromes (Golji) and as *neurilemmoblastosis* (Inglis) consisting of developmental anomalies in tissues of ectodermal origin, such as the brain, retina, skin, and nails. It is considered congenital and may be hereditary or familial.

The term *tuberous sclerosis* was given to the disease because of the characteristic potato-like sclerotic patches scattered indiscriminately over the surface of the cerebral cortex. These patches are composed largely of neuroglial proliferations. Not infrequently the ventricular system of the brain is dilated and tumors of the lateral ventricles can be demon-

strated by pneumoencephalography. Most of the patients described in the literature are inmates of mental institutions because of mental retardation. Taylor and Genters suggested in 1958 that a mild form of the disease may go undiagnosed in a large group of persons.

Associated benign tumors and cysts of mesenchymal tissues are frequently encountered, the commonest organs involved being the lungs, kidneys, heart, liver, pancreas, and thyroid. The three most commonly involved sites in order of decreasing frequency of occurrence are: (1) brain, (2) face, and (3) kidney. Moolten stated that the clinical diagnosis of tuberous sclerosis can be made if two or more of the following findings can be demonstrated: (1) mental retardation, (2) epilepsy, (3) sebaceous adenoma of the face, (4) benign tumors of the retina or of the optic nerve, and (5) multiple mixed tumors of the kidneys. Periungual and subungual fibromas involving the toenails are seen occasionally.

Bony changes are roentgenographically demonstrable in a substantial percentage of cases (66% of 43 cases in Holt and Dickerson's series). They consist of (1) thickening of the periosteum, (2) calcification of the bones and joints, (3) increased density of the bones of the skull, vertebrae, and pelvis, and (4) generalized osteoporosis of the metacarpal and metatarsal bones and their phalanges. Holt and Dickerson stated: "Cyst-like foci can be seen in the phalanges with a rather destructive type of periosteal new bone formation along the shafts of the metatarsals and metacarpals."

Renal Lesions

Benign renal tumors are common accompaniments of tuberous sclerosis. In most cases they are small, multiple, and bilateral and are recognized only at necropsy. Their incidence has been variously estimated from 50 to 89% (Bel

Bernstein and Pitegoff; Golji; Wechsler). The majority of the renal tumors encountered in tuberous sclerosis are hamartomas (angiomyolipomas), but almost every type of benign tumor of connective tissue has been encountered. It is estimated that approximately 50% of all hamartomas occur in patients with various stigmata of tuberous sclerosis (Lucké and Schlumberger).

Clinical Data

As mentioned previously, most of the tumors remain small and are not recognized clinically. A few, however, enlarge and become palpable and a few cause pain. If the tumor is a hamartoma (angio-myolipoma), infarction or hemorrhage into the tumor is not uncommon and may cause severe renal colic as illustrated by the cases reported by Taylor and Genters; Rusche; Morgan, Straumfjord, and Hall; and Heckel and Penick. Hematuria is not a consistent symptom.

Urography

The roentgen characteristics of the lesions of significant size have been discussed above. Taylor and Genters have called attention to the similarity of the appearance of the urograms with those of polycystic disease when the lesions are bilateral, which is often the case (Figs. 10-23, 10-24, and 10-25).

(*Text continued on page 1068.*)

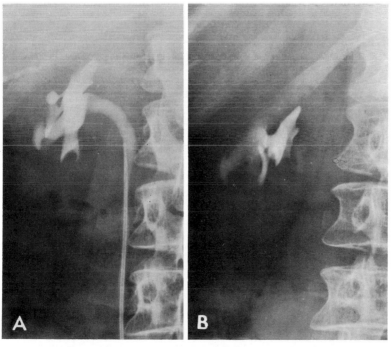

Figure 10–1.   Degenerating cystadenoma in solitary right kidney. Left kidney had been removed 5 months previously elsewhere for grade 2 hypernephroma which grossly appeared as almost pedunculated tumor that did not extend very deeply into renal cortex. *Retrograde pyelograms.* **A,** *Anteroposterior view.* **B,** *Oblique view.* These suggest lesion in middle of kidney. Tumor was removed surgically.

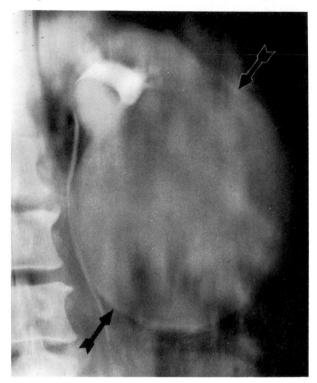

Figure 10–2. Benign papillary adenoma of left kidney with areas of hemorrhagic necrosis. *Nephrotomo-gram, nephrographic phase.* Large relatively translucent mass. Thick capsule (*arrows*) differentiates it from renal cyst. (From Rabinowitz, J. G., Wolf, B. S., and Goldman, R. H.)

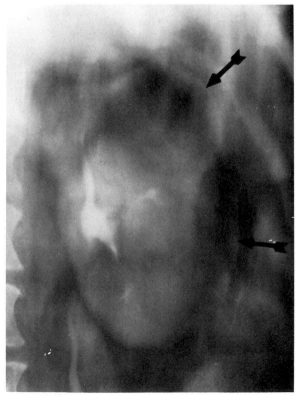

Figure 10–3. Benign tubular adenoma in upper pole of kidney. *Nephrotomogram, nephrographic phase.* Large, relatively translucent mass in upper pole. Capsule (*upper arrow*) is well outlined and appears thickened. Elongated translucent area along outer aspect of renal outline below upper-pole mass; at operation this proved to represent subcapsular hematoma. Capsule of hematoma is visible (*lower arrow*). (From Rabinowitz, J. G., Wolf, B. S., and Goldman, R. H.)

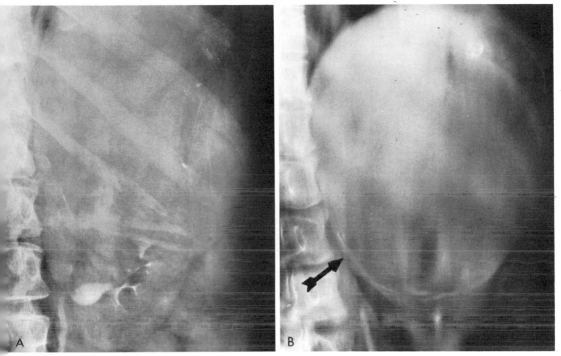

Figure 10-4. Benign tubular adenoma in upper pole of left kidney. **A,** *Excretory urogram.* Large mass in upper pole. **B,** *Nephrotomogram, nephrographic phase.* Mass relatively translucent. Note thick capsule (*arrow*). (From Rabinowitz, J. G., Wolf, B. S., and Goldman, R. H.)

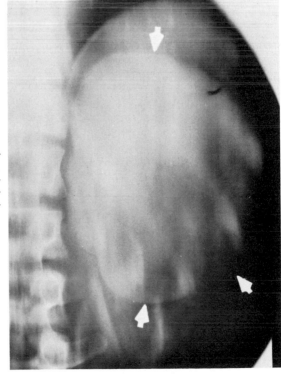

Figure 10-5. Benign (solid) vascular tubular adenoma. *Nephrotomogram, nephrographic phase.* Mass is homogeneously opacified and sharply demarcated. Preoperative diagnosis was hypernephroma. (From Rabinowitz, J. G., Wolf, B. S., and Goldman, R. H.)

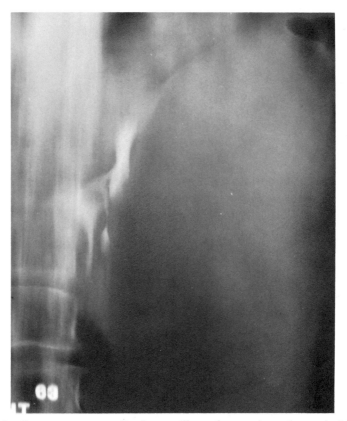

Figure 10–6.   *Excretory urogram.* Benign papillary adenoma (cystadenoma) of left kidney.

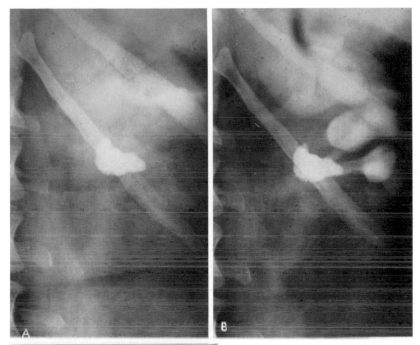

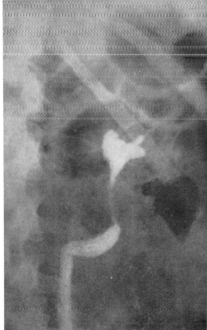

Figure 10-7. Compression of ureter by peripelvic adenoma simulates ureteral stricture. Stone in pelvis. A, *Plain film.* Calcific shadow over midleft renal area. B, *Excretory urogram.* Marked calycectasis. Stone apparently in pelvis, which is not outlined. C, *Left retrograde pyelogram.* Apparent stricture of proximal 3 cm of ureter. Pelvis contracted tightly around stone. No medium entering calyces. Surgical exploration revealed cause of "stricture" to be peripelvic adenoma surrounding pelvis and adjacent ureter and causing marked constriction. (Courtesy of Dr. A. Arnold, Dr. S. Immergut, and Dr. Z. R. Cottler.)

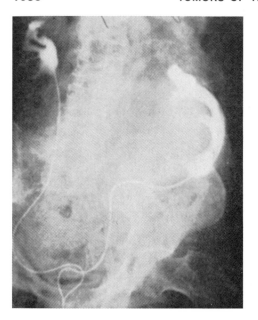

Figure 10–8. Primary fibromyxolipoma of kidney in woman, 78 years of age. *Bilateral retrograde pyelogram.* Left kidney rotated on vertical axis and displaced laterally by huge intrarenal mass. Elongation, flattening, and irregularity of pelvis and calyces. Large soft-tissue mass appears to cross midline. (From Spillane, R. J., Singiser, J. A., and Prather, G. C.)

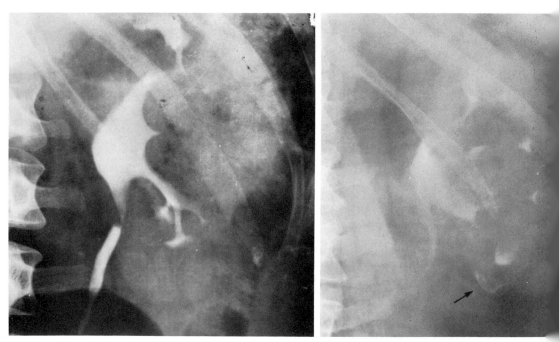

Fig. 10–9   **Fig. 10–10**

Figure 10–9. *Left retrograde pyelogram.* **Cavernous hemangioma of renal cortex** involving pyramidal portion of kidney. Impossible to distinguish from hypernephroma or other malignant tumor. (From River, H. F., and Pool, T. L.)

Figure 10–10. *Excretory urogram.* **Lymphangioma,** 4 cm in diameter, in lower pole of left kidney, with small calcareous infarct (*arrow*). Patient, man 49 years of age, complained of severe pain in left flank of weeks' duration. There were also multiple peripelvic cysts. Nephrectomy.

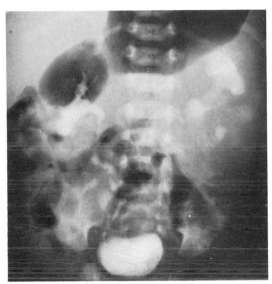

Figure 10–11.   Leiomyoma of left kidney in boy aged 15 days. Palpable mobile mass in left loin. *Excretory urogram.* Enlargement and spreading of calyces. *Operation: left nephrectomy.* Gross specimen showed large, solid, smooth tumor which replaced pelvis. Microscopic diagnosis: "Leiomyoma probably taking origin from renal pelvis." (From Addison, N. V., and Peach, B.)

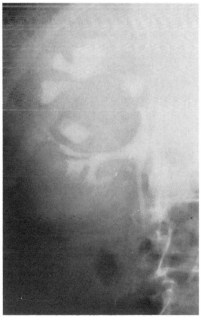

Figure 10–12.   *Preoperative excretory urogram.* Myxoma of renal sinus. (From Appel, S. D., and Schoenerg, H. W.)

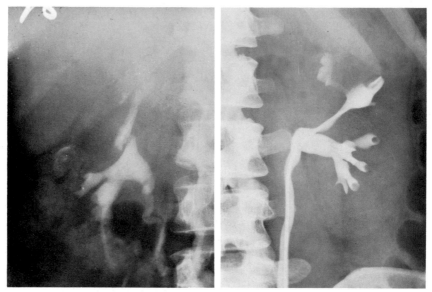

Fig. 10–13   Fig. 10–14

Figure 10–13. *Excretory urogram.* Hamartoma (hemangiolipofibroma) of cortex of right kidney, which had invaded pelvis and produced hematuria. Impossible to distinguish from hypernephroma.

Figure 10–14. *Retrograde pyelogram.* Hamartoma (angiolipomyoma) in woman, 27 years of age. Attacks of severe renal pain 7 years previously during first pregnancy, associated with renal mass (hemorrhage into tumor?). Recent pain. No mass palpable. Nephrectomy.

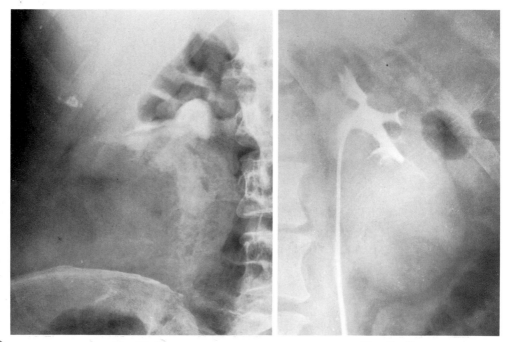

Fig. 10–15   Fig. 10–16

Figure 10–15. Hamartoma (angiolipoleiomyoma) in woman, 58 years of age. Recent severe renal pain in right upper quadrant. Nephrectomy.

Figure 10–16. *Retrograde pyelogram.* Hamartoma (angiolipomyoma) in lower pole of kidney of woman 53 years of age, examined because of nondescript lower abdominal pain. No palpable mass. Lesion discovered accidentally from excretory urogram.

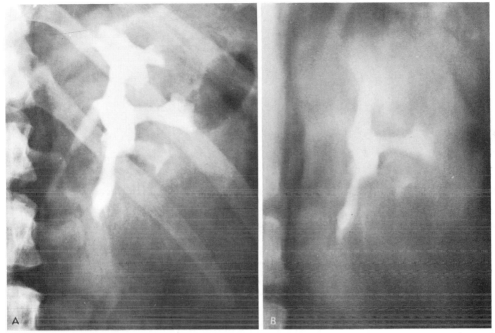

Figure 10–17. Hamartoma (angiolipomyoma) of left kidney with hemorrhage in man, 44 years of age. Previous right nephrectomy elsewhere for "benign tumor." Exploration and biopsy. A, *Excretory urogram.* B, *Nephrotomogram.* Irregular radiolucent area interspersed with dense areas suggests cysts; these actually were areas of hemorrhage and infarction.

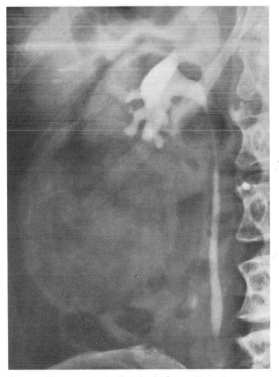

Figure 10–18. Angiomyolipoma (hamartoma) of right kidney. *Excretory urogram.* Large mass arising from lower pole of kidney. Note homogeneous radiolucency within mass but also thick capsule. Moderate distortion of calyces and rotation about its horizontal (transverse) axis. (From Adelman, B. P.)

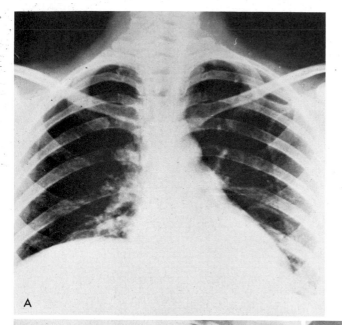

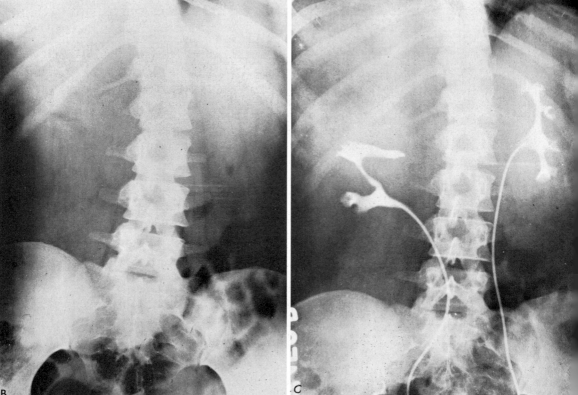

Figure 10–19. Hamartoma with spontaneous rupture and massive retroperitoneal hemorrhage. Woma aged 31. Sudden severe right flank pain and mass. **A,** *Chest roentgenogram.* Elevated right hemidiaphrag **B,** *Plain film.* Large soft-tissue mass filling right side of abdomen. Scoliosis of lumbar spine with concavi toward mass. **C,** *Retrograde pyelogram.* Distortion of pelvis and calyces with some lateral and downwa displacement of kidney and marked medial displacement of ureter. *Operation:* Retroperitoneal hematom 2,500 ml of clots evacuated. Necrosis of tumor in upper pole. *Nephrectomy.* (From Keshin, J. G.)

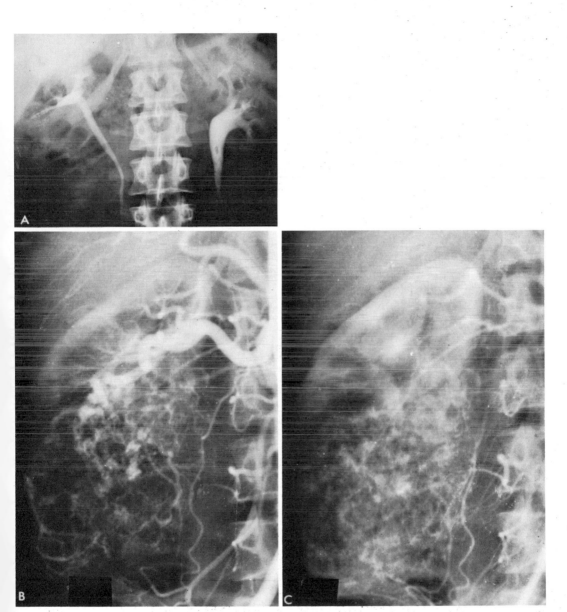

Figure 10–20. Angiomyolipoma (hamartoma) of right kidney. Woman aged 34 with intermittent right-upper-quadrant pain and palpable mass. **A,** *Excretory urogram.* Mass in lower pole of right kidney distorting pelvis and calyces and displacing lower pole of kidney laterally and upward. *Angiogram* at 1½ seconds (**B**) and at 2½ seconds (**C**). Abnormal vascularization in lower-pole mass with puddling and tumor "stain." Preoperative diagnosis was hypernephroma. (From Love, L., and Frank, S. J.)

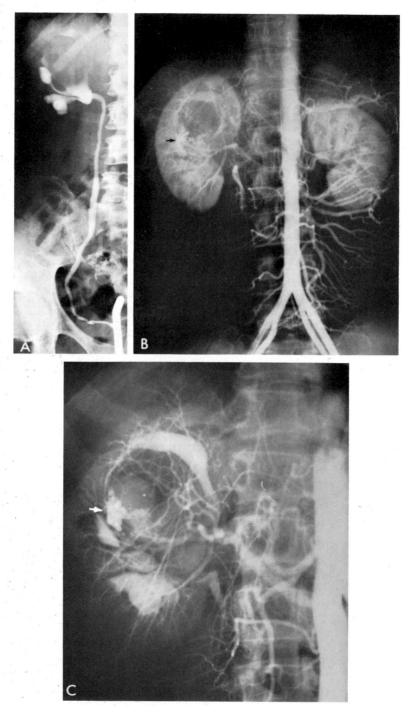

Figure 10–21. Angiomyolipoma (hamartoma) of right kidney. Woman aged 40. Mass and pain in right flank. **A,** *Retrograde pyelogram.* Filling defect in upper half of right kidney. **B** and **C,** *Retrograde femoral arteriograms.* Neovascularization and puddling of contrast medium in region of filling defect suggest malignant tumor. (From Seabury, J. C., Jr., Ensor, R. D., and Wolfe, W. G.)

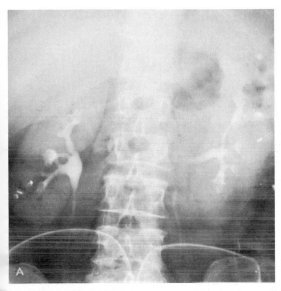

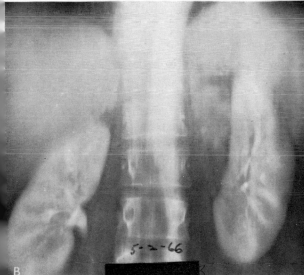

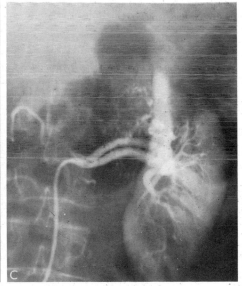

Figure 10–22. Angiolipoleiomyoma (hamartoma). Woman aged 67 being investigated because of polythemia vera. **A**, *Excretory urogram.* Indeterminate upper pole of left kidney. **B**, *Nephrotomogram.* Ill-defined vascular mass medial to upper pole of kidney. **C**, *Arteriogram.* Mass medial to upper pole of kidney is well defined and vascular. "Pathologic type" of tumor vessels suggests malignant tumor. *Exploration.* Hamartoma 8 by 7 by 4 cm attached to medial portion of upper pole of kidney by "meaty" stalk 1.5 cm in diameter. Second 1.5-cm lesion found in lower pole of kidney.

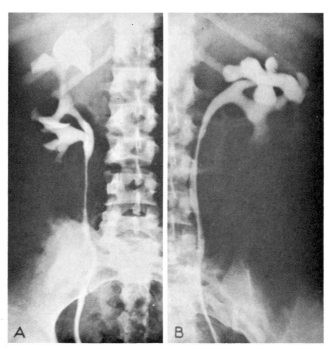

Figure 10–23. Bilateral hamartomas associated with tuberous sclerosis. Suggest polycystic disease. (From Deming, C. L.) **A,** Right kidney. **B,** Left kidney.

Fig. 10–24

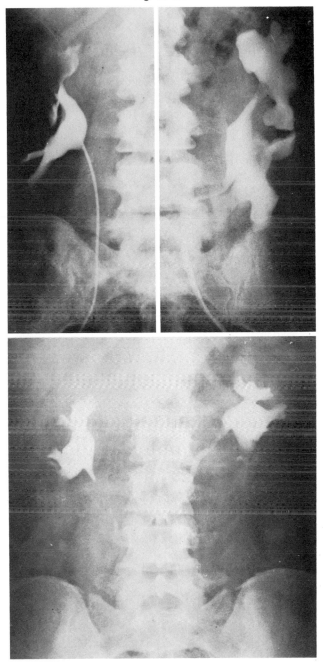

Fig. 10–25

Figure 10–24. *Bilateral retrograde pyelogram.* Bilateral hamartoma (angiolipomyoma) simulating poly-
ystic disease in woman, 40 years of age, with **tuberous sclerosis.** Note increased density of lumbar vertebrae.
From Taylor, J. N., and Genters, K.)

Figure 10–25. *Bilateral retrograde pyelogram.* Bilateral hamartoma (angiolipomyoma) simulating poly-
ystic disease in woman, 42 years of age, with **tuberous sclerosis.** (From Taylor, J. N., and Genters, K.)

Malignant Tumors of the Renal Cortex (Parenchyma)

EPITHELIAL TUMORS (ADENOCARCINOMA; HYPERNEPHROMA)

Epithelial cell tumors are generally considered to arise from the renal tubules and are spoken of as *renal cell tumors*. They comprise approximately 85% of all renal tumors. Many names besides hypernephroma or adenocarcinoma have been given to these tumors, among which may be mentioned Grawitz's tumor, hypernephroid carcinoma, alveolar carcinoma, clear cell adenocarcinoma, dark cell carcinoma, granular cell carcinoma, papillary cystadenocarcinoma, and parenchymal carcinoma.

The tumor cells may be large and clear or small with scant darkly stained basophilic cytoplasm containing many granules. These characteristics are responsible for the descriptive terms *clear cell, dark cell*, or *granular cell adenocarcinoma*. Grawitz in 1883 noted the similarity of the tumor cells to the cells of the adrenal cortex and postulated that the tumors arose from adrenal rests, which are so common in the kidney. He coined the term *hypernephroma*. The terms *hypernephroma* and *Grawitz's tumors* are used most commonly to this day.

Histogenesis

Most pathologists agree that adenocarcinoma of the kidney arises from tubular cells, but the mechanism is by no means clear. Cohnheim's theory of embryonic rests and more specifically Grawitz's theory of adrenal rests are not in current favor. In recent years the theory that adenocarcinoma arises from small benign adenomas has gained increased acceptance (Cristol, McDonald, and Emmett; deVeer and Hamm; Kozoll and Kirshbaum). The high incidence of adenomas in kidneys containing hypernephroma plus the difficulty of accurately distinguishing (microscopically) an adenoma from a low-grade hypernephroma supports this postulate. There are two main theories concerning the origin of the benign adenoma: (1) development in sclerotic kidneys in association with cysts and (2) development in association with embryologic abnormalities.

Clinical Considerations

Adenocarcinoma of the kidney occurs twice as frequently in males as in females. The common triad of symptoms is gross hematuria, flank pain, and palpable mass. In an occasional case persistent fever of unknown origin is the only symptom. Extension of tumor into the renal vein is a common surgical finding and portends a serious prognosis. McDonald and Priestley found such extension in 54% of their cases. It also explains the high incidence of early metastasis. The most common sites of metastasis in decreasing order of frequency are lungs, lymph nodes, liver, bones, and adrenal glands.

Urographic Diagnosis; "Conventional" Urograms
(Figs. 10–26 through 10–56)

Before the advent of modern tomograms, nephrotomograms, and arteriograms, which permit an almost three-dimensional visualization of the renal parenchyma, diagnosis depended on the two-dimensional "conventional" pyelogram. The outline of the renal parenchyma in that era left much to be desired, but if it could be seen it was of diagnostic help. Let us first consider the "conventional" pyelogram.

The most common general types of deformity encountered in hypernephroma are (1) enlargement or irregularity, or both, of the renal outline, (2) elongation of one or more calyces, with an abnormal termination, (3) narrowing or complete obliteration ("cut off") of a calyx or group of calyces, (4) encroachment on the pelvis to cause flattening, elongation, narrowing, irregular filling defects, or complete obliteration, (5) deformity or complete occlusion at the ureteropelvic juncture, (6) secondary pyelectasis, (7) calcification, (8) abnormal position of the renal pelvis, and (9) complete disruption of the gross architectural composition of the kidney. It should be helpful to consider these urographic changes in greater detail.

Renal Outline. Evidence of a tumor involving the renal cortex often may be obtained by observing closely the contour of the kidney in the plain film. Irregularity of outline or unilateral enlargement must always be regarded with suspicion, although it is by no means a diagnostic finding and must be substantiated by means of urography. In the case of a long-standing extensive tumor the plain film may show a huge "soft tissue" mass in the region of the kidney with no renal outline remaining.

Calyces. As the tumor enlarges toward the periphery, it tends to stretch or draw the calyx or calyces in the vicinity with it. In this process the calyx may be considerably elongated. Although elongation of the calyx is the most characteristic deformity seen in cortical tumor, it may also be the cause of many diagnostic errors. The reason for this is that elongated calyces occur with relative frequency in normal kidneys (Fig. 10–26). The important differential point to be remembered is that the termination of the elongated calyx in cases of tumor is nearly always abnormal (Figs. 10–27 through 10–36), in contrast to the normal terminal irregularity of the minor calyces in normal kidneys. Also, elongated calyces in normal kidneys usually are symmetrical; thus urographic visualization of the other kidney will be of great help in interpretation. The tip of the calyx in a case of tumor usually is narrowed, tapered, bulbous, or connected with an area of cortical necrosis, or it may be partially or completely obliterated.

The extent or number of calyces involved does not necessarily indicate the size of the tumor, although it usually is regarded as being somewhat indicative. The elongated calyces often present unusual outlines. A calyx may be narrowed uniformly throughout its entire length, or there may be irregular areas of narrowing and dilatation. In some cases the calyces may be stretched to unusual lengths and may extend in different directions, producing a bizarre appearance in the urogram, which has been described by the term *spider-leg deformity.*

As growth progresses, changes in the calyces become more marked. Portions of the calyces may not be visualized, so that irregular, detached patches of contrast medium are all that can be seen of the calyx. In more advanced cases one or more calyces may become completely obliterated from invasion of the growth (Figs 10–37, 10–38, and 10–39). Occasionally cases are seen in which the growth apparently has occluded the distal portion of the calyx so that retrograde medium does not enter it, yet an excretory urogram will visualize the deformed proximal portion if some function remains.

Invasion of Renal Pelvis. There is a tendency for cortical tumors to extend into and invade the renal pelvis. It is obvious that in such cases almost any type of deformity could result, such as flattening, narrowing, elongation, or dilatation of the pelvis. Filling defects from masses of tumor projecting into the pelvis or calyces *may be difficult to distinguish from primary epithelial tumors of the renal pelvis or from blood clots* (Figs. 10–40 through 10–45). Associated calyceal deformity or deformity of the renal outline, however, usually assists one in making the proper interpretation. Crater-like deformity of the renal pelvis is not uncommon and, in advanced cases, the pelvis may be completely obliterated, the outline of the retrograde medium terminating abruptly in the region of the ureteropelvic juncture. Such a lesion might be confused with nonfunctioning hydronephrosis with obstruction at the ureteropelvic juncture. Tumors large enough to produce external pressure on or to invade the adjacent ureter may produce similar urographic changes (Figs. 10–46 and 10–47).

Displacement and Rotation of Kidney. Displacement of the involved kidney from its normal position may be of diagnostic value. Especially is this true if the lesion involves the lower pole and becomes large enough to displace the ureter. It is obvious that the renal pelvis may be displaced in almost any direction, depending on the contour which the neoplasm assumes. However, displacement of the pelvis may occur in many conditions, so that it is unwise to place much reliance on this finding unless it is accompanied by other urographic evidence of greater significance (Figs. 10–48 through 10–52).

Calcification. The presence of calcification in a renal neoplasm, as with other such lesions, usually indicates that the tumor is of long standing. Though calcification is not common, it occurs with sufficient frequency that one must think of the possibility of tumor whenever it is encountered. It may simulate renal lithiasis or calcification of a renal cyst (Figs. 10–53 through 10–56).

Resemblance to Extrarenal Tumors and to Subcapsular and Perirenal Hematomas (Figs. 10–57 through 10–64). A hypernephroma may simulate an extrarenal or perirenal tumor which is displacing the kidneys (Figs. 10–57A and B and 10–58).

Subcapsular and Perirenal Hematomas; Differentiation From Hypernephroma and Extrarenal Tumor. Hematomas may simulate renal tumor (Figs. 10–59 through 10-62) but a nephrotomogram may clarify the situation and demonstrate the relation of the renal parenchyma to the mass. In the case of perirenal hematoma the renal parenchymal outline is not compromised. Gerota's fascia distended contains the extravasated blood. If the hematoma is subcapsular the renal capsule, being rigid, gives very little so that the pressure distorts and compresses the renal substance (Figs. 10–63 and 10–64).

In all fairness, it must be admitted that many urograms in cases of tumor of the renal parenchyma are difficult to fit into any classification or description given in previous paragraphs. In such cases, about all that can be said is that the *architecture of the kidney is completely disrupted.* When such cases are encountered, the presence of a renal tumor must be seriously considered (Figs. 10–65 and 10–66).

Hypernephroma With No Urographic Abnormality. Also, it must not be forgotten that it is possible, although unusual, to encounter an *extensive tumor of the renal parenchyma when the urogram seems almost normal* (Fig. 10–67). Apparently the only explanation for this phenomenon is that the tumor has grown in such a manner that it has replaced the normal parenchyma with tumor cells without disturbing the normal contour of the pelvis and calyces.

(Text continued on page 1087.)

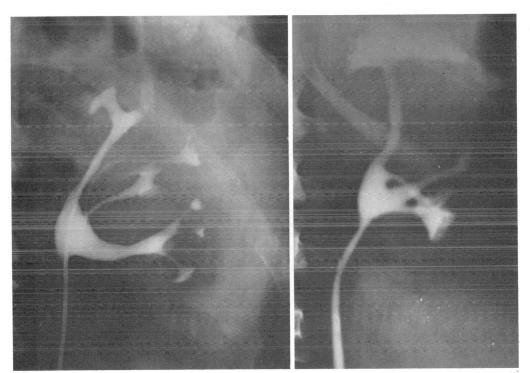

Fig. 10-26   Fig. 10-27

Figure 10-26. *Left retrograde pyelogram.* **Normal. Elongated type of calyx which might be confused with** adenocarcinoma (hypernephroma). Distinguishing factor here is that terminal irregularities of all calyces are normal.

Figure 10-27. *Left retrograde pyelogram.* **Adenocarcinoma** (hypernephroma) of left kidney. Elongated upper calyx with abnormal termination in cortical pocket.

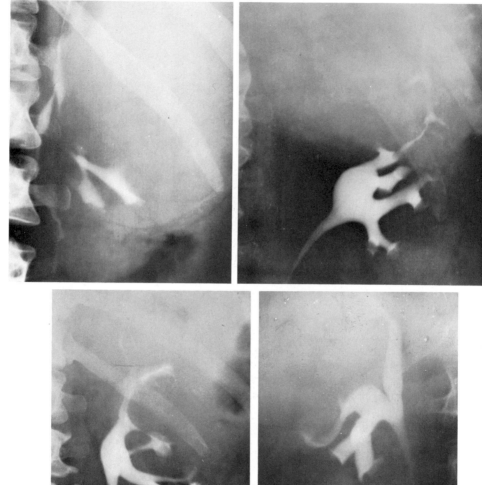

Fig. 10-30   Fig. 10-31

Figure 10-28. *Excretory urogram.* **Adenocarcinoma (hypernephroma)** of left kidney. Marked elongation of upper calyx, with abnormal termination.

Figure 10-29. *Left retrograde pyelogram.* **Adenocarcinoma (hypernephroma).** Huge tumor of upper pole with elongation of branch of upper calyx, which extends up as irregular tract of medium into tumor.

Figure 10-30. *Left retrograde pyelogram.* **Adenocarcinoma (hypernephroma).** Marked elongation of branches of middle and upper calyces, which have abnormal terminal irregularities.

Figure 10-31. *Right retrograde pyelogram.* **Adenocarcinoma (hypernephroma).** Elongated calyces of rather bizarre contour, and abnormal terminal irregularities.

Fig. 10-32

Fig. 10-33

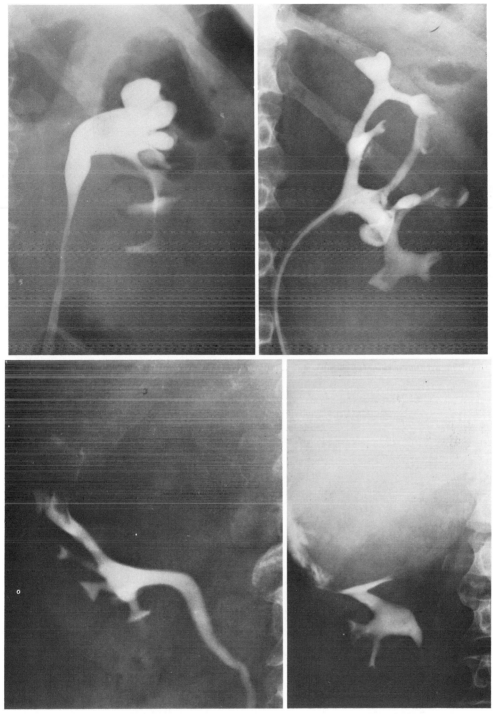

Fig. 10-34

Fig. 10-35

Figures 10–32 and 10–33.   *Left retrograde pyelograms.* Adenocarcinoma (hypernephroma).
Figures 10–34 and 10–35.   *Right retrograde pyelograms.* Adenocarcinoma (hypernephroma) involving upper pole.

Fig. 10–36

Fig. 10–37

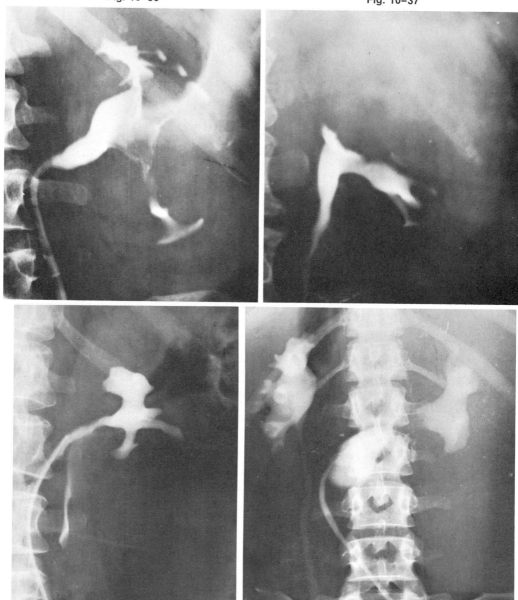

Fig. 10–38

Fig. 10–39

Figure 10–36. *Left retrograde pyelogram.* **Adenocarcinoma (hypernephroma).** Complete obliteration of middle calyx, partial obliteration of lower.

Figure 10–37. *Left retrograde pyelogram.* **Adenocarcinoma (hypernephroma).** Complete destruction and obliteration of upper and middle calyces from extensive tumor in upper half of kidney.

Figure 10–38. *Left retrograde pyelogram.* **Adenocarcinoma (hypernephroma).** Marked medial displacement of lower calyx.

Figure 10–39. *Bilateral retrograde pyelogram.* **Huge adenocarcinoma (hypernephroma)** involving bifid left kidney. At operation, tumor and kidney weighed 3,300 gm.

Fig. 10–40   Fig. 10–41

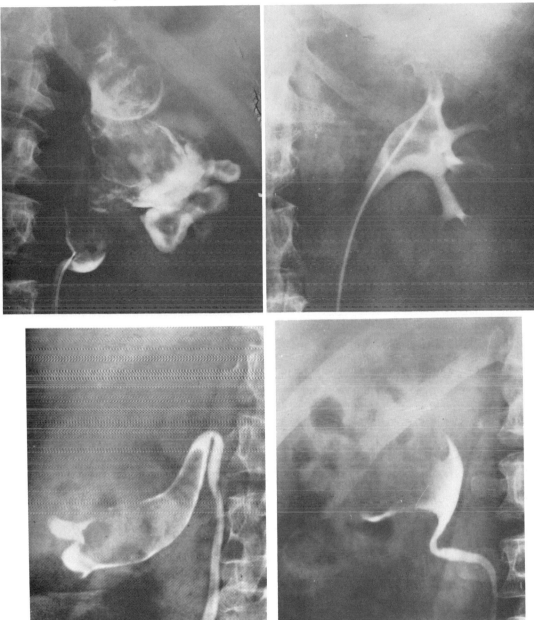

Fig. 10–42   Fig. 10–43

Figure 10–40. *Left retrograde pyelogram.* **Extensive adenocarcinoma (hypernephroma) which invaded** pelvis and ureter. Could be confused with papillary tumor of renal pelvis.

Figure 10–41. *Left retrograde pyelogram.* **Adenocarcinoma (hypernephroma) invading pelvis and upper** calyx, simulating solid epithelial tumor of renal pelvis.

Figure 10–42. *Right retrograde pyelogram.* **Adenocarcinoma (hypernephroma) invading pelvis and upper** calyx, simulating solid epithelial tumor of renal pelvis.

Figure 10–43. *Right retrograde pyelogram.* **Adenocarcinoma (hypernephroma).** Destruction of middle and upper calyces and invasion of pelvis. Would be difficult to differentiate from extensive epithelial tumor of renal pelvis.

Fig. 10–44

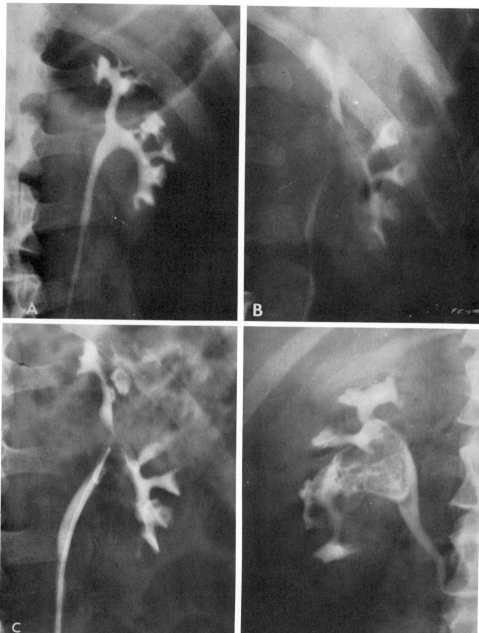

Fig. 10–44

Fig. 10–45

Figure 10–44. Rapidly growing adenocarcinoma (hypernephroma) in young man. **A**, *Left retrograde pyelogram,* made at onset of hematuria. Left kidney appeared urographically normal. **B** and **C**, *Excretory urogram and left retrograde pyelogram* made on same date, 2 months later than **A.** Inability to fill infundibulum of upper calyx of left kidney by either retrograde or excretory urography suggested tumor of renal pelvis. Operation disclosed grade 2 adenocarcinoma (hypernephroma). Left nephrectomy. Patient died from metastasis 2 months later.

Figure 10–45. *Right retrograde pyelogram.* Adenocarcinoma (hypernephroma) of renal cortex simulating epithelioma of renal pelvis. Preoperative diagnosis was epithelioma of renal pelvis. At operation, grade 2 adenocarcinoma (hypernephroma type) was found.

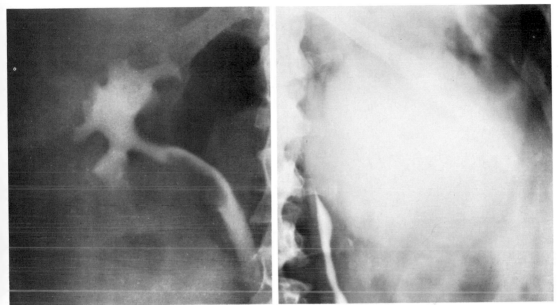

Fig. 10-46   Fig. 10-47

Figure 10-46. *Right retrograde pyelogram.* **Adenocarcinoma (hypernephroma)** of renal cortex. Middle and lower group of calyces completely obliterated. Partial involvement of upper calyx. Growth has eroded and almost obliterated renal pelvis. Could be confused with epithelial tumor of renal pelvis.

Figure 10-47. *Left retrograde pyelogram.* **Advanced adenocarcinoma (hypernephroma)** of renal cortex with complete obstruction at ureteropelvic juncture. Could easily be confused with hydronephrosis with obstruction at ureteropelvic juncture.

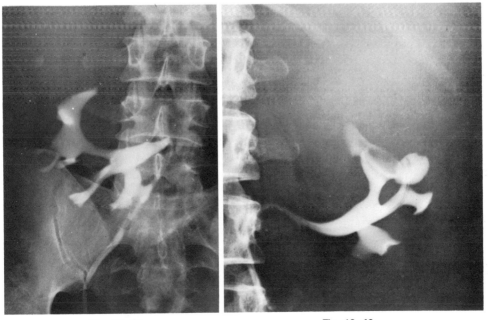

Fig. 10-48   Fig. 10-49

Figure 10-48. *Right retrograde pyelogram.* **Adenocarcinoma (hypernephroma)** of renal cortex. Marked deformity of pelviocalyceal system, associated with downward displacement of kidney resulting from tumor in upper pole.

Figure 10-49. *Left retrograde pyelogram.* **Adenocarcinoma (hypernephroma)** of renal cortex. Marked deformity of pelviocalyceal system, associated with downward displacement of kidney from tumor in upper pole.

Fig. 10–50

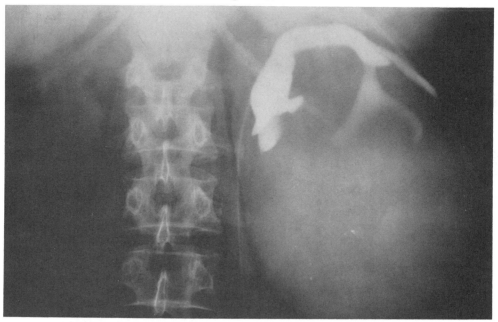

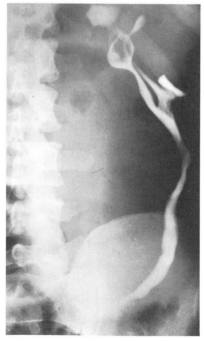
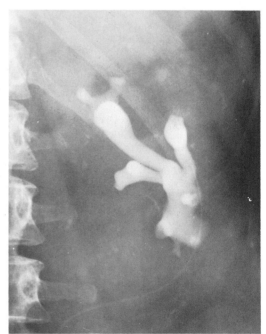

Fig. 10–51   **Fig. 10–52**

Figure 10–50. *Left retrograde pyelogram.* **Adenocarcinoma (hypernephroma)** of renal cortex. Marked deformity of pelvis and calyces, with upward displacement and rotation from tumor.

Figure 10–51. *Left retrograde pyelogram.* **Extensive adenocarcinoma (hypernephroma)** of renal cortex, producing marked deformity of pelviocalyceal system and lateral displacement of kidney and ureter.

Figure 10–52. *Left retrograde pyelogram.* **Extensive adenocarcinoma (hypernephroma)** of renal cortex, producing marked deformity of pelviocalyceal system and malrotation of kidney and ureter.

Fig. 10–53

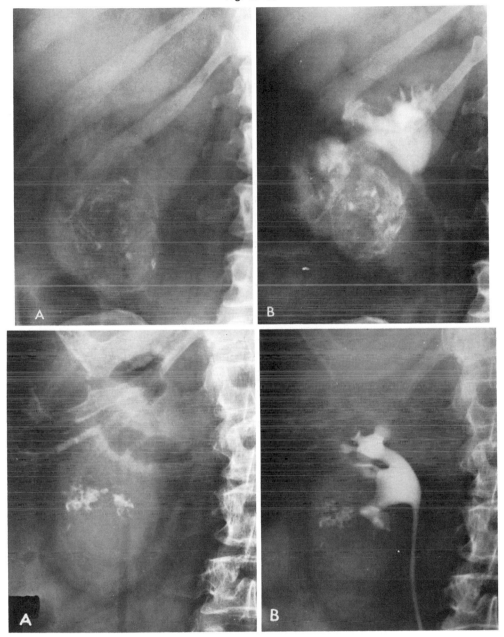

Fig. 10–54

Figure 10–53.   Adenocarcinoma (hypernephroma) of renal cortex with calcification. **A,** *Plain film.* Irregular diffuse area of calcification overlying lower pole of right kidney, and projecting beyond lower pole and medial margin. **B,** *Excretory urogram.* Irregular deformity of lower calyx of right kidney, typical of tumor, which surrounds calcific area. At operation, large hypernephroma of lower pole of right kidney, with calcification.

Figure 10–54.   Adenocarcinoma (hypernephroma) of renal cortex with calcification. **A,** *Plain film.* Diffuse area of calcification over right midrenal area. **B,** *Right retrograde pyelogram.* Irregular deformity of middle and lower calyces, which overlie and surround calcific shadow. Could easily be confused with renal tuberculosis with calcification.

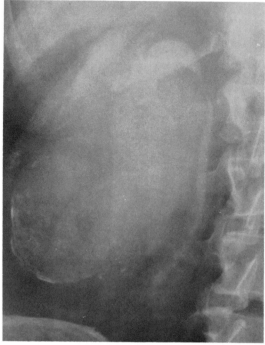

Figure 10–55.   Renal carcinoma with curvilinear calcification. *Excretory urogram.* Carcinoma of lower pole of right kidney partly outlined by calcification. (From Simpson, W.)

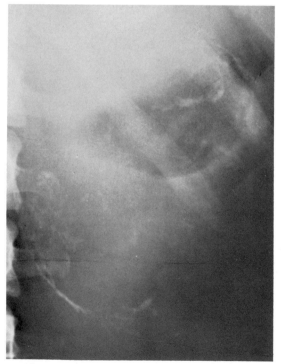

Figure 10–56.   Renal carcinoma with curvilinear calcification. *Excretory urogram.* Carcinoma of lower pole of left kidney almost completely outlined by calcification. (From Simpson, W.)

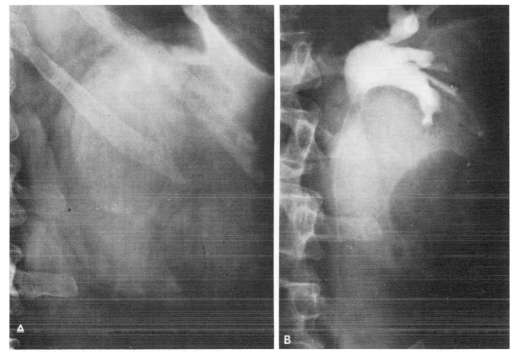

Figure 10-57. Adenocarcinoma (hypernephroma) of renal cortex, simulating extrarenal tumor. **A,** *Plain film.* Huge mass occupying left side of abdomen. **B,** *Left retrograde pyelogram.* Mass has displaced kidney upward and medially, with little or no deformity of pelviocalyceal system. Suggests extrarenal tumor. Exploration revealed hypernephroma.

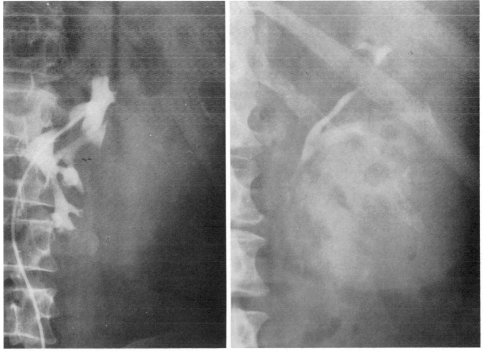

Fig. 10-58   Fig. 10-59

Figure 10-58. Adenocarcinoma of renal cortex (hypernephroma) simulating extrarenal tumor. *Left retrograde pyelogram.* Huge mass occupying left side of abdomen, which has displaced kidney medially and has produced little or no deformity of pelviocalyceal system. Suggests extrarenal tumor. Exploration revealed grade 2 adenocarcinoma.

Figure 10-59. *Excretory urogram.* Perirenal hematoma suggests hypernephroma.

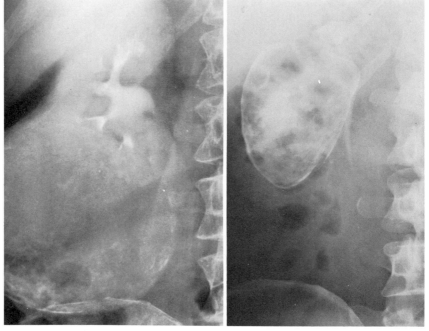

Fig. 10–60   Fig. 10–61

Figure 10–60. *Excretory urogram.* Calcified subcapsular hematoma.
Figure 10–61. *Retrograde pyelogram.* Calcified subcapsular hematoma which overlies lower half of duplicated kidney. Nephrectomy. Pathologic diagnosis: subcapsular, cystic, calcified hematoma.

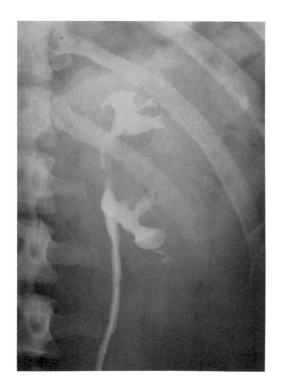

Figure 10–62. *Retrograde pyelogram.* Subcapsular hematoma in male, 18 years of age, who had been in automobile accident 9 months previously. There were gross hematuria and renal pain for 4 days following accident.

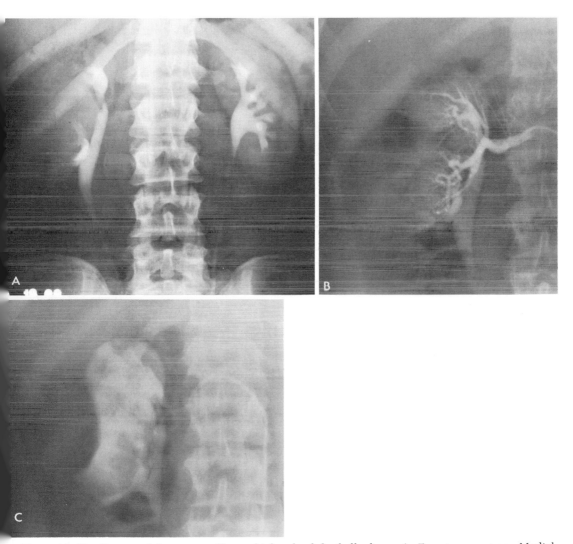

Figure 10–63.   Intrarenal hematoma. Young high school football player. **A,** *Excretory urogram.* Medial displacement of pelvis and calyces of right kidney by mass. **B,** *Arteriogram.* Mass appears to be subcapsular. Lateral margin of bulge well defined. Vessels displaced medially and mass is avascular. **C,** *Nephrographic phase.* Renal substance opacified, showing concavity of lateral margin from pressure of subcapsular hematoma.

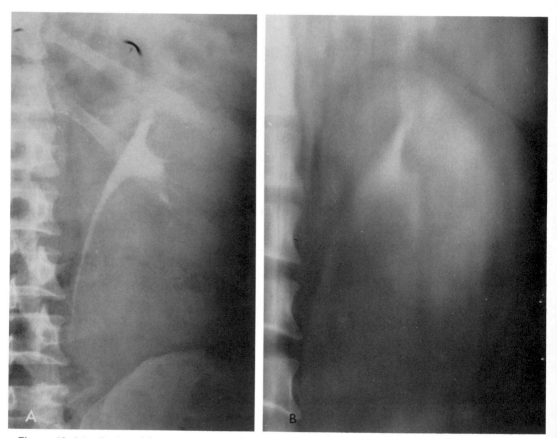

Figure 10–64.   Perirenal hematoma (caused by hemorrhage from small hypernephroma which cannot be seen). **A,** *Excretory urogram.* Mass of indeterminate limits involving left kidney. Ureter displaced slightly toward midline. **B,** *Nephrotomogram.* Renal outline appears normal. There is large soft-tissue mass (hematoma) which encases kidney but does not compress or distort it. Mass appears most extensive around lateral margin and below lower pole of kidney.

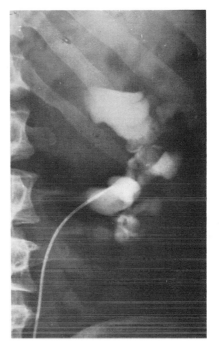

Figure 10–65. *Left retrograde pyelogram.* **Adeno-carcinoma** (**hypernephroma**) with almost complete destruction of architecture of kidney.

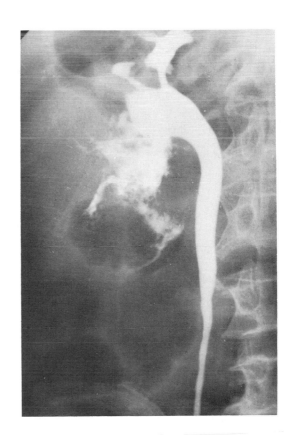

Figure 10–66. *Retrograde pyelogram.* **Hyper-nephroma** with extravasation of contrast medium into tumor.

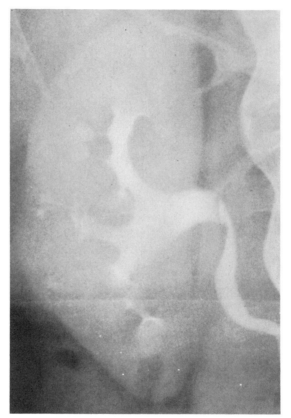

Figure 10–67.   Hypernephroma with normal *excretory urogram* and *tomogram*. Man, aged 62, presented
with symptoms related to widespread metastasis. Primary lesion discovered only at autopsy. Growth was on
medial aspect of kidney growing away from renal parenchyma.

Nephrotomography and Arteriography;
Differentiation of Tumor and Cyst
(Figs. 10–68 through 10–98)

The differentiation of tumor and cyst by means of conventional urograms has always been difficult or impossible (Figs. 10–68 through 10–71). Accuracy in differentiating tumors from cysts has been greatly increased with the use of intravenous nephrotomography and arteriography. As pointed out in Chapter 9, intravenous nephrotomography has been reported as accurately differentiating cyst from tumor in up to 95% of the cases (Chynn and Evans), and arteriography has detected renal carcinoma in 97% of cases (Watson, Fleming, and Evans). Selective renal arteriography is more effective than aortography in demonstrating vascular changes in tumors and both are more effective in this regard than nephrotomography. Nephrotomography, however, has the advantage of simplicity and safety and because of the dense nephrogram produced by this technique it is more effective than arteriography for demonstrating demarcation of the lesion from surrounding normal renal parenchyma and for indicating the thickness of the wall of the lesion. Consequently these techniques should not be considered competitive but rather complementary techniques which can be used singly or in combination to best serve the needs of the clinical situation.

In our own experience at the Mayo Clinic with more than 4,000 patients studied by intravenous nephrotomography, accuracy has been high if renal anatomy is well demonstrated and if rigid diagnostic criteria are adhered to. In 15 to 20% of our cases renal anatomy was not adequately demonstrated and the classic signs of cyst or tumor were not present; therefore differential diagnosis was not attempted and further study by renal arteriography, percutaneous aspiration, or exploration was employed. The criteria for differentiation of renal cyst from tumor are listed in Table 10–3. These criteria are essentially the same for both nephrotomography and arteriography (Figs. 10–72 through 10–98).

Renal carcinoma (hypernephroma) is usually a highly vascular tumor (Boijsen and Folin; Edsman; Folin; Olsson), though wide variation occurs. The tumor

Table 10–3. **Criteria for Differentiating Renal Cyst From Neoplasm by Nephrotomography and Arteriography**

PHASE	CYST	NEOPLASM
Arteriographic	Mass avascular Surrounding vessels displaced and stretched by mass	Mass vascular Abnormal "tumor type" vessels within mass Arteriovenous fistula often present Microaneurysms often present
Nephrographic	Mass radiolucent throughout	Irregular opacification of mass with pooling or puddling of medium
	Mass of homogeneous density throughout	Density of mass greater than, same as, or slightly less than that of adjacent renal cortex
	Wall thin and well defined Distinct, sharp margin between mass and adjacent renal cortex	Wall thick and irregular Margins poorly defined, fade into adjacent normal renal parenchyma
	Acute crescentic angle formed by renal cortex at junction with cyst wall	

is supplied by branches of the renal artery, the capsular arteries, and perforating branches. In advanced lesions, especially when the tumor has extended beyond the capsule, an accessory blood supply may be developed from the lumbar, intercostal, adrenal, or other regional arteries in the area of tumor invasion. The renal artery supplying the affected kidney is often larger than the artery to the normal kidney because of increased blood flow.

The carcinoma itself contains numerous irregular and distorted "tumor" vessels which are opacified during the arterial phase of the examination. **Arteriovenous fistula** may be present, producing early filling of veins draining the tumor. In some instances, **microaneurysms** are demonstrated in the tumor vessels. A diffuse "tumor blush" is seen during the nephrographic phase and "pooling" or "puddling" of contrast medium in the tumor produces an irregular mottled appearance. The prominence of the tumor vessels and the intensity of the tumor blush may be increased in some cases by the injection of small amounts of epinephrine directly into the renal artery just prior to injection of contrast medium (Abrams, Boijsen, and Borgström; Kahn and Wise) (Figs. 10–87 and 10–88). The margins of the tumor as seen during the nephrographic phase are rarely sharply defined but rather fade into the adjacent normal parenchyma with no clear demarcation between normal and abnormal tissue.

Vascularity of renal carcinomas varies widely and tumor vessels may not be a prominent feature in some tumors (Becker and associates). Watson, Fleming, and Evans found that the tumor was either avascular or minimally vascular in 22 of 100 consecutive cases (Table 10–4). Avascular tumors may be solid or may exhibit all degrees of tumor necrosis and cystic change; some mimic cysts in roentgenographic appearance. Most of these avascular malignant lesions can be

Table 10–4. Classification of Renal Carcinoma According to Degree of Vascularity on Angiography*

GROUP	CHARACTERISTIC	CASES
0	Avascular	6
1	Minimal vascularity	16
2	Moderate vascularity	16
3	Marked vascularity	62
Total		100

*From Watson, R. C., Fleming, R. J., and Evans, J. A.

suspected, however, if careful attention is directed to other signs of tumor which are best shown on the nephrogram. The wall of the tumor is thickened (Bosniak and Faegenburg) (Figs. 10–89 and 10–91) in contrast to the paper-thin wall of a benign cyst. The margins of even a well-encapsulated tumor are poorly defined and appear to fade into the surrounding normal parenchyma, and the marginal lips where the mass protrudes through the cortex are absent or poorly demonstrated (Figs. 10–92 and 10–93).

Carcinoma arising within a cyst can be a source of diagnostic error since it mimics simple cyst in roentgenographic appearance (Watson, Fleming, and Evans). For practical purposes, however, these lesions do not present a significant problem in diagnosis since they are so rare as to constitute a pathologic curiosity. Emmett, Levine, and Woolner were unable to find an example of this lesion among 1,007 explorations of renal masses, and only isolated case reports describing tumor arising in a cyst are found in the literature (Khorsand).

In advanced carcinoma with renal vein or inferior vena caval obstruction by tumor thrombus, the kidney is usually nonfunctioning (Fig. 10–96). Despite this, the tumor is readily demonstrated by arteriography in most instances and the extent of the venous thrombosis may be demonstrated by inferior vena cavography (Figs. 10–93, 10–94, and 10–95). Tumor spread beyond the confines of the kidney as well as metastasis to adjacent structures is often visualized when present (Figs. 10–97 and 10–98).

Lindau–von Hippel Disease

It is well known that patients with von Hippel's disease (retinal angiomatosis) commonly have associated intracranial lesions. This observation was first made by Lindau in 1926. He described associated cerebellar cysts, cerebellar and medullary angioblastic tumors, pancreatic cysts, and cystic and hypernephroid tumors of the kidney. These associated lesions occur in approximately 20% of patients and when present the resultant syndrome is known as Lindau-von Hippel disease. Although Lindau described only cysts and benign tumors of the kidney, more recent reports (Greene and Rosenthal; Kaplan, Sayre, and Greene; Kernohan, Woltman, and Adson) have shown that the renal component of the disease may be malignant (hypernephroma). In the two cases reported by Kaplan, Sayre, and Greene, the adenocarcinomas were multiple and bilateral (Figs. 10–99 and 10–100A, B, and C). A subsequent communication (Levine, Witten, and Greene) reported one patient with a simple cyst and another with a hemangioepithelioma (Fig. 10–101)

(Text continued on page 1117.)

Fig. 10–68　　　　　　　　　　　　Fig. 10–69

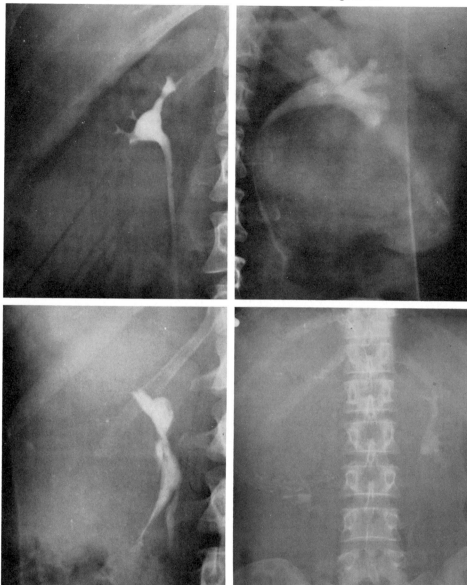

Fig. 10–70　　　　　　　　　　　　Fig. 10–71

Figure 10–68. Hypernephroma simulating cyst. *Right retrograde pyelogram.* Large circular soft-tissue mass involving lower pole of right kidney. Lower calyx incompletely outlined. Could be confused with simple cyst with poorly outlined lower calyx. Surgical exploration revealed grade 3 hypernephroma.

Figure 10–69. Hypernephroma simulating cyst. *Left retrograde pyelogram.* Large circular soft-tissue mass involving lower pole of left kidney, causing crescentic compression of pelvis and lower calyx, but little evidence of destruction of calyces.

Figure 10–70. Hypernephroma simulating cyst. *Right retrograde pyelogram.* Large circular, smooth soft-tissue mass involving midportion of right kidney, causing apparent compression and displacement of middle and lower calyces. Could easily be confused with cyst.

Figure 10–71. Ruptured necrotic cyst of right kidney with retroperitoneal hematoma. Cyst had been discovered urographically 6 years previously. Woman aged 54 with sudden onset of severe pain in right upper quadrant. *Excretory urogram.* Suggested large renal cyst. Preoperative diagnosis was "acute peritonitis; inconsequential cyst." *Nephrectomy* done. *Pathology:* Ruptured necrotic cyst arising from anterior surface of kidney and containing **small focus of grade 2 hypernephroma.** (From Thompson, G. J., and Culp, O. S.

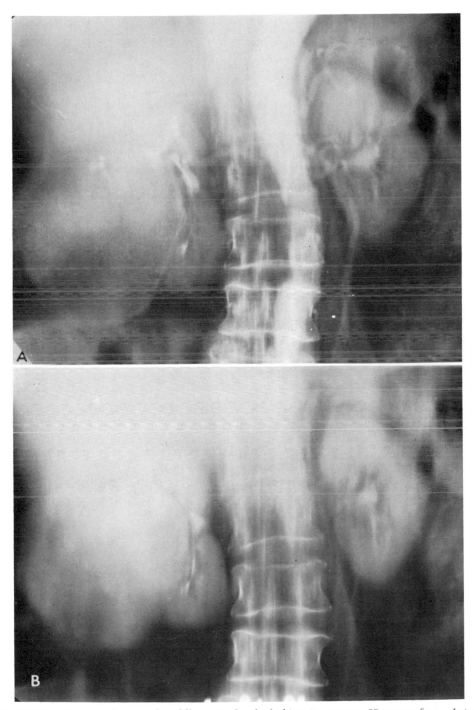

Figure 10–72. Hypernephroma of middle part of right kidney in woman, 69 years of age. *Intravenous nephrotomogram.* **A,** *Vascular phase.* Abnormal vascularization seen in upper part of mass suggests tumor. **, *Nephrographic phase.* Increased density of mass with areas of radiolucency indicates tumor with necrosis.

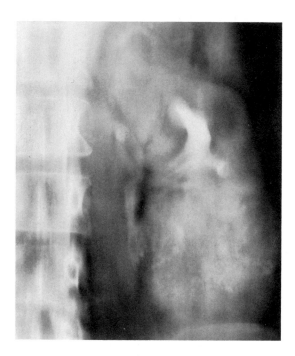

Figure 10–73. *Intravenous nephrotomogram.* **Hypernephroma of lower pole** of left solitary kidney. Note increased density of tumor as well as pathologic vascularization, puddling, and tumor staining. Right kidney removed elsewhere previously, apparently because of hydronephrosis and infection.

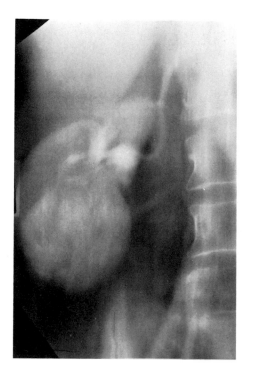

Figure 10–74. *Intravenous nephrotomogram, vascular phase.* **Hypernephroma** of lower pole of right kidney in woman, 56 years of age. Typical increased density of tumor with abnormal vascularization tumor stain, and puddling.

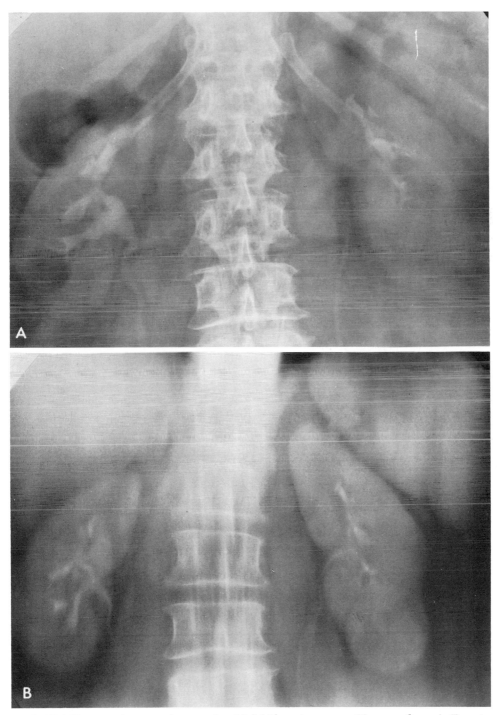

Figure 10–75. **Hypernephroma** at lower pole of left kidney in woman, 60 years of age. **A,** *Excretory uro-gram.* Poor outline of possible soft-tissue mass in lower pole of left kidney. Minimal (if any) deformity of wer calyx. **B,** *Intravenous nephrotomogram (nephrographic phase).* Solid tumor at lower pole, causing inimal changes in lower calyx.

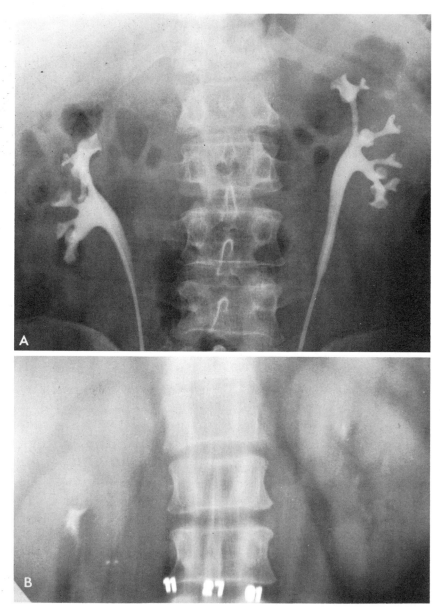

Figure 10–76. Hypernephroma with metastasis in man, 44 years of age. **A,** *Bilateral pyelogram* made because biopsy of suspected painful area in rib had shown metastatic carcinoma which suggested hypernephroma. Pyelogram normal, but renal outlines (especially on right) not well-delineated. **B,** *Intravenous nephrotomogram, nephrographic phase.* Hypernephroma, arising from upper pole of right kidney, which is growing away from kidney and is not distorting calyces.

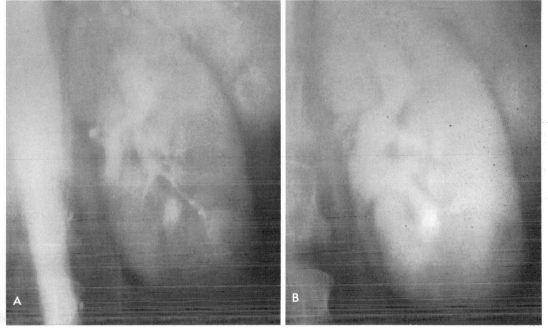

Figure 10–77. Renal carcinoma (hypernephroma). *Intravenous nephrotomograms.* **A,** *Vascular phase.* Tumor in lower pole of left kidney is highly vascular and of greater density than surrounding renal parenchyma. **B,** *Nephrographic phase.* Rapid washout of contrast medium has made tumor radiolucent as compared to renal parenchyma. Margins are sharply defined. If only nephrographic films were available, this tumor would be misdiagnosed as cyst.

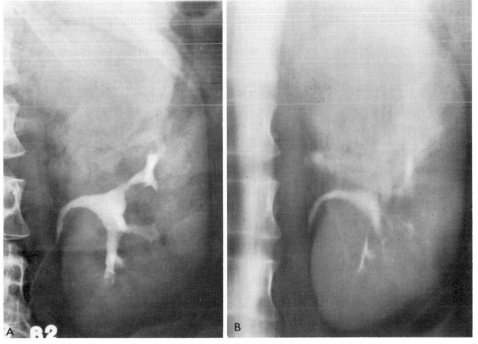

Figure 10–78. Hypernephroma of upper pole of left kidney with metastasis to lung. **A,** *Excretory urogram.* Mass in upper pole of kidney displacing calyces downward. **B,** *Intravenous nephrotomogram.* Large necrotic tumor with radiolucent center. Note pathologic vascularization of lower part of tumor with extensive puddling of contrast medium (tumor staining).

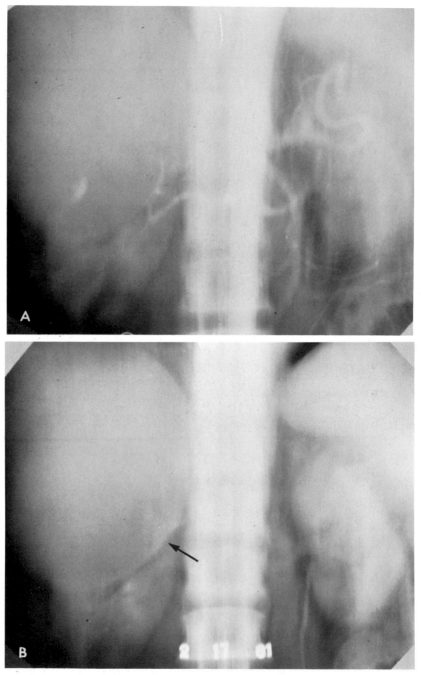

Figure 10–79. *Intravenous nephrotomograms.* **Hypernephroma** of right kidney in man, 62 years of age. **A,** *Vascular phase.* Vessels appear to skirt avascular mass. **B,** *Nephrographic phase.* Large round mass with radiolucent areas in lower and medial half, but increased density of upper half. Accentuation of lower and medial parts of capsule (*arrow*). Exploration revealed necrotic hypernephroma. Thickened capsule is pathognomonic of tumor rather than cyst.

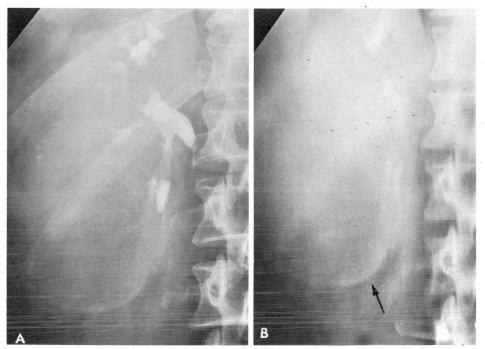

Figure 10–80. Hypernephroma in lower half of right kidney in man, 56 years of age. *A, Excretory urogram.* Large space occupying lesion compressing and distorting middle and lower calyces. **B,** *Intravenous nephrotomogram, nephrographic phase.* Large tumor with necrosis of lower half. Large radiolucent area in lower pole suggests cyst, but thickened capsule *(arrow)* and abnormal calyces suggest tumor.

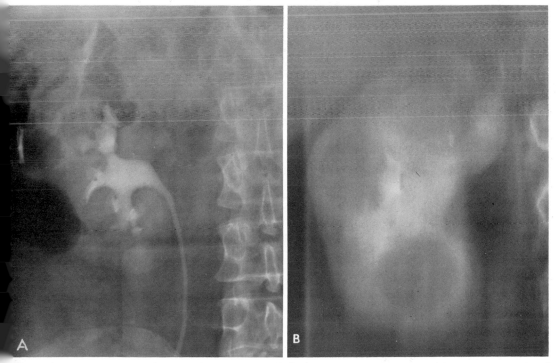

Figure 10–81. Cysts and hypernephroma in same kidney. **A,** *Excretory urogram.* Mass in upper pole of right kidney displaces upper pole laterally. Crescentic deformity in middle and lower pole calyces. **B,** *Intravenous nephrotomogram, nephrographic phase.* Typical simple cysts are present in mid and lower portions of kidney. Larger mass (hypernephroma) occupies upper pole. Tumor is opacified while cysts are lucent and sharply marginated.

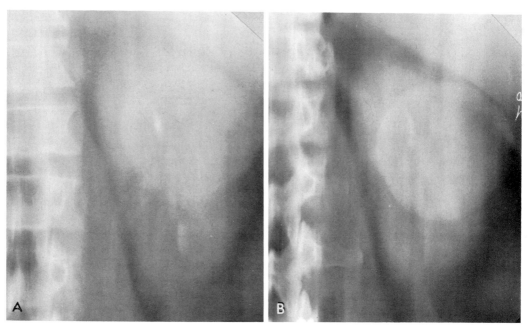

Figure 10–82.   Simple cyst of left kidney diagnosed erroneously as neoplasm. *Intravenous nephrotomo grams.* **A,** *Arterial phase.* Renal vessels not shown. **B,** *Nephrographic phase.* Shows apparent opacification o mass which suggested tumor. Surgical exploration revealed cyst.

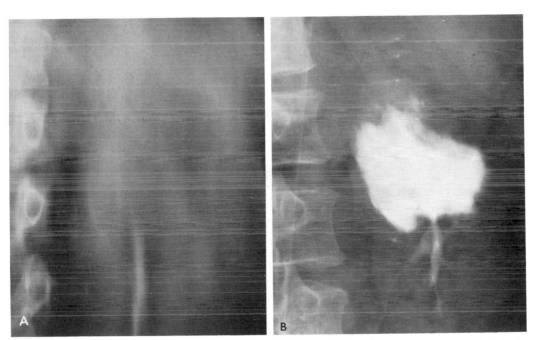

Figure 10–83. Hypernephroma. **A,** *Intravenous nephrotomogram.* Indeterminate mass in left kidney, possibly cyst. **B,** *Percutaneous needle puncture* yielded thick cloudy fluid typical of hypernephroma with cystic degeneration. *Injection of contrast medium* into mass showed marked irregularity of wall seen in cases of necrotic tumor.

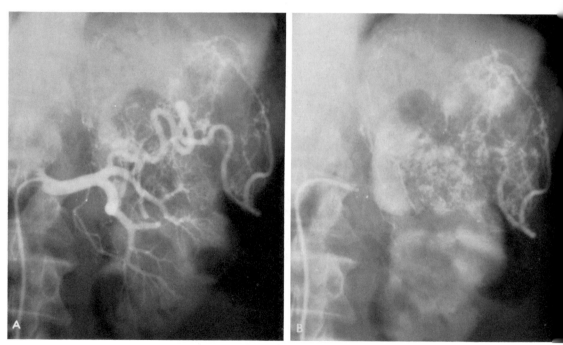

Figure 10–84.   Hypernephroma. *Selective renal arteriograms.* **A,** *Arterial phase.* Large mass containing irregular and distorted "tumor vessels" is present in upper pole of left kidney. Main arterial supply to tumor is from large branch of renal artery to upper pole. **B,** *Nephrographic phase.* "Tumor blush" is present and pooling or puddling of medium is seen.

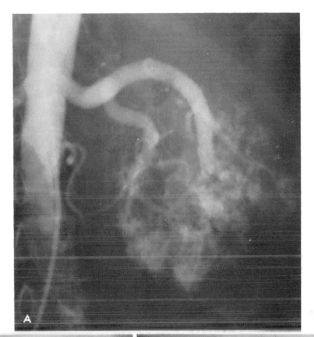

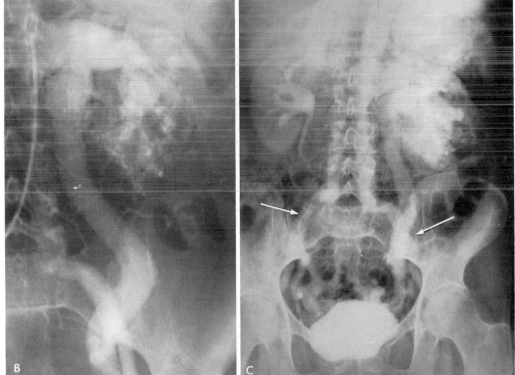

Figure 10-85. Hypernephroma with arteriovenous fistula. **A,** *Selective renal arteriogram, arterial phase.* Huge left renal artery with large irregular tumor vessels. **B,** *Late arterial phase.* Beginning opacification of enlarged renal vein. **C,** *Arterial phase of nephrotomogram* showing marked dilatation of both left and right ovarian veins (*arrows*) with opacification of uterine and ovarian vessels due to shunting and increased blood flow. No obstruction of renal vein or inferior vena cava was found at operation. (From De Weerd, J. H.: Arteriovenous Fistula in Hypernephroma. J. Urol. 93:666–668, 1965.)

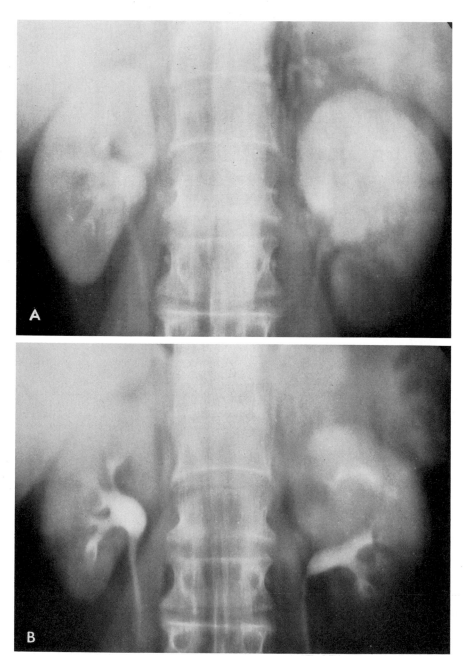

Figure 10–86.   *Intravenous nephrotomograms.* **A,** *Nephrographic phase.* **Solid tumor** (**hypernephroma**) in upper pole of left kidney. **B,** *Later nephrographic phase* showing deformity of upper calyx from tumor. **C** *Aortogram, vascular phase.* Typical abnormal vascularization of tumor with puddling (staining) and irregular diffusion of medium. (Courtesy of Dr. Hugh Williams.)

Figure continues on facing page

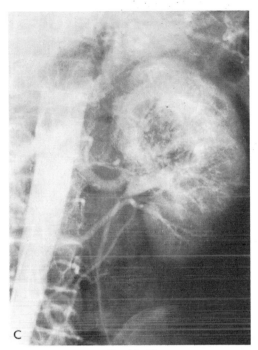

Fig. 10–86

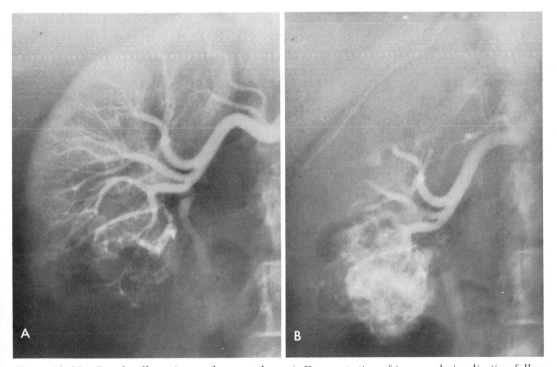

Figure 10–87.   Renal cell carcinoma (hypernephroma). Demonstration of improved visualization follow-ing epinephrine injection. **A,** *Selective right renal arteriogram* shows absence of nephrogram at right lower pole and abnormal vessel distribution. **B,** *After injection of 10 μg of epinephrine* directly into renal artery. Note general renal vasoconstriction and intense tumor blush. (From Kahn, P. C., and Wise, H. M., Jr.)

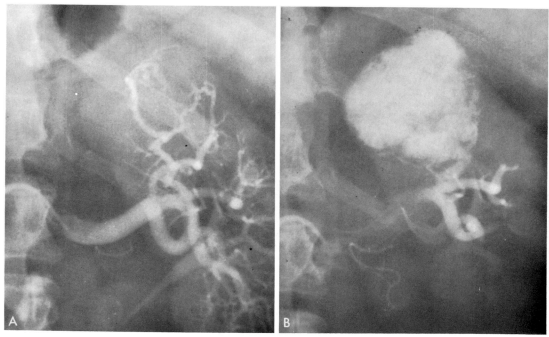

Figure 10–88. Renal cell carcinoma (hypernephroma). Demonstration of improved visualization following epinephrine injection. **A,** *Selective renal arteriogram.* Somewhat sparse tumor vessels are present in upper pole of left kidney. **B,** *After injection of epinephrine* directly into renal artery. Note intense opacification of tumor with little opacification of renal parenchyma. (From Kahn, P. C., and Wise, H. M., Jr.)

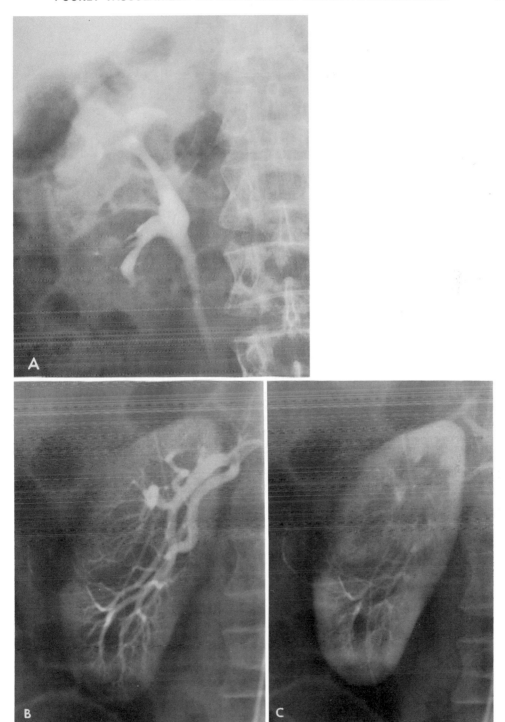

Figure 10–89.   Poorly vascularized hypernephroma. **A,** *Excretory urogram.* Some displacement of calyces in mid right kidney suggesting possible mass. **B,** *Selective renal arteriogram, arterial phase.* Poorly vascularized mass is present in midportion of kidney. Capsular arteries extend over surface of tumor. **C,** *Nephrographic phase.* No tumor blush is seen. Medium remains in capsular vessels. Irregular disruption of renal cortex is seen with no sharp margin between tumor and normal cortex.

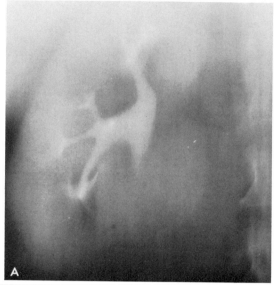

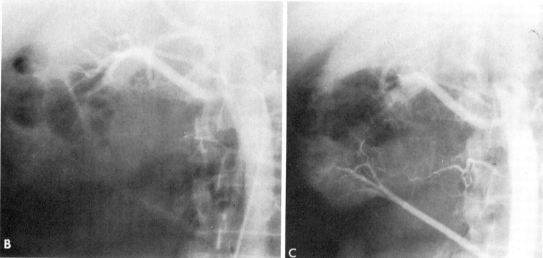

Figure 10–90.   Hypovascular hypernephroma in kidney with two renal arteries. A, *Tomogram made at time of excretory urography* shows mass in medial portion of right kidney. B, *Selective renal arteriogram* fails to demonstrate tumor. C, *Midstream injection* fills both renal arteries. Tumor, present in central part of kidney, is filled from lower renal artery. This case illustrates importance of examination of entire arterial supply to kidney when tumor is suspected.

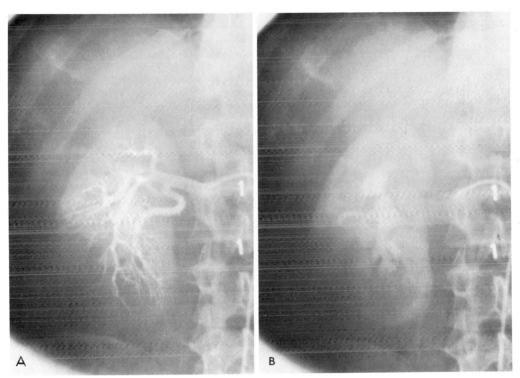

Figure 10–91. Papillary adenocarcinoma (hypernephroma). Patient presented with signs of prostatism. On an admission intravenous urogram, mass of lower pole of right kidney was identified. *Arteriogram* (**A**) shows avascular mass that does not opacify on *nephrographic phase of arteriogram* (**B**). Interface with kidney is irregular, but not typical of cyst in single radiographic projection. Solid tumor encountered at operation. Nephrectomy performed. In this case nephrotomography with "thick wall" might have proved diagnostic but unfortunately it was not performed. (From Becker, J. A., Fleming, R., Kanter, I., and Melicow, M.)

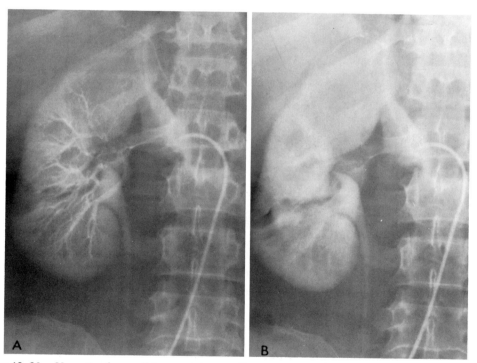

Figure 10–92.   **Necrotic clear cell hypernephroma.** Patient presented with hematuria. *Intravenous pyelogram* demonstrated mass in upper pole of right kidney. Diffuse metastatic disease in lung. **A,** *Arteriogram.* Poorly vascularized lesion, with several small irregular vessels at margin of kidney and mass. **B,** *Nephrographic phase* reveals lack of opacification and irregular interface with normal kidney. Kidney was removed; tumor proved to be necrotic clear cell carcinoma. (From Becker, J. A., Fleming, R., Kanter, I., and Melicow, M.)

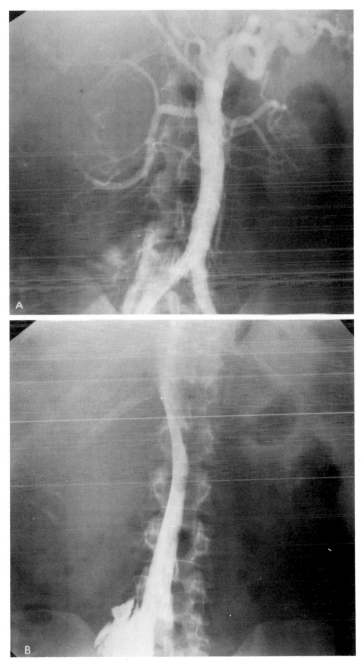

Figure 10–93. Huge, partially necrotic hypernephroma. **A,** *Arteriogram* shows tumor vessels and distortion of branches of right renal artery by mass. Much of tumor is avascular due to necrosis. **B,** *Inferior vena cavogram.* Inferior vena cava is displaced by tumor but no tumor thrombus is present. Lesion was still operable.

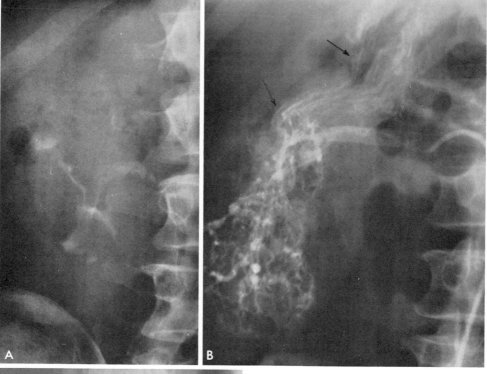

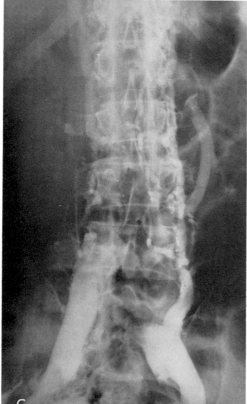

Figure 10–94. Vascular hypernephroma. **A,** *Excretory urogram.* Poorly functioning right kidney is seen with mass distorting collecting system. **B,** *Renal angiogram.* Huge vascular tumor occupies lower pole of right kidney. Striated pattern of vessels overlying upper pole at level of renal vein is evident (*arrows*). **C,** *Inferior vena cavogram.* Inferior vena cava is completely obstructed from fourth lumbar vertebra to hemidiaphragm. Large collateral veins are outlined by medium. (From Ferris, E. J., Bosniak, M. A., and O'Connor, J. F.)

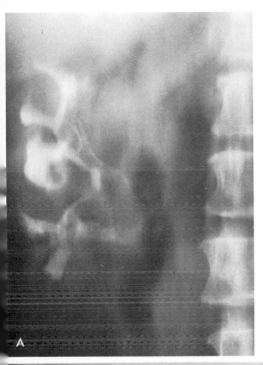

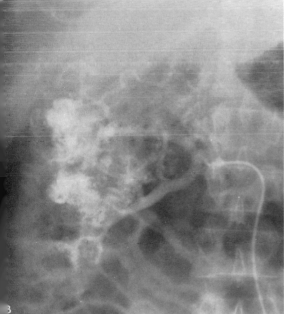

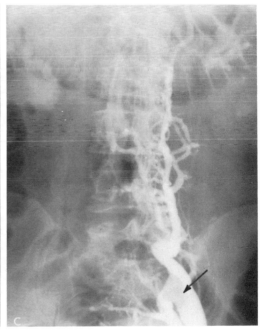

Figure 10–95.   Hypernephroma with obstruction of inferior vena cava. **A,** *Excretory urogram.* Functioning
ght kidney with tumor and blood clot in renal pelvis. **B,** *Selective renal arteriogram.* Huge vascular tumor
volves upper two thirds of right kidney. **C,** *Inferior vena cavogram.* Inferior vena cava is filled with tumor
wn to left iliac veins (*arrow*). Massive collateral circulation is present with filling of spinal and perispinal
eins.

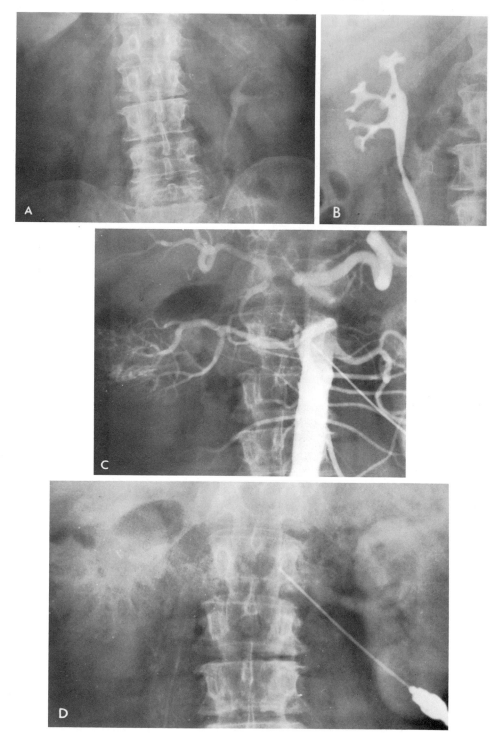

Figure 10–96.   Hypernephroma with occlusion of renal vein by tumor. **A,** *Excretory urogram.* Nonfunctio of right kidney. **B,** *Retrograde pyelogram.* Minimal distortion of middle calyceal group with little other ev dence suggesting the presence of tumor. **C,** *Aortogram, early film.* Hypernephroma involving midportion kidney. **D,** *Aortogram, delayed film.* No nephrogram is seen. At operation, right renal vein was completel occluded by tumor thrombus.

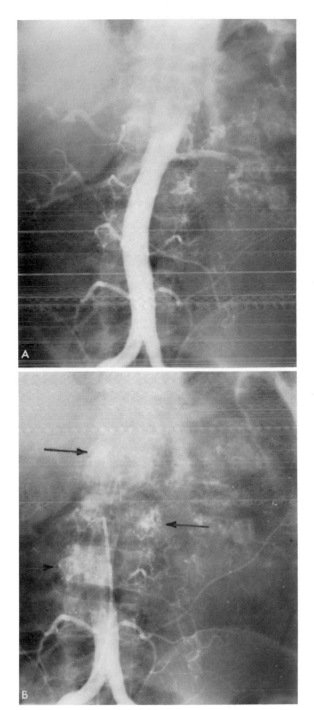

Figure 10–97.   Inoperable **hypernephroma** of left kidney **with metastasis to lungs and spine.** *Arteriogram.* ‸uge hypernephroma of left kidney with metastasis rich in vascular supply in lumbar spine. **A,** *Early phase.* ‸umor vessels and tumor stain visible throughout large mass. **B,** *Later phase.* Metastasis to bodies of lumbar ‸rtebrae 2, 3, and 4 is demonstrated by abnormal tumor-type vessels in areas of metastasis (*arrows*).

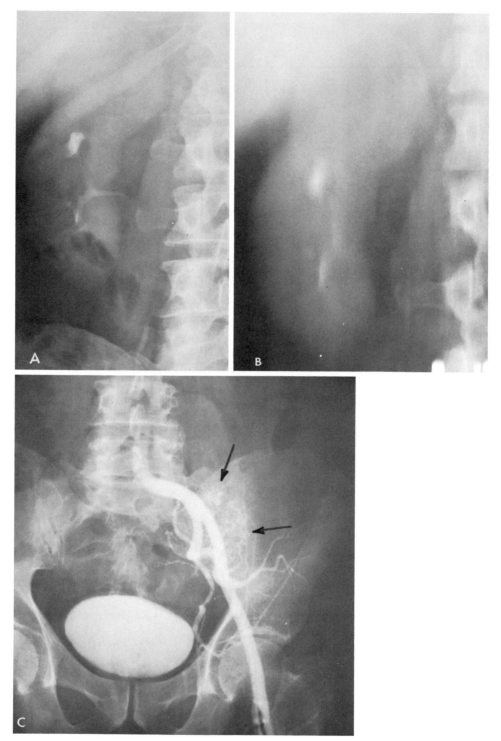

Figure 10–98. Unsuspected **hypernephroma** of right kidney. (Patient presented with pulsating mass o
buttock.) **A,** *Excretory urogram.* Mass in upper pole of right kidney. **B,** *Nephrotomogram, nephrographi*
phase. Thick walled, partially necrotic tumor. **C,** *Left iliac arteriogram.* Highly vascular metastasis to le
ilium (*arrows*).

Fig. 10–99   **Fig. 10–100**

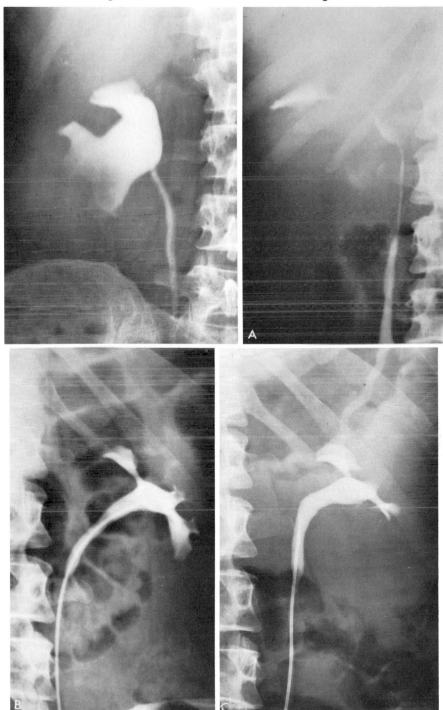

Fig. 10–100

Figure 10–99. Woman, 62 years of age, with **Lindau-von Hippel disease.** *Retrograde pyelogram.* **Hyper-** **nephroma.** Nephrectomy. Patient died 9 years later. Necropsy revealed multiple hypernephromas in remain- g kidney, with metastasis to lungs. (From Kaplan, C., Sayre, G. P., and Greene, L. F.)

Figure 10–100. Woman, 38 years of age, with **Lindau-von Hippel disease. A** and **B,** *Bilateral excretory* *elograms* (1956). **A,** *Right:* **hypernephroma. B,** *Left:* **normal.** Right nephrectomy done. **C,** *Left retrograde* *elogram* (1958). Lesion of lower pole of solitary kidney. Surgical exploration revealed **multiple hyper-** **nephromas associated with multiple small cysts.** (From Kaplan, C., Sayre, G. P., and Greene, L. F.)

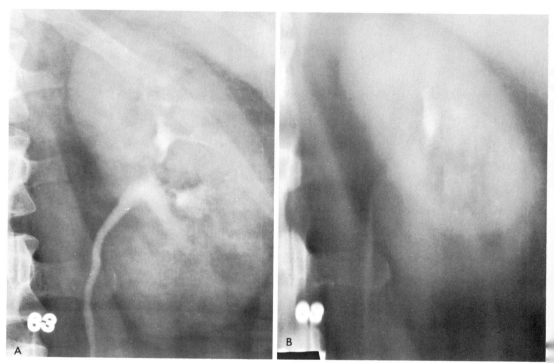

Figure 10–101.   Hemangioendothelioma of kidney in patient **with Lindau-von Hippel disease. A,** *Excretory urogram.* Filling defect in infundibulum of upper calyx and also some downward displacement of middle calyx. **B,** *Nephrotomogram.* Highly vascular lesion between middle and upper calyx. At operation, lesion was "shelled out" after biopsy which showed lesion to be benign hemangioendothelioma. (From Levine S. R., Witten, D. M., and Greene, L. F.)

MESENCHYMAL (CONNECTIVE TISSUE) TUMORS (FIBROSARCOMA; LIPOSARCOMA; LEIOMYOSARCOMA; RHABDOMYOSARCOMA)

Fibrosarcoma, liposarcoma, leiomyosarcoma, and rhabdomyosarcoma are the malignant variants of the benign tumors fibroma, lipoma, leiomyoma, rhabdomyoma, and angioma). As mentioned previously these tumors may arise from fibrous tissue in the renal capsule or renal parenchyma (Weisel, Dockerty, and Priestley) or from smooth muscle rests in the renal pelvis and calyces, parenchyma, and blood vessels. In 1966 Bazaz-Malik and Gupta found 31 cases of leiomyosarcoma of the kidney reported in the literature and added 1 of their own. In the case of benign tumors the origin may be clear, but it may be impossible (even on gross and microscopic examinations) to determine the site of origin of a malig-

nant mesenchymal tumor such as a fibrosarcoma. The difficulty in diagnosis is further compounded by the many malignant connective tissue tumors that originate from retroperitoneal tissue in the vicinity of the kidney. The tumor and the kidney may be so intimately related that it is often impossible to decide (even at surgical exploration) whether the tumor is of renal or perirenal (retroperitoneal) origin. It goes without saying that urographic diagnosis is not definitive (Figs. 10–102 through 10–105). (See also "Retroperitoneal Tumors" later in this chapter.)

Generally speaking, *fibrosarcomas* arise most frequently from the renal capsule. *Liposarcomas* are rare in the kidney but are the most commonly encountered retroperitoneal tumor. Although extremely rare, *osteogenic sarcomas* arise with almost equal frequency from the renal capsule and the cortex.

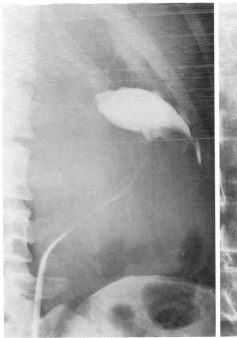

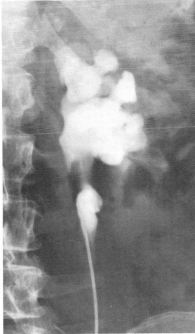

Fig. 10–102   **Fig. 10–103**

Figure 10–102. Leiomyosarcoma of left kidney in woman, 52 years of age. Nephrectomy. Tumor probably originated from capsule.

Figure 10–103. *Retrograde pyelogram* of woman, 66 years of age. Polypoid fungating sarcoma, grade 3, middle and lower portions of left kidney and projecting into lumen of pelvis. Associated transitional cell epithelioma, grade 2, of pelvis and calyces is invading kidney. Capsule perforated. Perirenal fat involved.

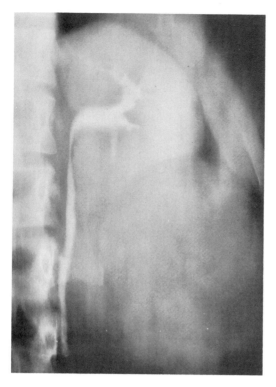

Figure 10–104. *Nephrotomogram.* **Lipomyxosar-coma associated with lower pole of left kidney** Woman aged 46. Liposarcoma removed from lef thigh 8 months previously. Patient now has mass in left side of abdomen. *Operation.* Tumor "adjacent" and attached to lower pole of left kidney. Impossible to be sure whether tumor arose from renal capsule or retroperitoneal space.

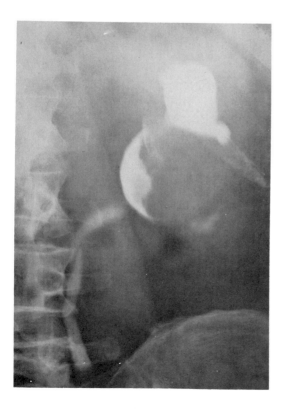

Figure 10–105. *Retrograde pyelogram.* **Fibrosar-coma of lower pole of left kidney, simulating tumo of renal pelvis** in man, 71 years of age. Adjacer peritoneum is involved. Nephrectomy.

EMBRYONAL TUMORS; WILMS' TUMOR (OLD TERMS: EMBRYONAL ADENOSARCOMA; ADENORHABDOMYOSARCOMA; NEPHROBLASTOMA; MALIGNANT NEPHROMA; MALIGNANT MIXED EMBRYOMA; MIXED CONGENITAL TUMOR; MESOBLASTIC NEPHROMA)

Origin

Wilms' tumors, described by Wilms in 1899, are considered to arise from the metanephrogenic renal blastema. The renal blastema is a part of the nephrogenic line which contains the most primitive mesoderm (mesenchyme) and carries with it certain elements of all cell layers (Culp and Hartman). Bell (1946) expressed the view that these cells may retain multipotential properties. The metanephrogenic renal blastema should be distinguished from the mesonephric or wolffian duct. Culp and Hartman divided embryonal tumors of the kidney into two classifications: (1) those of *mesoblastic origin* (renal cortex) and (2) those of *mesonephric origin* (renal pelvis). Embryonal tumors of the cortex (Wilms' tumor or embryonal adenosarcoma) are the most common, and these authors have suggested the term *mesoblastic nephroma* as the name of choice rather than Wilms' tumor. These tumors contain both epithelial and connective tissues with, of course, various degrees of cellular differentiations. Culp and Hartman stated that some of the embryonal carcinomas and poorly differentiated sarcomas may be mesoblastic nephromas in which one type of primitive cell has "completely dominated."

Wilms' tumor is usually *unilateral*; the incidence of *bilateral* tumors has been reported to vary from 1 to 10% (Bishop and Hope; Scott; Williams and Young). At present it is not clear whether the bilateral tumors reported represent separate primary lesions or metastasis from a primary lesion in the opposite kidney (Gyepes and Burko).

Pathology

Wilms' tumor tends to be encapsulated and may remain so for a considerable period, but as it enlarges the capsule is perforated, permitting invasion of the renal parenchyma and perinephric tissues. The tumor may arise in any part of the kidney and may reach an enormous size. *On cut section* it is usually sharply demarcated from the rest of the kidney by its "pseudocapsule."

Microscopically an abundant embryonic type of malignant connective tissue surrounds some gland-like tubules of variable size and shape. Solid cords and strands of epithelial cells may be present. Structures resembling abortive glomeruli may be seen as well as smooth or striated muscle, myxomatous tissue, fat, and cartilage.

Metastasis is principally by the hematogenous route, the lungs being the most frequent site and the liver next. The *bones are rarely involved*, in contradistinction to neuroblastoma,* in which bone is the most common site of metastasis. Less common and rare sites for metastasis include peritoneum, brain, spleen, adrenal gland, ipsilateral ureter, and bladder (Ferris and Beare).

Clinical Data: Symptoms and Findings

The presenting complaint is most often an *abdominal mass* or a general enlargement of the abdomen discovered by the mother. Pain is present in not more than 20 to 30% of cases. In contradistinction to malignant renal tumors in adults, *hematuria* (either gross or microscopic) is not a common finding. Some authors (Caffey; Hope and Borns; Scott) say that it is rare; others, however, have found that it occurs more frequently (Kinzel and associates, 12%; Williams and

---

*Neuroblastoma is considered under the heading of retroperitoneal tumors, pages 1212–1214.

Young, one third of cases; Lalli and associates, 14 of 31 cases). *Fever* has been reported in 10 to 20% of cases.

Although Wilms' tumor is occasionally encountered in adults, it is considered to be chiefly a disease of infants and children. More than 90% of cases are encountered before the eighth year of life. It is extremely important that the lesion be discovered and treated as early as possible because the length of survival and "cures" are infinitely superior when the tumor is diagnosed and treated in children less than 2 years of age. One important reason for this is the observation that the incidence of metastasis "on presentation" in children less than 2 years of age is approximately 25% whereas in older children it is nearer 50% (Rubin and associates, 1968b).

Diagnosis

When confronted with an abdominal mass or enlargement in an infant, the physician should remember that there is at least a 50% chance that it is related to the urinary tract (Lattimer, Melicow, and Uson), the most common renal lesion being hydronephrosis, the next being Wilms' tumor. The most common "nongenitourinary" tumor is neuroblastoma. Neuroblastoma occurs more frequently than Wilms' tumor. Of the abdominal masses presenting in a series of 285 children (Lattimer, Melicow, and Uson), half were of renal origin. Almost one third were Wilms' tumor; a third were neuroblastoma. It is important that the urologist consider the possibility of hydronephrosis in each case, as it is surprising how many children are still subjected to abdominal exploration for possible Wilms' tumor or neuroblastoma only to have hydronephrosis found. The hydronephrosis may be unilateral, involving a single kidney, but more often it involves the upper pelvis of a duplex kidney associated with an ectopic ureter or ectopic ureterocele. (See Figs. 12-250,

12-254, and 12-255, and pages 1452-1453.) The fact that an abdominal mass is firm and indurated does not exclude hydronephrosis, as a distended, tense renal pelvis or hydronephrotic sac may feel very firm to palpation.

In most cases an excretory urogram, done with meticulous technique and employing reinjection and delayed films of several hours when necessary, will differentiate a tumor involving the kidney, either intrinsically (Wilms') or extrinsically (neuroblastoma), from hydronephrosis. At times visualization may be poor because of the large overlying tumor, but some contrast medium can usually be seen. In the complete absence of visualization one must consider obstructive hydronephrosis as a likely possibility, but an extensive tumor with a tumor thrombus in the renal vein or inferior vena cava or both is also a possibility. This may be detected with an inferior vena cavogram. It has been suggested (Hope and Borns; Rubin and associates, 1968b) that in infants suspected of having a Wilms tumor the excretory urogram be initiated as an inferior vena cavogram by injecting the contrast medium into the saphenous or femoral vein. In this way one obtains both a cavogram and an excretory urogram with one procedure.

Urographic Data; Differentiation From Neuroblastoma (Figs. 10-106 through 10-121)

Wilms' tumor is an *intrinsic* lesion of the kidney so that one expects, and usually finds, distortion of the "internal architecture" (collecting system) of the kidney. This is in contrast to *extrinsic* neuroblastoma, which chiefly displaces the kidney (lateral angulation); at times however, this distinction is not too well defined. As mentioned previously, Wilms' tumor may remain encapsulated from some time so it may appear more like a cyst distorting the pelvis and calyces, or the mass may become so large that it displaces one pole of the kidney with minimal distortion of the pelvis and calyces suggesting displacement from a neuroblastoma. In some cases the tumor appears to grow "away from" rather than "into" the kidney so that one may encounter a huge tumor and at some place on its periphery a tiny, almost normal-appearing kidney is attached. Following roentgen therapy it is not unusual to see the urographic appearance in such a case return almost to normal. To illustrate difference of opinion, Caffey stated that neuroblastoma cannot be conclusively differentiated from Wilms' tumor on the basis of the roentgen picture; on the other hand, Hope and Borns stated "These two lesions can be correctly diagnosed with a high percentage of accuracy by intravenous urography." In our experience the true situation lies somewhere between these two statements. Inasmuch as surgical exploration and biopsy are indicated in either case, an absolute preoperative differentiation does not appear imperative.

Among the urographic changes that have been described, the following may be mentioned: an enlarged renal shadow or renal mass with indistinct borders, obliteration of the psoas muscle outline, and displacement of abdominal viscera (bowel); flattening, elongation, or bizarre distortion of pelvis or calyces or both; obliteration of one or more calyces; and displacement of one pole or the entire kidney. Anterior displacement of the kidney (as seen in lateral-view films) has been emphasized by Lalli and associates; displacement and compression of the ureter may occur but this is more characteristic of neuroblastoma. Wilms' tumor may at times be confused with polycystic disease, especially if the disease is bilateral. It may also be confused with leukemic infiltration of the kidney or lymphoma. The descriptions given above are, of course, common to almost any variety of malignant renal tumor.

An important factor in differentiation may be the *absence of calcification* in the tumor; calcification is common in neuroblastoma (see Fig. 10–246) but rare in Wilms' tumor. The *absence of bony metastasis* is another important diagnostic factor; it is common in neuroblastoma but exceedingly rare in Wilms' tumor. The presence of catecholamines in the urine of patients with neuroblastoma is another important feature in differential diagnosis.

The situation of a renal mass with no visualization in the excretory urogram has already been discussed, and the possibility of hydronephrosis as the diagnosis was mentioned. Such a situation is also possible in an extensive tumor that has invaded the pelvis and adjacent ureter and/or has extended into the renal vein and vena cava. This occurs in approximately 10% of cases (Lalli and associates). In differential diagnosis one must also consider spontaneous renal thrombosis, especially in the newborn infant. In both cases a cavogram may reveal the obstruction. It has been suggested that the presence of either microscopic or gross hematuria in such a case suggests thrombosis instead of tumor; if there is no hematuria the Wilms tumor is the more probable diagnosis (Rubin and associates, 1968b). In the newborn infant with an enlarged nonfunctioning kidney and a patent vena cava, the possibility of a multicystic kidney must be kept in mind.

Treatment

Treatment of Wilms' tumor consists of surgical removal (if feasible), irradiation, and chemotherapy, especially dactinomycin (actinomycin D) (Farber, 1955; Farber and associates, 1956; 1960). At the present writing, *preoperative* irradiation is not considered unless the tumor is so large that surgical removal is impossible until it has first been shrunk by irradiation.

Operation as soon as the diagnosis is

made is imperative. Excessive preoperative palpation of the tumor is to be avoided. Most often, treatment of Wilms' tumor consists of immediate surgical removal plus subsequent irradiation or chemotherapy (dactinomycin) or both. There seems to be general agreement that dactinomycin should be given intravenously on the day of operation—as soon as the diagnosis is confirmed while the patient is on the operating table and before excessive manipulation of the tumor has been begun. The transperitoneal approach is preferred so that the renal pedicle can be ligated early; the renal vein and vena cava must be carefully inspected for tumor thrombosis. There is much disagreement as to the amount and type of postoperative chemotherapy and as to whether or not irradiation should be given.

Articles in the literature by some competent observers favor no postoperative irradiation, especially if the patient is less than 1 or 2 years of age and if metastases are not demonstrated. Other equally competent workers feel that both irradiation and chemotherapy should be used despite the minimal risk of irradiation damage to normal tissue such as the spinal column, spinal cord, and blood vessels (Fig. 10–121). The reason for such difference of opinion is, of course, that no one person or group has enough cases from which to draw firm conclusions.

To obviate this deficiency, national study groups have been set up with standard protocols of treatment so that treatment may be objectively evaluated. This should eventually provide answers not presently available. A description of one such protocol (no. 6512) currently being investigated may illustrate present trends. According to this protocol, patients are arbitrarily placed in two groups: A and B.

Group A. Patients are given a "combination" treatment of (1) surgery, (2) dactinomycin at operation and for 10 days after operation, (3) postoperative irradiation, and (4) vincristine weekly for 6 weeks.

Group B. Patients are given postoperative irradiation and immediate dactinomycin therapy followed by intensive courses of dactinomycin therapy given at 6-week intervals for 1 year. No vincristine is given to this group.

Whereas previously the outlook has been considered almost hopeless, results with modern treatment are now most encouraging as evidenced by Farber's (1966) report of survivals of 2 years or more in 58% of 31 children with proven metastasis. It should be pointed out here that a 2-year survival of an infant corresponds to at least a 5-year survival of an adult. Collins' hypothesis (Collins, 1955, 1958; Collins, Leffler, and Tivey) of the "period of risk," which is equal to the age of the patient at the time of the original diagnosis plus 9 months (gestation period), forms the basis of this concept. His "safe period," then, is twice the age of the child at original diagnosis plus 9 months. Statistical data of results seem to support Collins' hypothesis, as 95% of deaths from Wilms' tumor appear to occur within 2 years after treatment (Garcia, Douglass, and Schlosser; Klapproth;

(Text continued on page 1131.)

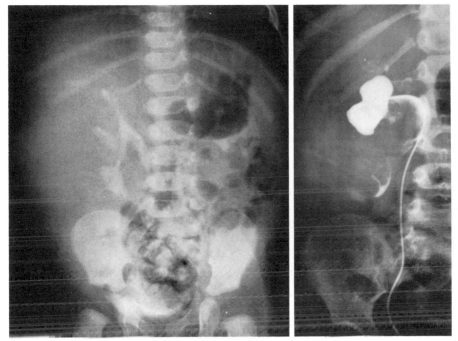

Fig. 10–106   Fig. 10–107

Figure 10–106. Wilms' tumor in boy, 3 months of age. Presenting symptom. large, smooth mass in right side of abdomen. *Excretory urogram.* Medial displacement of right kidney and ureter, with marked elongation and flattening of lower calyx. Middle and upper calyces incompletely outlined. Left kidney normal. Exploration revealed Wilms' tumor 30 cm in diameter. Right nephrectomy done.

Figure 10–107. Wilms' tumor in boy, 3 years of age. *Retrograde pyelogram.* Marked disruption of collecting system with dilatation of upper calyces. Medial displacement of ureter.

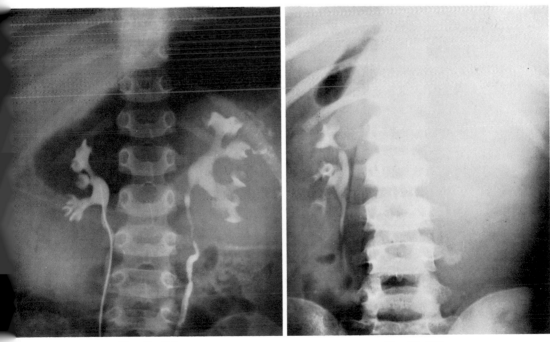

Fig. 10–108   Fig. 10–109

Figure 10–108. *Bilateral retrograde pyelogram.* Wilms' tumor of left kidney in boy, 5 years of age. Right kidney normal.

Figure 10–109. *Excretory urogram.* Wilms' tumor of left kidney in girl, 7 years of age. **No function.**

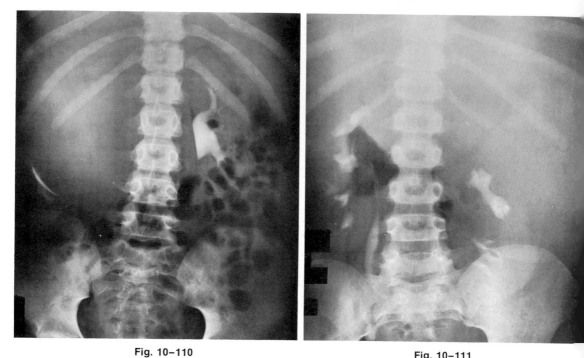

Fig. 10–110   Fig. 10–111

Figure 10–110. *Excretory urogram.* **Wilms' tumor** of right kidney in girl, 8 years of age.

Figure 10–111. *Excretory urogram.* **Wilms' tumor** of left kidney in boy, 9 years of age. Large tumor involving upper pole of kidney. Left nephrectomy.

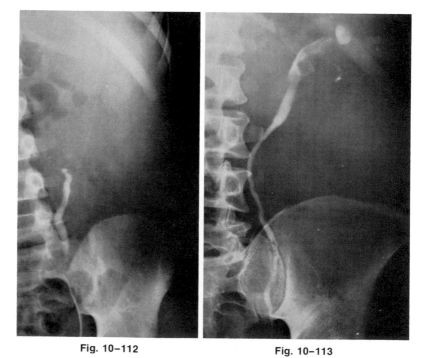

Fig. 10–112   Fig. 10–113

Figure 10–112. *Left retrograde pyelogram.* Complete obstruction of upper part of ureter (no function evidenced in excretory urogram) caused by **Wilms' tumor** in boy, 9 years of age.

Figure 10–113. *Retrograde pyelogram.* **Wilms' tumor** in man, 45 years of age.

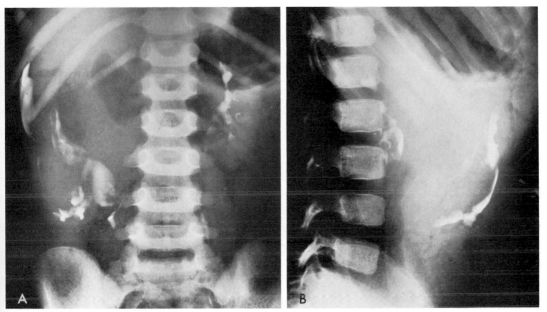

Figure 10–114. Wilms' tumor (right kidney) in boy aged 3 years, 9 months. *Excretory urograms.* **A,** *Antero-posterior view.* Marked distortion of pelves and calyces from extensive infiltrating lesion. **B,** *Lateral view.* Marked anterior displacement of involved kidney. (From Lalli, A. F., Åhström, L., Ericsson, N. O., and Rudhe, U.)

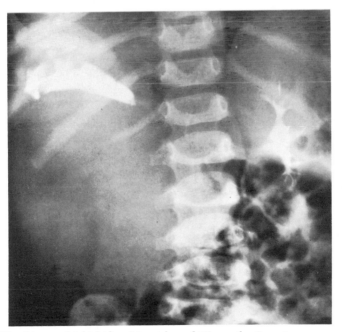

Figure 10–115. Wilms' tumor (right kidney) in girl aged 15 months. *Excretory urogram.* Lower-pole mass splacing pelvis and calyces cephalad. Normal nephrographic effect in upper pole but absent in lower pole. rom Lalli, A. F., Åhström, L., Ericsson, N. O., and Rudhe, U.)

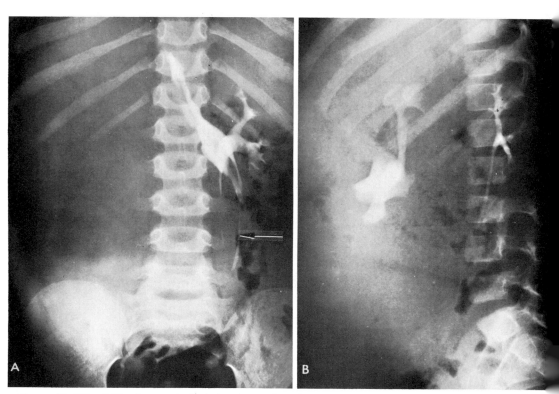

Figure 10–116.   Wilms' tumor (right kidney) in girl aged 4½ years. *Excretory urograms.* **A,** *Anteroposterior view.* Distortion of pelvis and calyces by tumor so large it is displacing kidney across midline and partially obscuring left kidney. *Arrow* indicates displaced right ureter. **B,** *Lateral view.* Marked anterior displacement of involved right kidney. (From Lalli, A. F., Åhström, L., Ericsson, N. O., and Rudhe, U.)

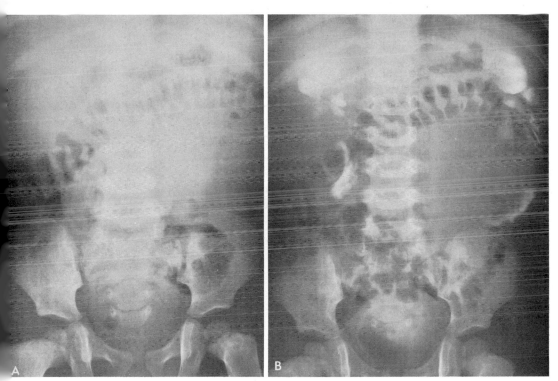

Figure 10–117.   Bilateral Wilms' tumor in boy aged 2½ years. Proved by exploration and biopsy. **A,** *Plain* *m.* **B,** *Excretory urogram.*

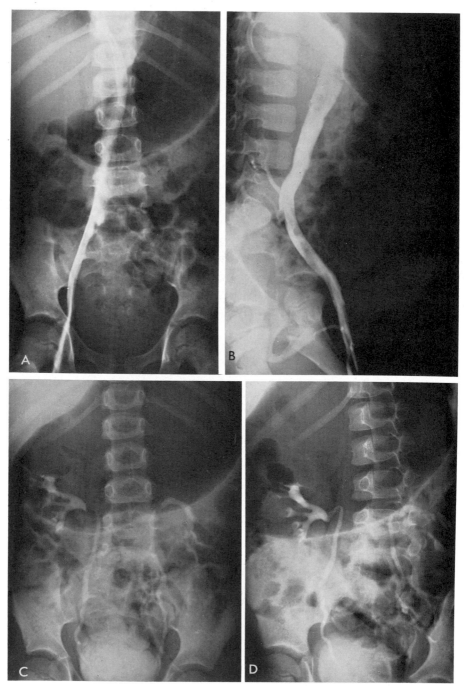

Figure 10–118. Bilateral Wilms' tumor in boy aged 5. **A,** *Inferior vena cavogram, anteroposterior view.* Cava is patent but displaced medially. **B,** *Lateral view.* Cava in upper lumbar region abnormally broad in anteroposterior diameter. **C** and **D,** *Excretory urograms. Anteroposterior and oblique views.* Mass involving upper pole of each kidney. Seems definitely intrinsic with distortion of collecting system on left, but questionable on right. (From Hope, J. W., and Borns, Patricia F.)

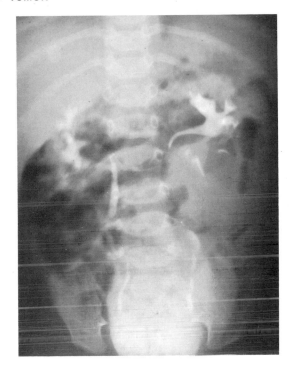

Figure 10–119. *Excretory urogram.* Wilms' tumor (left) in boy aged 6 months.

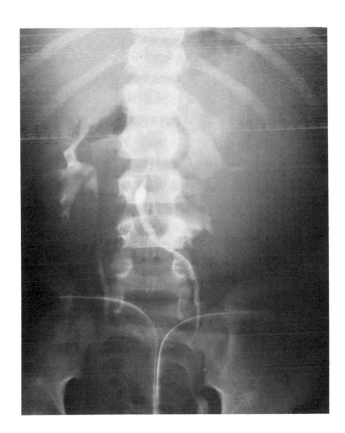

Figure 10–120. *Excretory urogram.* Wilms' tumor (left) in boy aged 9 years.

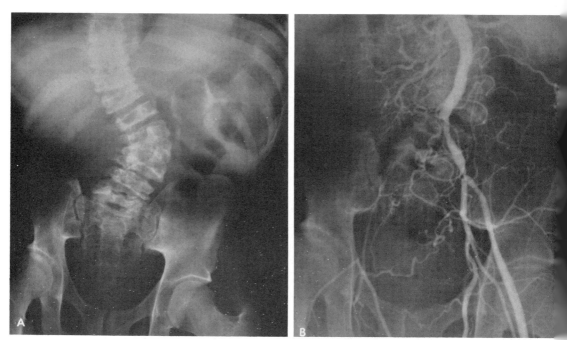

Figure 10–121.   Effect of irradiation of Wilms' tumor on spinal column and major vessels. A, *Plain film* Arrested development of right ilium with deformity of lumbar vertebra and lower right ribs. B, *Aortogram* Aorta is hypoplastic. Right iliac artery is not patent and left is irregularly narrowed. Patient died of hyper tension and vascular occlusion at age 28.

SECONDARY INVOLVEMENT OF RENAL CORTEX

Diseases of White Blood Cells; Tumors of Lymph Nodes and Reticuloendothelial System (Leukemia, Lymphoma, Malignant Lymphoma, Lymphoblastoma, Hodgkin's Disease, Lymphosarcoma, Reticulum Cell Sarcoma, Plasmacytoma [Myeloma and Multiple Myeloma])
(Figs. 10–122 through 10–135)

The above names are used for a rather poorly understood neoplastic disease complex that involves primarily the hemopoietic organs such as bone marrow, lymph nodes, spleen, and liver. Secondarily almost any tissue or organ in the body may become involved. It occurs in both children and adults. It has been estimated that 56% of all childhood tumors are in the "leukemia-lymphoma" category (Hope and Borns).

Leukemic Infiltration of Kidney. Leukemic infiltration of the kidney is manifested by general renal enlargement. The pelvis and calyces appear to be "stretched out" or elongated without real deformity (Gowdey and Neuhauser) as a result of parenchymal infiltration; the deformity is not unlike that seen in polycystic disease and if bilateral may easily be mistaken for it (Figs. 10–122, 10–123, and 10–124).

Malignant Lymphoma. As concerns the *malignant lymphoma group* of lesions, in a large autopsy series Richmond and colleagues found the kidneys involved in 13% of cases in *Hodgkin's disease,* in 33.5% in *malignant lymphoma,* in 38.5% in *lymphosarcoma without bone marrow involvement,* in 53% in *lymphosarcoma with bone marrow involvement,* and in 46% in *reticulum cell sarcoma.* In the entire group, bilateral disease was the rule (ratio of 3 to 1).

It is quite generally agreed that all cases represent secondary involvement; in the few reported cases of primary lymphoma of the kidney the diagnosis has been questioned. The type of renal involvement varies from that of a large, bulky, single tumor to that of multiple nodules (Martínez-Maldonado and Ramírez de Arellano), or to that of simply diffuse symmetrical infiltration of the renal parenchyma in which the kidney is greatly enlarged but usually retains its normal shape. The most common type of involvement is the nodular one (61%). Although most renal involvement is considered to be metastatic, direct extension from neighboring disease in the retroperitoneal space is not uncommon. In many cases, renal involvement may be discovered only by microscopic examination of the tissue, no gross lesions being apparent. Although a few patients may present with an abdominal or flank mass with or without pain, in most instances the lesions are discovered during an investigation for general symptoms of the disease. Only about 0.5% of the deaths from lymphoma are due to lymphomatous involvement of the kidneys.

Urography. An excretory urogram may show generalized diffuse enlargement of one or both kidneys or a localized expanding lesion or lesions causing distortion of the collecting system (Richmond and associates; Shapiro and associates) (Figs. 10–125 through 10–129). As with any renal tumor, if it becomes large enough the kidney or ureter or both may be displaced and the ureter obstructed.

Seltzer and Wenlund have listed the characteristics of arteriograms in renal lymphoma as follows: (1) displacement of vessels around the mass, (2) typical tumor vessels, (3) irregular capillary stain of a portion of the tumor, and (4) irregular junction of the tumor with the normal kidney. They also noted a peculiar "palisade of tumor vessels" which occupied the proximal portion of the periphery of the tumor (Fig. 10–130).

The ureters and bladder may also be involved, displaced, or deformed by retroperitoneal lymphadenopathy or by primary malignant lymphoma, originating either in the retroperitoneal space or in pelvic organs (Farrell) (Figs. 10–131 through 10–135).

Metastasis to the Kidney
(Figs. 10–136, 10–137, and 10–138)

It will no doubt surprise even experienced urologists to realize that metastatic tumors of the kidney are encountered twice as frequently as primary tumors (Newsam and Tulloch). They are of relatively minor clinical importance, however, because they rarely cause symptoms and usually are found only at autopsy. Willis in a study of 500 consecutive autopsies after death from malignant disease found metastasis to the kidneys in 8%. Involvement is more commonly bilateral than unilateral (85 of 118 cases reported by Klinger).

By far the most common site of the primary lesion (if lymphoma is excluded) is the bronchus (in all of Newsam and Tulloch's 13 cases), the next most common being the breast and stomach; however, almost any organ can be the site of the primary lesion. Metastasis usually occurs via the bloodstream but also occurs by direct extension from adjacent organs or via the lymphatics. Patrick, Norton, and Dacso reported a case of metastatic **choriocarcinoma** to the kidney in a 24-year-old woman, the mother of two children, who had delivered her second child just 4 months before the renal lesion was discovered (Fig. 10–138). Of 516 cases of choriocarcinoma studied by Park and Lees, metastasis was demonstrated in 295, with renal involvement in 34. Metastatic involvement of the urinary tract from **melanoma** is also occasionally seen (Das Gupta and Grabstald). (See Figs. 10–197 and 10–198.)

In addition, it must not be forgotten that a malignant lesion of one kidney may metastasize to the other. In such a case, one cannot be sure whether the lesions are both primary or one is metastatic (Fig. 10–136).

(*Text continued on page 1145.*)

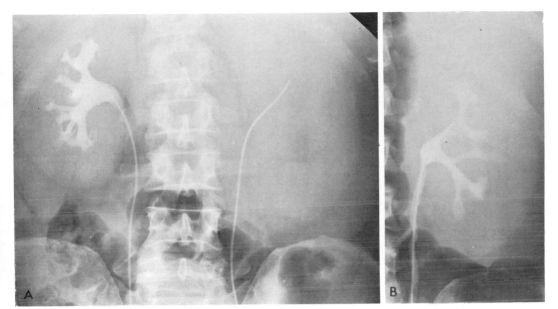

Figure 10–122. Chronic myelogenous leukemia with leukemic infiltration of both kidneys. (Patient died of leukemia.) **A** and **B**, *Bilateral retrograde pyelograms.* Both kidneys enlarged (left larger than right). Note "stretched out" appearance of calyces especially in left kidney.

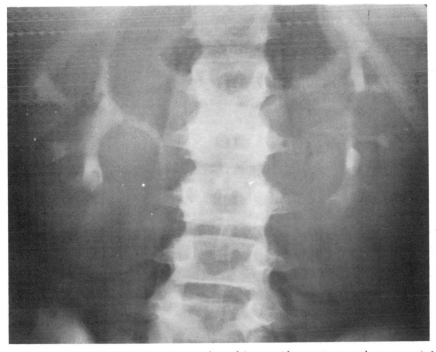

Figure 10–123. Acute lymphatic leukemia in girl aged 9 years (diagnosis proved at autopsy). Note greatly enlarged kidneys and "stretched out" calyces. (Courtesy of Dr. C. W. Latchem.)

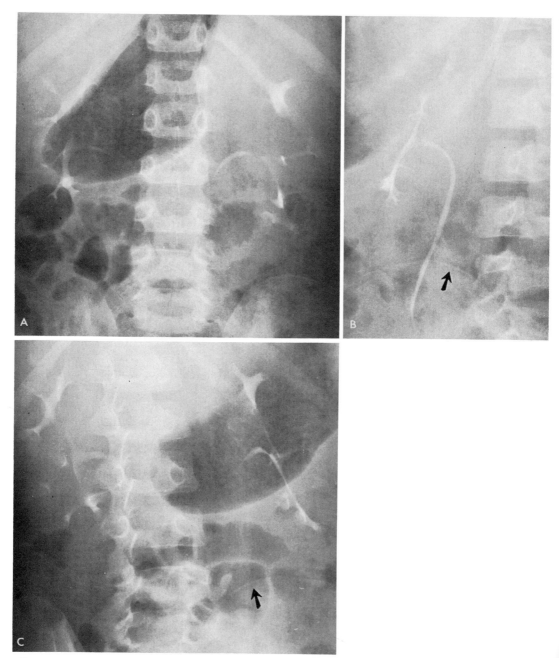

Figure 10–124. Leukemic infiltration of kidneys in 4-year-old boy with lymphocytic leukemia. **A,** *Excretory urogram. Anteroposterior view.* Symmetrical enlargement of both kidneys with "stretching" and distortion of pelves and calyces. **B,** *Right posterior oblique view* showing "stretching" in right kidney. **C,** *Left posterior oblique view* showing similar deformity in left kidney. (From Hope, J. W., and Borns, Patricia F.

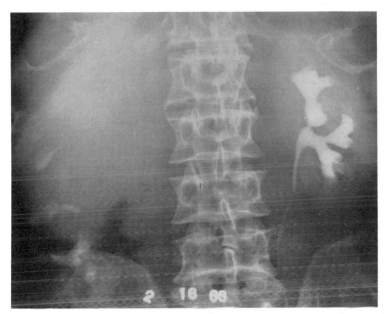

Figure 10–125. *Excretory urogram.* Lymphoma (lymphosarcoma type) involving right kidney.

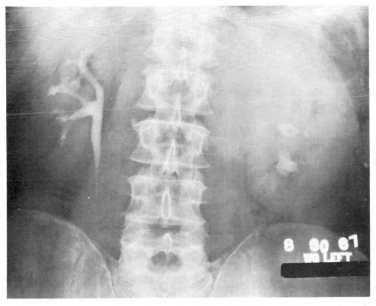

Figure 10–126. *Excretory urogram.* **Lymphoma involving left kidney.** Note greatly enlarged renal outline with no filling of collecting system in upper half of kidney. *Operation.* Extensive abdominal involvement. Mass in head of pancreas, hard nodules in mesentery of small bowel; sheet of small nodules scattered up and down on anterior surface of aorta which obscured its pulsation.

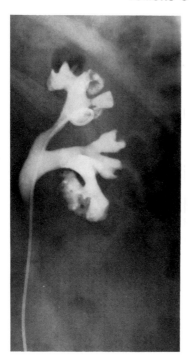

Figure 10–127. Retroperitoneal lymphosarcoma. *Left retrograde pyelogram.* Marked destruction of upper and lower calyces. Would suggest hypernephroma rather than sarcoma. Exploration revealed infiltrating tumor 12.5 cm in diameter involving mesocolon of descending colon and extending to vicinity of tail of pancreas. Also two secondary tumors found. Lesion inoperable. Tissue from peritoneum and region of tail of pancreas was reported as necrotic lymphosarcoma.

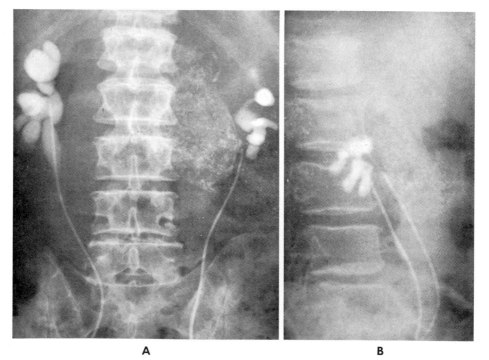

A   B

Figure 10–128. Retroperitoneal lymphoblastoma with calcification. **A,** *Bilateral retrograde pyelogram.* Lateral displacement and evidence of obstruction of both kidneys caused by calcified lymphoblastoma overlying lumbar portion of spinal column. **B,** *Lateral view.* Calcified tumor projected anteriorly.

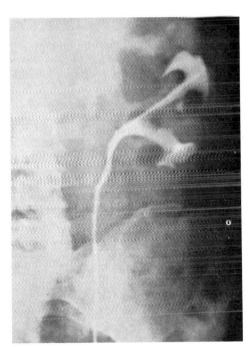

Figure 10–129. *Left retrograde pyelogram.* Lymphosarcoma invading the upper pole of left kidney, distorting left kidney. (From Gibson, T. E.)

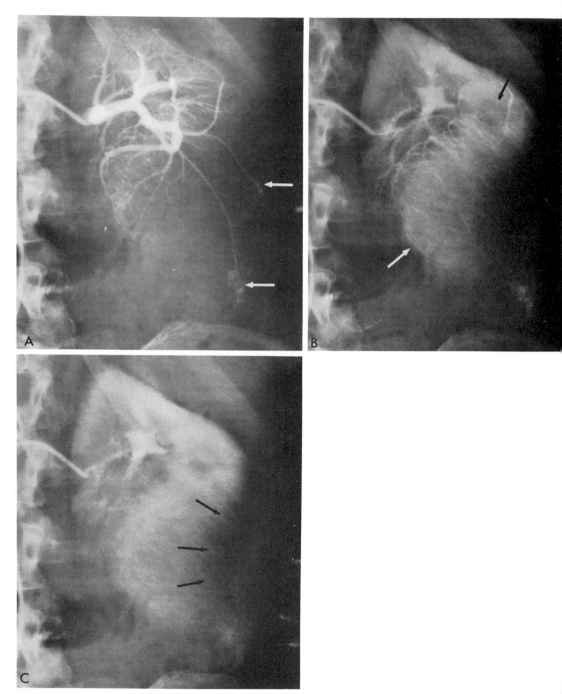

Figure 10–130. Malignant lymphoma involving left kidney. *Selective left renal arteriograms.* **A,** *Early arterial phase* shows arteries displaced about mass. Two clusters of large tumor vessels are supplied by branches of renal artery (*arrows*). **B,** In *late arterial phase*, dense collection of tumor vessels is seen to course toward avascular portion of mass in palisade-like arrangement (*arrows*). **C,** In *capillary phase* there is irregular capillary stain in proximal periphery of mass with more distal area of avascularity (*arrows*). Note irregular junction of tumor with renal parenchyma. (From Seltzer, R. A., and Wenlund, D. E.)

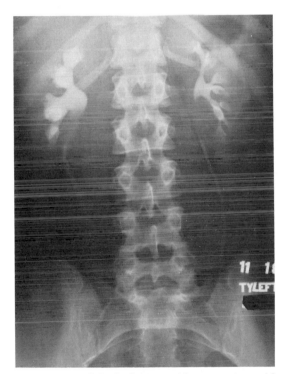

Figure 10–131. *Excretory urogram.* Hodgkin's disease with retroperitoneal lymphadenopathy displacing both ureters with early obstruction of right ureter.

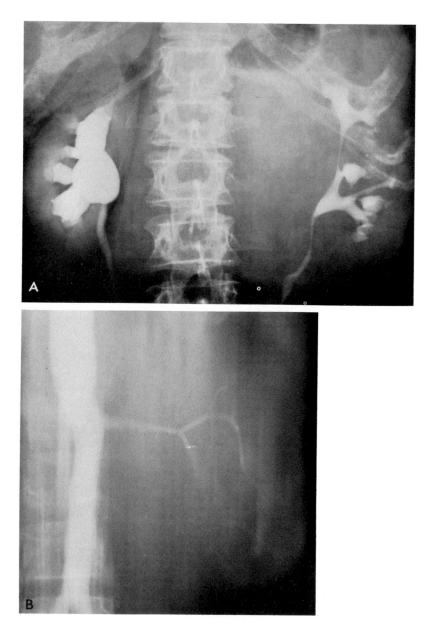

Figure 10–132. A, *Excretory urogram.* Invasion of left kidney by myeloma. B, *Arteriogram.* Renal artery stretched over tumor to reach kidney.

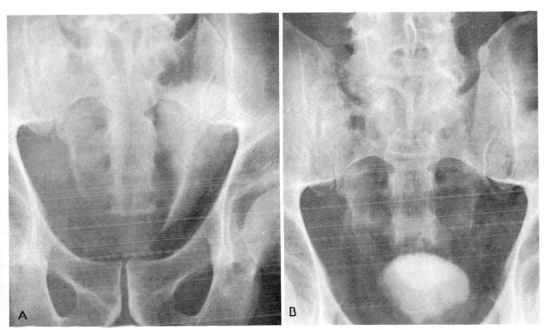

Figure 10–133.   Retroperitoneal lymphoma displacing bladder to left of midline. A, *Preirradiation excretory urogram*. B, *Postirradiation excretory urogram*, 95 days later. Bladder has returned to normal position.

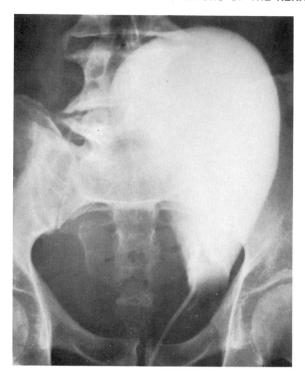

Figure 10-134. *Cystogram.* **Lymphoma (lymphosarcoma type)** causing marked displacement of bladder.

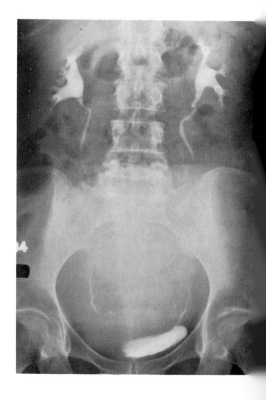

Figure 10-135. *Excretory urogram.* **Huge lymphoma arising from left ovary** and encroaching on bladder. At operation it was attached to posterior surface of uterus and also right ovary.

Fig. 10–136

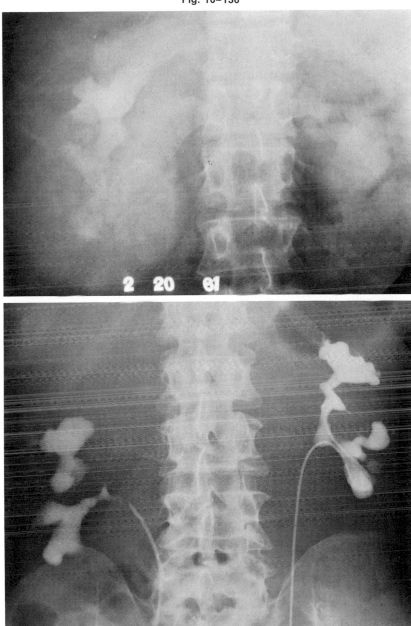

Fig. 10–137

Figure 10–136. *Nephrogram.* **Hypernephroma** of lower pole of solitary right kidney in man, 46 years of age. Left kidney had been removed 3 years previously for hypernephroma. Note abnormal vascularization of recurring tumor in left renal fossa. Question arises whether tumor in right kidney is primary or metastatic.

Figure 10–137. **Bilateral secondary involvement of kidneys from bronchogenic carcinoma** with extensive retroperitoneal metastasis which involved renal sinuses bilaterally, obstructing calyces, with resulting anuria. Peritoneal dialysis used twice before patient died. (Courtesy of Dr. George Nagamatsu and Dr. F. J. Borrelli.)

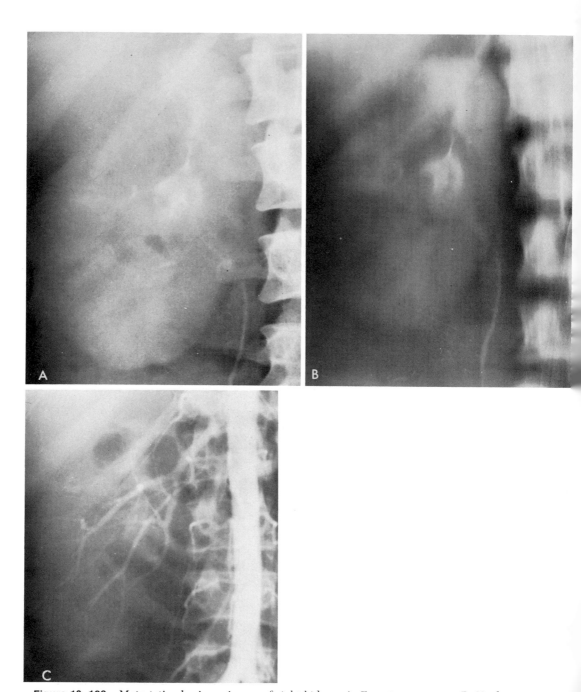

Figure 10–138. Metastatic choriocarcinoma of right kidney. **A,** *Excretory urogram.* **B,** *Nephrotomogram.* Multiple radiolucent areas. **C,** *Arteriogram.* Some spreading of vascular tree with poor vascularization of upper pole but no "tumor vessels" or "tumor staining." (From Patrick, C. E., Norton, J. H., and Dacso, M. R.)

TUMORS OF RENAL PELVIS AND URETER

Benign Tumors
(Figs. 10–139 through 10–148)

Tumors of the renal pelvis and ureter will be considered together because they have a common (mesodermal) origin (from the wolffian ducts) and are lined by the same type of transitional cell epithelium. The only detectable difference in this lining is that the epithelium increases in thickness from the renal pelvis to the bladder. Parenthetically it should be mentioned that the bladder (except for the trigone) has essentially the same embryologic origin and is also lined by the same type of epithelium.

In this discussion all benign tumors are considered to be of nonepithelial origin. At the Mayo Clinic we subscribe to the growing tendency to classify all epithelial tumors as potentially malignant. Thus, we classify so-called benign papilloma as papillary transitional cell epithelioma, grade 1, Broders' classification. *For the purpose of this discussion benign tumors of the renal pelvis and ureter, therefore, will be limited to tumors derived from nonepithelial elements of the walls of the pelvis, calyces, and ureter.*

Renal Pelvis

Benign tumors of the renal pelvis are rare. They consist primarily of such lesions as *hemangiomas, fibromas,* and *fibrolipomas.* Lucké and Schlumberger concluded that in reality most such tumors have arisen from the renal parenchyma and bulged into the renal pelvis. However, they may arise from the subepithelial connective tissue of the renal pelvis. Immergut and Cottler reported a case of polypoid type of fibroma 7 cm long and 1.5 cm thick attached to the wall of the renal pelvis by a thin pedicle. Urographically it presented a mottled "negative" filling defect (Fig. 10–139). Hemangiomas frequently cause gross hematuria. Urographically it is difficult or impossible to distinguish them from malignant epithelial tumors (Fig. 10–140).

Ureter

As mentioned, all benign tumors of the ureter arise from the nonepithelial elements of the wall of the ureter. They are rare. It is difficult to estimate their incidence from the literature because most benign tumors reported are the so-called benign papilloma, which is an epithelial tumor and which for the purposes of this discussion is classified as papillary transitional cell epithelioma, grade 1.

Almost any type of mesenchymal tumor is possible, such as fibroma, fibrolipoma, hamartoma, myoma, hemangioma, and neurofibroma; "granulomatous" tumors also have been reported. A review of the world literature in 1968 by Bustos, Lichtwardt, and Lichtwardt turned up 76 cases of benign nonepithelial tumor of the ureter to which they added 2 cases of their own, in both of which the tumors were polyps (Fig. 10–141).

Ureteral Polyps. Judging from the literature, the most common benign tumor is the benign polyp, but this may be due to the fact (1) that the polyp becomes large and mobile enough to cause obstruction, and (2) that it provides rather dramatic urograms and operative findings which seem worthwhile reporting. The long bifid polyp reported by Schneiderman, Simon, and Sedlezky is a case in point (Fig. 10–142). One limb of the polyp was 14 cm long; the other, 6.5 cm. Most polyps are composed of a thick *core of fibrous connective tissue* covered with a layer of normal transitional epithelium. The polyp in Howard's case is probably the largest yet reported on the basis of total volume. It measured 10 by 3 cm and was composed of fibrous tissue stroma covered with a thin layer of normal transitional epithelium (Figs. 10–143A and B and 10–144A and B). Brock in 1960 reported finding a polyp which was 9 cm long and was composed of a core of fibroangiomatous tissue covered by normal transitional epithelium. Brodny and Hershman in 1954 found a polyp 6.5 cm long which could be seen protruding from the ureteral orifice. On microscopic examination it was found to be a *hemangioma*. The surface of the polyp contained no epithelium. Palmer and Greene reported on a polyp which protruded from the ureteral orifice (Fig. 10–145). It was composed of a core of fibromucous tissue covered with normal transitional epithelium. Auerbach, Lewis, and McDonald reported a polypoid hamartoma in the ureter and renal pelvis of an adolescent (Fig. 10–146). Compere and associates reported two cases in which operation was being done for correction of what was considered to be an obstruction at the ureteropelvic juncture with hydronephrosis. Ureteral polyps were found adjacent to the ureteropelvic junction and were the true cause of the obstruction.

Nonpolypoid Tumors. Reports of nonpolypoid benign tumors are more difficult to find. Cooney described a *fibroma* of the midureter which was 2 cm long. Forssman's case of a fibroma 2 cm long which pointed toward the renal pelvis seems similar to Cooney's case. Roen and Kandalaft's case was that of a "teardrop"-shaped tumor about 1 cm long attached by a small stalk to the wall of the midureter. It produced a typical negative filling defect. The body of the lesion was composed of fibrous tissue covered by normal transitional epithelium. Ravich's

neurofibroma of the ureter was on gross examination difficult to distinguish from a periureteral tumor constricting the ureter. When removed, the tumor could not be dissected from the ureter, so it was considered to be primary in the ureter. At the Mayo Clinic we have encountered one case of small sessile *hemangioma* of the upper part of the ureter (Fig. 10–147). Wöller also reported a small broad-base *hemangioma* measuring 0.5 by 0.5 cm of the upper part of the ureter. It obstructed the ureter, causing hydronephrosis. Galbraith reported a somewhat similar case. Several lipomatous or fibrolipomatous tumors of the ureter have also been reported (Robertson and Hand; Spillane, Singiser, and Prather; Tahara and Hess).

Urographic Diagnosis. Pedunculated tumors (polyps) are difficult to visualize urographically because complete filling of the ureter with contrast medium is difficult. A space-occupying negative filling defect with more or less smooth contour is the pathognomonic finding. A thin rim or outline of contrast medium lining the dilated ureteral wall is characteristic; it represents contrast medium which is surrounding the tumor and demonstrates that the lesion is not attached to the ureteral wall except by a thin pedicle. At times a filling defect is almost impossible to demonstrate, and one must make the diagnosis more or less by deduction from such factors as pyelectasis and ureterectasis (Compere and associates; Evans and Stevens) (Fig. 10–148). This is particularly true when the lesion is near the ureteropelvic juncture. Nonpolypoid lesions produce either a simple filling defect or complete obstruction.

(Text continued on page 1152.)

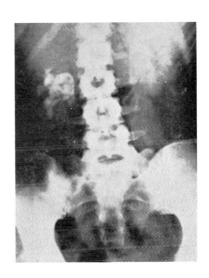

Figure 10–139. Benign polypoid fibroma of renal pelvis. *Excretory urogram.* Mottled negative filling defect in renal pelvis. (From Immergut, S., and Cottler, Z. R.)

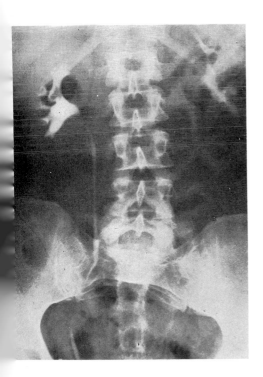

Figure 10–140. Hemangioma of renal pelvis in woman, 47 years of age. *Retrograde pyelogram.* Negative filling defect in pelvis at juncture with upper calyx. Repeat pyelogram 10 days later showed defect still present. Nephroureterectomy. Two small hemangiomas found, each 4 mm in diameter. (From Anderson, J. B., Lee, J. J., Hancock, R. A., and Black, S. R.)

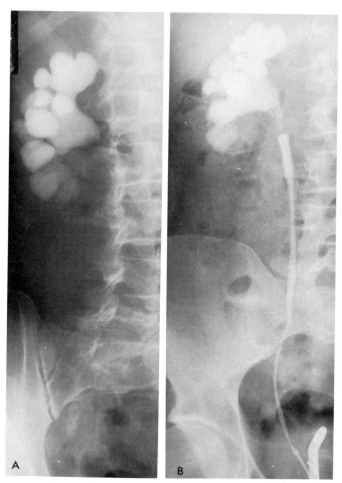

Figure 10–141. Obstruction from **multibranched benign ureteral polyp** in right upper ureter. Man aged 30. **A,** *Excretory urogram.* Right pyelocaliectasis looks like obstruction of ureteropelvic junction. **B,** *Retrograde pyelogram* (using bulb catheter). Filling defect in ureter immediately distal to ureteropelvic junction. *Operation.* Multibranched polyp, the longest measuring 5 cm. Excised. *Pathology:* Benign stroma-type tumor. (From Bustos, F., Lichtwardt, J. R., and Lichtwardt, H. E.)

Figure 10–142.   Ureteral polyp in woman, 37 years of age. *Retrograde pyelogram.* Markedly dilated and tortuous left ureter with smooth filling defect caused by long, pedunculated, bifid fibrous polyp approximately 15 cm in length. Previous excretory urogram showed no function. (From Schneiderman, C., Simon, M., and Sedlezky, I.)

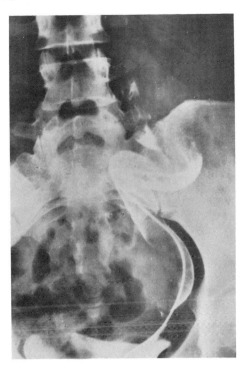

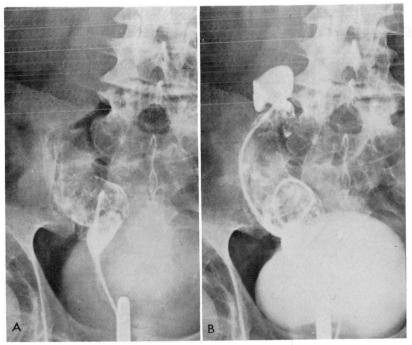

Figure 10–143.   Giant ureteral polyp in man, 60 years of age. **A**, *Retrograde pyelogram* with bulb catheter n lower part of ureter. Large filling defect in dilated ureter. **B**, *Retrograde pyelogram* made with two ureteral :atheters. Typical coiling of catheters in dilated ureter at site of polyp. (From Howard, T. L.)

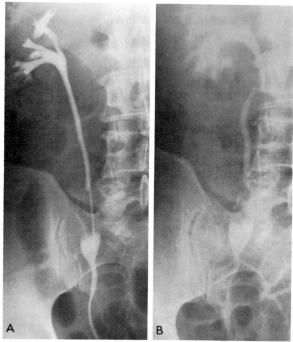

Figure 10–144. Large benign ureteral polyp. **A,** *Retrograde pyelogram.* Filling defect in midureter with typical dilatation below tumor and irregular meniscus-like filling defect. **B,** *Same,* 1 month later. Ureter is more completely filled. Thin rim of medium outlines medial and lateral borders of polyp, pedicle of which is attached at level of superior border of fifth lumbar vertebra. (Courtesy of Dr. D. B. Connery.)

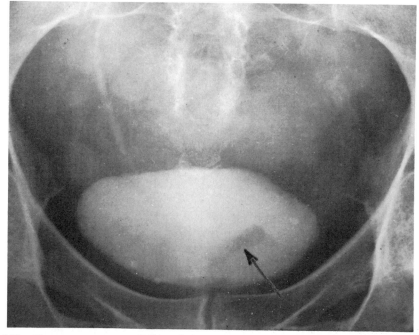

Figure 10–145. *Excretory urogram.* Filling defect in left side of bladder from **ureteral polyp,** attached within intramural portion of ureter and projecting into bladder. (From Palmer, J. K., and Greene, L. F.)

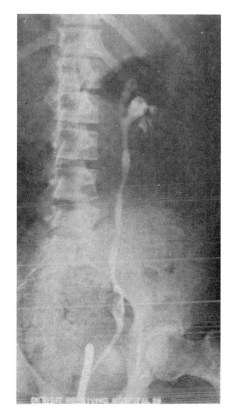

Figure 10–146. *Retrograde pyelogram.* "Secondary" polypoid hamartoma of ureter with "primary" at ureteropelvic juncture. Long filling defect in lower third of left ureter suggests benign polyp which proved to be secondary polypoid hamartoma with "primary" lesion being at ureteropelvic juncture, but not demonstrated in this film. Nephroureterography was done. (From Auerbach, S., Lewis, H. Y., and McDonald, J. R.)

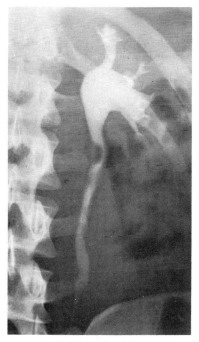

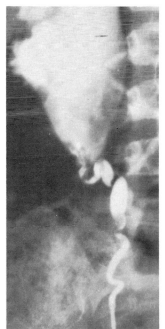

Fig. 10–147   **Fig. 10–148**

Figure 10–147. *Left retrograde pyelogram.* Hemangioma involving ureter just below ureteropelvic junction. Simulates epithelial tumor of ureter.

Figure 10–148. Multiple small fibrous polyps of upper part of ureter, projecting into pelvis of boy, 4 years f age. *Retrograde pyelogram.* Advanced obstructive pyelectasis from polyps. Difficult to visualize typical egative shadows of polyps, but suggestion of slight signet-ring deformity at ureteropelvic juncture. (From vans, A. T., and Stevens, R. K.)

Malignant Epithelial Tumors (Transitional Cell Epithelioma; Transitional Cell Carcinoma; Squamous Cell Epithelioma; Squamous Cell Carcinoma; Epidermoid Carcinoma)

The overwhelming majority of malignant tumors of the renal pelvis and ureter are epithelial tumors. Malignant mesenchymal tumors such as sarcoma are exceedingly rare.

General Considerations

Epithelial carcinoma is primarily a disease of males (four males to one female). As previously stated, at the Mayo Clinic we now routinely classify all epithelial neoplasms of the renal pelvis, ureter, and bladder as malignant tumors. The so-called benign papilloma is classified as a papillary transitional cell epithelioma, grade 1 (Broders' classification). It should be emphasized that the term "papillary" is a microscopic rather than a gross term. Tumors which may appear sessile or solid on gross or cystoscopic inspection may be papillary on microscopic examination. There are two main types of epithelial tumors: (1) *transitional cell epithelioma* (carcinoma), and (2) *squamous cell epithelioma* (epidermoid carcinoma). In addition, *primary mucinous adenocarcinomas*, although rare, have been observed (Lucké and Schlumberger).

Transitional cell tumors are divided into papillary and nonpapillary lesions. **Squamous cell tumors** are almost entirely nonpapillary growths. For many years the term "squamous cell epithelioma" was employed for both types of tumors so that in reading the literature one must be discerning as to which type of tumor is being discussed. Squamous cell epitheliomas may be distinguished from transitional cell epitheliomas by their tendency to reproduce the structure of stratified squamous epithelium and may show epithelial "pearls," keratin, or intercellular bridges. The papillary noninfiltrating

Table 10–5. Incidence of the Various Types of Epithelial Tumors of Renal Pelvis and Ureter in Two Mayo Clinic Series

TYPE	TUMORS, %	
	Primary in ureter (33 tumors)[*]	Renal pelvis (133 tumors)[†]
Papillary		
Noninfiltrating	54.9	39.9
Infiltrating	29.0	40.6
Nonpapillary		
Infiltrating	16.0	19.5

[*]Reported by Whitlock, McDonald, and Cook in 1955.
[†]Reported by Kaplan, McDonald, and Thompson in 1951.

tumor is least lethal; the papillary infiltrating is next, and the nonpapillary infiltrating tumor is the most lethal. For practical purposes all nonpapillary solid tumors are infiltrating. *Almost all squamous cell epitheliomas are nonpapillary and infiltrating;* these are the most malignant neoplasms of the entire group.

Approximately 80 to 85% of all epithelial tumors are papillary (Table 10–5).

Nonpapillary in situ carcinomas of either cell type may be encountered at times, particularly in the mucosa adjacent to an infiltrating carcinoma or as a multicentric tumor. Since in situ carcinoma may be asymptomatic per se and not demonstrable roentgenographically or cystoscopically, it is rarely diagnosed until a grossly indentifiable lesion has developed.

Only about 40% of papillary tumors are infiltrative as contrasted to almost 100% of the nonpapillary (solid) tumors. To illustrate the comparative lethal potential of the various types of lesions, the Mayo Clinic series of tumors of the renal pelvis (McDonald and Priestley) and ureter (Whitlock, McDonald, and Cook) may be cited (Table 10–6).

Multiplicity of Tumors: Implants

Papillary tumors have a distinct tendency to be multiple (in more than 40

| | % OF CASES | |
TYPE OF TUMOR	Primary ureteral tumors, 33 cases (1911-1945), 5-year survival*	Tumors of renal pelvis, 59 cases (1904-1940), 5-year survival†
Papillary	66.7	52.0
Papillary and infiltrating	14.3	16.7
Nonpapillary but infiltrating	0	7.1

*Data from Whitlock, McDonald, and Cook.
†Data from McDonald and Priestley.
Experience with substantial series of cases from clinical centers has recently been reported by Newman and colleagues and Grace and colleagues.

of Kaplan, McDonald, and Thompson's series), whereas nonpapillary (solid) tumors are almost always single lesions. When tumors are single (solitary), the renal pelvis is involved more than twice as frequently as the ureter. When multiple papillary tumors involve both the pelvis and the ureter, the lesion of the pelvis has always been considered the primary lesion, and the ureteral lesion, the secondary lesion or implant. This assumption is no longer considered valid, or multicentric origin of growth is now considered a more likely concept.* The old concept, however, still is used in descriptive terminology since tumors which occur *only* in the ureter are still spoken of as *primary ureteral tumors* in contrast to the term *secondary tumors* when there is a primary lesion in the renal pelvis on the same side. Similarly, if tumors are also present in the bladder and there is a lesion in the pelvis or ureter, the bladder lesions are spoken of as *secondary lesions* or *implants*. It goes without saying that whenever an epithelial tumor is encountered anywhere in the renal pelves, ureters, or bladder, the entire urinary tract must be visualized urographically or cystoscopically, or by both methods, before one can be sure that other lesions are not present. Only too often a papillary tumor of the bladder is treated for months or years only to have a "primary" lesion discovered in the renal pelvis or ureter which has progressed to the point of inoperability.

Multiple papillary lesions are almost always *ipsilateral*, that is, the pelvis and ureter of the same side and the half of bladder on the same side are involved. Kaplan, McDonald, and Thompson found the ipsilateral wall, dome, and trigone involved in 86% of their cases and the contralateral wall in only 14%.

Multiple papillary lesions (so-called implants or secondary lesions) may be present at the time of the initial examination or may develop months or years later. For instance, papillary lesions in the bladder may appear months or years after nephroureterectomy for a lesion of the renal pelvis or ureter or both.

Bilateral primary tumors of the renal pelves have been reported by Colston and Arcadi, Thompson and associates, Colston, and Potampa and Schneider. The first report of *bilateral ureteral tumors* was made by Ratliff, Banum, and Butler in 1949. Since then, cases have been reported by Barroso, Florence, and Scott; Crassweller; Gracia and Bradfield; Perlmutter, Retik, and Harrison; and Utz, Brunsting, and Harrison. Some of these cases represented simultaneous (synchronous) tumors—found at the same time. Others were encountered some time later than the original lesion.

EPITHELIAL TUMORS OF THE RENAL PELVIS
(Figs. 10–149 through 10–171)

Symptoms and Findings

The typical triad of signs and symptoms mentioned for tumors of the renal

---

*Other concepts include (1) direct extension along the mucous membrane and (2) metastasis from one area to another by way of the lymph vessels.

cortex (parenchyma) also applies here; that is, flank pain, gross hematuria, and a palpable mass. *Pain* is most often the result of obstruction of the ureteropelvic juncture or of a calyx by the tumor. Calculi are not uncommonly associated (especially with the nonpapillary tumors) and may obstruct and cause pain. This situation is a common cause of diagnostic error; a diagnosis of nephrolithiasis only may be made and the tumor may go unsuspected for several months (Fig. 10–169). In high-grade infiltrating tumors, pain may be the result of malignant extension and metastasis. *Hematuria* is common in the papillary tumors, fairly uncommon in the nonpapillary tumors. A *palpable mass* may be the result of obstructive hydronephrosis or a large perirenal extension of the tumor.

Urographic Diagnosis

When hydronephrosis is encountered in men past 40 years of age, the possibility of obstruction from a tumor of the renal pelvis or ureter should always be considered (Fig. 10–149A and B). This is especially true if gross hematuria has been present. Negative filling defects in a hydronephrotic kidney that has been bleeding can be due to blood clots or tumor (Fig. 10–150). It should also be remembered that tumors may be only an incidental finding in hydronephrosis, discovered accidentally during operation. *The pathognomonic urographic finding,* however, is a negative filling defect in a more or less normal-appearing renal pelvis.

Papillary Tumors (Figs. 10–151 through 10–164). In the case of *papillary tumors* the negative filling defects may be of irregular, mottled appearance, and in some cases some mottled calcification of the tumor may be apparent on the plain film and mistaken for a calculus (Fig. 10–151A and B). If the tumor is small and situated in a calyx, it may be extremely difficult to demonstrate; localized hydrocalyx may be the only finding. Differential diagnosis

must include (1) blood clots, (2) nonopaque calculi, and (3) parenchymal (cortical) tumors which have invaded the renal pelvis. Even with the kidney removed and available for examination, the pathologist may have difficulty in determining on gross examination whether the lesion is primary in the renal pelvis and invading the cortex secondarily or vice versa (Figs. 10–152 through 10–166).

Nonpapillary Solid Tumors (Figs. 10–165 through 10–169). Urographic diagnosis of *nonpapillary solid tumors* may be considerably more difficult. When the lesion is well-localized with moderate projection into the lumen of the renal pelvis, diagnosis is not difficult; a smooth-contoured, negative filling defect may be easily identified. The difficult problem, however, concerns the highly malignant nonpapillary infiltrating tumors which infiltrate the wall of the renal pelvis and invade the renal parenchyma and perirenal tissues with minimal or essentially no intraluminal intrusion. Associated calculi or calcification in the tumor may further confuse diagnosis.

Squamous Cell Epithelioma (Figs. 10–170 and 10–171). The most malignant variety of epithelial tumors is the squamous cell epithelioma. Utz and McDonald reviewed the Mayo Clinic cases of this lethal tumor in 1957 and also reviewed the literature; the interested reader is referred to their informative study for a detailed account. In brief, of 175 cases of carcinoma of the renal pelvis encountered from 1904 through 1954, 23 (13%) were cases of squamous cell epithelioma. These tumors are of insidious onset without any pathognomonic syndrome. They are frequently associated with chronic infection, leukoplakia, or stones (Figs. 10–170 and 10–171), so much so that irritation of the renal pelvis from calculi and infection has seriously been considered as a possible cause of the carcinoma. In 13 of the 23 cases (57%) calculi were associated. This compares favorably to the estimate of other authors: 52% by Gilbert an

MacMillan and 48% by Gahagan and Reed. Gross extension of the tumor beyond the pelvis and parenchyma with infiltration of the hilar structures was observed in 19 of 23 cases (83%).

The discouraging aspect of this problem is the inaccuracy of the preoperative urographic diagnosis because of the insidious infiltration of the pelvic wall and *minimal intraluminal intrusion.* For example, although urograms disclosed abnormalities in all 23 cases reported by Utz and McDonald, actual preoperative diagnosis of tumor of the renal pelvis was made in only 3 cases. Other diagnoses were as follows: indeterminate type of renal neoplasm, eight cases; pyonephrosis, eight cases; nephrolithiasis, seven cases; hydronephrosis, three cases; and tuberculous pyonephrosis, one case.

More than one diagnosis was made in some instances.

Adenocarcinoma (Mucinous Adenocarcinoma). Lucké and Schlumberger stated in 1957 that there were four cases of mucinous adenocarcinoma (Ackerman; Plaut; Ragins and Rolnick; Stone and Baer) reported in the literature. In each case the pelvis and calyces were filled with a massive staghorn calculus and extensive infection was associated. Urography was of no value in diagnosis "because the calculi and hydronephrosis obscured the changes in the pelvic epithelium." Suzuki and Siminovitch reported what they considered to be the ninth case in the literature. The kidney (of a woman aged 52) was hydronephrotic (2,000-ml capacity) with no function evident on the excretory urogram.

(Text continued on page 1169.)

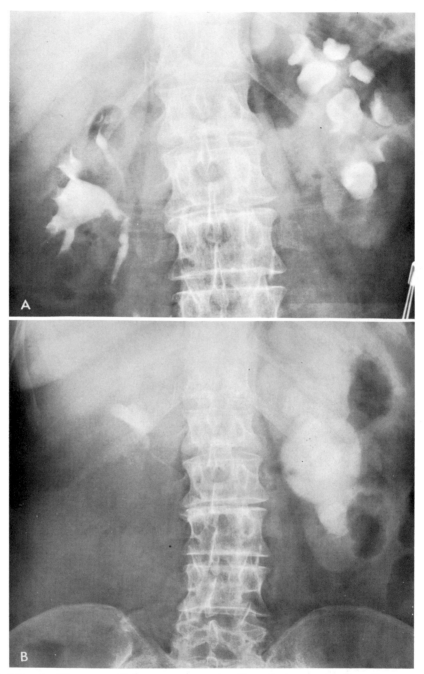

Figure 10–149. Papillary noninfiltrating transitional cell epithelioma of right renal pelvis in a duple kidney. **A,** *Excretory urogram* made before hemicolectomy for perforating carcinoma of right colon. Lef pyelectasis from obstruction of ureteropelvic juncture. Right: duplication. Question of negative filling defe at ureteropelvic juncture of lower pelvis. Did not return for exploration. **B,** *Excretory urogram* 4 years late Huge nonfunctioning hydronephrosis of lower segment of duplicated right kidney. Exploration reveale obstruction from papillary noninfiltrating transitional cell epithelioma, grade 2, measuring 5 by 4 by 3 cm ureteropelvic juncture. Right nephrectomy. Plastic repair of left ureteropelvic juncture.

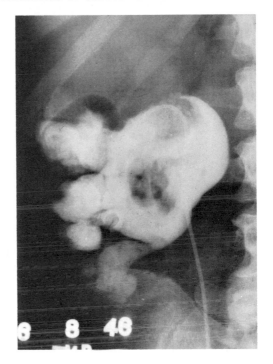

Figure 10–150. Papillary transitional cell epithelioma in hydronephrotic pelvis of solitary right kidney (previous left nephrectomy). *Right retrograde pyelogram.* Irregular filling defect in center of pelvis. Impossible to say whether this represented blood clot or tumor (hematuria was presenting symptom). At operation, grade 2 papillary transitional cell epithelioma of renal pelvis and pelvis filled with organized blood clot were found. Lesion was electrocoagulated and nephrostomy was established.

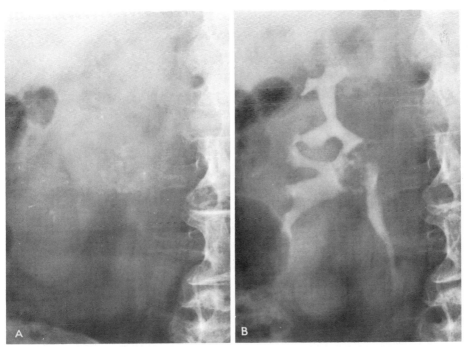

Figure 10–151. Papillary transitional cell epithelioma of renal pelvis with calcification and minimal filtration of pelvic wall. **A,** *Plain film.* Mottled calcification. Could be mistaken for stone. **B,** *Excretory urogram.* Negative filling defect. Reveals tumor of renal pelvis.

Fig. 10–152

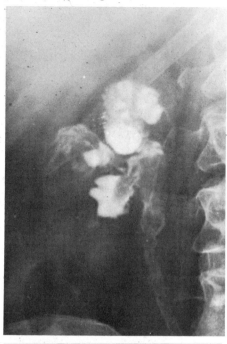

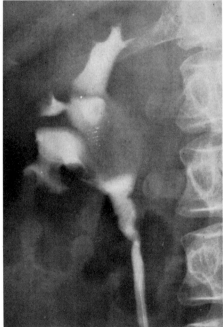

Fig. 10–153

Figure 10–152. *Right retrograde pyelogram.* **Extensive papillary transitional cell epithelioma** of rena
pelvis with "implants" in ureter and bladder. Plain film was negative. Extensive negative filling defects i
pelvis and calyces, associated with moderate pyelectasis. Filling defects along ureter caused by combinatio
of "implants" and blood clots.

Figure 10–153. *Right retrograde pyelogram.* **Filling defect from blood clot simulating tumor of ren**
pelvis. Mild pyelocaliectasis with filling defect involving almost entire pelvis. Diagnosis made of tumor
renal pelvis. Exploration revealed that filling defect was caused by blood clot. **Source of bleeding was throm**
bosis of vein, with infarct, in pyramid of upper pole of kidney.

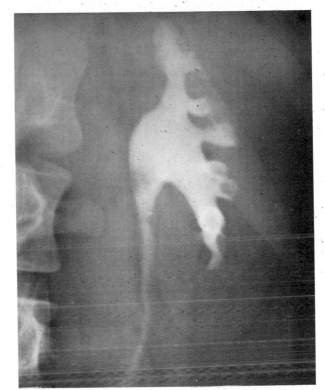

Fig. 10–154

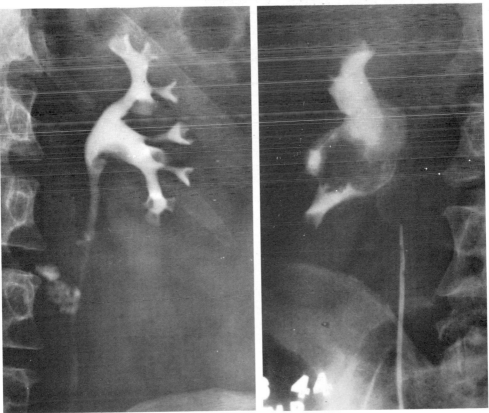

Fig. 10–155   Fig. 10–156

Figures 10–154 and 10–155. *Left retrograde pyelograms.* Papillary transitional cell epithelioma of renal pelvis. Negative shadow (filling defect) at ureteropelvic juncture from grade 1 papillary transitional cell epithelioma.

Figure 10–156. *Right retrograde pyelogram.* Papillary transitional cell epithelioma of renal pelvis. Filling defect in right renal pelvis from tumor. At operation, grade 2 papillary transitional cell epithelioma.

Fig. 10–157

Fig. 10–159

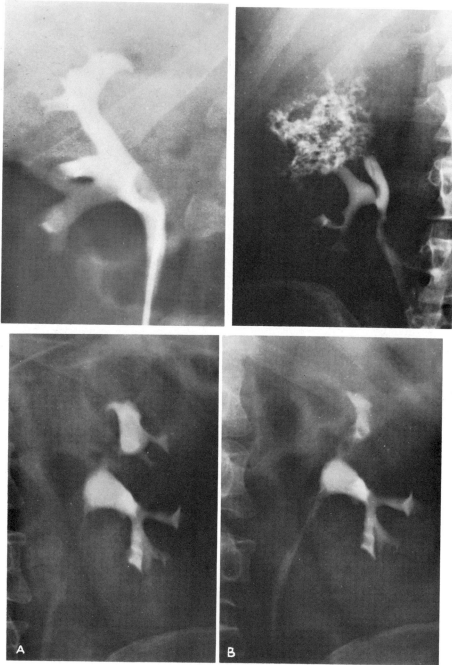

Fig. 10–158

Figure 10–157. *Retrograde pyelogram.* **Papillary tumor (transitional cell epithelioma) of renal pelvis** (Courtesy of Dr. Robert Pearman.)

Figure 10–158. **Papillary tumor of renal pelvis involving infundibulum of upper calyx.** **A,** *Left retrograd pyelogram.* Infundibulum of upper calyx is not filled with contrast medium. Type of lesion is not apparer in this film. Could be stricture or nonopaque stone. **B,** *Left retrograde pyelogram* (*second attempt*). Infundibulum of upper calyx is now filled and shows filling defect. Differential diagnosis includes papillary tumo in infundibulum of upper calyx and soft stone. Exploration revealed grade 1 papillary transitional cell ep thelioma.

Figure 10–159. *Right retrograde pyelogram.* **Tumor of renal pelvis.** Bifid pelvis with mottling of entire upper pole of kidney caused by extensive papillary epithelioma of upper calyx. At operation, grade 3 papillar transitional cell epithelioma with infiltration was found.

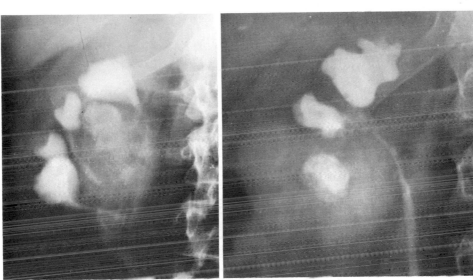

Fig. 10-160   Fig. 10-161

Figure 10-160. *Excretory urogram.* Papillary transitional cell epithelioma of renal pelvis. Right pyelectasis and calycectasis. Pelvis not well-filled because of papillary tumor which is partially filling it and obstructing ureteropelvic junction.

Figure 10-161. *Right retrograde pyelogram.* Papillary tumor (transitional cell epithelioma) of renal pelvis. Obliteration of pelvis and obstruction of calyces, with grade 2 calycectasis, caused by papillary, grade 4 transitional cell epithelioma of right renal pelvis.

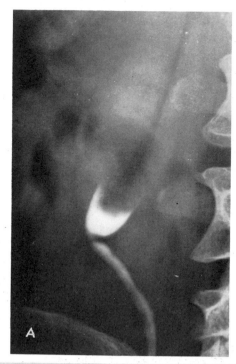

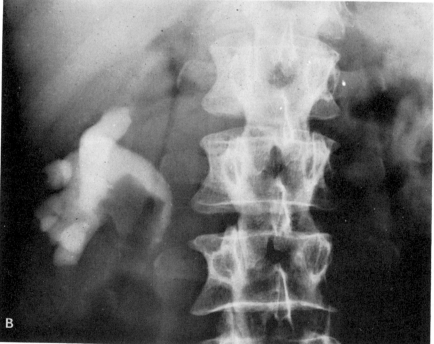

Figure 10–162. Papillary transitional cell epithelioma, grade 3, of renal pelvis requiring both excretory and retrograde urography to visualize upper and lower portions. **A,** *Right retrograde pyelogram.* Only lower portion of pelvis outlined, which delineates filling defect above from tumor. Medium does not enter calyces. **B,** *Excretory urogram.* Pyelocaliectasis, grade 2, with large filling defect in pelvis, which outlines upper margin of growth.

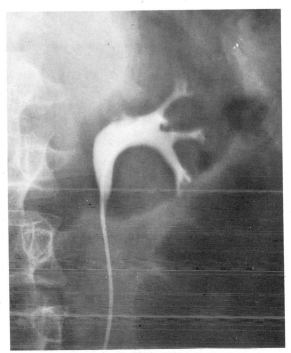

Figure 10–163. *Left retrograde pyelogram.* **Papillary tumor of upper calyx** of left kidney, causing complete obliteration of calyx. Papillary transitional cell epithelioma, grade 2, found in upper calyx.

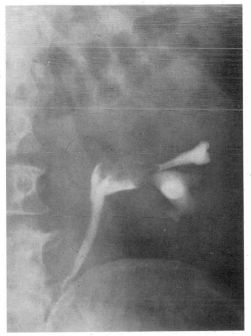

Figure 10–164. Extensive papillary transitional cell epithelioma of renal pelvis simulating hypernephroma. *Left retrograde pyelogram.* Extensive filling defect of pelvis. Complete obliteration of calyces of upper half of kidney. Growth apparently pushes middle calyx downward. Impossible to say from this film whether lesion was tumor of renal pelvis invading renal cortex or cortical tumor invading pelvis. *Exploration* revealed grade 3 papillary transitional cell epithelioma of upper portion of renal pelvis.

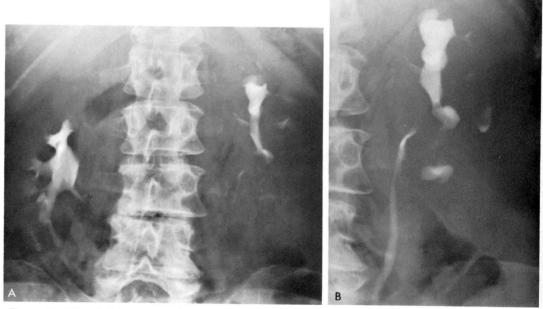

Figure 10–165. Solid transitional cell epithelioma of pelvis (and lower calyces) of left kidney in woman aged 62. Demonstrable widespread metastasis present. **A,** *Excretory urogram.* **B,** *Retrograde pyelogram* (Courtesy of Dr. T. R. Montgomery.)

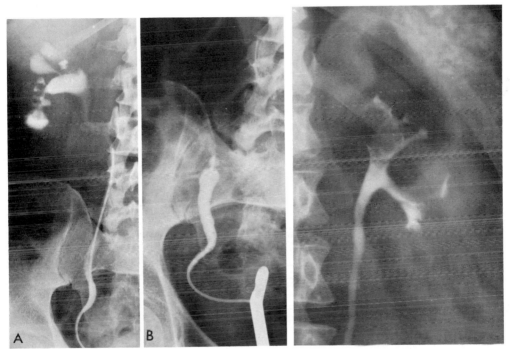

Fig. 10–166   Fig. 10–167

Figure 10–166. Infiltrating papillary tumor of renal pelvis with implant in stump of ureter 10 months following nephrectomy. **A,** *Retrograde pyelogram.* Tumors arising in lower calyx and pelvis. Poor surgical risk—only nephrectomy done as palliative procedure. Tumor had perforated capsule and involved perirenal fat. **B,** *Ten months later* (gross hematuria). *Right ureterogram.* Tumor involved most of stump of ureter except intramural portion. Ureter removed.

Figure 10–167. *Left retrograde pyelogram.* **Solid, nonpapillary transitional cell epithelioma** of renal pelvis. At operation nonpapillary (solid) transitional cell epithelioma, grade 2, was found arising from one of middle calyces. Deformed middle calyx apparently was superimposed on upper calyx in pyelogram.

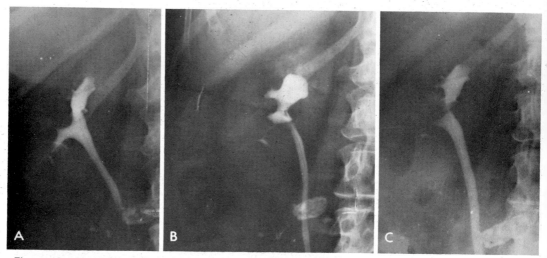

Figure 10–168. Progressive changes (over 7-month period) in grade 4 nonpapillary (solid) transitional cell epithelioma which began in lower calyx of right kidney. *Right retrograde pyelograms.* **A,** Incomplete filling of lower calyx, suggesting cicatricial deformity rather than classic filling defect. **B,** *Four months after* **A.** Increase in obliteration of lower calyx. **C,** *Three months after* **B.** Almost complete obliteration of lower calyx and portion of pelvis.

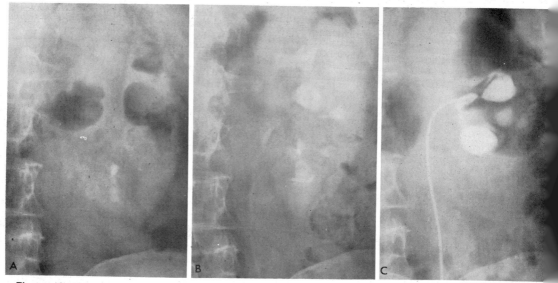

Figure 10–169. Nonpapillary transitional cell epithelioma of renal pelvis associated with nephrolithiasis. Diagnosis missed on first examination. Adult male with complaint of gross hematuria and pain. **A,** *Plain film.* Multiple calculi in lower pole of kidney. **B,** *Excretory urogram.* Calculi caused negative filling defects in lower calyx. One dilated calyx in upper group is seen "head on." Note that renal pelvis is not well filled. Diagnosis of nephrolithiasis made. **C,** *Retrograde pyelogram* 3 months later. Pain and hematuria had continued. Considerable distortion of pelviocalyceal system. Tumor suspected. *Left nephrectomy.* Infiltrating grade 3 transitional cell epithelioma 2 cm in diameter at ureteropelvic junction with perineural invasion. Multicentric lesions occupy majority of calyces. Multiple calyceal calculi.

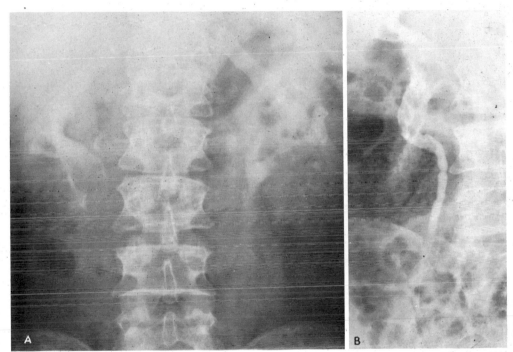

Figure 10-170.   Leukoplakia and squamous cell epithelioma of right renal pelvis. Man aged 48 with 20-year history of chronic pyelonephritis and leukoplakia. Passes debris and calcified material in urine. A, *Excretory urogram.* Moderately reduced function with poor visualization. Evidence of pyelonephritis on left with calycectasis and cortical atrophy. Apparent filling defect of right renal pelvis and obliteration of middle and lower calyces. B, *Right retrograde pyelogram.* Filling defects of pelvis and adjacent ureter. No filling of middle and lower groups of calyces. *Operation.* Right nephrectomy. Extensive leukoplakia associated with squamous cell epithelioma.

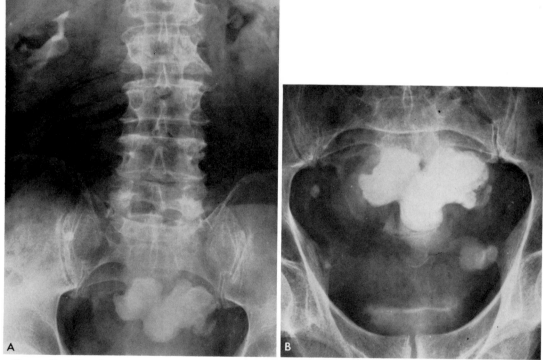

Figure 10–171.   Squamous cell carcinoma associated with staghorn calculus in ectopic (pelvic) left kidney. Man, aged 67, complained of gross hematuria and suprapubic pain. **A,** *Excretory urogram.* Normal right kidney. Absent left renal shadow; large irregular opacity in pelvis. **B,** *Excretory urogram* (postmicturition film). Note reflux up dilated left ureter; staghorn calculus demonstrated at operation for ectopic (pelvic) kidney. *Nephrectomy.* Specimen showed large branched calculus with solid tumor involving one pole of kidney. (From Charlton, C. A. C., and Richardson, W. W.)

PRIMARY EPITHELIAL TUMORS OF THE URETER
(Figs. 10–172 through 10–192)

As mentioned earlier, when a tumor involves the ureter (but not the renal pelvis), it is spoken of as a primary ureteral tumor. Multiple papillary tumors in a ureter are fairly common (Whitlock, McDonald, and Cook). This is not the case with solid, infiltrating nonpapillary tumors. As mentioned previously, bilateral ureteral tumors are rare (Figs. 10–172 and 10–187). "Implants" into the bladder are found in approximately half of the cases of papillary tumors either at the initial examination or months or years following nephroureterectomy. In about half of the cases the tumor involves the lower third of the ureter. In 10 of 33 Mayo Clinic cases the tumor could be seen cystoscopically, protruding from the ureteral orifice (Whitlock, McDonald, and Cook). The next most common site is the upper third of the ureter.

Gross hematuria is a common symptom. *Pain* or *palpable mass* or both may be present when the tumor causes ureteral obstruction or when there is infiltration through the ureteral wall with periureteral extension and metastasis.

Diagnosis; Reason for Inaccuracy

Diagnostic accuracy is poor, probably the poorest for any urologic lesion. The reason is that the ureters seldom completely fill with contrast medium during either excretory or retrograde urography (Fig. 10–173).* As a matter of fact if a ureter fills completely in the excretory urogram, one suspects possible obstruction at the ureterovesical juncture. Lack of visualization of parts of the ureter is too often dismissed with the comment that it is the result of "peristaltic waves."

---

*With modern up-to-date urographic technique using larger amounts of contrast medium and "infusion" technique when necessary, better filling of the ureters is being obtained. (See discussion in Chapter 1.)

In routine retrograde pyelography, it may be exceedingly difficult and time-consuming to attain complete and adequate filling of a ureter unless an acorn or bulb catheter is used and the ureter is filled from below upward (with the bulb positioned just inside [and occluding] the ureteral meatus). This procedure does not lend itself for use in routine cystoscopy because the urologist usually wants to obtain a specimen of urine from the kidney for study; the easiest way to accomplish this is to pass a 4- or 5-F ureteral catheter to the renal pelvis. When the conventional ureteral catheter is used, attempts to completely fill the ureter with contrast medium by means of a "down and out" film often fail.

Because of these factors, urologists are content to settle for incomplete visualization of the ureters in the average case. The rarity of primary ureteral tumors aids and abets this laxity. As a result the majority of ureteral tumors are not diagnosed at the first urologic examination (Fig. 10–174). The urologist may suspect a ureteral tumor only when the patient returns repeatedly because of recurring bleeding, and only then does he make an effort to visualize the ureters. Profuse bleeding when a catheter is passed up a ureter is a suggestive finding which may lead the urologist to suspect a ureteral tumor.

Because of this same low index of suspicion a recurrent papillary tumor of the bladder may be treated for months or years before a primary tumor in the ureter (or renal pelvis) is found. Every urologist, therefore, should adhere to the rigid rule: *Treat no papillary tumor until both kidneys and ureters have been completely and adequately visualized urographically.*

Urographic Diagnosis

The object in urographic diagnosis is to demonstrate a space-occupying lesion which appears as a negative filling defect. In the case of papillary tumors, differential diagnosis should include non-opaque calculi (see Fig. 6–153) and blood clots. In the case of nonpapillary (solid) tumors, it should include non-opaque calculi, ureteral stricture, and extraureteral compression from retroperitoneal tumors and retroperitoneal fibrosis, and other conditions.

Papillary Tumors (Figs. 10–172 through 10–187). In the presence of papillary tumors the ureter is often dilated locally to accommodate the expanding bulk of the tumor. In 1961 Bergman, Friedenberg, and Sayegh observed that in the case of an expanding ureteral tumor the ureter is dilated immediately below the growth in contradistinction to the condition in mechanical obstruction from stone in which case the ureter is collapsed below the stone (Fig. 10–175A and B). They made use of this observation in differential diagnosis and called attention to the frequency with which the ureteral catheter tends to coil in this dilated area below the tumor. (This observation is often called *Bergman's sign.*) They indicated that even if the catheter manages to pass by the tumor to the renal pelvis, a widely coiled portion may still lie in the region of the tumor. They concluded that this is pathognomonic (Figs. 10–176A and B and 10–177).

Either the upper or lower margin of the negative filling defect of the tumor may be outlined, but it is usually difficult to demonstrate both in any one film. For instance, an excretory urogram may reveal the upper margin of the growth while the retrograde pyeloureterogram may outline the lower (Figs. 10–178, 10–179, and 10–180). The contour of the lower margin has been variously described as simulating a meniscus, goblet, or wineglass (Wood and Howe).

A ureteral tumor may or may not be obstructive. If obstruction is present, pyeloureterectasis will call attention to the lesion and demand careful urographic investigation of the ureter. In the cases in which neither obstruction nor pyelectasis is present, however, the diagnosis is frequently missed.

Nonpapillary (Solid) Tumors (Figs. 10–188 through 10–192). Nonpapillary tumors present a more formidable diagnostic problem. Because of minimal intraluminal protrusion the negative filling defect is less pronounced than in papillary tumors, and the lesion is more likely to suggest a ureteral stricture, nonopaque stone (see Fig. 6–154, page 712), or extraureteral constriction from an adjacent retroperitoneal tumor, or retroperitoneal fibrosis (periureteritis plastica). A common error is to make a diagnosis of ureteral stricture. Abeshouse in 1956 emphasized this problem when he made the following statement: "It is important for the urologist to remember that stricture of the ureter with accompanying hydronephrosis is rare in patients of the cancer age. *For all intents and purposes, stricture of the lower third of the ureter in this group of patients should be regarded as malignant until proved otherwise.*"

(Text continued on page 1184.)

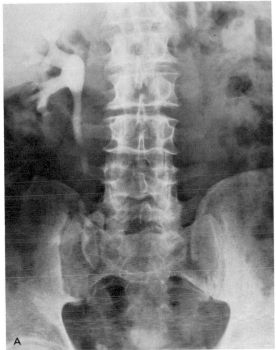

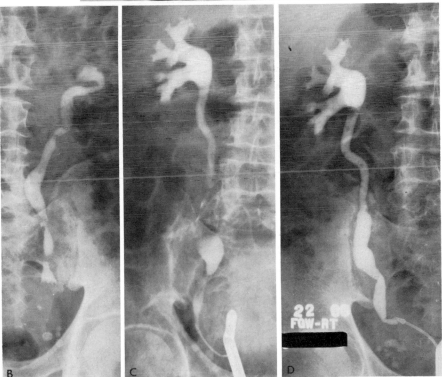

Figure 10–172.   Bilateral (synchronous) papillary ureteral tumors (transitional cell epithelioma, grade 1) in man aged 63. **A,** *Excretory urogram.* No function on left; normal right kidney but suggestion of filling defect with some dilation of ureter overlying wing of sacrum. **B,** *Left retrograde pyelogram.* Filling defect of lower third of ureter typical of tumor. **C,** *Right retrograde pyelogram.* Filling defect in ureter overlying fifth lumbar transverse process with typical dilation of ureter immediately below. *Operation.* Left nephro-ureterectomy and segmental resection of right ureter. **D,** *Right retrograde pyelogram.* One and one half years postoperatively. No recurrence of tumor. Minimal postoperative dilation of lower half of ureter.

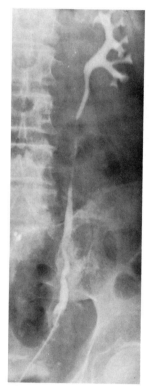

Figure 10–173.   Left ureteral papillary tumor missed on excretory urogram (not shown here). No obstruction. Ureters were incompletely filled. *Retrograde pyelogram.* Small papillary transitional cell epithelioma just below sacro-iliac joint. Terminal ureter is still incompletely filled. Calcification of adrenal.

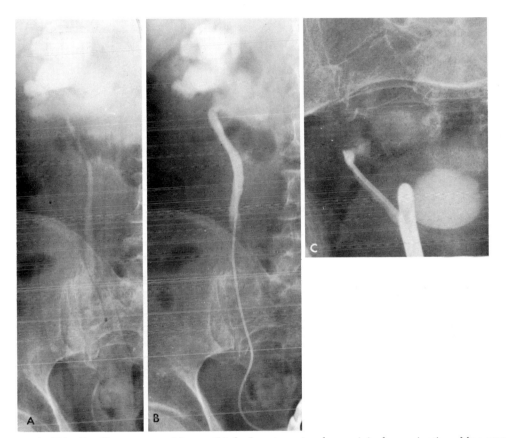

Figure 10–174. Papillary tumor of lower third of ureter missed on original examination. Man aged 66 with mild, intermittent gross and microscopic hematuria for 1 year. Excretory urogram had been reported negative except that ureters were "only fractionally visualized." Cystoscopic examination negative. Returned 3 years later with same complaint. **A**, *Excretory urogram.* Pyelocaliectasis on right. **B**, *Retrograde pyelogram.* Angulation of ureter below pelvis; minimal dilation of upper half of ureter; lower half not visualized even with "down and out" film. *Operation.* Right nephrectomy. Cause of hydronephrosis not apparent. **C**, *Retrograde pyelogram* 3 months later (because of continuing hematuria). Irregular filling defect in lower one third of ureter from tumor. *Operation.* Ureterectomy. *Pathology.* Papillary transitional cell epithelioma, grade 2. No infiltration.

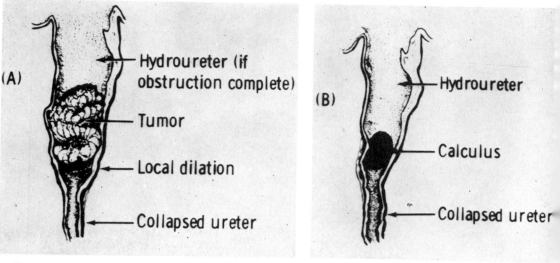

Figure 10-175. A, Localized dilatation of ureter below tumor, allowing space for coiling of catheter. B, Collapsed ureter below calculus. (From Bergman, H., Friedenberg, R. M., and Sayegh, V.)

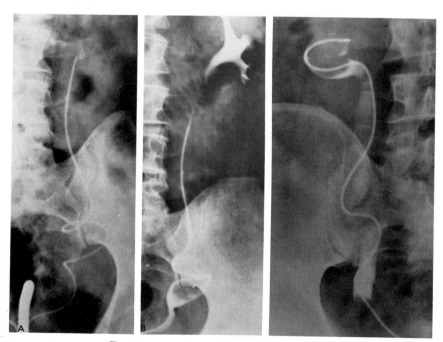

Fig. 10-176   **Fig. 10-177**

Figure 10-176.   Ureteral tumor. A, *Plain film.* **Typical coiling of catheter** in dilated ureter at site of tumor. B, *Retrograde pyelogram.* Negative filling defect of tumor in dilated segment of ureter. (From Bergman, H., Friedenberg, R. M., and Sayegh, V.)

Figure 10-177.   *Retrograde pyelogram.* **Multiple primary papillary tumors of ureter** in man, 58 years of age. Tumor in lower part of ureter with upper margin demonstrated, as in inverted goblet or wineglass deformity. Large tumor in upper third with typical Bergman sign with coiled catheter.

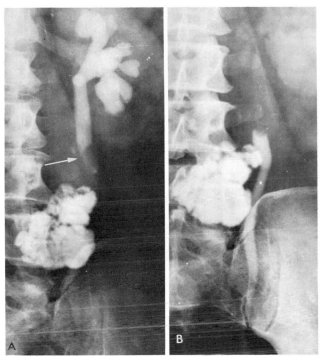

Figure 10–178.   Primary papillary tumor of middle portion of left ureter. **A,** *Excretory urogram.* Upper margin of growth only is outlined and is situated opposite second lumbar vertebra. This could be confused with ureteral stricture in this area. **B,** *Left retrograde pyelogram.* Lower margin of growth revealed opposite lower margin of third lumbar transverse process. Definite filling defect produced by lower margin of growth clarifies diagnosis. Illustration of necessity of both excretory and retrograde urography to outline upper and lower margins of tumor. *Exploration* revealed grade 2 papillary transitional cell epithelioma. (Calcific shadow overlying lumbosacral area is produced by large calcified mesenteric lymph node.)

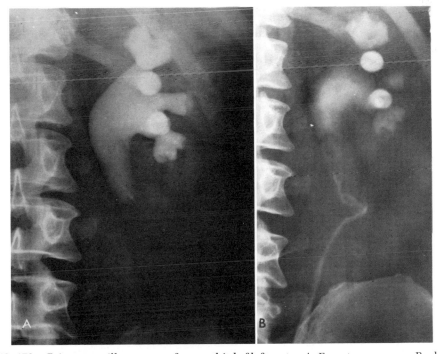

Figure 10–179.   Primary papillary tumor of upper third of left ureter. **A,** *Excretory urogram.* Pyelocaliectasis with dilatation and abrupt termination of adjacent portion of ureter, suggesting irregular filling defect from upper margin of ureteral tumor. **B,** *Left retrograde pyelogram.* Diagnosis of ureteral tumor confirmed. Extensive mottling and filling defects caused by tumor of upper part of ureter. Grade 2 papillary transitional cell epithelioma of ureter found.

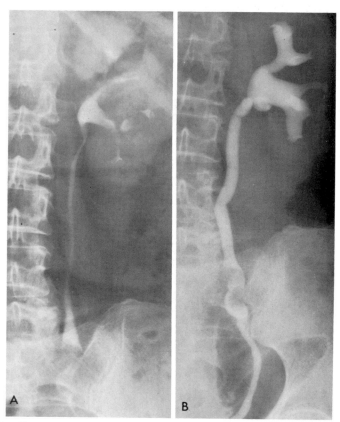

Figure 10–180.   Papillary tumor of left ureter. **A,** *Excretory urogram.* Upper margin of tumor well delineated but lower is indistinct. **B,** *Retrograde pyelogram.* Entire tumor is delineated as negative filling defec overlying wing of sacrum.

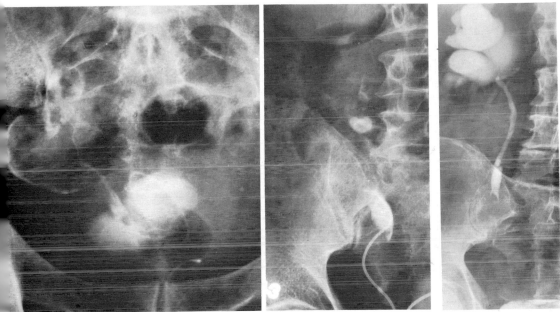

Fig. 10–181   Fig. 10–182   Fig. 10–183

Figure 10–181. Extensive primary papillary tumor of lower third of right ureter. *Right retrograde pyelo-*
ram. Opaque catheter in lower third of ureter outlines large circular area, mottled in appearance, from nega
ive shadows caused by tumor in dilated lower portion of ureter. Kidney showed absence of function with
xcretory urography. *Exploration* revealed papillary transitional cell epithelioma, grade 2.

Figure 10–182. *Right retrograde pyelogram.* **Extensive papillary transitional cell epithelioma, grade 1,**
involving almost entire ureter. Irregular splotches of medium caused by tumor which is producing typical
egative shadows, filling defects, and mottling.

Figure 10–183. **Low grade papillary ureteral tumor of 4 years' duration** in man, 65 years of age. Gross
ematuria 4 years before this examination. Excretory urogram (not shown) had been considered normal,
lthough ureters were only fractionally visualized. Cystoscopic examination had been negative. Intermittent
ross hematuria continued. *Retrograde pyelogram.* Right hydronephrosis with suggestion of obstruction of
reteropelvic juncture. Negative filling defect in lower third of ureter. Only upper margin of tumor visual-
zed as irregular defect. *Nephroureterectomy.* Papillary noninfiltrating grade 1 transitional cell epithelioma,
cm long.

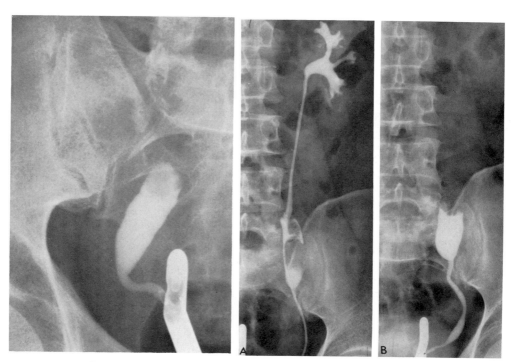

Fig. 10–184   **Fig. 10–185**

Figure 10–184. Low grade papillary ureteral tumor in man, 56 years of age. *Retrograde bulb pyelogram.* Goblet or wineglass deformity from tumor in lower third of right ureter. *Nephroureterectomy.* Papillary transitional cell epithelioma, grade 1 (1.5 by 1.5 by 1 cm).

Figure 10–185. Large papillary ureteral tumor causing no obstruction. **A,** *Conventional retrograde pyelogram* with 5-F ureteral catheter. Long filling defect over brim of pelvis. **B,** *Retrograde pyelogram,* using bulb catheter in ureteral meatus. Goblet or wineglass deformity outlining lower margin of tumor with typical dilated ureter below as described by Bergman, Friedenberg, and Sayegh.

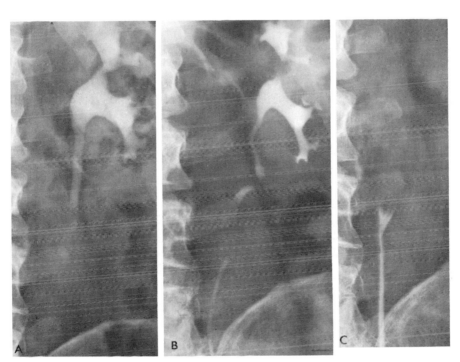

Figure 10–186. Papillary ureteral tumor in man, 52 years of age. Illustration of how easily ureteral tumors can be missed because of fractional visualization of ureter. **A,** *Excretory urogram.* Questionable filling defect n upper part of ureter. **B,** *Retrograde pyelogram* made with conventional ureteral catheter. **C,** *Retrograde pyelogram* made with bulb catheter. Goblet or wineglass deformity from lower margin of tumor. *Nephroureterectomy.* Papillary transitional cell epithelioma, grade 2.

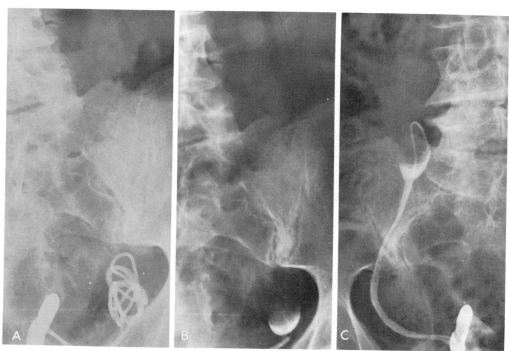

Figure 10–187. Bilateral papillary ureteral tumors occurring asynchronously in man, 69 years of age. **A,** *Plain film.* Ureteral catheter coiled in dilated ureter below tumor. **B,** *Left bulb ureterogram.* Goblet deformity indicating lower margin of ureteral tumor. Previous excretory urogram showed normal right kidney and ureter but no function on left. *Nephroureterectomy.* Papillary transitional cell epithelioma, grade 2, with superficial infiltration. **C,** *Five months later than* **A** *and* **B.** Patient had had gross hematuria. Excretory urogram (not shown here) revealed mild right hydronephrosis and hydroureter. Cystoscopy showed multiple papillary tumors of bladder. *Retrograde pyelogram.* Typical coiling of ureteral catheter in dilated part of ureter below lower margin of tumor with goblet or wineglass deformity. Ureter was opened and polyp-like papillary tumor was excised. Papillary transitional cell epithelioma, grade 2. (From Utz, D. C., Brunsting, C. D., and Harrison, E. G., Jr.)

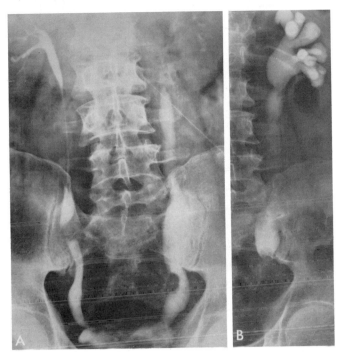

Figure 10–188.   Solid nonpapillary carcinoma of ureter in man, 66 years of age. **A,** *Excretory urogram.* Peculiar indentations in lower part of both ureters—over promontory of sacrum on right, below sacro-iliac joint on left. Considered to be from extraureteral pressure. **B,** *Left retrograde pyelogram* 6 months later than A. Advanced dilatation of upper two thirds of ureter with inverted goblet deformity indicating upper margin of large ureteral tumor. *Nephroureterectomy.* **Nonpapillary, solid, transitional cell epithelioma, grade 4,** infiltrating wall of ureter.

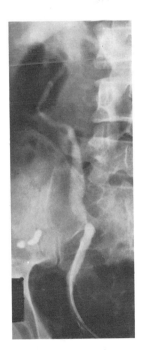

Figure 10–189.   *Right retrograde pyelogram.* **Primary solid (nonpapillary) tumor of ureter simulating ureteral stricture.** Tumor situated opposite second sacral vertebra, and catheter would not go beyond it. Urographically it suggests narrowing from stricture rather than primary tumor. *Exploration* revealed tumor, and *nephroureterectomy* was done. Pathologic diagnosis was **nonpapillary (solid) transitional cell epithelioma, grade 4,** 2 cm long. Compare with Figure 6–154 in which similar ureteral deformity was caused by nonopaque stone.

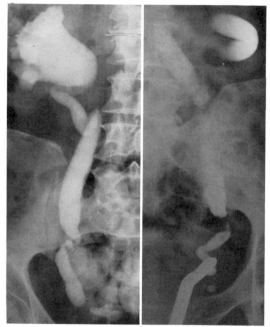

Fig. 10-190   Fig. 10-191

Figure 10-190. Papillary ureteral tumor mistaken for carcinoma of bladder. Gross hematuria. Excretory urogram (not shown) revealed tumor simulating stricture in woman, 66 years of age, and moderate dilatation of lower part of right ureter. *Cystoscopy showed broad-based papillary tumor of bladder* involving lower part of right lateral wall and obscuring ureteral orifice (which could not be identified). Fulgurated. Returned 6 months later; papillary tumor could be seen projecting from right ureteral orifice. *Retrograde pyelogram at second visit.* Pyeloureterectasis. Narrowing and angulation over promontory of sacrum simulate stricture, but are caused by tumor. Tumor also present in dilated terminal ureter. Papillary transitional cell epithelioma, grade 2.

Figure 10-191. Solid (nonpapillary) carcinoma of ureter simulating stricture in woman, 56 years of age. *Retrograde pyelogram* made with bulb catheter in ureteral meatus, filling ureter from below upward. Short, narrowed area at lower margin of left sacro-iliac joint appears to be stricture with marked ureterectasis above. *Nephroureterectomy.* Lesion was nonpapillary, solid, squamous cell epithelioma, grade 3, which had infiltrated through muscular wall of ureter.

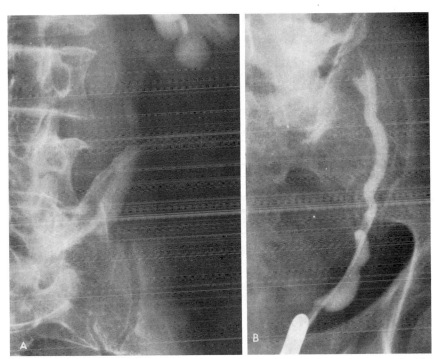

Figure 10–192.   Ureteral tumor. Solid, nonpapillary, infiltrating, grade 3 transitional cell epithelioma with obstruction. **A,** *Excretory urogram.* Pyeloureterectasis with obstruction at level of lumbosacral junction. Patient also had aortic aneurysm which was considered as possible cause of obstruction. **B,** *Retrograde ureterogram.* Complete obstruction. *Exploration.* Solid tumor involving 2.5 cm of ureter. It infiltrated through full thickness of ureteral wall and involved periureteral fat.

MALIGNANT NONEPITHELIAL TUMORS OF THE RENAL PELVIS AND URETER

Primary Tumors

Renal Pelvis. Reports of malignant nonepithelial tumors of the renal pelvis are extremely rare. The reason for this is, no doubt, that even though a sarcoma arose from the connective tissue in the wall of the renal pelvis or calyces, it would be practically impossible for the pathologist to be sure that it did not arise from the kidney proper or peripelvic or periureteral tissues. Harbaugh reported a case of botryoid sarcoma of the renal pelvis in a 7-year-old girl (Fig. 10–193).

Ureter. Malignant nonepithelial tumors of the ureter are rare. The ones reported have been some variety of sarcoma, and an occasional case of "carcinosarcoma" has appeared in the literature (Renner). A search of the literature for these rare tumors was made by d'Aunoy and Zoeller in 1930, Smith in 1935, and Rademaker in 1943. Rademaker found five cases and added one of his own. In 1953, Senger and Furey stated that only two additional cases had been reported since 1943, making a total of eight. In 1955, Alznauer added the ninth, a case of leiomyosarcoma which he believed to be the third authentic case of leiomyosarcoma in the literature. The cases of Kraus reported in 1944 and of Rossien and Russell in 1946 also are of interest. Fein and Hamm in 1965a reported a case of hemangiosarcoma of the terminal portion of the right ureter in a woman aged 76. They reviewed the literature and found only an occasional report of malignant mesodermal tumors of the ureter.

In most cases, diagnosis has been made at either abdominal exploration or necropsy. As might be surmised, it is always open to question whether the growth actually arose from the connective tissue in the wall of the ureter or from periureteral tissue. In Rademaker's and Fein and Hamm's cases, preoperative diagnosis was made urographically.

Secondary Tumors

Ureter (by Direct Invasion) (Figs. 10–194, 10–195, and 10–196). The pelvis and ureter may become involved by direct extension and invasion from malignant tumors of almost any abdominal organ. Lesions arising from retroperitoneal tumors such as lymphoma or from carcinoma of the pancreas are the common offenders. In the case of carcinoma of the pancreas, the upper part of the right ureter should be involved most frequently because of its proximity to the head of the pancreas (Putschar and Irwin). For some reason, however, most examples of this condition that we have encountered in the Mayo Clinic cases have involved the left ureter (Figs. 10–194, 10–195, and 10–196). Carcinoma of the cervix commonly involves the ureter; carcinoma of the colon does so less often (see Figs. 5–113 through 5–115).

Ureter (by Metastasis) (Figs. 10–197 and 10–198). Metastasis to the ureter can result from primary tumors located almost anywhere in the body. The relative frequency of primary sites is shown in Table 10–7 compiled by Lucké and Schlumberger.

Table 10–7.   Primary Site of Metastatic Tumors of the Ureter in 62 Cases[*]

SITE OF PRIMARY TUMOR	CASES
Renal parenchyma	15
Stomach	11
Prostate	9
Breast	7
Lung	5
Lymphoma	5
Colon	4
Uterus	2
Ovary	1
Testis	1
Urethra	1
Skin	1
Total	62

[*]Compiled from review of literature in 1957 by Lucké and Schlumberger.

It is of interest that malignant lesions of the renal cortex (that is, adenocarcinoma or hypernephroma) rank highest on the list. This subject was extensively reviewed by MacAlpine in 1948 at which time he found 12 cases reported in the literature. Since then, other cases have been reported by Hovenanian; Howell; and Heslin, Milner, and Garlick. In 1967 Young found 34 cases reported in the literature. It has been suggested (Deming; Hovenanian) that such lesions are downstream implants of tumors that could have resulted from manipulation of the hypernephroma during nephrectomy. It has been suggested also that, if there are any papillary elements in the hypernephroma, a complete nephroureterectomy should be done as in the case of epithelial tumors of the renal plevis.

The general subject of metastatic growths in the ureter has been reviewed by Presman and Ehrlich, Porras, McCrea and Peale, and Klinger. There appear to be less than 50 case reports in the literature. As might be expected, many of the lesions are discovered accidentally during abdominal operation or at necropsy. Interesting cases in which preoperative urograms were available have been reported by Mirabile and Spillane from bronchogenic carcinoma of the lung, by Robbins and Lich from carcinoma of the cervix, and by Stearns, Farmer, and Gordon from carcinoma of the stomach. Samellas and Marks reported a case of metastasis to the ureter from a melanoma of the scalp (Fig. 10–197) Richardson encountered a case of metastatic melanoma (from the eye) which involved both the pelvis and ureter (Fig. 10–198).

(Text continued on page 1189.)

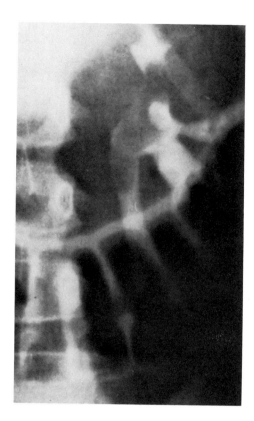

Figure 10–193. Botryoid sarcoma of renal pelvis in girl aged 7. *Excretory urogram.* Nonopaque filling defect of upper calyx and pelvis. At operation freely movable mass could be palpated within renal pelvis. Nephrectomy done. *Gross pathology.* Pelvis filled with long polypoid structure attached within upper calyx. It protruded into pelvis and into upper part of ureter. (From Harbaugh, J. T.)

Figure 10–194. *Excretory urogram.* Carcinoma of pancreas causing upward and lateral displacement of kidney and lateral displacement of ureter.

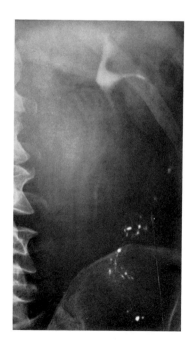

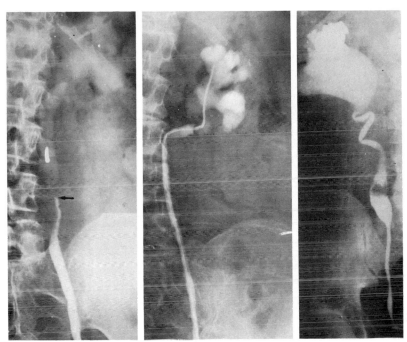

Fig. 10–195   Fig. 10–196   Fig. 10–197

Figure 10–195. Metastatic carcinoma involving left ureter. *Left retrograde pyelogram.* Irregular narrowing of middle third of left ureter, associated with filling defects and pyeloureterectasis above. Ureteral stricture and primary carcinoma of ureter considered in differential diagnosis. *Exploration* revealed metastatic tumor invading ureter. **Primary origin not accurately determined,** but probably in uterine fundus. Uterus previously removed for low-grade carcinoma.

Figure 10–196. Carcinoma of pancreas involving left ureter. *Left retrograde pyelogram.* Marked displacement and angulation of upper third of left ureter, with ureteropyelectasis above. No function in the excretory urogram.

Figure 10–197. *Retrograde pyelogram.* Melanoma which has metastasized to kidney and ureter. Primary lesion was pigmented nevus removed from right side of scalp 18 months previously. Necropsy showed pedunculated mass of friable metastatic tumor attached to pelvis just above ureteropelvic juncture, and similar lesion in upper part of ureter (shown by filling defect in pyelogram). Pyelectasis apparently resulted from lesion in pelvis obstructing ureteropelvic juncture. (From Samellas, W., and Marks, A. R.)

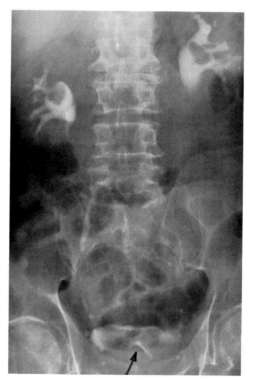

Figure 10–198.   Metastasis from melanoma of eye to urinary tract in man aged 76. Eye had been removed 5 years previously. *Excretory urogram.* Negative filling defects in both renal pelves from metastatic tumor; also small lesion in trigone of bladder (*arrow*). (Courtesy of Dr. E. J. Richardson.)

RETROPERITONEAL TUMORS AND CYSTS

Retroperitoneal tumors (and cysts) are of interest to the urologist because they frequently compromise the urinary tract by displacement, obstruction, and in-vasion. Ackerman in 1954 defined the retroperitoneal space as "that indefinite area in the lumbar and iliac region which lies between the peritoneum and the posterior parietal wall of the abdominal cavity. It extends upward to the twelfth rib and twelfth thoracic vertebra and downward to the base of the sacrum and the iliac crest."

Classification of Retroperitoneal Tumors

A practical classification of retroperitoneal tumors has been suggested by Ackerman (Table 10–8).

Incidence of Retroperitoneal Tumors

Primary retroperitoneal tumors are relatively rare. An estimate of the comparative incidence of the various retroperitoneal tumors can be made from the 340 tumors tabulated by Stout (cited in Ackerman) (Tables 10–9 and 10–10).

Table 10–8. Classification of Retroperitoneal Tumors by Ackerman

| TISSUE OF ORIGIN | TUMORS | |
	Benign	Malignant
I. Tumors of mesodermal origin		
Adipose tissue	Lipoma	Liposarcoma
Smooth muscle	Leiomyoma	Leiomyosarcoma
Connective tissue	Fibroma	Fibrosarcoma
Striated muscle	Rhabdomyoma	Rhabdomyosarcoma
Lymph vessels	Lymphangioma	Lymphangiosarcoma
Primitive mesenchyme	Myxoma	Myxosarcoma
Blood vessels	Hemangioma and angiosarcoma	
	Hemangiopericytoma (benign and malignant)	
Uncertain origin	Xanthogranuloma	
II. Tumors of neurogenous origin		
Nerve sheath	Nonencapsulated neurofibroma	
	Encapsulated neurilemmoma	
	Malignant schwannoma	
Sympathetic nervous system	Ganglioneuroma	
	Sympathicoblastoma (ganglioneuroblastoma)	
	Neuroblastoma	
Heterotopic cortical adrenal and chromaffin tissue	Carcinoma arising from cortical adrenal tissue	
	Malignant nonchromaffin paraganglioma	
	Paraganglioma	
	Functioning pheochromocytoma	
III. Tumors arising from embryonic remnants or notochord		
	Benign and malignant teratomas	
	Chordomas	

Table 10–9. Benign Retroperitoneal Tumors in 75 Cases[*]

	TUMORS
Cyst of caudal gut	17
Pheochromocytoma (active)	14
Granular cell myoblastoma	11
Neurofibroma	6
Leiomyoma	6
Xanthogranuloma	5
Ganglioneuroma	4
Lipoma	4
Papillary cystadenoma	2
Paraganglioma (inactive)	2
Dermoid cyst	2
Adenoma	1
Neurilemmoma	1
Lymphangioma	0

[*]Data from Stout, A. P., Laboratory of Surgical Pathology, Columbia University, 1905 to 1951 Inclusive. Taken from Ackerman (1954), p. 10.

Table 10–10. **Malignant Retroperitoneal Tumors: 265 Tumors***

	TUMORS
Lymphosarcoma	51
Liposarcoma	35
Leiomyosarcoma	29
Hodgkin's disease	26
Embryonal carcinoma	24
Sympathicoblastoma	18
Hemangiopericytoma	18
Undiagnosed tumor	18
Metastatic carcinoma of unknown origin	13
Teratoma	6
Mesenchymoma	5
Rhabdomyosarcoma	5
Fibrosarcoma	4
Malignant schwannoma	3
Myxoma	3
Leukemia	2
Chordoma	2
Dysgerminoma	1
Malignant melanoma (metastatic)	1
Suprarenal cortical carcinoma	1
Plasmacytoma	0
Total	265

*Data from Stout, A. P., Laboratory of Surgical Pathology, Columbia University, 1905 to 1951. Taken from Ackerman (1954), p. 11.

Tumors and Cysts of Mesodermal Origin

Malignant Lesions
(Figs. 10–199 through 10–213)

Liposarcomas are probably the most common retroperitoneal neoplasms (DeWeerd and Dockerty), and leiomyosarcomas are probably next. As mentioned in the section on malignant mesenchymal tumors of the renal cortex, it is often difficult even at operation or necropsy to tell whether a sarcoma in the region of the kidney originates primarily from the renal cortex or renal capsule, or from perinephric connective tissue or muscle and has invaded the kidney secondarily.

These tumors do not lend themselves well to accurate urographic diagnosis and about all that can be determined is that the kidney or ureter or both are displaced, distorted, obstructed, or invaded by an adjacent soft-tissue mass. Accurate diagnosis can be made only by exploration and biopsy.

Benign Lesions
(Figs. 10–214 through 10–226)

Benign retroperitoneal tumors may reach enormous size and cause marked displacement of the kidney and ureter. At times a kidney may be completely displaced across the vertebral column so that it overlies the opposite kidney. *Lipomas* and *retroperitoneal cysts* are especially likely to produce this marked distortion (DeWeerd and Dockerty; Greene; Windholz).

(*Text continued on page 1205.*)

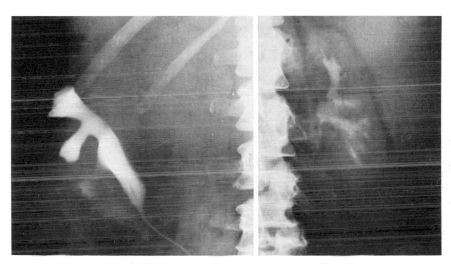

Fig. 10–199 Fig. 10–200

Figure 10–199. *Retrograde pyelogram.* **Retroperitoneal sarcoma. Enormous lymphosarcoma.** Exploration revealed huge retroperitoneal tumor which was inoperable. Specimens were removed for microscopic examination only.

Figure 10–200. *Excretory urogram.* **Retroperitoneal lymphosarcoma** surrounding and compressing left kidney. Diagnosis made by sternal biopsy; no exploration. Roentgen therapy given. Patient died of lesion.

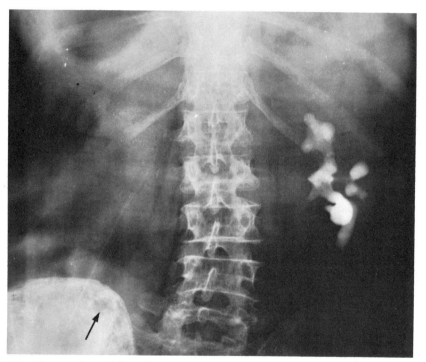

Figure 10–201. **Retroperitoneal lymphosarcoma.** *Left retrograde pyelogram.* Bizarre deformity of pelv and calyces of left kidney suggests tumor, but diagnosis from this film would be difficult. Excretory urogra showed no function on left side. Primary complaint: tumor of right ilium. Some osteoclastic metastasis right ilium (*arrow*). Inguinal nodes palpable; were excised and examined microscopically. Diagnosis mac of **grade 4 lymphosarcoma.** Five years later patient was still alive. Epitrochlear node excised elsewhere ar sent to Mayo Clinic for examination. Diagnosis of lymphosarcoma.

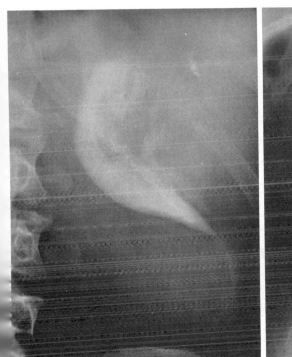
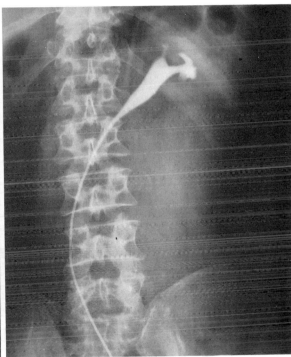

Fig. 10-202   **Fig. 10-203**

Figure 10-202.   Retroperitoneal tumor. *Excretory urogram.* Large tumor in region of lower pole of left kidney, displacing lower pole upward and laterally, and causing marked deformity of pelviocalyceal system. Impossible to say from film whether intrarenal or extrarenal tumor. Surgical exploration revealed large retroperitoneal tumor situated in front of kidney. Surgeon felt it was probably arising from renal capsule. Tumor and kidney removed. **Pathologic diagnosis: grade 1 leiomyosarcoma** attached loosely to kidney in hilar region. Tumor had compressed ureter in upper third and produced hydronephrosis.

Figure 10-203.   Retroperitoneal lipomyxosarcoma. *Left retrograde pyelogram.* Huge soft-tissue mass filling entire left side of abdomen, pushing left kidney upward, its lower pole laterally, and ureter medially across midline. Does not compromise pelvis and calyces; seems to be connected with lower pole of left kidney. Surgical exploration through left rectus incision. Large retroperitoneal tumor, 20 cm in diameter, situated in region of renal pedicle and lower pole of kidney. Tumor removed without removal of kidney. **Pathologic diagnosis: grade 2 lipomyxosarcoma.**

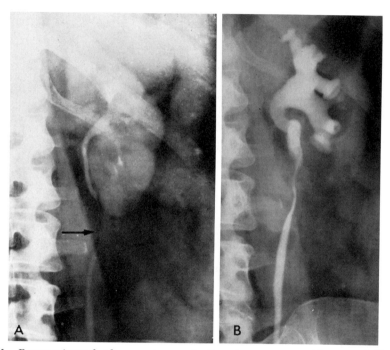

Figure 10–204. Retroperitoneal adenocarcinoma. **A,** *Excretory urogram.* Absence of filling of localized segment of ureter between third and fourth transverse processes of the lumbar vertebrae. **B,** *Left retrograde pyelogram.* Marked narrowing and constriction of localized segment of ureter suggest periureteric compression or ureteral stricture rather than filling defect from primary tumor of ureter. Surgical exploration revealed retroperitoneal mass involving connective tissue adjacent to ureter and constricting ureter in its upper third. Tumor, kidney, and upper third of ureter removed. **Pathologic diagnosis: periureteric tumor grade 3 adenocarcinoma. Primary origin unknown.** Kidney not involved.

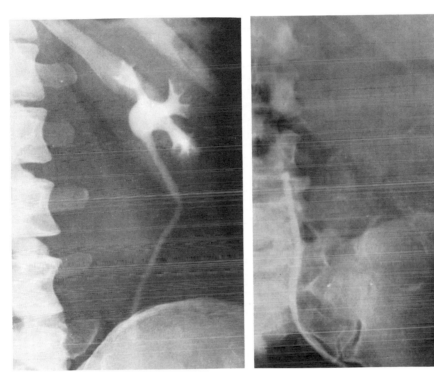

Fig. 10-205   Fig. 10-206

Figure 10-205.   Retroperitoneal tumor. *Left retrograde pyelogram.* Marked lateral displacement of lower pole of left kidney and upper part of ureter from apparently extrarenal mass. Surgical exploration revealed large retroperitoneal tumor filling entire pelvis and extending along spinal column almost to diaphragm. Bladder was pushed high into abdomen. Mass filled entire true pelvis. Tissue removed for microscopic examination showed **grade 3 malignant neoplasm.** Impossible to say whether sarcoma or adenocarcinoma.

Figure 10-206.   Retroperitoneal tumor. *Left retrograde pyelogram.* Large soft-tissue mass filling left side of abdomen. Complete obstruction of ureter, apparently at site of ureteropelvic juncture. *Excretory urogram* showed no function of this kidney. Huge hydronephrosis with complete obstruction at ureteropelvic juncture was suspected. Surgical exploration revealed huge retroperitoneal tumor which involved left kidney and adrenal gland. Tumor, adrenal gland, and kidney removed. **Pathologic diagnosis: grade 3 osteochondrofibrosarcoma,** with complete destruction of renal substance.

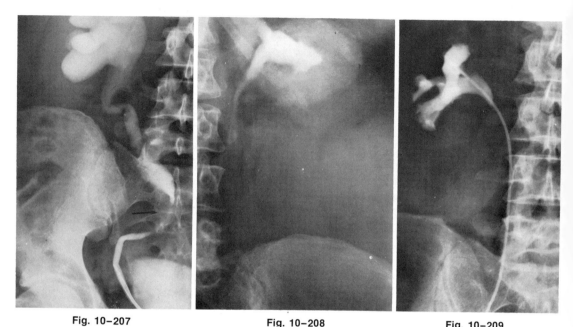

Fig. 10–207   **Fig. 10–208**   **Fig. 10–209**

Figure 10–207. Retroperitoneal rhabdomyosarcoma. Ganglioneuroma was suspected preoperatively. *Right retrograde pyelogram.* Marked medial displacement of middle part of ureter in region of promontory of sacrum. Definite constriction of ureter at this point (*arrow*), with ureteropyelectasis above. Surgical exploration revealed extensive tumor attached to right psoas muscle, deep in pelvis. Specimen removed for microscopic examination showed **grade 4 malignant neoplasm, probably rhabdomyosarcoma.**

Figure 10–208. Retroperitoneal fibromyxosarcoma. *Excretory urogram.* Huge soft-tissue mass filling left side of abdomen, displacing left kidney upward and laterally, and causing malrotation of kidney. Renal outline seems intact and there is no characteristic deformity of pelviocalyceal system. Large cyst and retroperitoneal tumor were considered in differential diagnosis. Surgical exploration showed large retroperitoneal tumor which was adjacent to but not attached to kidney. Tumor removed. **Pathologic diagnosis: grade 1 fibromyxosarcoma, possibly originating in adventitia of blood vessels.**

Figure 10–209. Retroperitoneal liposarcoma, simulating renal cyst. *Right retrograde pyelogram.* Large, round soft-tissue shadow with smooth outline, superimposed over outline of kidney. Minimal deformity of calyces. Some pressure on lower and medial borders of pelvis, producing crescentic deformity. Solitary cyst and retroperitoneal tumor considered in differential diagnosis. Surgical exploration revealed large retroperitoneal tumor mass, 12 cm in diameter, adherent to lower pole of right kidney. Tumor and kidney removed. **Pathologic diagnosis: cystic grade 1 liposarcoma, attached to lower pole of right kidney** and infiltrating its substance at two points. Minimal destruction of renal substance.

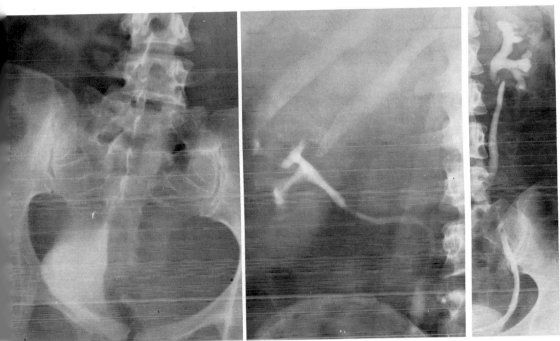

Fig. 10-210   Fig. 10-211   Fig. 10-212

Figure 10-210. Retroperitoneal hemangioendothelioma (hemangiopericytoma subgroup). *Excretory urogram.* Marked displacement of bladder to right side of bony pelvis with similar distortion of left ureter. Surgical exploration through left rectus incision; huge multilocular cystic type of retroperitoneal tumor invading almost entire pelvis. Incision into mass evacuated large quantities of what had gross appearance of chyle. Specimen removed showed low-grade malignant neoplasm which appeared to be low-grade hemangioendothelioma (hemangiopericytoma subgroup). This type of tumor has been described by Zimmerman, Stout, and Murray.

Figure 10-211. Retroperitoneal leiomyosarcoma. *Excretory urogram.* Soft-tissue mass in region of upper pole of right kidney, which apparently is displacing right kidney downward and laterally. Some distortion of upper calyces. Surgical exploration through right midrectus incision. Retroperitoneal tumor found, closely attached to renal capsule and right renal vein. Tumor, kidney, and adrenal gland removed. **Pathologic diagnosis: grade 2 leiomyosarcoma arising from region of right kidney and attached to capsule** of kidney. Kidney practically normal, except for few small cysts. Adrenal gland normal.

Figure 10-212. *Retrograde pyelogram* of woman, 48 years of age, with left abdominal pain. **Retroperitoneal leiomyosarcoma encircling left ovarian vein,** displacing left ureter medially at level of fifth lumbar vertebra and producing some ureteral obstruction. Excretory urogram (not shown) showed delayed visualization. Surgical removal; ureter freed easily from tumor. Would be difficult to distinguish from retroperitoneal fibrosis.

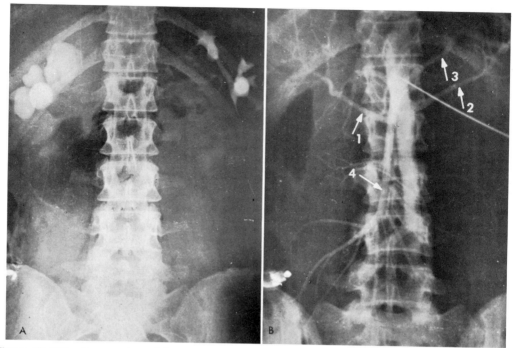

Figure 10–213. Retroperitoneal lymphosarcoma in woman, 26 years of age. **A,** *Excretory urogram.* Both kidneys displaced upward and laterally, with moderate calycectasis on right. **B,** *Aortogram* shows right (1) and left (2) renal arteries well visualized. Both kidneys show good blood supply, with displacement caused by retroperitoneal mass which is symmetrically placed. Splenic (3) and superior mesenteric (4) arteries seen. Comment: Primary lesion in kidneys was excluded with aortogram. Surgical exploration substantiated diagnosis of extensive retroperitoneal lymphosarcoma. (Courtesy of Dr. A. K. Doss.)

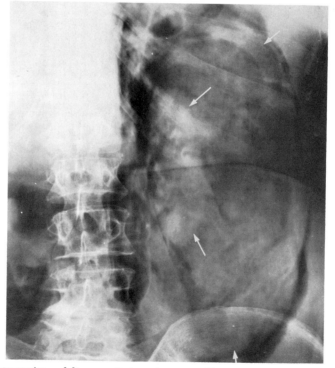

Figure 10–214. Retroperitoneal lipoma. *Perirenal air insufflation* which outlines huge perirenal lipoma that is compressing but not displacing left kidney. (Courtesy of Dr. S. J. Arnold and Department of Urology and Radiology, The Jewish Hospital of Brooklyn.)

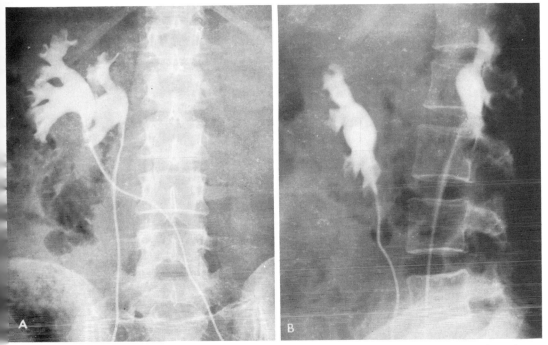

Figure 10–215.   Retroperitoneal lipoma which has displaced left kidney across midline. A, *Bilateral retrograde pyelogram.* Left kidney is seen to be farther lateral than right kidney. **B,** *Lateral view.* Right kidney in normal position and in same plane as spinal column. Left kidney is lying considerably anterior. Exploration revealed multiple retroperitoneal lipomas, the largest 40 cm in diameter and weighing 22 lb (about 10 kg). In addition, there were numerous other lipomas varying in size from 6 to 10 cm in diameter.

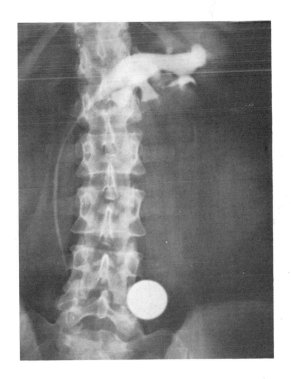

Figure 10–216.   Retroperitoneal lipoma. *Left retrograde pyelogram.* Medial and upward displacement of left kidney, with marked medial displacement of ureter across midline. Malrotation of kidney. Pelvis and calyces otherwise intact. Transabdominal exploration revealed huge retroperitoneal lipoma; removed surgically without removal of kidney.

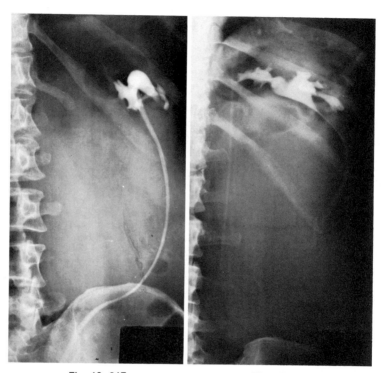

Fig. 10–217   Fig. 10–218

Figure 10–217. Retroperitoneal cystadenoma. *Left retrograde pyelogram.* Large soft-tissue mass in le
side of abdomen. Marked upward and lateral displacement of left kidney and ureter, with malrotation. Pelv
and calyces apparently not involved with lesion. Surgical exploration through left rectus incision reveale
large multilocular cystic mass arising from retroperitoneal area and not involving kidney. Mass excise
Pathologic diagnosis: multilocular cystadenoma.

Figure 10–218. Retroperitoneal cyst. *Excretory urogram.* Malrotation and marked upward and later
displacement of left kidney and ureter from huge soft-tissue mass filling left side of abdomen. Surgical e
ploration through left posterolumbar incision; large retroperitoneal cyst found and removed, without remov
of kidney.

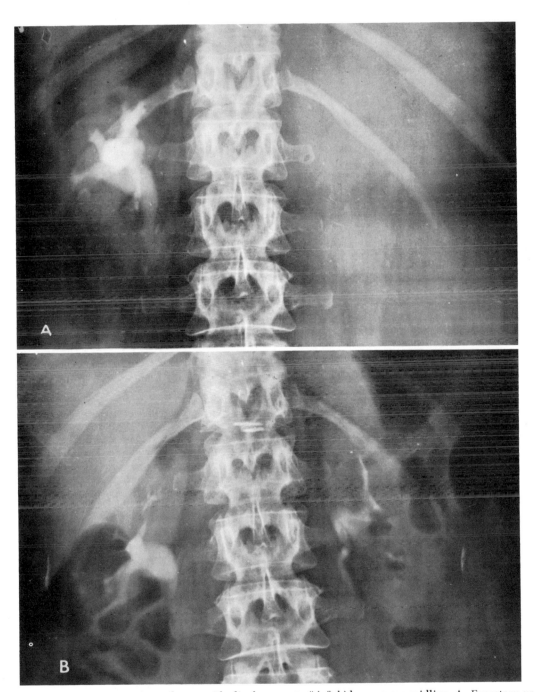

Figure 10–219.   Retroperitoneal cyst with displacement of left kidney across midline. A, *Excretory uro-gram*. Left kidney has been pushed across midline and its pyelogram is superimposed over right kidney. Surgical exploration revealed large retroperitoneal cyst which displaced kidney. Cyst was removed. B, *Postoperative excretory urogram*. Left kidney has returned to normal position.

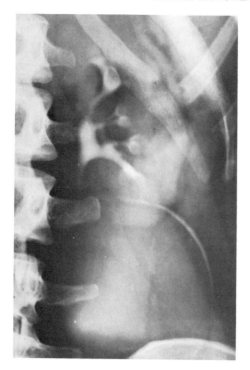

Figure 10–220. Retroperitoneal cyst displacing left ureter. *Left retrograde pyelogram.* Marked lateral displacement of left ureter. Surgical exploration revealed cyst, 8 cm in diameter; ureter passed directly over cyst. Cyst removed.

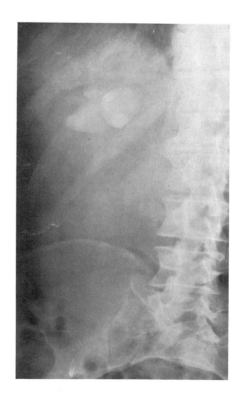

Figure 10–221. *Excretory urogram.* Man aged 58 with large **retroperitoneal chylous cyst** which obstructed right ureter and produced right hydronephrosis with poor function. At operation, cyst contained 2,500 ml of milky fluid. (From Thompson, G. J., and Culp, O. S.)

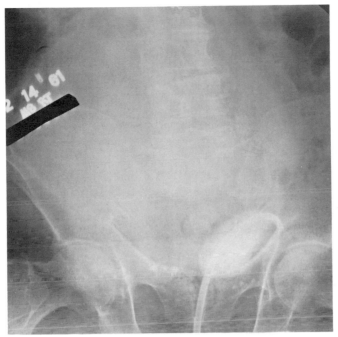

Figure 10–222.   Huge retroperitoneal cyst which displaced bladder to left and completely obstructed right ureter. Man aged 82 with large abdominal mass and frequency of urination but no residual urine. At operation, cyst of 3,000-ml capacity removed. *Pathologic diagnosis.* Cystic lymphangioma. (From Thompson, G. J., and Culp, O. S.)

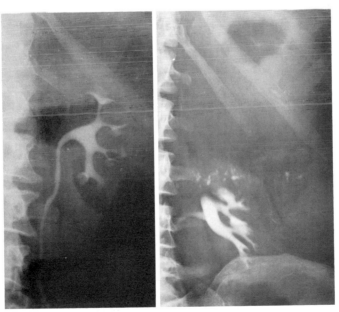

Fig. 10–223   **Fig. 10–224**

Figure 10–223.   Large pancreatic cyst. *Left retrograde pyelogram.* Normal. No displacement or deformity of kidney, despite the fact that pancreatic cyst was so large that it filled upper three fourths of abdomen and was visible, protruding against abdominal wall.

Figure 10–224.   Small pancreatic cyst. *Left retrograde pyelogram.* Downward displacement of left kidney from moderate-sized pancreatic cyst, involving tail of pancreas. Extrarenal shadow is residual barium in colon.

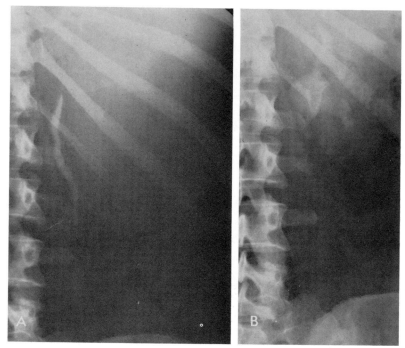

Figure 10–225. **Pancreatic cystadenoma** in woman aged 47. Large asymptomatic mass in left upper quadrant of abdomen. **A,** *Excretory urogram.* Compression and medial displacement of upper part of ureter and kidney suggested renal cyst. **B,** *Postoperative excretory urogram* after lesion had been removed. Left kidney has returned to normal position. (From Thompson, G. J., and Culp, O. S.)

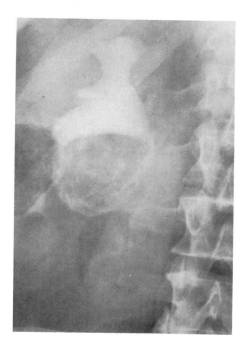

Figure 10–226. *Excretory urogram.* **Retroperitoneal fibrolipoma, with mottled calcification,** closely attached to kidney, mostly around lower pole but nodule also in region of upper pole. At operation lesion was firmly adherent to pelvis and upper part of ureter.

Differential Diagnosis; Intra-abdominal Lesions Which Displace Kidneys and Ureters
(Figs. 10–227 through 10–240)

That retroperitoneal tumors cause displacement of the kidneys and ureters is well documented (Greene; Sweetser; Windholz). However, it must not be forgotten that similar displacement may occur, although much less frequently, from tumors of intra-abdominal organs, such as the gallbladder, liver, spleen, bowel, and mesentery (Schulte and Emmett).

(Text continued on page 1211.)

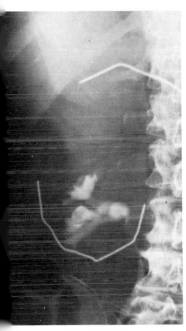

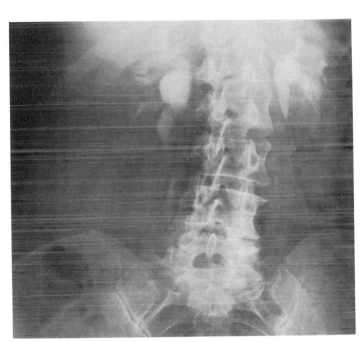

Fig. 10-227   **Fig. 10-228**

Figure 10-227. Hydrops of gallbladder. *Right retrograde pyelogram.* Downward displacement of right kidney from hydrops of gallbladder.

Figure 10-228. Hydrops of gallbladder producing upward and medial displacement of kidney and minimal pyelectasis. Woman aged 50 with asymptomatic, movable, fluctuant mass in right upper quadrant of abdomen. *Excretory urogram.* Large circular soft-tissue mass visible below kidney but kidney with normal outline can be seen through mass. (From Thompson, G. J., and Culp, O. S.)

Fig. 10–229   Fig. 10–230

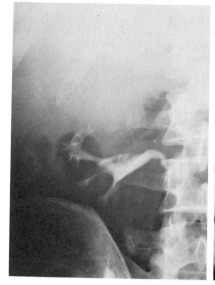
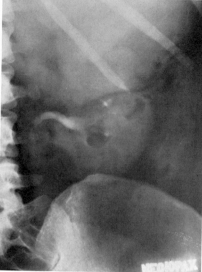

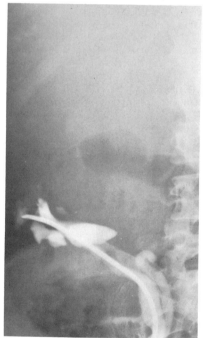

Fig. 10–231

Figure 10–229. Carcinoma of liver. *Right retrograde pyelogram.* Downward displacement of right kidney from carcinoma of liver.

Figure 10–230. Cyst of left lobe of liver. *Excretory urogram.* Downward and lateral displacement of left kidney from large cyst of left lobe of liver; proved surgically.

Figure 10–231. Cyst of liver. *Right retrograde pyelogram.* Incomplete duplication of ureter. Kidney displaced downward. Upper pelvis not visualized. Exploration revealed cause of displacement to be enormous cyst of liver.

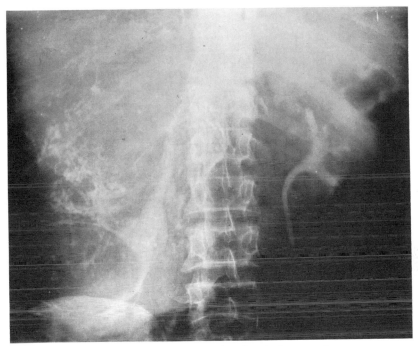

Figure 10–232. Polycystic disease of liver associated with calcification. *Excretory urogram.* Medial and downward displacement of right kidney, with some pelviocalyceal deformity

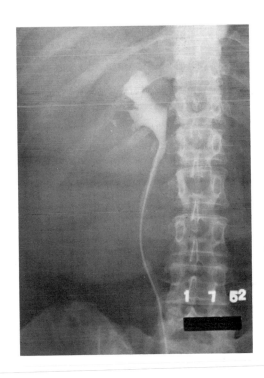

Figure 10–233. Hepatic cyst displacing right kidney upward and medially. Woman aged 56 with smooth, movable, cystic mass in right upper part of abdomen. Only vague discomfort. Cholecystogram was normal. *Right retrograde pyelogram.* Large, soft-tissue mass below kidney displacing kidney upward and medially. *Operation* (through right rectus incision) revealed large cyst of right lobe of liver. Cyst was excised. Postoperative excretory urogram (not shown here) showed right kidney had returned to normal. (From Thompson, G. J., and Culp, O. S.)

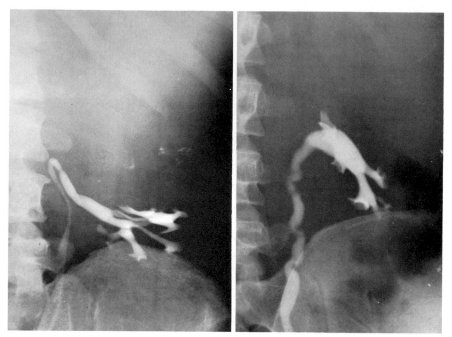

Fig. 10–234   Fig. 10–235

Figure 10–234. **Banti's disease.** *Left retrograde pyelogram.* Downward displacement of left kidney caused by **enlarged spleen.** Splenectomy done.

Figure 10–235. **Splenomegaly.** *Left retrograde pyelogram.* Downward displacement of left kidney, with rotation on anteroposterior axis, from enlarged spleen.

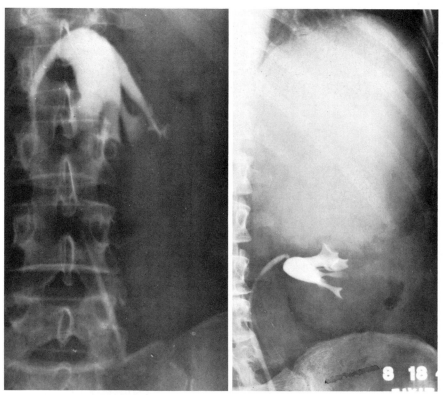

Fig. 10–236   Fig. 10–237

Figure 10–236. **Splenomegaly.** *Left retrograde pyelogram.* Downward and medial displacement of left kidney, with rotation on anteroposterior axis, from enlarged spleen.

Figure 10–237. **Carcinoma of spleen.** *Left retrograde pyelogram.* Downward displacement of left kidney from carcinoma of spleen, which involved kidney and stomach. Impossible to say where lesion originated

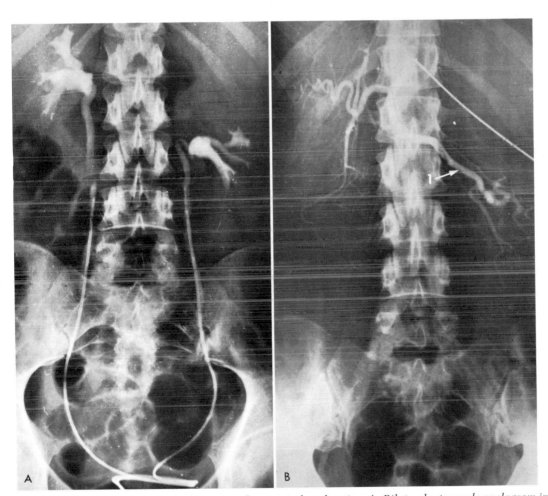

Figure 10–238.   Simple cyst of spleen proved at surgical exploration. **A,** *Bilateral retrograde pyelogram* in woman, 32 years of age. Marked downward displacement of left kidney; cause indeterminate. **B,** *Aortogram.* Not too satisfactory technically because complete filling of aorta was not obtained. However, splenic artery (1) is well-outlined, which shows downward displacement of spleen. There is concentric deformity, saucer-fashion, of smaller splenic vessels, which is characteristic of cyst of spleen. (Courtesy of Dr. A. K. Doss.)

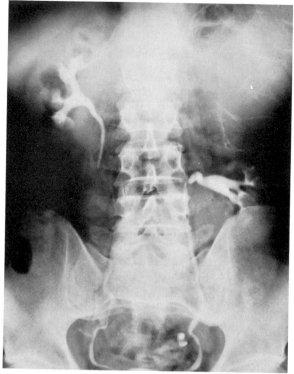

Figure 10–239. **Displacement of left kidney by primary tumor of spleen.** *Excretory urogram.* Bizarre linear calcification of splenic tumor. Kidney displaced downward and descending colon displaced medially (demonstrated by colon roentgenogram not shown here). (Courtesy of Dr. H. W. ten Cate.)

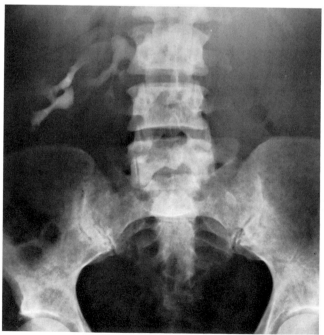

Figure 10–240. *Excretory urogram.* Displacement of left kidney across midline from enlarged spleen caused by "agnogenic myeloid metaplasia with myelosclerosis."

Tumors of Neurogenic Origin
(Figs. 10–241 through 10–250)

TUMORS ORIGINATING IN THE NERVE SHEATH

Neurofibroma

Neurofibromas are rare in the retroperitoneal region. This *benign tumor* is characterized by diffuse proliferation of the peripheral nerve elements in contradistinction to the neurilemmoma, which is an encapsulated tumor. A neurofibroma arising in a solitary kidney was reported by Freund, Crocker, and Harrison. It was thought to have arisen from a nerve in the renal pelvis. Although the neurofibroma may occur as a solitary lesion (Fig. 10–241), its common manifestation is in the syndrome known as *von Recklinghausen's disease.*

Neurilemmoma (Schwannoma)

This *encapsulated benign* tumor may arise from peripheral, cranial, and sympathetic nerves. It originates from the sheath of Schwann. Ordinarily these tumors are small and rarely attain a size greater than 6 cm. In the retroperitoneal area, however, they have been known to grow to huge proportions. According to Stout (1935), *if the nerve of origin is small* and can be found, it will be located in the capsule of the tumor. *If the nerve of origin is large,* the tumor develops inside the epineural sheath, and as it expands, the component nerve fascicles spread out over the surface of the tumor and are attached to its capsule. Fein and Hamm (1965b) reported a case of a low-grade malignant schwannoma of the renal pelvis in a 51-year-old women. They searched the literature and found three additional cases of schwannoma involving the kidney.

Neurilemmomas are not often found in the retroperitoneal area, but when they do occur there they may be found in strange and unusual places (Ackerman). Examples of such locations include: (1) obturator nerve projected into obturator canal (Erb), (2) sacral plexus, mistaken clinically for ectopic gestation (Frank), (3) behind the rectum and pressing against it (Krekeler; Krumbien), (4) crural nerve in pelvis (Moreau and Van Bogaert), and (5) behind the bladder and prostrate (Pana). Deming reported the case of a 25-year-old woman in whom the neurilemmoma displaced the upper two thirds of the left ureter laterally (Fig. 10–242).

Malignant neurilemmomas and schwannomas have been encountered but are extremely rare.

TUMORS ARISING FROM THE SYMPATHETIC NERVOUS SYSTEM

There is a close embryologic relationship between the cells that develop into the sympathetic nervous system and those that become the medullary portion of the adrenal gland. Explanations of this complicated developmental process vary, as can be appreciated from the following examples.

Karsner's position is that the primitive neuroectoderm gives rise to two main lines of cells as follows:

The *first line of descent* includes (1) the neuroblasts (sympathoblasts), from which the highly malignant neuroblastomas arise and (2) the sympathetic ganglion cells (differentiated neuroblasts or sympathoblasts) which make up the sympathetic nervous system and from which benign ganglioneuromas arise (Bielschowsky; Dockerty). The *second line of descent* gives rise to the chromophil cell (chromaffin cell) which forms the medullary portion of the adrenal gland (see below under "Tumors of the Adrenal Gland" and "Pheochromocytoma").

Robbins states:

The adrenal medulla is derived from the primitive cells of the neural crest, which migrate into the center of the fetal adrenal cortex and form the medulla with its complement of mature cells—pheochromocytes. In the fetus similar collections of cells are found along the abdominal aorta, mainly in relation to the origin of the inferior mesenteric artery, and constitute the organs of Zuckerkandl. Other groups are scattered throughout the sympathetic nervous system in relation to the cervical and thoracic ganglia, the gastrointestinal system, the bladder, the heart and the gonads. These islands are usually replaced by lymphatic tissue shortly after birth, but may persist and lead to extra-adrenal pheochromocytomas in later life.

The cells of the neural crest are also capable of forming the ganglion cells of the sympathetic nervous system, which are produced by way of the intermediate cell—the neuroblast.

Sjoerdsma has put it this way:

The cells of the adrenal medulla and other portions of the sympathetic nervous system are of ectodermal origin and arise from the primitive neural crest. The parent cells or sympathogonia may differentiate to form sympathoblasts or neuroblasts and finally mature ganglion cells, or, alternatively, they may give rise to chromaffin cells. The latter are so named because of intracellular granules that give a brown color on treatment with chromium salts.

This interrelationship has also been described somewhat like this; the sympathetic ganglion cells and adrenal medulla have a common embryologic origin as follows: The neural crest produces two types of cells: (1) *stationary* and (2) *migratory.* The stationary cells become the dorsal root ganglia whereas the migratory cells become the sympathetic ganglion cells and the chromaffin cells of the adrenal medulla.

From a practical standpoint, however, the important point is to appreciate the close relationship of the cells that make up the sympathetic nervous system and the adrenal medulla. The group of tumors under discussion may therefore arise anywhere in the chain of the sympathetic ganglia, which extends from the base of the skull (cribriform plate in the nose) to the coccyx; thus these tumors may arise from the sympathetic ganglia

in the retroperitoneal area such as the celiac ganglion or organ of Zuckerkandl at the bifurcation of the aorta, and from the adrenal medulla. They may be located, therefore, either *retropleurally* or *retroperitoneally.* When retroperitoneal, they are most often in the vicinity of the adrenal, kidney, and ureters and tend to spread down the retroperitoneal gutters. Between 40 and 50% of all neuroblastomas are found in the adrenal gland (Robbins).

Neuroblastoma (Sympathicoblastoma) (Figs. 10–243 through 10–249)

The neuroblastoma is by far the most common malignant abdominal tumor in infants and children. (Wilms' tumor is the second most common, see page 1120.) Rubin and associates (1968a) state that "The term 'neuroblastoma' is an umbrella covering a variety of histologic types of tumor which arise from cells in the neural crest to form the sympathetic ganglia and the adrenal medulla." The lesion varies from the highly malignant sympathicoblastoma through the partly differentiated ganglioneuroblastoma finally reaching the stage of the differentiated (benign) ganglioneuroma.

Formerly neuroblastoma was regarded as a hopeless situation with an almost 100% mortality regardless of treatment. In recent years, however, this attitude has changed, the chief reason being the observation that highly malignant neuroblastomas may proceed through a "maturation" phase in which the highly malignant sympathicoblastic cells develop into more benign ganglioneuroma types (Bodian and White; Cushing and Wolbach; Ladd and Gross; Wyatt and Farber). *Neuroblastoma is therefore a rare example of a malignant tumor which can mature to a fully differentiated form (benign ganglioneuroma) either spontaneously or while being treated.* Factors that have been considered as possibly stimulating maturation include partial surgical removal, exploration with biopsy, and irradiation. The use of vitamin B_{12} (cyanocobalamin) to hasten this maturation process was suggested in 1950 by Bodian but its effectiveness has not been confirmed in the United States.

In 60 to 75% of cases, *metastasis* is already present when the patient is first seen; as a matter of fact, it is often the symptoms from the metastatic lesion that bring the patient to the physician. The metastatic spread may be hematogenous, lymphatic, or by direct extension. **The most common site for metastasis is bone, which is an important point in its differentiation from Wilms' tumor,** in which the lungs are the most common site while metastasis to bone is rare.

Diagnosis. Neuroblastoma was formerly considered to be a "nonfunctioning" tumor (in contrast to "functioning" tumors such as medullary pheochromocytoma with paroxysmal hypertension or cortical tumors with Cushing's syndrome). In 1957 it was discovered (Armstrong and associates; Mason and associates) that neuroblastomas may excrete catecholamines and their metabolites as do pheochromocytomas, except that there is usually no associated hypertension. This discovery has provided a new diagnostic aid. Biochemical assays of the urine for the metabolites of the catecholamines (metanephrines [MN] and vanillylmandelic acid [VMA] now provide great help in diagnosis). (See discussion below under "Pheochromocytoma.") A rapid and reasonably accurate test is possible by using a single random specimen of urine. It is stated that the diagnosis should be 95% accurate if "the correct materials are estimated" (Bell, 1963; 1966; Crout, Pisano, and Sjoerdsma; Gifford and associates, 1964; Kelleher and associates; Sheps and associates; Voorhess and Gardner; Williams and Greer; Young and associates).

As in Wilms' tumor, one of the most common presenting complaints is abdominal mass or abdominal enlargement or distention. In contrast to Wilms' tumor, however, is the frequency of symptoms related to the metastatic spread (Willis). Metastasis to bone may cause pain in the extremities and severe anemia. Aspiration biopsy of the bone marrow in suspected cases may often provide the diagnosis. Metastasis to mesenteric or aortic lymph nodes and the liver may contribute to the abdominal distention. **Proptosis and periorbital ecchymosis** indicate metastasis to the base of the skull and walls of the orbital cavity.

Urographic Data (Figs. 10–243 through 10–249). As mentioned previously in the discussion of Wilms' tumor, neuroblastoma is essentially an *extrinsic* rather than an *intrinsic* renal tumor. The typical urographic appearance therefore is the "angular displacement" of the kidney (upward and lateral displacement of the lower pole or downward and lateral displacement of the upper pole) without distortion of the pelvis and calyces. However, in some cases the distortion may be so great that it is impossible to distinguish from "intrinsic" Wilms' tumor. **Calcification in the tumor** is helpful in differential diagnosis as it is relatively common (about 50%) in neuroblastoma but rare in Wilms' tumor. Ross has called attention to the "stippled" characteristic of the calcification which may also be present in the metastatic lesions in the liver. The presence of *bony metastases* (lytic, blastic, or both) may indicate the diagnosis. Destructive and reactive lesions of the skull with separation of the sutures are almost pathognomonic. Positive biochemical tests of the urine or aspiration biopsy of bone marrow or both may provide conclusive evidence.

Treatment and Prognosis. In the past both neuroblastoma and Wilms' tumor were considered hopeless situations. As mentioned above (page 1122), the prognosis of Wilms' tumor has now greatly improved. There has also been some improvement in the outlook for patients with neuroblastoma, but not as much as for those with Wilms' tumor. One reason for optimism in treating neuroblastoma is that the tumor may regress in an occasional case, either spontaneously or during treatment. Although highly radiosensitive, the tumor tends to recur rapidly after irradiation. The average length of survival in untreated patients is considered to be about 4 months.

The addition of chemotherapy (vincristine and cyclophosphamide [Cytoxan]) has yielded some encouraging results (James and associates), and presently national study groups are attempting to evaluate its efficacy and toxicity at various dosage levels. One such group is presently evaluating two methods of administration, namely in high dosage and in low dosage.

At the present writing, opinion seems to favor surgical removal, if feasible, followed by both irradiation and chemotherapy. If the lesion cannot be removed surgically, irradiation and chemotherapy are used. If the lesion is moderately well localized, surgical removal may be considered after its size has been reduced by irradiation and chemotherapy. As in Wilms' tumor, early diagnosis is imperative, as the results of treatment are best in patients less than 2 years old. As is also true in Wilms' tumor, 2-year survival in children is considered equal to 5-year survival in adults. (For a discussion of Collins' "period of risk" and the "safe period" in evaluating malignant tumors of infancy and childhood, the reader is referred to the discussion under Wilms' tumor, page 1122.)

Differentiated Ganglioneuroma (Benign)

The ganglioneuroma is a well-differentiated tumor composed of sympathetic ganglion cells. It occurs predominantly in young adults in contrast to the undifferentiated highly malignant neuroblastoma, which occurs principally in children. Ganglioneuromas may grow large and cause marked displacement of both retroperitoneal and intra-abdominal organs. Of lesions in 250 cases collected by Stout (1947), 44 were located in the lumbar region (Fig. 10–250), 32 in the pelvis, 31 arose from the adrenal gland, and 5 were in the mesentery. The most common location is the posterior mediastinum.

Pheochromocytoma (Chromaffin Paraganglioma; Chromocytoma)

See below under "Tumors of the Adrenal Gland."

(Text continued on page 1222.)

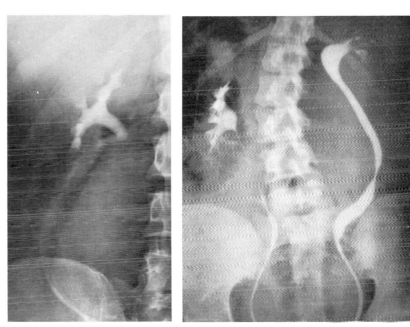

Fig. 10–241   Fig. 10–242

Figure 10–241. Retroperitoneal neurofibroma. *Excretory urogram.* Marked lateral displacement of right ureter from soft-tissue mass lying lateral to lumbar part of spinal column. Surgical exploration revealed neurofibroma, which was completely enucleated. **Pathologic diagnosis: hemorrhagic lipoid degenerating neurofibroma.**

Figure 10–242. *Bilateral pyelogram.* **Schwannoma (neurilemmoma)** in pregnant woman, 25 years of age. Displaces and obstructs left ureter. Pregnancy completed normally. (From Deming, C. L.)

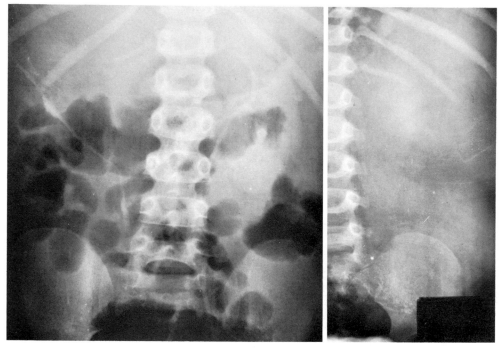

Fig. 10–243
Fig. 10–244

Figure 10–243. Neuroblastoma in girl, 3½ years of age. *Excretory urogram.* Marked lateral displacement of right kidney and upper part of ureter. Left kidney and ureter normal. Transabdominal surgical exploration revealed huge retroperitoneal tumor arising from region of right kidney and spreading retroperitoneally behind pancreas and across vertebral column. Inoperable. Specimen removed for microscopic examination and reported grade 4 malignant neoplasm, probably neuroblastoma.

Figure 10–244. **Neuroblastoma of kidney.** *Excretory urogram.* Large left abdominal tumor with little or no function in girl, 22 months of age. Surgical exploration revealed huge tumor of left kidney. Kidney removed. **Pathologic diagnosis was grade 4 necrotic malignant neoplasm, probably neuroblastoma.** Destruction of 70% of renal substance. Tumor was perforating renal capsule in region of renal pelvis.

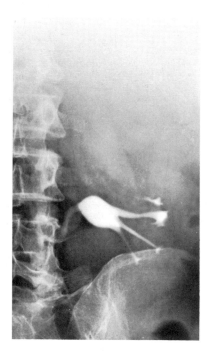

Figure 10–245. **Adrenal medullary tumor (sympathicoblastoma).** *Left retrograde pyelogram.* Large soft-tissue mass lying above left kidney and pushing it downward. Upper calyx incompletely visualized in this film. In lateral view it was well filled and appeared to be normal. Surgical exploration through left rectus incision revealed retroperitoneal encapsulated tumor 20 cm in diameter lying beneath the pancreas and depressing left kidney. Tumor removed without removal of kidney. **Pathologic diagnosis was adrenal medullary tumor grade 2 (sympathicoblastoma);** weight 2,340 gm. (From Kaplan, J. H., and Greene, L. F.)

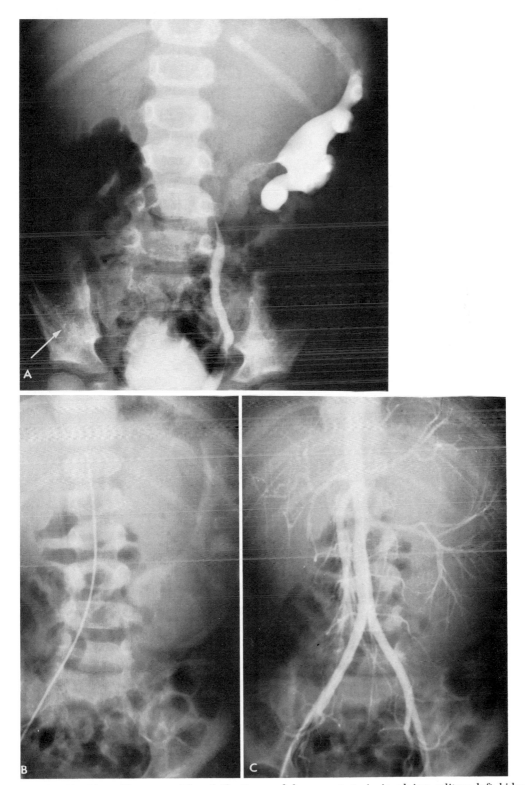

Figure 10–246. Neuroblastoma with calcification and bony metastasis involving solitary left kidney. Boy aged 4 years. **A,** *Excretory urogram.* Mass with area of calcification medial to upper pole of solitary left kidney displacing upper pole laterally and downward (lateral angulation). Note metastasis to right innominate bone (*arrow*). **B,** *Plain film.* Catheter in place in aorta to make arteriogram. Renal outline can be seen displaced laterally and inferiorly. **C,** *Arteriogram.* Normal vascularization of kidney. No evidence of excessive vascularity of neuroblastoma.

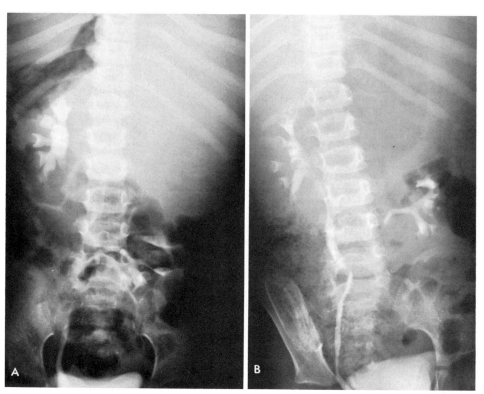

Figure 10–247. Inoperable **neuroblastoma** involving left kidney in girl aged 5. Excretory urogram an biopsy. **A,** *Excretory urogram.* Before irradiation. Large mass in left upper quadrant of abdomen depressin left kidney. **B,** *Postirradiation.* Kidney has returned almost to normal level.

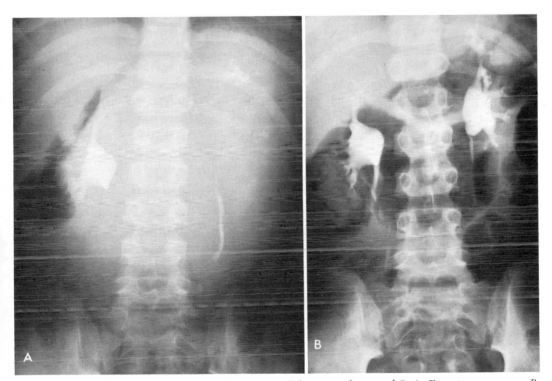

Figure 10–248. Huge neuroblastoma in left upper abdomen in boy aged 9. **A,** *Excretory urogram. Pre-operation.* Soft-tissue mass in left upper quadrant of abdomen compressing pelvis, calyces, and ureter, with fractional visualization. At operation, tumor surrounded and compressed kidney and ureter but did not invade kidney. Attachment was to retroperitoneal region near tail of pancreas. Tumor removed including tail of pancreas and spleen. Postoperative irradiation. **B,** *Excretory urogram* 2 months postoperatively. Kidney still little closer to spine than normal but is normal in appearance.

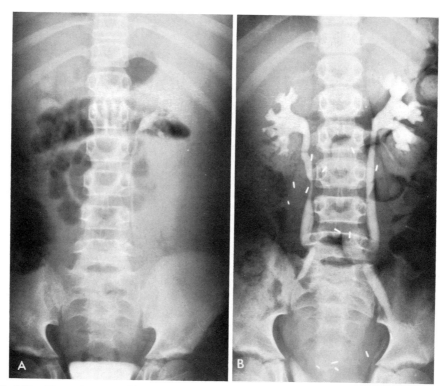

Figure 10–249.   **Extensive neuroblastoma with obstruction** of right kidney in girl aged 10 years. **A,** *Excretory urogram.* Large soft-tissue mass in abdomen appears more on left than right. Pyelocaliectasis of *right* kidney. *Exploration.* Huge mass replacing almost entire greater omentum. Origin of tumor could not be ascertained but appeared to be primarily on *right* side with some extension across vertebral column. Right ureter freed from mass up to hilum of kidney. Silver clips put on limits of tumor for identification. Irradiation. **B,** *Excretory urogram* 6 months postoperatively. Kidneys functioning normally. There still appears to be some tumor in pelvis causing some spreading and mild compression of lower ureters.

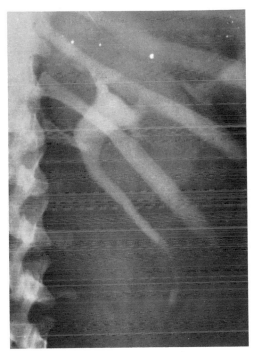

Figure 10–250.   Retroperitoneal ganglioneuroma in woman, 24 years of age. Presenting symptom was abdominal mass. *Excretory urogram.* Soft-tissue mass lying medially and below left kidney, displacing left kidney and ureter upward and laterally. Surgical exploration through left posterolumbar incision revealed encapsulated tumor, 20 cm in diameter, attached to lower pole of left kidney and to two lumbar nerves. Kidney and tumor removed. **Pathologic diagnosis: degenerating ganglioneuroma. Kidney attached to tumor.**

Tumors Arising From Embryonic Remnants

Teratoma (Cystic and Solid) and Dermoid Cyst

Teratoma is a tumor that contains fetal remains. It is often composed of multiple tissues foreign to the parts in which it arises and all three germinal cell layers, namely the ectoderm, the mesoderm, and the endoderm, are represented in various combinations. In some cases, however, the tumor may be composed mostly of cells from only one germinal layer.* It occurs most commonly in infants and children and is more frequent in females than in males. Grossly the tumors are cystic and may contain well-organized tissue such as segments of intestine and bronchi with cartilaginous rings. Microscopically almost every conceivable type of tissue may be found, such as lung, respiratory epithelium, adrenal, thyroid, smooth and striated muscle, sympathetic ganglia, salivary gland, fibrous tissue, fat, hair, and teeth. Most teratomas contain well-differentiated tissue and are benign, but malignant change with invasion and metastasis may occur.

Such tumors may arise almost anywhere in the retroperitoneal space (Fig. 10–251) but *are most frequently located in the pelvis between the rectum and sacrum* where they are called *presacral* or *Middeldorpf tumors.* They are also encountered in the ovaries and testes. Gross, Clatsworthy, and Meeker's concept of origin (suggested by F. L. Bremer) is accepted by many workers as the most logical explanation. It suggests that teratomas arise from "totipotent" primordial cells. These cells are most concentrated and exist for the longest period in the area of the primitive knot (Hen-

son's node) located at the caudal end of the neural tube; its final location is in the region of the coccyx. The anlage of the reproductive glands is another source of these totipotent primordial cells (Gwinn, Dockerty, and Kennedy). Teratomas vary greatly in size; they may become so large that if located in the presacral region they may partially obstruct the rectum, displace and obstruct the bladder, and (in the adult female) interfere with delivery. In contrast to other presacral tumors, destruction of bone (sacrum and coccyx) is uncommon. In Gross, Clatsworthy, and Meeker's series of 40 cases the coccyx was involved and partially destroyed in only 2 cases. Calcification of the tumor was demonstrated in 43% of their cases.

Dermoid cysts are varieties of cystic teratomas which are predominantly ectodermal in origin and are lined with epithelium which is constantly desquamating. They have also been considered to be the result of faulty inclusion of ectoderm when the embryo coalesces. They are filled with an oily radiolucent fluid and may contain ectodermal derivatives such as hair and teeth. The capsule is fairly radiopaque in contrast to the radiolucent fluid inside. Although 95% of *these tumors arise from the ovary or testes,* a few arise from the retroperitoneal area (see Fig. 3–192).

The incidence of malignancy in presacral teratomas has been variously reported as 11% (Hatteland and Knutrud), 20% (Gross, Clatsworthy, and Meeker), 22% (Gwinn, Dockerty, and Kennedy), and 52% (Bodian). Apparently the incidence of malignancy increases sharply after the first 3 months of life so that immediate surgical removal is necessary.

Chordomas*

The chordoma arises from remnants of the fetal notochord, which lie entirely

---

*Derivatives of all three germinal layers were found in all of the 18 Mayo Clinic cases of presacral teratomas in infants reported by Gwinn, Dockerty, and Kennedy.

---

*See also discussion Chapter 3 (Figs. 3–189 and 3–190).

within the vertebrae and intervertebral disks. Most of these tumors arise from within the bone rather than from within the disk (Harvey and Dawson). They are found most commonly in the sacrococcygeal region* (approximately 70% of cases), are the most common presacral tumor in adults (Adson, Moersch, and Kernohan), and are most common in middle or later life. They affect males oftener than females. Chordomas are definitely malignant tumors; they destroy the sacrum by expansion, especially in the anteroposterior dimension, by erosion, and by invasion (see Figs. 3–189 and 3–190).

Miscellaneous Tumors

Among other retroperitoneal tumors including those encountered in the presacral area) may be mentioned ependymomas, Ewing's giant cell tumors, and anterior spina bifida cystica.

Presacral Tumors (Middeldorpf Tumors, Retrorectal Tumors)
(Figs. 10-252 through 10-257)

Classification and General Considerations

Obviously many of the tumors that occur in the retroperitoneal area also occur deep in the pelvis, ventral to the sacrum. When they occur in this area, diagnosis may be extremely difficult because of their inaccessibility both with regard to biopsy and surgical exploration. Owing to their location they become urologic problems because of displacement and obstruction of the ureters, displacement of the bladder, and obstruction of the bladder neck and urethra. Also, interference with innervation of the bladder may result in neurogenic vesical dysfunction. Tumors located in the presacral region

have been rather loosely called *Middeldorpf tumors* since Middeldorpf first reported his case of teratoma in a 1-year-old child in 1885. By strict definition of the term, only teratomas should be labeled as *Middeldorpf tumors;* other tumors should be described as *presacral* or *retrorectal.* By common usage, however, the term *Middeldorpf* has come to mean any tumor located in the presacral area.

As a group, presacral tumors (retrorectal) have received considerable attention and study. Jackman, Clark, and Smith in 1951 found 82 Mayo Clinic cases (encountered between 1935 and 1948) in which tissue was available for study. Mayo, Baker, and Smith reviewed the literature in 1953 and found 161 reported cases of tumors located "ventral to the sacrum." Their classification of the lesions and that of Jackman, Clark, and Smith were practically the same. They are indicated in Table 10-11. Mayo, Baker, and Smith mentioned previous reviews of this subject by Whittaker and Pemberton, Camp and Good, MacCarty and associates, Dahlin and MacCarty, and Young.

As can be seen from the classifications, *the most common presacral tumors are of the congenital type: namely, chordomas, dermoid cysts, and teratomas* (39% in Jackman, Clark, and Smith's series, 61% in Mayo, Baker, and Smith's series). Chordomas account for approximately half of the congenital tumors. Inflammatory lesions come next in frequency (22% in Jackman, Clark, and Smith's series and 11% in Mayo, Baker, and Smith's). Jackman, Clark, and Smith discussed the inflammatory lesions in detail. Although most are associated with anal and rectal fistulas, they encountered a few cases of "chemical tumors" (oleomas) that had resulted from the previous injection treatment of hemorrhoids. They also called attention to the fact that many small inflammatory lesions and anorectal fistulas are in reality small infected dermoid cysts that require excision for relief.

---

*They also occur in the craniopharyngeal region.

Table 10–11. Classification of Presacral Tumors by Two Groups of Authors

	JACKMAN, CLARK, AND SMITH CASES	MAYO, BAKER, AND SMITH CASES
I. Congenital tumors	32	99
Cartilaginous (chordoma)	14	51
Teratoma	7	19
Dermoid cyst	5	29
Meningocele	6	
II. Inflammatory lesions	18	18
III. Neurogenic tumors	12	18
Ependymoma	6	12
Neurofibroma	5	5
Neurilemmoma	1	1
IV. Osseous tumors	5	14
Osteogenic sarcoma	2	4
Chondroma	2	4
Giant cell tumor	1	5
Osteoma*		1
V. Miscellaneous tumors	15	12
Metastatic tumor	4	4
Lipoma	2	
Plasma cell myeloma	3	3
Hemangioendothelioma	2	
Fibrosarcoma and leiomyosarcoma	3	
Unclassified or other	1	5
Total	82†	161

*Not in Jackman, Clark, and Smith's group.
†Mayo Clinic cases.

Clinical Findings

Presacral tumors large enough to become clinically apparent can almost always be palpated on digital rectal examination. The *sacrococcygeal teratomas in infants* are usually apparent on external examination as they present in the region of the coccyx and often extend into and cause enlargement of the buttocks. Large tumors may be palpated abdominally. The bladder may be displaced anteriorly and to either side depending on the location of the tumor. The tumor may be firm, or cystic degeneration may be present so that the tumor may feel fluctuant and suggest a deep pelvic cyst or cyst of the seminal vesicle.* Symptoms, if present, may consist of lower abdominal pain from expansion of the tumor, or pain referred to the lower part of the back, perineum, gluteal region, and legs from involvement of the sacral nerve roots.† Urinary manifestations usually consist of urinary obstruction varying from mild to complete retention, frequency, dysuria, and occasionally hematuria. These symptoms may result either from displacement of the bladder and obstruction of the urethra and bladder outlet or from neurogenic dysfunction caused by involvement of the nerves supplying the bladder.

Roentgen and Urographic Diagnosis

The Plain Film. The plain film is helpful in diagnosis, especially if bony changes caused by the tumor are present (see Figs. 3–189 through 3–194). *Tumors arising within the sacral canal,* such as ependymomas and neurofibromas, may cause erosion of the bone by pressure and expansion. The margins of such bone defects tend to be sharp and well defined. *Tumors which arise from the sacral body* (such as chordomas) cause expansion of the sacrum by an infiltrative process which best can be seen in the anteroposterior dimension. Remnants of bone (simulating sequestra or calcification) may be seen to be free in the tumor.

Tumors that arise adjacent to the sacrum (such as teratoma or dermoid cyst) do not produce changes in the bone except in rare instances. If the tumor

---

*Roberts, Coppridge, and Hughes in 1958 reported a large cystic neurilemmoma which arose from the sheath of a sacral nerve as it emerged from a foramen on the right side of the sacrum (see Fig. 10–255).
†Pain and vesical dysfunction resulting from pressure on nerve roots are most commonly seen with chordomas. These symptoms were present in almost all of the chordomas in Jackman, Clark, and Smith's series of cases.

large, however, sacral erosion may be present from pressure of the tumor. In infants with large teratomas, the large soft-tissue mass anterior to the sacrum is usually easily visible in the plain film, and often anterior displacement of the gas-filled rectum may be seen. Backward tilting of the coccyx is pathognomonic of such tumors; destruction of the coccyx is uncommon (Hanbery, Senz, and Jeffrey). Erosion of the ventral surface of the sacrum from pressure of the tumor is also uncommon. In Gross, Clatsworthy, and Meeker's series of 40 cases of presacral teratoma in infants, erosion or destruction of bone was present in only 2 cases. Dermoid cysts (and occasional teratomas) may contain teeth or bone which may be recognized in the plain film (see Figs. 3-101 through 3-104).

A rather unusual lesion is *spina bifida cystica*, which presents anteriorly (into the pelvis) rather than posteriorly. This lesion may be recognized because of a defect in the sacrum with separation of the laminae (see Fig. 3-194).

The Urogram (Figs. 10-252 through 10-256). Urography may be of value to demonstrate (1) displacement and obstruction of the ureters, (2) anterior displacement of the bladder as well as some lateral displacement, as the tumor is usually predominantly on one side of the midline, and (3) distention of the bladder from obstruction of the vesical neck or urethra. In infants, because the bladder lies high in the pelvis (it is really an intra-abdominal structure in infants), the anterior displacement may not be great unless the tumor is large enough to encroach on the abdominal cavity also.

Differential Diagnosis

Probably the greatest problem in differential diagnosis is presented by the *deep pelvic cysts;* these are usually congenital and of müllerian-duct origin, but they occasionally arise from the seminal vesicles. Needle aspiration through the perineum or rectum plus injection of contrast medium may permit the diagnosis. Cystoscopic insertion of a ureteral catheter through the utricle into the cyst may achieve the same result. (This subject is considered more fully in Chapter 12, Figs. 12-290, 12-291, 12-292, and 12-301.) Sarcoma (and occasionally carcinoma) of the bladder may cause unusual forward displacement of the bladder that could simulate a presacral tumor (Roberts, Coppridge, and Hughes) (Fig. 10-257). *Carcinoma of the seminal vesicle* is extremely rare but must be considered (Smith). A large vesical diverticulum with a small neck which does not fill with contrast medium must be considered in the differential diagnosis (see Chapter 5). Ectopic kidneys lying over the sacrum also have been mistaken for presacral tumors. In addition to the plain film, urography, and needle aspiration, transrectal biopsy has been most helpful in diagnosis (Jackman, Clark, and Smith). Surgical exploration, however, may be necessary before the true nature of the lesion is ascertained.

(Text continued on page 1230.)

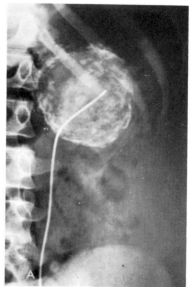

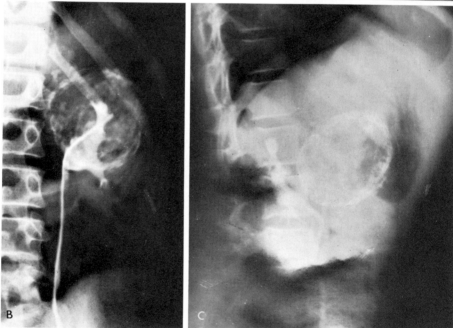

Figure 10–251.   Pararenal teratoma. A, *Plain film.* Large calcific shadow over left renal area. Lead catheter in ureter. **B,** *Left retrograde pyelogram.* Pelvis seems to occupy position over calcified mass. Pelviocalyceal system apparently not compromised by lesion. **C,** *Lateral film.* Calcific mass is seen to be lying against anterior surface of kidney. *Surgical exploration* showed retroperitoneal tumor intimately adherent to renal pedicle and anterior surface of left kidney. Tumor and kidney removed together. On sectioning mass, partially cystic structure was exposed. Wall of cyst was up to 1 cm thick. Section of cyst wall showed round cell infiltration, bundles of smooth muscle fibers and nests of dilated blood vessels, cellular structures suggestive of bronchial mucosa, hyaline cartilage, and mucinous and serous glands. Some small acinar structures resembled serous secreting salivary glands. Some other areas revealed acini suggestive of convoluted tubules of renal cortex. Myelinated nerve fibers and fat were also seen. **Diagnosis: pararenal teratoma.** (Courtesy of Dr. W. J. Baker. From Baker, W. J., and Ragins, A. B.: Pararenal Teratoma: Case Report. Tr. Am. A. Genito-Urin. Surgeons *41*:93–101, 1949.)

Fig. 10–252

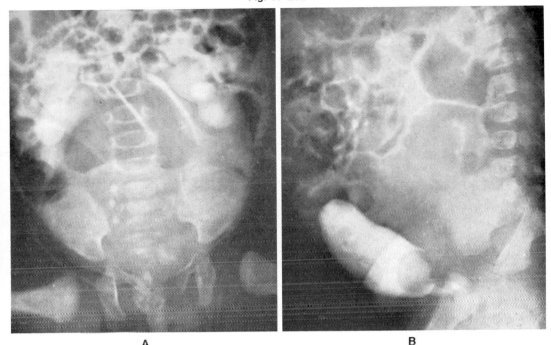

A   B

Figure 10–252. Sacrococcygeal teratoma (Middeldorpf tumor) in baby girl, 2½ months old, with large abdominal mass and difficulty in voiding. Strains and cries when trying to void. **A,** *Excretory urogram.* Bilateral hydronephrosis from ureteral obstruction. **B,** *Retrograde cystogram, lateral view.* Bladder displaced forward against abdominal wall by tumor. *Exploration* revealed cystic and solid tumor, abdominal portion showing cyst and pelvic portion solid tumor. Lesion completely enucleated and removed. Microscopic examination showed cystic tridermic teratoma with various types of epithelium, smooth and striated muscle, connective tissue, fat, glial tissue, ganglionic tissue, nerve tissue, bone, and calcium.

Figure 10–253. Sacrococcygeal teratoma in girl aged 1 year. *Retrograde cystogram, lateral view:* forward and upward displacement of bladder and rectum) with dilatation from urethral obstruction. (From Willox, G. L., and MacKenzie, W. C.: Sacrococcygeal Teratomas. Arch. Surg. 83:11–16 [July] 1961.)

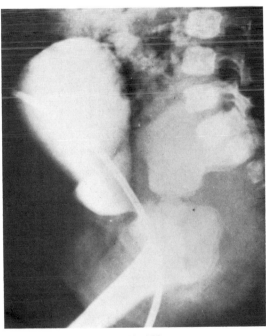

Fig. 10–253

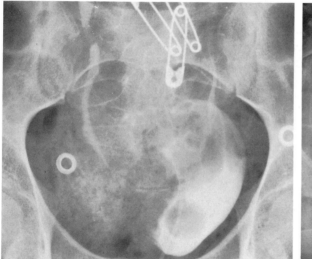 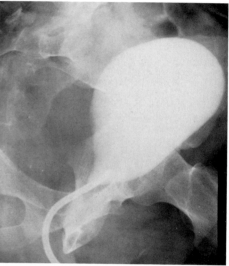

Fig. 10-254   Fig. 10-255

Figure 10-254. *Excretory urogram.* **Ganglioneuroma** in youth, 21 years of age. Large retroperitoneal pelvic mass arising from right side of pelvis and extending anteriorly to left between rectum and bladder and downward to upper level of prostate. Base of bladder rotated markedly to left. Right ureter and vas displaced to left. It was difficult to remove tumor from posterior wall of bladder.

Figure 10-255. **Presacral neurilemmoma** in man, 40 years of age, with acute urinary retention and large palpable mass above prostate. *Retrograde cystogram, oblique view.* Displacement of bladder upward and to left. Exploration revealed degenerating cystic tumor attached to right side of sacrum. Pathologist's report: neurilemmoma. (From Roberts, L. C., Coppridge, W. M., and Hughes, J.)

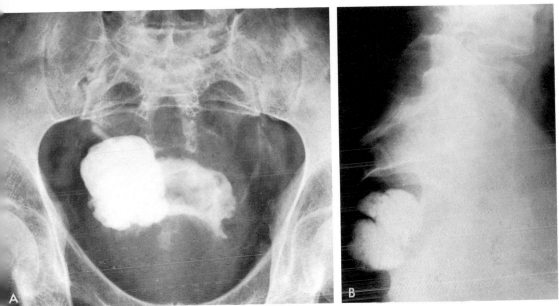

Figure 10–256.   Highly malignant, undifferentiated retroperitoneal (presacral) tumor (either carcinoma or sarcoma) containing large calculus (dystrophic calcification). Lesion extended from right side of sacrum to undersurface of prostatic capsule and displaced rectum to left. *Excretory cystograms.* **A,** *Anteroposterior view.* **B,** *Lateral view* showing calculus adjacent to sacrum. (**A** from Albers, D. D., Milla, A. E., and Vickers, P. M.)

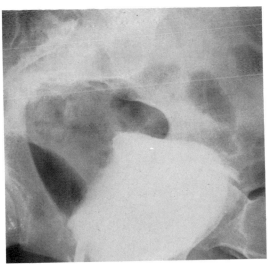

Figure 10–257.   *Retrograde cystogram, left oblique view.* **Encapsulated leiomyosarcoma of bladder simulating deep pelvic cyst or presacral tumor** in man, 40 years of age. On cystoscopy, posterolateral wall of bladder was pushed inward but covered with normal mucosa. Preoperative diagnosis: probable müllerian cyst. Segmented resection of encapsulated tumor in wall of bladder. (From Roberts, L. C., Coppridge, W. M., and Hughes, J.)

TUMORS OF THE ADRENAL GLAND
(Figs. 10–258 through 10–289)

The adrenal gland is made up of two parts: (1) the medulla (10%) and (2) the cortex (90%).

The medulla is of ectodermal origin derived from neuroectodermal tissue, which is closely associated in site of origin with the sympathetic ganglion cells. It secretes epinephrine and norepinephrine (pressor amines, catechols, and catecholamines).

The cortex is of mesodermal origin, derived from cells near the mesonephron which are near the primitive sex gland. In spite of the mesodermal origin, the cells have an "epithelial appearance." They secrete many steroid hormones, some of which have been well-studied, others not. There are four principal groups of cortical hormones: (1) glucocorticoids (for example, hydrocortisone); (2) mineralocorticoids (for example, aldosterone); (3) androgens (for example, androstenedione and dehydroepiandrosterone), and (4) estrogens (for example, estradiol, estriol, and estrone).

Classification

Tumors of the adrenal gland may be classified as follows:

    I. *Stromal tumors (nonfunctioning)*
      A. Nonfunctioning only
        1. Fibroma, lipoma, neuroma, neurofibroma, myoma, osteoma, hemangioma, sarcoma, lymphangioma, melanoma, and others
    II. *Tumors of the medulla*
      A. Nonfunctioning
        1. Ganglioneuroma and neuroblastoma*
      B. Functioning
        1. Pheochromocytoma (chromaffinoma)

---

*Neuroblastoma is now considered to be a functioning tumor. See previous discussion, page 1213.

III. *Tumors of the cortex*
    A. Both functioning and nonfunctioning
      1. Adenoma and carcinoma
    B. Functioning
      1. Bilateral cortical hyperplasia

Stromal Tumors

The extremely rare stromal tumors are recognized only because of symptoms and signs resulting from enlargement of the lesion or metastasis or both. They are hormonally inactive.

Tumors of the Medulla

Under the heading "Tumors Arising From the Sympathetic Nervous System," page 1211, the common origin of the cells of the sympathetic nervous system and of the adrenal medulla from the neural crest was discussed (see pages 1211 and 1212). *Two lines of descent* were postulated. The neuroblastoma (malignant) and ganglioneuroma (benign) arise from the *first line of descent.* Formerly they were considered to be "nonfunctioning" or hormonally inactive tumors but in recent years it has been found that neuroblastomas may cause increased excretion of catecholamines (see page 1213).

PHEOCHROMOCYTOMA (CHROMAFFINOMA)

The pheochromocytoma (chromaffinoma) arises from the *second line of descent.* This is a functioning tumor* that excretes pressor amines (catecholamines). As mentioned previously under "Tumors Arising From the Sympathetic Nervous System," page 1211, the cell that makes up this tumor is characterized by the

---

*The rare nonfunctioning "nonchromaffin paraganglioma" will be mentioned farther on.

development of cytoplasmic granules possessing an affinity for chromium salts. Tumors which arise from these cells retain their affinity for chromium salts and can thus be identified by staining. There is considerable confusion in the profession regarding terminology of the hormones that are excreted by the adrenal medulla, so the following brief discussion may be helpful.

Hormones of the Adrenal Medulla

The pathway for the synthesis of hormones of the adrenal medulla is as follows: **Tyrosine** is hydroxylated to form **dopa** which is then decarboxylated to form **dopamine** which in turn is hydroxylated (on the beta position of the side chain) to form **norepinephrine** which is N-methylated to form **epinephrine**. The last three compounds (dopamine, norepinephrine, and epinephrine) are classified as **catecholamines** (CA),[*] though in common usage the term refers only to norepinephrine and epinephrine. Epinephrine was the first hormone of man to be isolated in crystalline form. In 1929 Rabin demonstrated that a pheochromocytoma contained increased amounts of epinephrine. Later on, norepinephrine was demonstrated in the adrenal medulla and also in pheochromocytomas. Subsequently it was shown that both of these CA are increased in amounts in both blood and urine of patients with pheochromocytoma.

In 1957, Armstrong, McMillan, and Shaw demonstrated the fate of the CA (norepinephrine and epinephrine) after they are excreted. Small amounts are excreted unchanged but a large share is metabolized by O-methylation into **metanephrine** and **normetanephrine**. An even larger share undergoes further oxidation of the amine group to **vanillylmandelic acid**. The discovery of these metabolites has done much to simplify the diagnosis of pheochromocytoma because they may be identified and determined quantitatively in urine (and plasma) much more easily than the CA.

Approximately 90% of pheochromocytomas arise in the adrenal gland, 10% are extra-adrenal, and 5% are multiple (Sheps). When extra-adrenal (heterotopic), they have been called **chromaffin paragangliomas**. Extra-adrenal lesions may occur anywhere along the length of the sympathetic nervous system, ventral to the abdominal aorta in the organ of Zuckerkandl and in the chemoreceptor tissue (carotid body and glomus jugulare). They have even been found in such places as the wall of the urinary bladder[*] and may produce episodes of paroxysmal hypertension when the bladder contracts during micturition (Figs. 10–258 and 10–260). In rare instances such lesions may prove to be **nonfunctioning nonchromaffin paraganglioma (chemodectoma or carotid body type tumors)** (Fig. 10–261). Involvement of the kidney and ureter has also been observed (Fig. 10–262).

Clinical Problem

Pheochromocytoma is important because of the secretion of pressor amines which may cause either sustained or paroxysmal hypertension. It is a disease of young adults (usually aged 20 to 40). Of 71 Mayo Clinic cases reported by Gifford and associates in 1961, 9 (13%) were malignant. Harrison and Jenkins estimated the incidence of malignancy as about 10%.

In the case of typical intermittent paroxysmal hypertension, diagnosis is not difficult, but in about half the cases it is persistent although somewhat fluctuant. In the latter cases it may be difficult clinically to distinguish from essential hyper-

---

[*]Catechol = dihydroxybenzene.

[*]Twenty-four such cases have now been reported (Bourne and Beltaos; Moloney, Cowdell, and Lewis).

tension, and **biochemical** or so-called **pharmacologic** tests or both types of tests are important.

Biochemical Tests

Plasma. During or after an attack of paroxysmal hypertension or at any time in the patient with sustained or persistent hypertension from pheochromocytoma, the plasma CA (norepinephrine and epinephrine) are usually increased to at least twice their normal value. The rise may be as high as 80 μg per liter.

Urine. Examination of the urine is now considered preferable to examination of the plasma because the determination is simpler to carry out and elevated urinary levels of pressor substances are often demonstrable even during normotensive periods. In urine the CA may be measured, but it is easier and more practical to measure the *metabolites* of the catecholamines, namely normetanephrine and metanephrine (MN) and vanillylmandelic acid (VMA), because as Crout, Pisano, and Sjoerdsma pointed out they appear in the urine in much larger amounts than the parent amines.

The development of more specific techniques for assaying CA, MN, and VMA levels in the urine has greatly simplified the screening of large numbers of hypertensive patients for pheochromocytoma. It has been shown (Sheps; Sheps and Maher, 1966; Sheps, Tyce, and Flock; Sheps and associates) that CA determinations may be falsely normal in 25% and VMA falsely normal in 20% of tumor patients. Determination of MN appears to be most accurate, as they found that a normal value for MN is rare in the presence of a functioning pheochromocytoma. For this reason the *determination of total urinary MN has become the preferred screening test for pheochromocytoma.* Positive tests should be confirmed by repetition and by the determination of other metabolites.

Pharmacologic Tests

The resting or basal values are diagnostically high in all tumor patients with sustained hypertension and in about half who have paroxysmally functioning tumors. In these cases the **cold pressor histamine test** or the **cold pressor glucogen test** (Sheps and Maher, 1968) may be necessary. Since the advent of the improved biochemical tests of urine for MN and VMA the **phentolamine (Regitine) suppression test** is no longer necessary and is seldom employed.

Localization of Tumor

It would be helpful to the surgeon if the site of the tumor could be determined before operation. Because the tumor may be located either in one of the adrenals or ectopically it is the custom to do a transabdominal exploration, so that the entire retroperitoneal area (on both sides) can be examined. Even so, at times it may be difficult or even impossible to find the tumor if it is in a heterotopic position.

Differential Assay

Recently attempts have been made to localize the tumor by so-called differential assay of the urine for epinephrine and norepinephrine (or metanephrine or normetanephrine). It has been shown that the enzyme required to form epinephrine from norepinephrine is highly localized to the mammalian adrenal medulla (Wurtman). Therefore if the differential urinary assay indicates an abnormally high value for epinephrine, it suggests that the tumor is located either in an adrenal gland or in the organ of Zuckerkandl.

Blood sampling at various points in the nervous system to find the point of greatest concentration of plasma CA is being tried to localize the approximate site of heterotopic tumors.

Roentgenographic Localization

The purpose of roentgen diagnosis is principally to "lateralize" the tumor if it is located in an adrenal gland, that is, to determine on which side the tumor is located. It should be emphasized that the diagnosis is a clinical and laboratory one, so that a negative roentgen examination means nothing. The use of excretory urography, nephrotomography, pneumography, and arteriography will be considered below under the heading "Roentgenographic and Urographic Diagnosis."

Tumors of the Cortex

by

Randall G. Sprague

Tumors of the adrenal cortex are divided into functioning (hormonally active) or nonfunctioning (hormonally inactive). Functioning tumors, owing to their hormonal activity, produce a variety of striking clinical syndromes. As with adrenal medullary tissue, cortical tissue is occasionally not confined to the adrenal gland; adrenal rests may occur in such extra-adrenal locations as kidney, broad ligament, vas deferens, and epididymis, and rarely such ectopic adrenal tissue is the site of a tumor.

NONFUNCTIONING (HORMONALLY INACTIVE) TUMORS: ADENOMA AND CARCINOMA

Nonfunctioning tumors may be either benign (adenomas) or malignant (carcinomas). Small adenomas are common; they are found in approximately 5% of autopsies and are frequently multiple and bilateral. The carcinomas are usually well-encapsulated, but approximately 20% recur after removal. They become clinically apparent because of symptoms or signs resulting from expansion (palpable mass and pain) or metastasis, or both. Urographic demonstration will be described farther on.

FUNCTIONING (HORMONALLY ACTIVE) LESIONS: ADENOMA, CARCINOMA, AND BILATERAL CORTICAL HYPERPLASIA

Functioning tumors also include both adenomas and carcinomas, but the patient usually seeks medical advice not because of a mass or pain but because of symptoms resulting from excess secretion of cortical steroids. Certain clinical syndromes may be identical whether caused by tumor or by bilateral hyperplasia of the glands; indeed, in Cushing's syndrome hyperplasia is more common than tumor (ratio of 4 to 1), and in the adrenogenital syndrome the preponderance of hyperplasia is even greater. For this reason, bilateral cortical hyperplasia must be considered as a third type of hyperfunctioning lesion of the adrenal cortex. The term "hyperplasia" is used in a physiologic sense to indicate hyperfunctioning adrenal glands that are not the site of a tumor; such glands may be only slightly increased in size or not at all, and often are not roentgenographically demonstrable.

The clinical problem of functioning (hormonally active) adrenal tumors or hyperplasia of the adrenal cortex represents one of the most complicated and fascinating chapters of modern medicine. Although a detailed discussion of this large subject is not within the province of a book of this kind, a few brief statements may help clarify the position of urography in diagnosis and place it in proper perspective.

As a result of excess cortical function (from either tumor or hyperplasia), five main clinical syndromes are recognized:

1. *Cushing's syndrome* is the most common in the adult. It is caused by *excess secretion of the glucocorticoids,* particularly hydrocortisone. Long-term

administration of hydrocortisone-like steroids in more than physiologic dosage may produce an identical syndrome. It is recognized clinically by obesity of the trunk, face, and neck; cervicodorsal hump; protuberant abdomen; thin extremities due to muscular wasting; thin skin with purplish striations and ecchymoses; hyperglycemia (steroid diabetes); hypertension; osteoporosis; amenorrhea or impotence; hirsutism; acne; and psychic changes.

2. *The adrenogenital syndrome* is caused by *excess secretion of androgenic hormones.* The syndrome may be either congenital, due to a cortical enzyme deficiency which leads to adrenal cortical hyperplasia, or acquired, usually due to adrenal cortical tumor. The congenital type in the genetic female is characterized by various manifestations of intersexuality, such as female pseudohermaphroditism, persistent urogenital sinus, and varying degrees of hypospadias. (See discussion in Chapters 11 and 12.) In the genetic male it is characterized by macrogenitosomia praecox with precocious isosexual and somatic development. Various manifestations of cortical insufficiency may be present because of deficient production of glucocorticoids or mineralocorticoids or both. The acquired type is characterized by virilism in females (masculine habitus, hypertrophy of the clitoris, growth of male type of sexual hair, amenorrhea, deep voice, acne, and loss of scalp hair). In boys there is precocious development of secondary sexual characteristics. There may be somatic precocity in children of both sexes. In the adult male there may be no readily recognizable endocrine manifestations.

3. *Mixed syndromes* combine features of both Cushing's syndrome and the adrenogenital syndrome. The adrenal lesion is usually a tumor and it is likely to be malignant.

4. *Primary aldosteronism* is caused by excess secretion of the mineralocorticoid

aldosterone by a tumor or tumors of the zona glomerulosa (Salassa and associates). It is characterized chiefly by hypertension, hypokalemia, and alkalosis.

5. *Feminizing syndrome* results from excessive secretion of estrogenic steroids by an adrenocortical tumor, usually malignant, and occurs chiefly in adult males.

Diagnosis of adrenogenital syndrome is supported by demonstrating an increase of the urinary 17-ketosteroids and pregnanetriol in the congenital form and 17-ketosteroids in the acquired form, and diagnosis of Cushing's syndrome is supported by an increase of the urinary ketogenic steroids or 17-hydroxycorticosteroids (Poutasse; Priestley and Salassa; Sprague; Sprague and Priestley; Sprague and associates) and by lack of diurnal rhythm of the plasma corticosteroids. After the disease has been diagnosed, a difficult problem is to decide whether the adrenal lesion is a tumor or bilateral hyperplasia. This is especially important in the adrenogenital syndrome, because if tumor is present surgical intervention should be carried out, whereas if bilateral hyperplasia is present suppression of adrenal cortical function with prednisone or dexamethasone is the treatment of choice. To provide this differentiation the dexamethasone suppression test is of great value. In Cushing's syndrome the most useful differential procedures are the dexamethasone suppression test (Liddle) and the metyrapone test (Liddle and co-workers).

Roentgenographic and Urographic Diagnosis

The Plain Film; Urograms and Pneumograms
(Figs. 10–263 through 10–277)

Generally speaking, roentgen demonstration of lesions of the adrenal gland has not been a brilliant success and opinions concerning its diagnostic value differ. Thus some workers such as Steinbach and Smith, Hinman, Steinbach, and Forsham, and Joelson, Persky, and Rose are favorably disposed whereas the Harvard-Massachusetts General Hospital group (Cope and Raker), and Columbia Presbyterian Hospital group (Platz, Knowlton, and Ragan), and Poutasse are not so enthusiastic. Before the widespread use of nephrotomography and arteriography, most workers seemed to agree that excretory urography was not adequate and that if any degree of accuracy were required perirenal insufflation (pneumography) was necessary. A few (Cope and Raker) were not too impressed with pneumograms and concluded that a plain film would usually supply as much information. There seemed to be general agreement, however, that only large tumors could be visualized roentgenologically, while small tumors and cortical hyperplasia did not lend themselves to roentgen demonstration. Iannaccone and associates tried to evaluate this problem statistically by studying 57 cases of Cushing's syndrome encountered at Mount Sinai Hospital. They concluded that carcinoma of the adrenal lends itself best to roentgenographic diagnosis because in most cases the tumor is large. In 12 of 15 such cases diagnosis was made from roentgenograms — 9 from either a plain film or excretory urogram and 3 after perirenal insufflation of gas (pneumogram). All nine of the benign adenomas were relatively small (6 to 24 gm), and none were diagnosed by means of a plain film or excretory urogram. Pneumography was employed in all cases, and the correct diagnosis was made in six. Bilateral hyperplasia was not diagnosed in any of the 34 cases from the plain film or excretory urogram; pneumography was done in 31 cases (tomography done in 24). The diagnosis of hyperplasia was suspected from 23 of the 27 satisfactory films.

The experience of Platz, Knowlton, and Ragan was not so encouraging. Of 26 pneumograms, 18 were regarded as suggestive of tumor; yet tumor was found in only 6. Of eight patients whose pneumograms were considered negative, three were explored but no tumor was found.

Most workers seem to agree that it is not too difficult to visualize the adrenals in thin individuals, but it is very difficult in obese patients (even with pneumograms). Roentgenographically the *normal adrenal glands* appear as triangular shadows lying immediately above each kidney (Figs. 10–263, 10–264, and 10–265). An oblique view may reveal this shadow when it cannot be seen in the anteroposterior view. Attempts have been made to evaluate their size so that a diagnosis of *bilateral hyperplasia* may be made on the basis of slight degrees of enlargement (Kaplan and Greene). Steinbach and Smith attempted to measure the size of the glands. In contradistinction to tumor, hyperplastic glands retain their normal shape (Figs. 10–266 and 10–267).

Small adenomas can best be visualized in oblique films and diagnosis is based on a rounded protuberant density projecting from one edge of the gland (Iannaccone and associates).

Large tumors (adenoma, pheochromocytoma, or carcinoma), as mentioned previously, may be easily recognized from plain films, urograms, or pneumograms (Figs. 10–268 through 10–273). Downward displacement of a kidney may result from a large tumor and provide the basis for roentgenographic recognition; this was the situation in 16 of 39 proved cases of adrenal tumor seen at the Mayo Clinic, reported by Kaplan and Greene (Figs. 10–274 and 10–275). Cysts of the adrenal glands may become sufficiently large to displace the kidneys as do other varieties of retroperitoneal cysts (Figs. 10–276 and 10–277).

(*Text continued on page 1247.*)

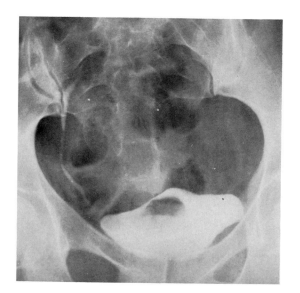

Figure 10-258. *Excretory cystogram.* **Pheochromocytoma of the bladder** in woman aged 34. Typical symptoms of paroxysmal hypertension induced by micturition. Tumor 3 cm in diameter in trigone removed surgically. (From Van Buskirk, K. E., O'Shaughnessy, E. J., Hano, J., and Finder, R. J.)

Figure 10-259. Malignant pheochromocytoma of bladder in man aged 26. *Excretory cystogram.* Filling defect of right lateral wall and dome from tumor. Typical symptom of paroxysmal hypertension on voiding. Subsequent widespread metastasis. (From Moloney, G. E., Cowdell, R. H., and Lewis, C. L.)

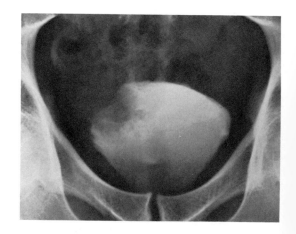

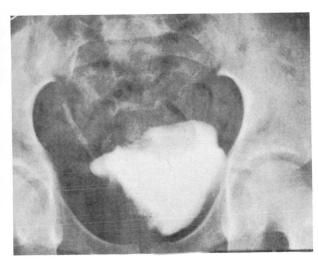

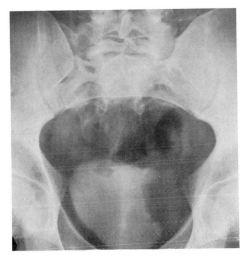

Fig. 10-260   Fig. 10-261

Figure 10-260. *Excretory urogram.* Pheochromocytoma involves right anterolateral wall of bladder near vesical neck. It produced symptoms of paroxysmal hypertension on voiding. Surgical removal (segmental resection) with relief of symptoms. (From Tan, T., and Young, B. W.)

Figure 10-261. *Excretory urogram.* Chemodectoma (nonchromaffin paraganglioma) involving left lateral wall of urinary bladder in man, 22 years of age. Nonfunctioning tumor. (Courtesy of Dr. Theodore Everett.)

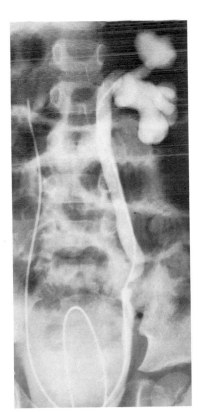

Figure 10-262. *Left retrograde pyelogram.* Malignant nonchromaffin paraganglioma with metastasis to kidney. Compression and obstruction of left ureter at brim of pelvis from 2-cm tumor which was firmly attached to ureter and could not be removed from it. Nephroureterectomy showed involvement of lymphatics of kidney. (From Cohen, S. M., and Persky, L.)

Fig. 10–263

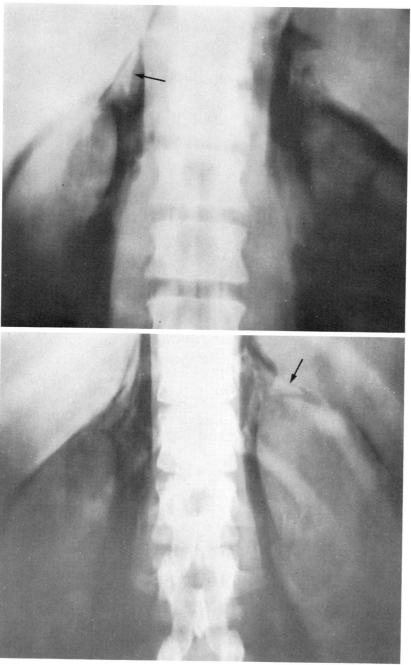

Fig. 10–264

Figure 10–263. *Pneumotomogram.* **Normal adrenal glands.** Right (*arrow*) is triangular; left is semilunar. Right seen more clearly than left. (Courtesy of Dr. D. R. Smith.)

Figure 10–264. *Pneumotomogram.* **Normal adrenals.** Left (*arrow*) is semilunar and more clearly seen than right. (Courtesy of Dr. D. R. Smith.)

Fig. 10–265

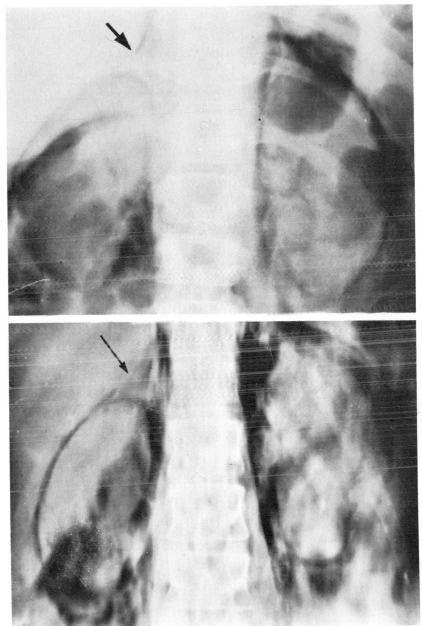

Fig. 10–266

Figure 10–265. *Pneumogram.* **Normal adrenals.** Right (*arrow*) more clearly seen than left. (Courtesy of Dr. D. R. Smith.)

Figure 10–266. **Bilateral adrenal hyperplasia in patient with Cushing's syndrome.** *Pneumotomogram.* Right adrenal well-outlined (*arrow*) (and enlarged?). Left badly obscured. (From Iannaccone, A., Gabrilove, L., Brahms, S. A., and Soffer, L. J.)

Fig. 10–267

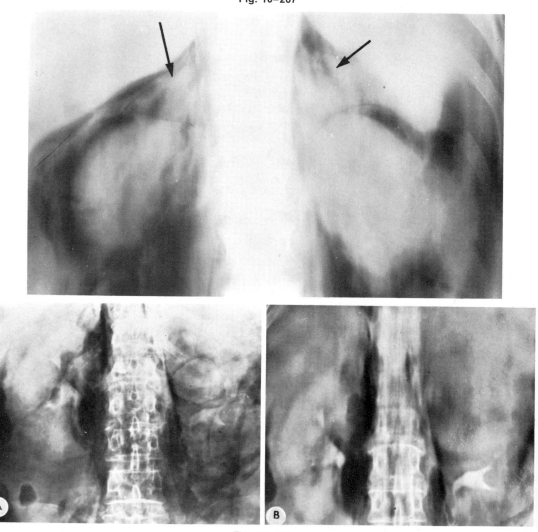

Fig. 10–268

Figure 10–267. *Pneumotomogram.* **Bilateral adrenal hyperplasia.** Adrenals have been emphasized with pencil line for better delineation (*arrows*). (Courtesy of Dr. D. R. Smith.)

Figure 10–268. **Cancer of left adrenal cortex in patient with Cushing's syndrome. A,** *Pneumourogram.* Tumor badly obscured by gas in intestine. **B,** *Tomogram.* Better delineation of large left adrenal tumor with some calcification. (From Iannaccone, A., Gabrilove, J. L., Brahms, S. A., and Soffer, L. J.)

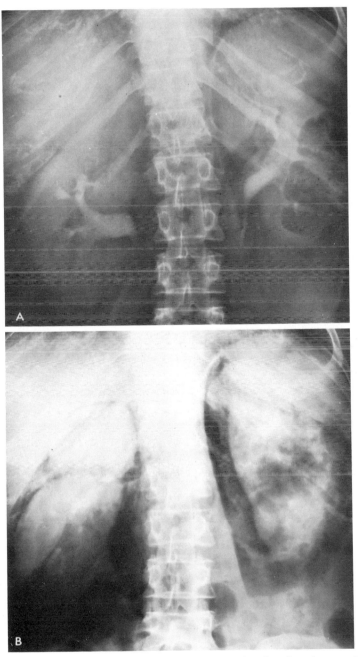

Figure 10–269.   Cushing's disease resulting from carcinoma of right adrenal cortex in woman, 27 years of age. **A,** *Excretory urogram.* Right kidney appears slightly displaced downward. Suggestion of faint soft-tissue shadow above. **B,** *Presacral pneumogram* (100% oxygen). Large adrenal tumor lying above right kidney. Surgical removal. (Courtesy of Drs. Lester Persky and F. A. Rose.)

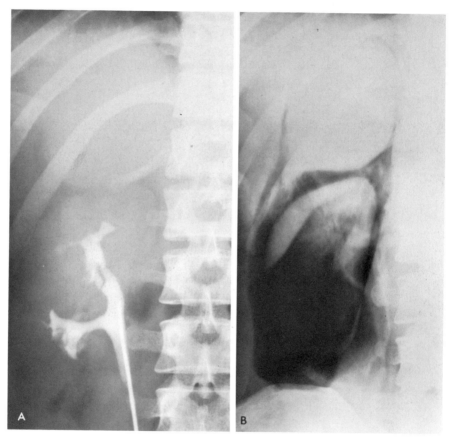

Figure 10–270.   Functioning cortical adenoma with signs of virilism in girl, 18 years of age. **A,** *Retrograde pyelogram.* Right kidney appears a little low, and there is dim outline of soft-tissue mass above it. **B,** *Perirenal pneumogram* using 100% oxygen. Large adrenal tumor above right kidney well-delineated. (Courtesy of Drs. Lester Persky and F. A. Rose.)

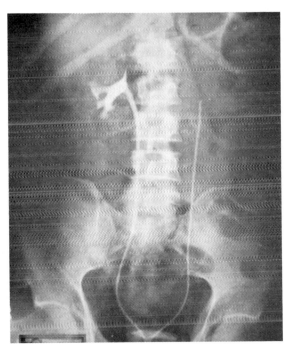

Figure 10–271. *Retrograde pyelogram.* Nonfunctioning carcinoma of right adrenal which had invaded kidney in man, 33 years of age. Hemorrhage into perinephric tissues from necrosis had resulted in sudden profound shock. (From Harrison, J. W., and Jenkins, D.)

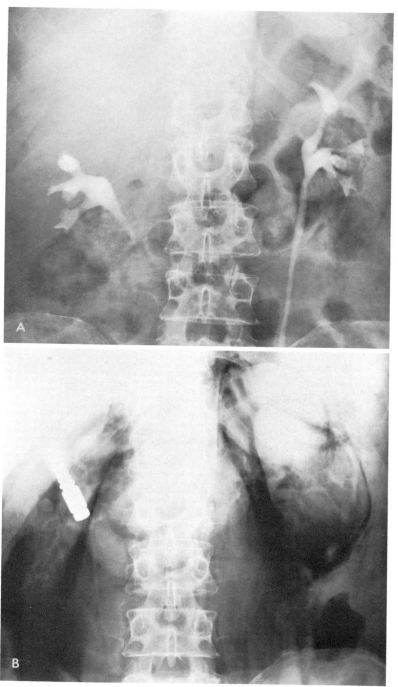

Figure 10–272. Pheochromocytoma of left adrenal in man, 58 years of age. **A,** *Excretory urogram.* Only suggestion of adrenal tumor is slight depression of right kidney. **B,** *Pneumogram (presacral technique)* using 100% oxygen. Excellent demonstration of adrenal tumor lying above left kidney. Surgical transperitoneal removal. Slight depression of kidney would suggest tumor on right side but pneumogram showed it to be on left. (Courtesy of Drs. Lester Persky and F. A. Rose.)

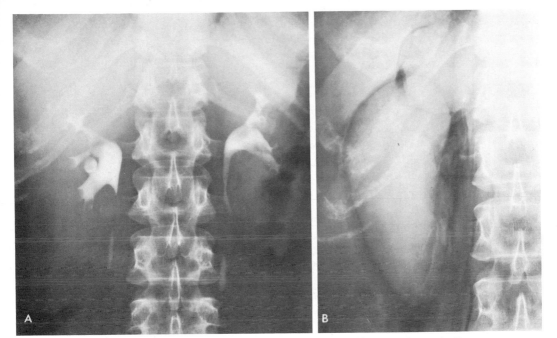

Figure 10–273. **Pheochromocytoma of right adrenal** in woman, 55 years of age. **A,** *Excretory urogram.* Normal. Nothing to suggest adrenal tumor. **B,** *Presacral pneumogram* using 100% oxygen, *anteroposterior view.* Excellent delineation of tumor lying above right kidney. Surgical removal. (Courtesy of Drs. Lester Persky and F. A. Rose.)

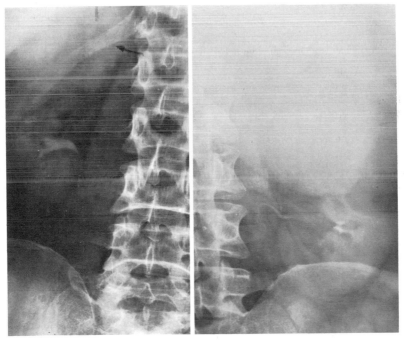

Fig. 10–274   Fig. 10–275

Figure 10–274. **Adenocarcinoma of right adrenal cortex.** *Excretory urogram.* Large soft-tissue mass adjacent to upper pole of right kidney, displacing right kidney downward. Surgical exploration revealed adrenal cortical tumor. (From Kaplan, J. H. and Greene, L. F.)

Figure 10–275. **Carcinoma of left adrenal cortex.** *Excretory urogram.* Large soft-tissue mass lying above left kidney and pushing it downward. Seems to be contiguous with, but not invading, kidney. Surgical exploration, through left posterolumbar incision, revealed adrenal tumor, 35 cm in diameter. Tumor removed without removal of kidney. Pathologic diagnosis was grade 3 adenocarcinoma of adrenal cortex; weight 2,695 gm.

Fig. 10–276

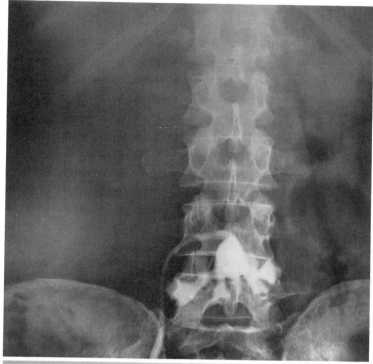

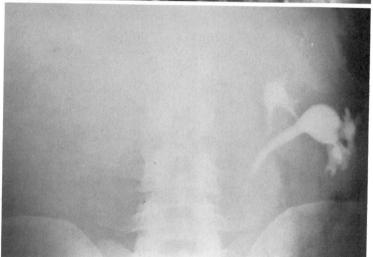

Fig. 10–277

Figure 10–276. Cyst of right adrenal gland. *Right retrograde pyelogram.* Large soft-tissue mass displacing right kidney medially and rotating it on its anteroposterior axis so that calyces are projected caudad. Surgical exploration, through posterolumbar incision, revealed huge cyst of adrenal gland. Cyst removed without removal of kidney.

Figure 10–277. Cystic necrotic adenoma of right adrenal gland. *Excretory urogram.* **Complete displacement of right kidney across midline** so that it overlies left kidney and projects farther laterally than left kidney. Huge soft-tissue mass filling almost entire abdomen. Surgical exploration revealed huge cystic tumor of adrenal gland. Four thousand milliliters of dark brown fluid aspirated before cyst was removed. Cyst extended across midline and down into pelvis. After aspiration, cyst was removed without removal of kidney. Pathologic diagnosis was cystic, necrotic adenoma of adrenal cortex.

INTRAVENOUS NEPHROTOMOGRAPHY, ARTERIOGRAPHY, AND VENOGRAPHY
(Figs. 10–278 through 10–289)

Nephrotomograms

At the Mayo Clinic an evaluation of nephrotomography in the diagnosis of adrenal tumors (Hartman, Witten, and Weeks) has brought out some interesting data. The series consisted of 125 consecutive patients with suspected adrenal disease* who were referred for nephrotomography from 1961 to 1966. It was concluded that nephrotomography was at least as reliable as retroperitoneal pneumography in demonstrating tumors in patients with Cushing's syndrome and pheochromocytoma. It was also felt that the examination was simpler to perform and safe. Nephrotomography is also important in excluding soft-tissue shadows in the adrenal areas accidentally discovered during routine excretory urography; often they are only the result of superimposition of shadows of some anatomic structure (see Fig. 10–283).

The study indicated that the size of the lesion is apparently the critical factor in roentgen visualization. Tumors 2 to 5 cm in diameter or larger were all demonstrated, whereas none smaller were identified. Adrenal carcinomas producing Cushing's syndrome are usually 4.0 cm or more in diameter and easily seen, whereas aldosteronomas are often less than 2 to 5 cm in diameter and cannot be demonstrated. Hyperfunctioning glands in Cushing's disease are usually of normal weight and only slightly enlarged, which makes their delineation difficult or impossible. It was concluded that the diagnosis of adrenal tumors should first be made by appropriate clinical and laboratory examination (steroid assays with suppression tests and metyrapone challenges in suspected Cushing's disease and chemical and pharmacologic tests in suspected pheochromocytoma); excretory urography and nephrotomography are then indicated to "lateralize" the tumor. Whether or not this is necessary or too dangerous in suspected pheochromocytoma is open to question, as in most of these cases transperitoneal exploration is performed so that both adrenal areas and the entire retroperitoneal area may be examined for both adrenal and extra-adrenal (heterotopic) tumors. In the series of patients under discussion, nephrotomography was performed on 25 patients suspected of having a pheochromocytoma; a tumor was found in 6 cases; no untoward reactions were encountered (Figs. 10–278 through 10–288).

Arteriography and Venography

The use of arteriography and adrenal venography for study of the adrenal glands and specifically for detection of adrenal tumors has increased rapidly as the techniques for demonstrating the adrenal vasculature have improved (Kahn and Nickrosz; Köhler and Holsti; Lang and associates, 1966). Aortography has probably had the widest use because of its long availability. This study demonstrates most of the larger, highly vascular tumors, but many of the smaller tumors and even some large ones go undetected by this technique. Selective injection of the renal and suprarenal vessels (Kahn and Nickrosz) has further improved the radiographic demonstration of the adrenal glands and makes it possible to study the normal adrenal as well as to demonstrate a tumor. As in nephrotomography, these techniques identify and localize the tumor and in most cases differentiate it from adrenal hyperplasia, but to the present time no radiographic criteria have been recognized which differentiate pheochromocytoma from adenoma or benign from malignant adrenal tumors.

---

*The "referral" diagnosis in the 125 cases was as follows: Cushing's syndrome, 46 cases; possible Cushing's syndrome, 9; possible pheochromocytoma, 25; primary aldosteronism, 5; possible adrenal mass on an excretory urogram, 33; miscellaneous, 7.

On the arteriogram (Fig. 10–289) abnormal vessels are observed within a mass located in the adrenal region or, in the case of extra-adrenal pheochromocytoma, outside this area along the sympathetic chain (Boijsen, Williams, and Judkins; Kahn and Nickrosz). The abnormal vessels may arise from any one or all of the suprarenal arteries (superior, middle, or inferior suprarenal arteries), and these vessels are stretched and displaced. Early filling of dilated veins is occasionally observed, suggesting arteriovenous shunting. On the late films, the tumor, if solid, acquires a diffuse tumor blush which clearly delineates the lesion but is usually not as intense as that seen in hypernephroma. The fact that the tumor does not arise from the upper pole of the kidney is apparent on the late films when both renal parenchyma and the adrenal tumor are opacified.

A number of fatal and nonfatal hypertensive crises have resulted from arteriography in pheochromocytoma. All of the deaths and many of the nonfatal episodes have occurred with translumbar aortography and some (Boijsen, Williams, and Judkins) recommend that this procedure not be used in suspected pheochromocytoma. Arteriography by the retrograde femoral technique appears to be much less hazardous, but the possibility of hypertensive crises should always be prepared for when arteriography is performed in these patients.

Adrenal venography has only recently been advocated for study of adrenal tumor (Reuter and associates). This technique is more successful for study of the left than the right adrenal since catheterization of the right adrenal vein is often difficult and may be impossible when the vein does not drain into the inferior vena cava. On the venogram the venous branches are distorted and spread around the tumor, and capsular veins are dilated and displaced (Reuter and associates). Tiny tumors probably cannot be detected by this technique. This technique appears promising but its place in the study of diseases of the adrenal glands must await evaluation of larger experiences.

(Text continued on page 1257.)

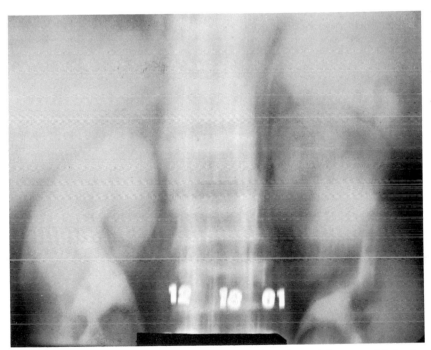

Figure 10–278. *Intravenous nephrotomogram, nephrographic phase.* **Adenoma of left adrenal gland in** woman, 49 years of age, with **Cushing's disease.** Surgical removal. Pathologist reported cellular cortical adenoma and marked cortical atrophy in associated portion of adrenal.

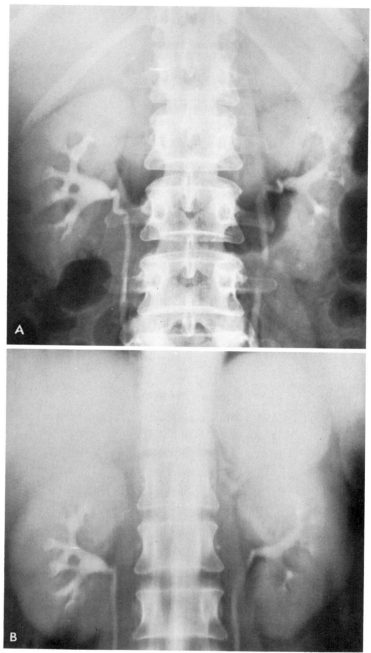

Figure 10–279. **Functioning cortical adenoma of left adrenal gland** in woman, 51 years of age, with mild adrenogenital syndrome, generalized hirsutism, and temporal recession of scalp hair. **A,** *Excretory urogram.* Circular soft-tissue outline of adrenal tumor can be dimly seen above left kidney. **B,** *Intravenous nephrotomogram, nephrographic phase.* Excellent visualization of tumor. Left adrenalectomy. Tumor measured 7 cm in diameter.

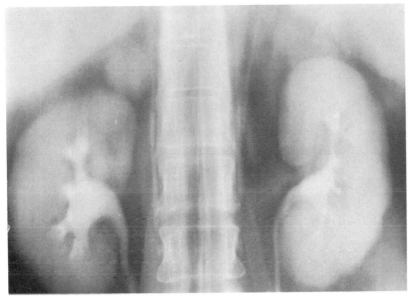

Figure 10–280. *Intravenous nephrotomogram.* Functioning right renal adenoma 3.5 cm in diameter. (From Hartman, G. W., Witten, D. M., and Weeks, R. E.)

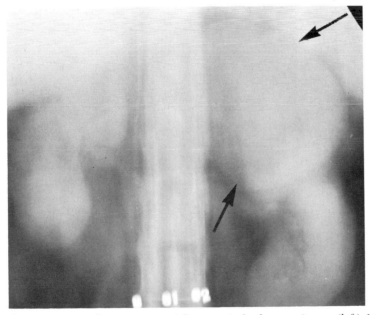

Figure 10–281. *Intravenous nephrotomogram.* Adrenocortical adenocarcinoma (left) 13 cm in greatest diameter. (From Hartman, G. W., Witten, D. M., and Weeks, R. E.)

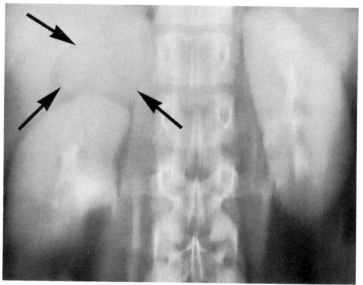

Figure 10–282.   *Intravenous nephrotomogram.* A 4.5-cm benign pheochromocytoma of right adrenal (From Hartman, G. W., Witten, D. M., and Weeks, R. E.)

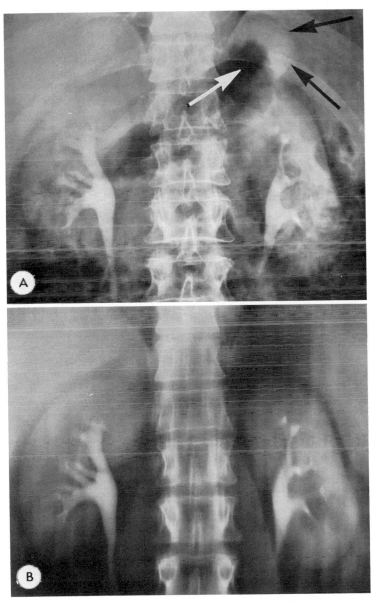

Figure 10–283. Fluid in gastric fundus simulating adrenal tumor. **A,** *Excretory urogram.* Density above left kidney simulates adrenal tumor. **B,** *Intravenous nephrotomogram.* Tumor excluded. (From Hartman, G. W., Witten, D. M., and Weeks, R. E.)

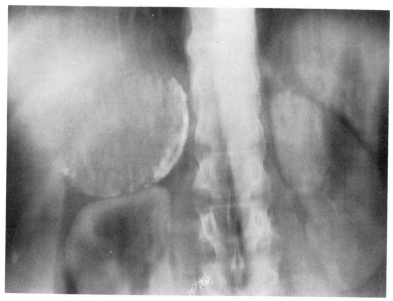

Figure 10-284. *Intravenous nephrotomogram, nephrographic phase.* Calcified cyst of right adrenal gland depressing right kidney. (From Hartman, G. W., Witten, D. M., and Weeks, R. E.)

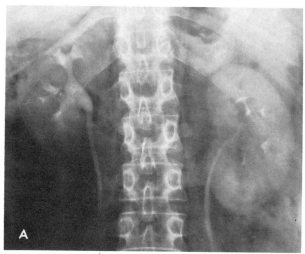

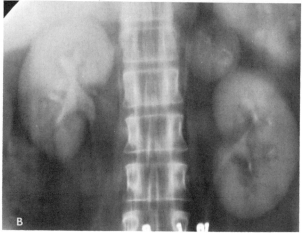

Figure 10-285. *Intravenous nephrotomogram.* Adenoma of left adrenal gland with calcification. **A**, *Excretory urogram.* Suggestion of mass (?) but poor detail. **B**, *Nephrotomogram.* Excellent visualization of tumor.

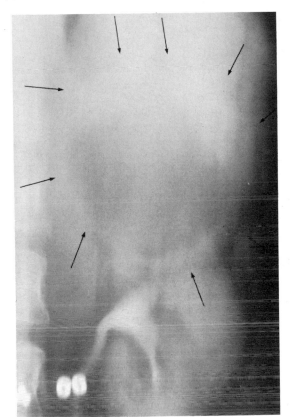

Figure 10–286. *Intravenous nephrotomogram.* Large, malignant, partially necrotic pheochromocytoma.

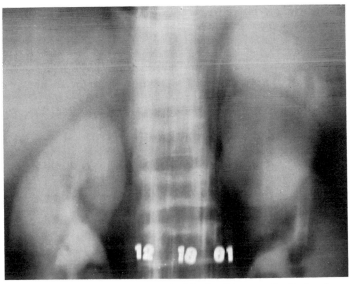

Figure 10–287. *Intravenous nephrotomogram.* Cushing's disease. Cortical adenoma in left adrenal gland.

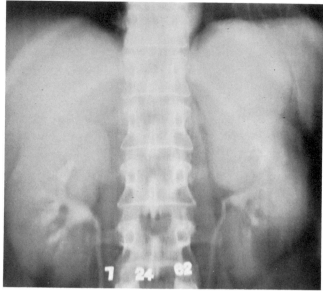

Figure 10–288. *Intravenous nephrotomogram.* **Adrenogenital syndrome in woman aged 51. Encapsu-lated cellular active cortical adenoma.**

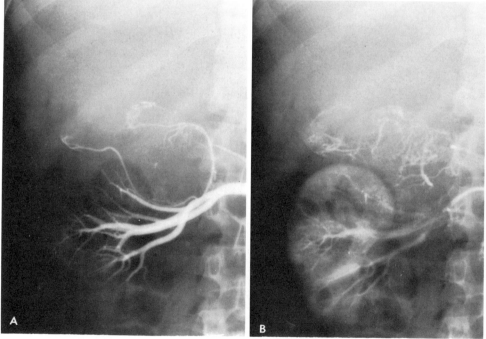

Figure 10–289. *Selective renal arteriogram.* **Carcinoma of right adrenal. A,** *Early film.* **Adrenal arteries** arising from right renal artery are stretched and displaced. Abnormal tumor vessels are seen within mass. Upper part of tumor is not supplied by inferior suprarenal artery. **B,** *Film at 2½ seconds.* There is faint tumor blush with abnormal vessels in tumor. Early filling of dilated veins is evident. Tumor is clearly separated from kidney.

MALIGNANT TUMORS OF THE BLADDER

Tumors of the urinary bladder are *principally a cystoscopic rather than a urographic diagnostic problem*. Urography, however, may supply helpful data that may be complementary to cystoscopy and bimanual palpation, such as (1) the recognition of asymptomatic tumors by excretory urography which is being done for other reasons, (2) the demonstration of ureteral obstruction from the tumor, and (3) information which may be helpful in assessing the degree of involvement (infiltration) of the bladder wall.

Epithelial Tumors: Transitional Cell Epithelioma (Transitional Cell Carcinoma) and Squamous Cell Epithelioma (Squamous Cell Carcinoma; Epidermoid Carcinoma)
(Figs. 10-290 through 10-323)

As stated previously in the discussion of epithelial tumors of the renal pelves and ureters (see pages 1152 and 1153), at the Mayo Clinic we regard all neoplasms of uroepithelium (transitional and squamous cell tumors) as malignant. So-called benign papillomas are classified by our pathologists as papillary transitional cell epitheliomas, grade 1 (Broders' classification). It is important to distinguish between papillary* and nonpapillary tumors because this is probably the greatest single factor in evaluating the seriousness and lethal potential of the tumor. *Papillary tumors* tend to grow into the lumen of the bladder; infiltration is not common and when present is usually of minor degree. Nonpapillary (solid) tumors, on the other hand, tend to grow into and through the bladder wall, and the incidence of infiltration is high. Almost all squamous cell tumors are nonpapillary and all are infiltrative (McDonald and Thompson); they are the most lethal of all epithelial tumors of the uroepithelium. The degree of infiltration of the bladder wall cannot be accurately determined until surgical exploration; helpful information, however, may be provided by (1) bimanual examination under general or spinal anesthesia, (2) cystoscopic observation, and (3) urography. The degree of infiltration and involvement of the bladder wall is of great importance in the decision on the type of therapy to be instituted.

UROGRAPHIC DIAGNOSIS*

Estimation of Thickness of Wall of Bladder

As can be surmised from the discussion thus far, it would be distinctly helpful if the thickness and limits of the wall of the bladder could be determined roentgenographically. Opinions differ as to whether this is possible and if so in what proportion of cases. Franksson, with Lindblom and with Lindblom and Whitehouse, and Nilson stated that the thickness of the wall of the bladder can be determined roentgenographically in a large proportion of cases. They described a more or less **radiolucent shadow (ring) of the perivesical (extraperitoneal) layer of fat which surrounds the bladder** except near the prostate and the region of the ureterovesical juncture. When this shadow is discernible, the thickness of the bladder wall is determined in the cystogram by the distance between the contrast medium

---

*The term *papillary* is used here as a microscopic rather than a gross term. Tumors which may appear *solid* on cystoscopy may be papillary on microscopic examination. Also, this term should not be confused with *pedunculated* or *nonpedunculated* which are gross descriptive terms.

*See Chapter 1, pages 58–71, for discussion of methods and techniques for obtaining various types of cystograms, such as conventional cystograms, double contrast cystograms, combined perivesical insufflation of oxygen and carbon dioxide cystograms, and polycystograms (also called fractionated or superimposition cystograms).

(which fills the bladder cavity) and the perivesical translucent shadow (see Figs. 10–304 through 10–308). In our experience at the Mayo Clinic we have not been impressed with the constancy of this perivesical shadow. It was visible in only 30% of Braband's cases of bladder tumors. Smith could not identify it in the majority of his cases. There seems little doubt, however, that more careful attention to roentgen technique and more critical examination of films should increase the percentage in which radiologic estimation of thickness of the bladder wall is possible.

Bartley and Eckerbom used **perivesical insufflation with oxygen combined with a cystogram,** using carbon dioxide to demonstrate the thickness of the bladder wall and the degree of infiltration in bladder tumors. They introduced a needle immediately above the symphysis pubis and directed it caudally and dorsally until its tip lay 1 cm behind and below the upper border of the symphysis. The position of the needle was checked roentgenographically. After aspiration, to be sure that the needle was not in a vessel, 700 to 800 ml of oxygen was injected around the bladder. Carbon dioxide was not used because it is absorbed too rapidly. From 200 to 300 ml of carbon dioxide was then injected into the bladder through a urethral catheter. Both conventional films and tomograms were exposed in various anteroposterior, oblique, and lateral positions (see below).

Gosalbez and Gil-Vernet also have introduced air both intravesically and perivesically for radiologic study of the bladder.

Papillary, Noninfiltrative Tumors
(Figs. 10–290 through 10–297)

Pedunculated, papillary tumors provide the most dramatic variety of filling defects seen in the **conventional cystogram.** They are well-delineated, and the lesion is almost completely surrounded by contrast medium so that the normal intact

bladder wall can be demonstrated to be uninvolved and of relatively normal thickness (Figs. 10–290, 10–291, and 10–292). Huge tumors may provide a negative filling shadow which may almost completely fill the lumen of the bladder; yet a thin layer of contrast medium remains to outline the bladder wall and shows the tumor to be of a noninfiltrating nature. Papillary tumors usually provide filigree or mottled shadows with infiltration of the contrast medium into the spaces between the papillary fronds of the tumor (Fig. 10–293).

A refinement in cystographic diagnosis was suggested by Bartley and Helander in 1960. They employed **a double contrast technique using a combination of carbon dioxide and contrast medium.** They first injected about 10 ml of 30% contrast medium (Urografin, Hypaque, or propyliodone [Dionosil aqueous]) and then carbon dioxide until the patient experienced the desire to void (usually 200 to 300 ml). The patient then was rotated to make sure that the contrast medium coated all parts of the tumor. Multiple films were exposed with the patient in different positions (prone, supine, and right and left lateral and oblique). An axial exposure (tangential to the base of the bladder) was made also. By this technique they have been able to project tumors in profile so that even small papillary tumors (that would be completely obscured in a conventional cystogram) may be visualized (Figs. 10–294 through 10–297). Whether it is practical or economically sound to go to this effort urographically when cystoscopy may provide the same information more simply and quickly seems open to question.

Nonpapillary (Solid) Infiltrating Tumors
(Figs. 10–298 through 10–316)

Although the practical importance of urography in papillary noninfiltrative tumors may be open to question, it is undoubtedly important in evaluating nonpapillary (solid) infiltrative tumors. **Ureteral obstruction** almost always indicates serious and extensive infiltration (Figs. 10–298 through 10–301). It is unusual for a papillary (noninfiltrative) tumor even in the region of a uretral orifice to produce obstruction.* Whereas papillary and pedunculated tumors produce well-circumscribed, negative filling defects, nonpapillary tumors produce flattened defects with ill-defined contours, sloping borders, and a tendency to minimal intraluminal projection (Braband; Franksson; Franksson and Lindblom). The bladder wall appears to be fixed and rigid in the area of the tumor and if the *radiolucent ring of the perivesical fat* is visible, the thickness of the tumor may be estimated. Absence of this negative shadow in the region of the tumor may be an indication of extensive involvement of the bladder wall and extravesical tissue (Franksson and Lindblom; Franksson, Lindblom, and

---

*Smith found evidence of ureteral obstruction associated with 39% of the *carcinomas* of the bladder in contrast to only 5% of the papillomas.

Whitehouse; Nilson) (Figs. 10–302 through 10–307). Demonstration of the degree of infiltration of the bladder wall by means of **perivesical insufflation of oxygen combined with a carbon dioxide cystogram** is shown in Figures 10–308, 10–309, and 10–310. Displacement of the bladder to the opposite side of the pelvis from a tumor is also a pathognomonic sign of extensive invasion of the bladder wall (Figs. 10–311 and 10–312). When this situation is present, however, one must exclude the possibility of a large vesical diverticulum with a small neck which does not fill with contrast medium (see Figs. 5–250 through 5–253). Rigidity and fixation of the bladder result in loss of contractility which may be demonstrated cystographically in the **postmicturition film** (Braband) or with the **polycystogram** (Figs. 10–313, 10–314, and 10–315). This is also called a "fractionated" or "superimposition" cystogram (Cobb and Anderson; Connolly and associates). (See Chapter 2, pages 60–61.) *Vesicoureteral reflux* rather than obstruction may result from fixation and distortion of the intramural portion of the ureter by the tumor (Fig. 10–316).

(Text continued on page 1273.)

Fig. 10-290

Fig. 10-291

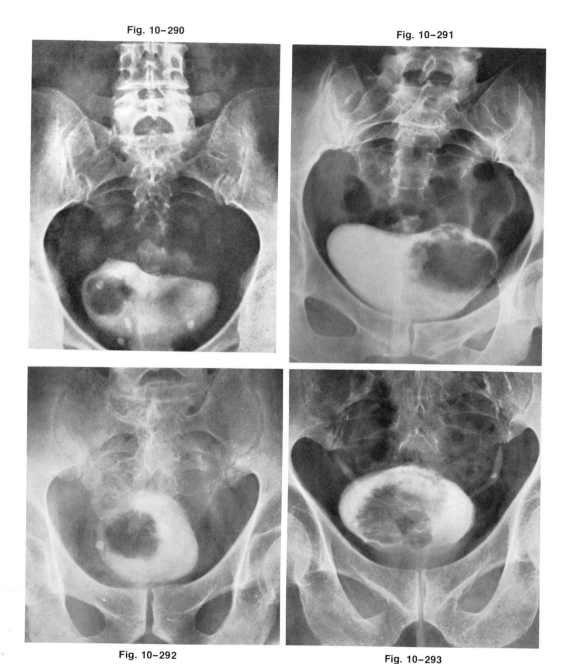

Fig. 10-292

Fig. 10-293

Figure 10-290. *Excretory cystogram.* **Pedunculated papillary neoplasm in right half of bladder.** Incomplete filling of left half.

Figure 10-291. *Excretory cystogram.* **Large pedunculated papillary neoplasm in left side of bladder.**

Figure 10-292. *Excretory cystogram.* **Filling defect from pedunculated papillary neoplasm.**

Figure 10-293. **Extensive, villous, papillary transitional cell epithelioma,** involving large area on right lateral and posterior wall of bladder. No infiltration of bladder wall. Note mottled, filigreed appearance of periphery of tumor from infiltration of contrast medium into spaces between papillary fronds of tumor.

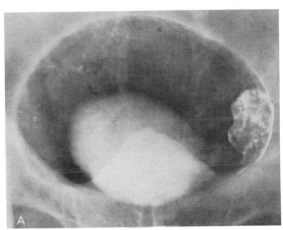
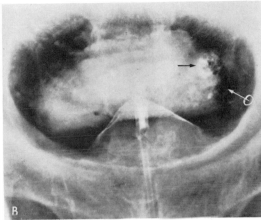

Figure 10-294. Vesical papilloma and prostatic hypertrophy. *Double contrast cystograms. A, Prone view.* Bulk of papilloma, situated posteriorly, is well shown because contrast medium has collected between papillae and because tumor is surrounded by gas. **B,** *Supine view.* Only small part of tumor is now outlined by gas (⟶) and has coating of opaque medium. Small contrast defect in anterior lateral part of base of bladder is caused by tumor(○⟶). Compare smooth, regular mucosal surface of prostatic adenoma with that of papilloma. (From Bartley, O., and Helander, C. G.)

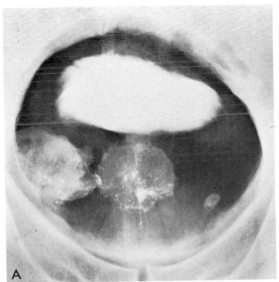
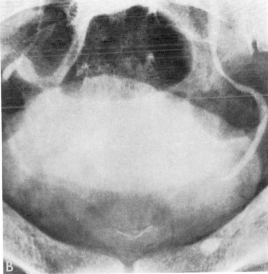

Figure 10-295. Two finely papillomatous tumors, one of them situated in anterior part of trigone. **A,** *Double-contrast cystogram, axial view.* Tumors well outlined. **B,** *Conventional retrograde cystogram.* Although tumors are relatively large, they are not well shown. Ureteral orifices are not involved. (From Bartley, O., and Helander, C. G.)

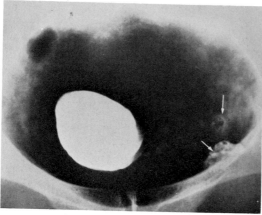
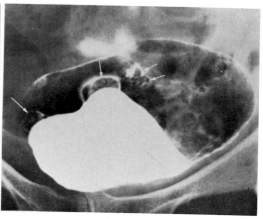

Fig. 10–296   Fig. 10–297

Figure 10–296. *Double contrast cystogram, prone view.* Two **papillomas, in left posterior part of bladder.** Larger one with accumulation of contrast medium between papillae, and smaller one about size of grain of rice (*arrows*). (From Bartley, O., and Helander, C. G.)

Figure 10–297. *Double contrast cystogram, prone view.* **Papillomatosis;** tumors range in size from grains of rice to half a hazelnut (*arrows*). (From Bartley, O., and Helander, C. G.)

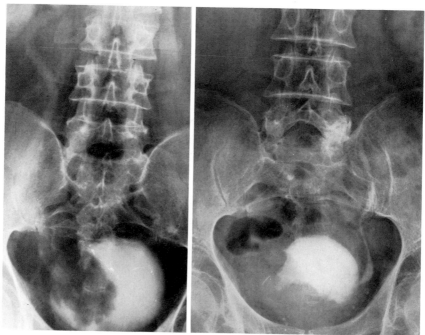

Fig. 10–298   Fig. 10–299

Figure 10–298. *Excretory cystogram.* Filling defect in right half of bladder from **infiltrating carcinoma of bladder causing pyeloureterectasis** above.

Figure 10–299. *Excretory urogram.* Extensive filling defect in right half of bladder from large, **solid, sessile, infiltrating carcinoma** which has completely **obstructed right ureter,** producing absence of visualization of right kidney. Large soft-tissue mass in right renal area from obstructive hydronephrosis.

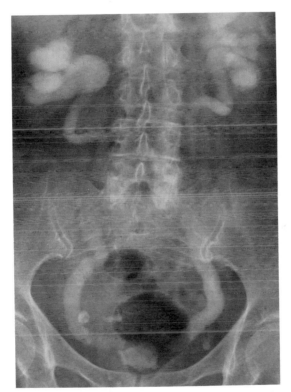

Figure 10–300. *Excretory urogram.* Bilateral ureteral obstruction from high-grade infiltrating carcinoma of trigone and contraction of bladder from external irradiation (cobalt).

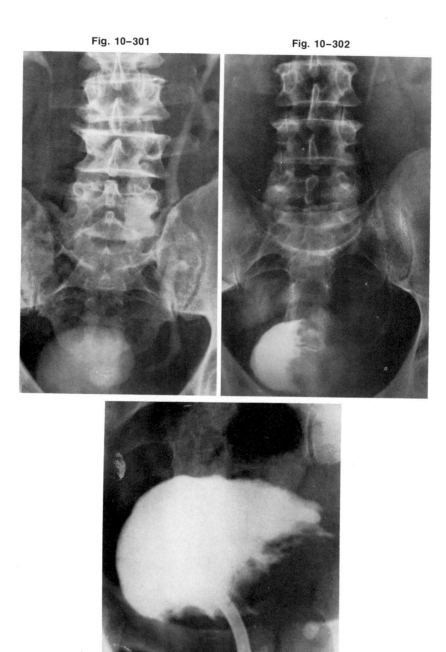

Fig. 10–301   Fig. 10–302

Fig. 10–303

Figure 10–301. *Excretory urogram.* Flattening and fixation of left half of bladder from **solid, sessile, infiltrating carcinoma of bladder** which is partially obstructing left ureter, producing ureterectasis above.

Figure 10–302. *Excretory cystogram.* Filling defect of left half of bladder from **infiltrating vesical tumor** which, however, has not obstructed left ureteral orifice.

Figure 10–303. *Retrograde cystogram.* Extensive filling defect of base and left half of bladder from **infiltrating vesical carcinoma.**

Fig. 10–304

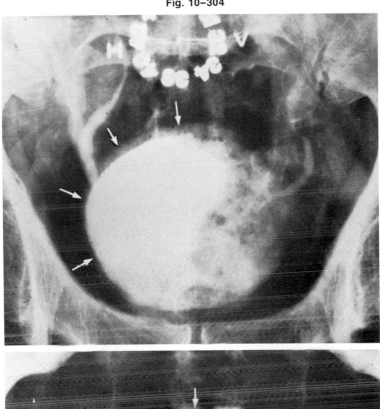

Fig. 10–305

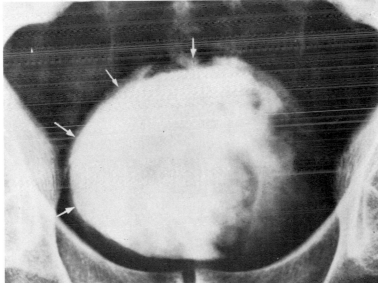

Figure 10–304. *Conventional retrograde cystogram.* Demonstration of thickness of bladder wall by radiolucent shadow of perivesical fat. **Broad-based tumor in left lateral wall of bladder infiltrating submucosa.** Slight local thickening of bladder wall. Ureter unobstructed. *Arrows* indicate outer surface of bladder wall which can be distinguished from inner surface (outlined by contrast medium). Note increased thickness of bladder wall as it approaches area of tumor (see text). (From Nilson, A. E.)

Figure 10–305. *Conventional retrograde cystogram.* **Broad-based tumor in left lateral wall of bladder which is infiltrating muscle.** Fairly pronounced local thickening of bladder wall (*arrows*). Ureter unobstructed. Note increase in thickness of bladder wall as it approaches tumor. (From Nilson, A. E.)

Fig. 10–306

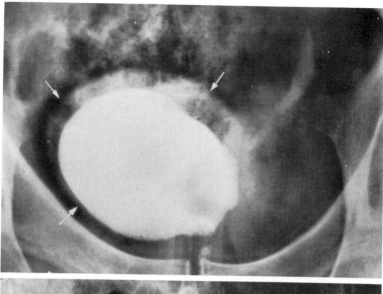

Fig. 10–307

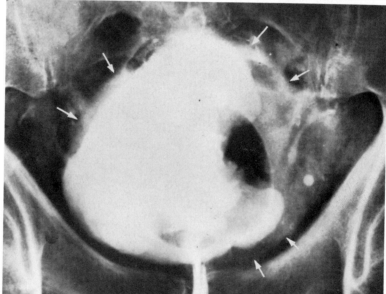

Figure 10–306. *Conventional retrograde cystogram.* **Infiltrating tumor of left wall of bladder** is involving perivesical tissues. Note marked thickening of bladder wall and smooth transition from tumor to vesical mucosa (*arrows*). In area of perivesical infiltration, contour of outer layer of bladder is diffuse and disappears. (Courtesy of Dr. A. E. Nilson.)

Figure 10–307. *Conventional retrograde cystogram.* **Broad-based tumor involving left wall of bladder and infiltrating perivesically.** Pronounced local thickening of bladder wall and smooth transition from tumor to inner vesical surface (*arrows*). Ureter unobstructed. Outer contour of bladder wall tends to disappear in region of perivesical infiltration. (From Nilson, A. E.)

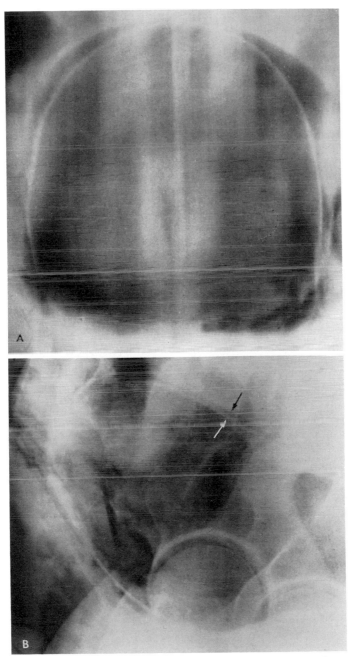

Figure 10–308.   Normal bladder. Gas (carbon dioxide) cystogram plus perivesical injection of gas (oxygen). **A,** *Tomogram, anteroposterior view.* **B,** *Conventional film, lateral view.* Thickness of bladder wall is defined by intravesical and perivesical gas (*arrows*). (From Bartley, O., and Eckerbom, H.)

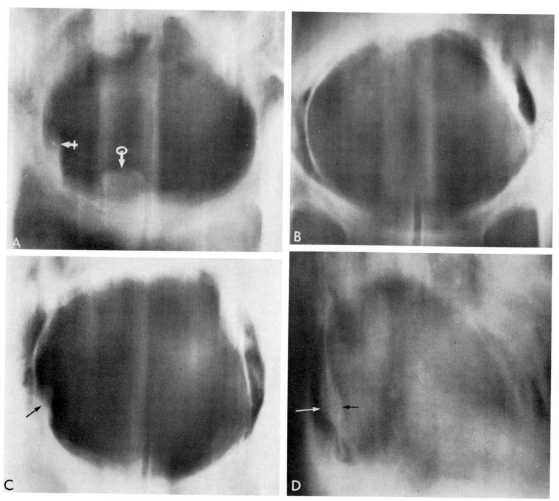

Figure 10–309. Two carcinomas of bladder, each about 1 cm in diameter. No tumor was demonstrable at cystography with positive contrast medium. **A,** *Tomocystogram* with intravesical (carbon dioxide) gas only. Two tumors were outlined, one in base of bladder near midline (○—→), the other anteriorly on right side (←—|—). Latter tumor had not been detected at cystoscopy. **B,** *Tomocystogram* using intravesical (carbon dioxide) gas and perivesical injection of oxygen. *Anteroposterior view.* Tomographic section lies behind tumors. Wall of bladder here is of normal thickness, and no tumor is discernible. **C,** Same as in **B** but with section through lateral tumor, which penetrates bladder wall (*arrow*). **D,** *Tomogram, lateral view.* Tumor growing through anterior bladder wall into perivesical fat (*arrows*). Wall above and below it is of normal thickness. (From Bartley, O., and Eckerbom, H.)

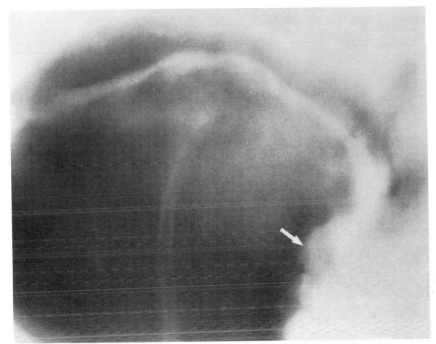

Figure 10–310. Sarcoma of left lower part of bladder (*arrow*). *Gas (carbon dioxide) cystogram plus perivesical injection of oxygen.* No perivesical gas at site of tumor which extends through bladder to pelvic wall (*arrow*). Entire bladder wall is somewhat thickened. (From Bartley, O., and Eckerbom, H.)

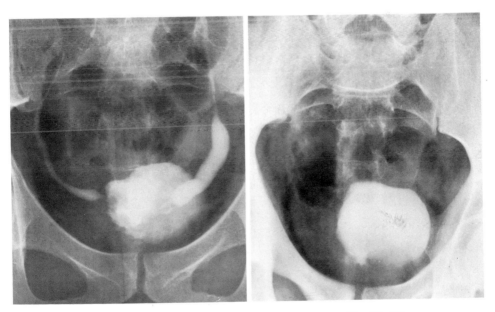

Fig. 10–311   Fig. 10–312

Figure 10–311. *Excretory urogram.* **Extensive, solid, sessile nonpapillary tumor** in trigone and right lateral and posterior walls of bladder. Bladder appears to be displaced to left side of pelvis. Note **dilatation of left ureter.** Total cystectomy. Tumor had extended into perivesical fat.

Figure 10–312. *Excretory urogram.* **Solid sessile, infiltrating transitional cell carcinoma, grade 3,** of right wall of bladder. Bladder appears displaced to left side of pelvis, which suggests extensive involvement and thickening of bladder wall. No ureteral obstruction.

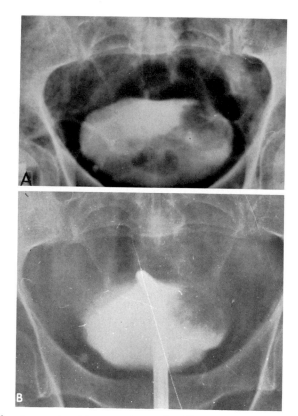

Figure 10–313. Bladder tumor (papillary transitional cell epithelioma, grade 2) without infiltration. A, *Excretory cystogram.* Filling defect of left lateral wall of bladder. No ureteral obstruction. B, *Superimposition cystogram.* Halo of contrast material around tumor indicates no infiltration. (From Cobb, O. E., and Anderson, E. E.)

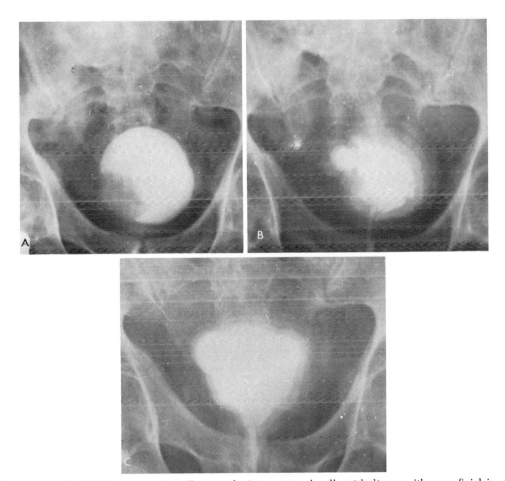

Figure 10–314. Bladder tumor (papillary grade 3 transitional cell epithelioma with superficial invasion of muscle). **A,** *Excretory cystogram.* Filling defect of right lateral wall with no ureteral obstruction. **B,** *Superimposition cystogram.* Halos of contrast medium around superficially invasive tumor. *Operation.* Suprapubic exploration and local excision of tumor. **C,** *Postoperative superimposition cystogram.* Absence of filling defect but diminution of halo formation along right lateral wall. (From Cobb, O. E., and Anderson, E. E.)

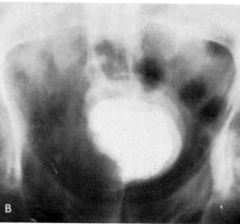

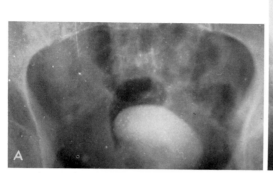

Figure 10–315. **Infiltrating bladder tumor** (high-grade deeply infiltrating squamous cell epithelioma). **A,** *Excretory cystogram.* Filling defect of right lateral wall. No ureteral obstruction. Bimanual examination shows extensive induration of base of bladder. *Biopsy.* Infiltrating squamous cell epithelioma. **B,** *Superimposition cystogram.* Absence of halo formation around deeply invasive tumor. (From Cobb, O. E., and Anderson, E. E.)

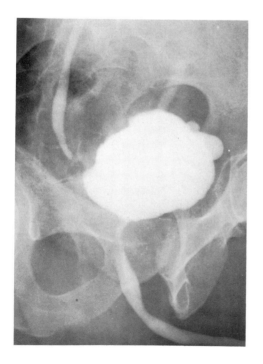

Figure 10–316. *Voiding cystourethrogram.* **Diffuse transitional cell epithelioma, grade 2 (in situ),** involving dome and anterior, posterior, and lateral walls and extending to vesicoprostatic juncture in man, 38 years of age. **Bilateral vesicoureteral reflux.** Note flattening of right posterolateral wall where tumor was most extensive. Total cystectomy and prostatectomy done.

Calcification of Tumors

Urinary salts may be deposited on the surface of almost any type of tumor. Necrosis of large tumors is often accompanied by extensive calcification (Figs. 10–317A and B and 10–318A and B).

Tumors in Vesical Diverticula

The possibility of tumors being present in vesical diverticula must always be kept in mind; in this location they are most serious because the wall of the diverticulum is thin and often contains no musculature. Even low-grade papillary tumors located in diverticula, therefore, can easily infiltrate and extend extravesically. If the interior of a diverticulum cannot be visualized cystoscopically, a retrograde cystogram may be of great help by demonstrating a negative filling defect within the diverticulum (Figs. 10–319, 10–320, and 10–321).

ARTERIOGRAPHY
(Figs. 10–322 and 10–323)

Boijsen and Nilsson first described the use of angiography in the diagnosis and staging of bladder tumors. They combined a carbon dioxide cystogram with the arteriogram. It was their opinion that important data concerning "staging" and the degree of infiltration of the tumor could be obtained in this manner. Subsequently favorable reports have been made by other authors (Cornell; Lang and associates, 1963; Wilchusky and Lewin; Wise and Fainsinger). Taylor and associates added a feature which they named the "triple contrast technique." This consisted of the perivesical insufflation of oxygen, in addition to obtaining the carbon dioxide cystogram.

The characteristics of the arteriogram in bladder tumor are quite similar to those in renal tumor (Figs. 10–322 and 10–323). The vessels supplying the tumor may be increased in number and caliber; if the tumor is pedunculated there may be massive vessels in the pedicle. The pathologic tumor vessels have a convoluted or "corkscrew" appearance and do not branch normally. They are usually best seen in the "late arterial phase" as is also the "tumor stain" appearance caused by the greatly increased number of capillaries in the tumor; there is arteriovenous shunting with early venous filling. These changes are more pronounced in high-grade poorly differentiated tumors. In extensive perforating tumors these neoplastic vessels are readily visible outside the bladder wall.

Estimates of the accuracy of staging with this modality have varied from 81% (Cornell) to 93% (Taylor and associates). These figures are the results of comparison with subsequent findings at either operation or necropsy. At present there is considerable difference of opinion as to whether the information obtained justifies the magnitude of this diagnostic procedure, especially if surgical exploration is to be done regardless of the results. So far at the Mayo Clinic we have not used this procedure.

(Text continued on page 1279.)

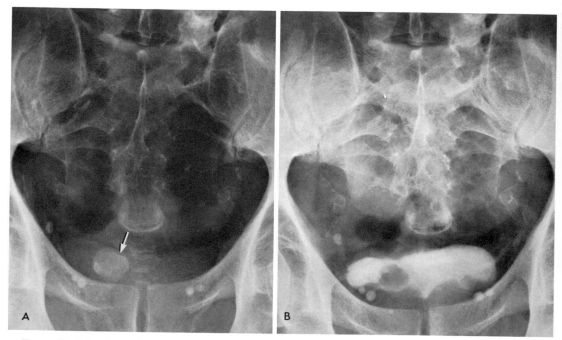

Figure 10–317.   Vesical tumor with calcification. A, *Plain film.* Calcific area, 2 to 3 cm in diameter, overlying right side of bony pelvis. Periphery is dense, with less dense center. **B,** *Excretory cystogram.* Filling defect of right side of bladder, which corresponds to calcific area. Cystoscopy showed vesical tumor covered with incrusted material.

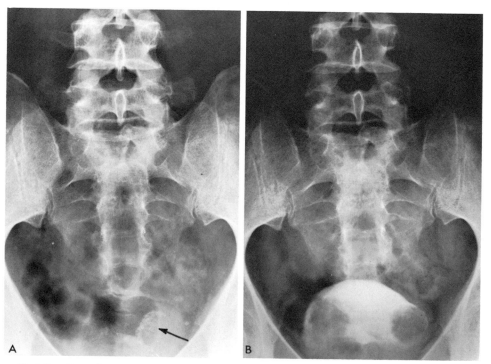

Figure 10–318.   Vesical tumor with calcification. A, *Plain film.* Mottled calcific shadow, 3 cm in diameter, in left side of bony pelvis. **B,** *Excretory cystogram.* Filling defect in left half of bladder corresponds to shadow. Proved to be vesical tumor with calcification. Shadow suggesting filling defect in right side of bladder was due to overlying gas.

Fig. 10–319

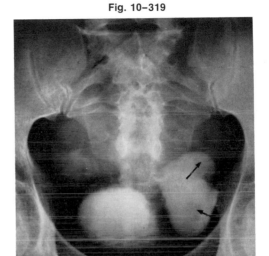

Figure 10–319. *Retrograde cystogram.* Vesical diverticulum arising from left side of bladder and connected with bladder by narrow neck. Filling defect in upper lateral aspect of diverticulum, and less distinct filling defect in lower portion of diverticulum. Cystoscopy showed these negative shadows to be caused by vesical tumor within diverticulum.

Figure 10–320. Vesical tumor with calcification situated in vesical diverticulum. A, *Plain film.* Triangular calcific shadow with indefinite mottled linear shadows extending cranially, adjacent to left ischial spine. B, *Excretory cystogram.* Vesical diverticulum arising from left side of bladder. Negative filling defects in diverticulum which correspond to areas of calcification. Cystoscopy revealed tumor covered with incrusted material situated in vesical diverticulum.

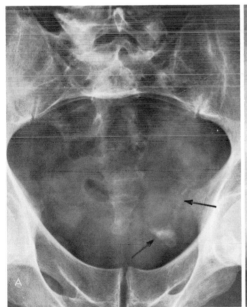

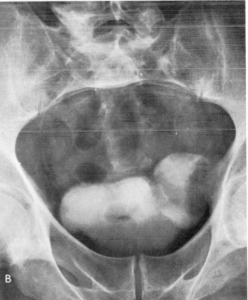

Fig. 10–320

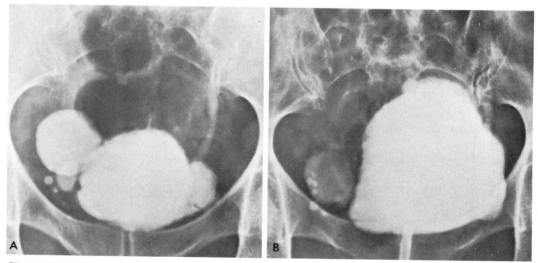

Figure 10–321. Tumor in vesical diverticulum. *Retrograde cystograms.* **A,** Multiple vesical diverticula; reflux up left ureter. **B,** Same case, 8 years later. Filling defect in diverticulum on right with displacement of right wall of bladder toward midline from tumor in diverticulum. (From Knappenberger, S. T., Uson, A. C., and Melicow, M. M.)

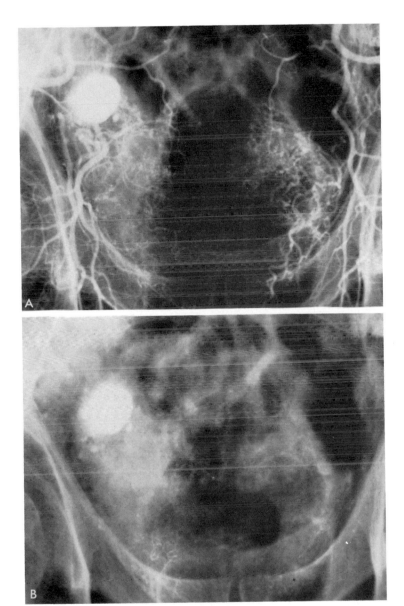

Figure 10–322. *Arteriogram* in **carcinoma of bladder. A,** *Arteriogram combined with carbon dioxide cystogram.* Highly vascular carcinoma. Tumor vessels on both sides are considerable distance away from gas-distended bladder, indicating spread of neoplasm into soft tissues of pelvis. **B,** *Film made several seconds later.* (Very dense areas in right upper part of illustration are residual barium from previous examination.) From Cornell, S. H.)

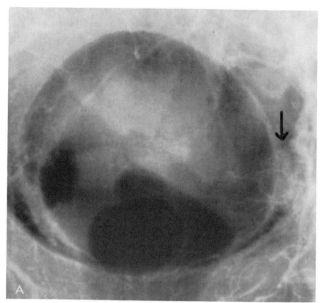

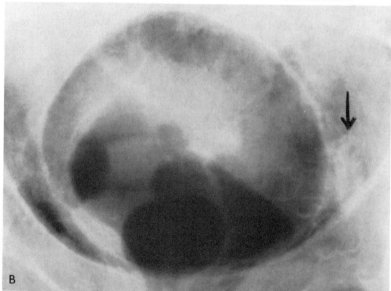

Figure 10–323. *Arteriogram* in **carcinoma of bladder. A,** *"Triple contrast" arteriogram* (combined with intravesical and perivesical injection of gas). *Arrow* points to neoplastic vessels which have extended through wall of bladder into perivesical space. **B,** *Film made several seconds later.* Capillary staining of tumor is more diffuse and dense. (From Cornell, S. H.)

Nonepithelial Tumors (Sarcoma of the Bladder and Prostate; Embryonal Rhabdomyosarcoma; Urogenital Rhabdomyosarcoma; Embryonal Sarcoma of the Urogenital Sinus; Polypoid Fibromyxosarcoma; Botryoid Sarcoma, Cellular Embryonic Sarcoma, etc.)

(Figs. 10–324 through 10–333)

Sarcoma of the bladder and sarcoma of the prostate are considered together here because, as will be pointed out in the subsequent discussion, the lesion appears to arise from remnants of the urogenital sinus and mesonephric (wolffian) ducts, located in the region of the trigone, bladder neck, prostatic urethra in the male, and the entire urethra in the female. It is often difficult or impossible to say whether the lesion is "primary" in the bladder or in the prostate; perhaps it is "primary" in neither organ.

Terminology and Histogenesis

The term *sarcoma of the bladder* is often used loosely and, as Khoury and Speer pointed out, often means nothing more than that the tumor is not of epithelial origin. In an excellent thesis on the subject, McFarland noted that 119 different names had been used in the literature for various types of sarcomatous tumors of the urogenital region. He concluded that they were embryonal tumors of dysontogenetic* origin. He pointed out that the four organs usually involved are the bladder, prostate, vagina, and uterus and that the tumor probably originated from or near those embryonal structures that enter into the formation of the urogenital sinus. Higgins also subscribed to this view. Khoury and Speer in 1944 and Smith in 1959 favored the theory of embryonal heterotopia occurring as an anomalous development of the wolffian duct system.

Batsakis has pointed out that it is the complex "trigonal area" of the bladder that is chiefly involved. This area is of mesodermal origin (the terminal portions of the mesonephric duct after it has "emitted the ureteric bud") and extends down the wall of the primitive urethra to the region of the müllerian tubercle. Included in this area therefore are the trigone, vesical neck, and prostatic urethra in the male, and the trigone and entire urethra in the female. Subepithelial extension of mesenchymal tissue upward on the adjacent walls of the bladder as the bladder elongates in growth may account for the occasional sarcomatous lesion, especially in the adult, which appears to be fairly well removed from the trigonal area.

It is unfortunate that the term "botryoid" has become so popular and that many believe it signifies a definite classification of sarcoma. It has been pointed out repeatedly (Batsakis) that this is simply a gross description of a sarcoma when it is located in a hollow organ where it has room to grow in an irregular polypoid or "botryoid" shape, which simply means a "bunch of grapes."

Mostofi and Morse stated that this variety of sarcoma arises from "embryonic tissue capable of differentiation into myxomatous or fibrous tissue and striated muscle," and they classified it as "polypoid" rhabdomyosarcoma.

Williams and Schistad commented on this subject, pointing out that although the term *rhabdomyosarcoma* implies the presence of striated muscle cells, fundamentally, as pointed out by White, these tumors are embryonic sarcomas consisting of immature mesenchyme which undergoes a variable degree of differentiation to striated muscle, to connective tissue, and possibly to smooth muscle. They stated,

It is a matter of speculation as to why tumours arising in these particular sites should show differentiation to striated muscle, but it seems

---

*Dysontogenesis: Abnormal development that may be followed by structural malformation or tumor.

clear that these embryonic sarcomata have little in common with rhabdomyosarcoma arising in voluntary muscle later in life.

Hunt suggested "heterotopic displacement of vagrant rhabdomyoblasts into the vesical submucosa from sites that normally contain striated muscle elements" (urogenital diaphragm, prostatic capsule, or others). Ober and associates (1954; 1958) suggested that the tumor arises from the mesenchyme of the urogenital ridge, in this way accounting for the great diversity of type and location. They nicely summarized the various theories of origin.

Dockerty favored a histologic classification which groups sarcomas into two broad categories. His first or dysontogenetic group includes such lesions as rhabdomyosarcoma, chondrosarcoma, osteogenic sarcoma, and the rare carcinosarcoma. These appear to arise from tissues which are not normally encountered in the bladder. Prognosis is grave, and treatment and outlook are little influenced by the various subtypes listed. His second category embraces such lesions as leiomyosarcoma, fibrosarcoma, and angiosarcoma, which contain native elements in the bladder. Prognosis in this group is somewhat more favorable. According to Legier it has been considered axiomatic that the older the patient, the better the prognosis regardless of cell type.

Incidence by Age and Sex

This tumor is most common in two ages of life: (1) youth and (2) late adulthood. Males are affected more frequently than females (ratio of about 3 to 1). It is the common tumor of the "lower urinary tract" in infants and children and is considered to be the second most common tumor of the genitourinary tract in children (Williams and Schistad). The term *botryoid sarcoma* has been used almost exclusively to designate the lesion in infants and children.

Because of the location of the lesion it has been difficult in some cases to be sure whether the lesion arises in the bladder, in the prostate, or in the urethra. This is especially true in infants. For this reason, one cannot be entirely sure of the accuracy of the case reports in the literature. In 1955 Longley collected 52 cases called "sarcoma of the bladder" and 41 called "sarcoma of the prostate." Of the bladder lesions, 24.5% were in children less than 5 years of age while 45.6% were in adults more than 50 years of age. Of the patients with prostatic lesions, 34% were less than 2 years of age, 48% less than 20, and only 18% more than 50. Approximately 250 cases of sarcoma of the *prostate* have been reported (Hamlin and Lund; Siegel). Siegel stated that it tends to be a disease of youth; the youngest patient in his collected series was 4 months of age, the oldest 89 years. He estimated that the disease appears before the age of benign prostatic hyperplasia in approximately 80% of cases.

Legier in 1961 reviewed the literature and found reports of 61 cases of sarcoma alleged to have arisen in the bladder, the great majority being in infants and children in the first 3 or 4 years of life. In 1964 Williams and Schistad reported a consecutive series of 14 personally observed rhabdomyosarcomas of the bladder; all were in children in the first 3 or 4 years of life; there were 9 males and 5 females. They stated that they had not experienced too much difficulty in distinguishing bladder from prostatic lesions.

Gross Appearance of Tumor

The typical **botryoid sarcoma** of the bladder seen in infants and children is a bulky, submucosal, pearly gray tumor composed of nodules or lobules which give the appearance of a polypoid lesion. The growth originates in the submucosa and superficial layers of muscle in the base of the bladder near the vesical neck. If the lesion is primary in the vagina it may protrude like a bunch of grapes. The same appearance may be produced if in little girl the bladder lesion is forced downward and extrudes through the urethra. Williams and Schistad have described the periphery of the tumor as a thin submucosal plaque with a clear-cut margin which gradually advances across the bladder or down the urethra to involve the entire urethra in the female and through the membranous urethra in the male.

Symptoms, Findings, and Diagnosis (the Pediatric Lesion — "Botryoid" Sarcoma)

Presenting symptoms are usually caused by obstruction of the bladder outlet and consist of frequency, poor stream, dysuria, and gross hematuria. Late symptoms include suprapubic pain, dependent edema, and obstipation because of obstruction of the rectum. Ureteral obstruction occurs relatively early, and when advanced, evidence of renal failure may be present Williams and Schistad have emphasized strangury as an important symptom. They compare it with the severe strangury caused by a stone impacted in the posterior urethra and feel that this is an important but differential point to distinguish it from sarcoma of the prostate, in which this symptom almost never occurs.

In infants and children the chief finding may be a large palpable suprapubic mass that may persist even after the vesical distention has been relieved by catheterization. Digital rectal examination may disclose a huge mass of rubbery consistency; in infant males it may be impossible on digital rectal examination to distinguish the prostate from the bladder. In adult males this lesion may simulate a huge benign or carcinomatous involvement of the prostate.

If renal function is adequate an *excretory urogram* may demonstrate ureteropyelectasis (Fig. 10–324). Angulation or "fish hook" deformity of the terminal ureters so common in cases of benign enlargement of the prostate may also be present. The excretory or retrograde cystogram will usually reveal negative lobulated filling defects in the lumen of the bladder. In the infant or child with the typical botryoid sarcoma multiple, smooth, roundish shadows that fill the lower half of the bladder and posterior urethra are typical and pathognomonic; they must not be confused with shadows of gas in the rectum or ectopic ureteroceles (Figs. 10–325 through 10–328). If the lesion becomes large it may appear to displace the bladder upward. In general, however, upward displacement of the bladder with displacement and stretching of the urethra suggests the lesion to be primary in the prostate (Figs. 10–329 and 10–330). Cystoscopy and cytoscopic biopsy should usually establish the diagnosis of sarcoma, but cystoscopy will often fail to settle the question of whether the growth is primary in the bladder or the prostate. The following two case abstracts are illustrative of the problem.

A boy, aged 13 years, was admitted to the Mayo Clinic on May 26, 1959. Urinary symptoms had appeared suddenly 2 weeks before admission. These consisted of urgency and frequency of urination. The severity of the symptoms rapidly increased so that within a few days the patient was voiding small amounts of urine every few minutes and suprapubic pain developed. The patient's home physician catheterized him and found 1,000 ml of residual urine. The catheter was left indwelling and the patient was sent to the Mayo Clinic.

On *digital rectal examination* a large hard mass was felt in the region of the prostate and the base of the bladder which caused marked posterior displacement of the rectum. *Proctoscopy* disclosed a large, firm, smooth, anterior extrarectal mass beginning just above the prostate. An *excretory urogram* showed normal kidneys and a huge filling defect in the base of the bladder which appeared to displace the bladder upward (Fig. 10–331). *Cystoscopy* with the panendoscope, with the patient under anesthesia, disclosed a huge fixed nodular mass which seemed to arise from the region of the prostate and vesical neck and protruded far into the lumen of the bladder. A small resectoscope was introduced and pieces of tissue were removed for microscopic examination. The pathologist diagnosed the lesion as a spindle cell sarcoma (grade 4) probably of the rhabdomyosarcoma type. No metastasis could be demonstrated and results of blood studies were normal.

In an effort to reduce the size of the lesion, preoperative irradiation was administered with the cobalt-60 bomb. One treatment was given daily for 14 days at the end of which time no change in the size or texture of the tumor could be detected on digital rectal examination.

On June 15, 1959, *total cystectomy, prostatectomy, and bilateral ureterosigmoidostomy were performed.* The large mass was easily palpable through the bladder wall and seemed to be fully movable even in the region of the vesical neck. There was a metastatic mass at the promontory of the sacrum. The pathologist reported the *specimen as encircling the bladder neck and diffusely invading the prostate gland.* Microscopic examination showed the lesion to be a grade 4 rhabdomyosarcoma. A node removed from the region of the right iliac vessels was involved with tumor. Immediate convalescence was excellent, but the patient died 13 months later from generalized metastasis.

A girl, aged 15 years, was admitted to the Mayo Clinic on Feb. 29, 1960. She stated that approximately 3 months previously she had noted blood when she urinated. At first she had thought this represented her period but later was sure that the blood was coming from the urethra. Frequency and urgency of urination developed gradually thereafter and occasionally there was some urgency incontinence. These symptoms were associated with intermittent low abdominal pain. The patient had been hospitalized elsewhere, and a mass protruding from the urethra was excised. The bleeding continued. Three weeks later cystoscopy was done and three nodular masses in the region of the bladder neck were removed with a resectoscope. The diagnosis was multiple benign papillomas.

Examination at the Mayo Clinic revealed the following: In the *excretory urogram* the kidneys appeared normal, but the *cystogram* revealed marked deformity of the base and left lateral wall of the bladder (Fig. 10–332). *Cystoscopy* revealed multiple, large, polypoid grape-like masses which seemed to arise from the entire circumference of the bladder neck and to protrude into the lumen of the bladder. This was especially pronounced on the left side where the growth seemed to invade a good portion of the left lateral wall of the bladder. The left ureteral orifice could not be identified. On bimanual examination the lesion could not be palpated. Tissue for examination

was removed with the resectoscope and was reported to be a grade 4 mesodermal (botryoid) sarcoma. A complete general examination was carried out and no metastasis could be demonstrated.

On Mar. 7, 1960, *total cystectomy and urethrectomy were performed* and the ureters were anastomosed to an *ileal conduit.* There was no evidence of local extension of the tumor through the bladder wall and no distant metastatic lesions could be demonstrated. The gross specimen when removed showed multiple polypoid masses, the largest being 6 cm in diameter. They surrounded the vesical neck and were most prominent in the region of the left ureteral orifice. Microscopic sections revealed polypoid (botryoid) rhabdomyosarcoma of grade 4. The patient was still living and in good health 9 years after operation.

Rhabdomyosarcoma of the Bladder in Adults

As mentioned previously, the lesion is more common in infants and children than it is in adults. In 1965, Evans and Bell reviewed the English literature and found 72 cases of rhabdomyosarcoma of the bladder. Only 10 of these (14%) were in patients more than 10 years of age. They added the three cases of their own, all in adults (ages 38, 51, and 84). Two of their cases were diagnosed "botryoid" type while one was associated with a squamous cell epithelioma. In 1966 Joshi and associates reviewed the literature and found only 13 cases in patients more than 20 years of age. Apparently they did not have access to Evans and Bell's report of three cases, as the time of the writing of their papers overlapped. This would bring the total to 16, to which they added 1 of their own for a total of 17 cases in adults. From a description of the cases it appears that, clinically, rhabdomyosarcoma of the bladder in the adult is quite similar to carcinoma, the distinction usually not being made until the results of biopsy are reported. Although "botryoid" characteristics on gross inspection are mentioned, the tumor does not present the dramatic appearance seen in infants and children. Also, although sarcoma of the bladder and sarcoma of the prostate do not pose the problem of differentiation as they do in children, still problem cases are encountered as illustrated by the following case abstract.

A man, 54 years of age, had had three transurethral resections elsewhere over a period of several months because of recurring urinary obstruction. A total of 130 gm of tissue had been removed. On digital rectal examination at the Mayo Clinic the right lobe of the prostate felt large, indurated, and fixed. On cystoscopic examination a structure that resembled a large right lateral intravesical prostatic lobe projected far into the bladder. An excretory cystogram revealed a large filling defect (Fig. 10–333). Transurethral prostatic resection was performed with the removal of 72 gm of tissue which came from this one "lobe." *The lesion appeared to be attached to the vesical neck at about the 8 o'clock position.* The pathologist's report on the tissue removed was pleomorphic sarcoma, grade 4, probably of rhabdomyosarcoma type. Postoperative digital rectal examination showed no change in size or consistency of the prostate, but the patient voided normally. After operation external radiation with cobalt-60 was given. Because of continued recurrence of tumor, multiple radon seeds were implanted into the prostate via the transvesical route. This eventually caused a urethrorectal fistula, but the patient remains well and free of metastasis now, 7 years since his first admittance.

Prognosis and Treatment

The last two decades have witnessed several "cures" as a result of early radical cystectomy and prostatectomy. Most of these have been in infants and children with the typical botryoid sarcoma. Since Kretschmer's case in 1947, several cures exclusive of those in cases of lymphosarcoma have been reported.* We have had two or three "cures" at the Mayo Clinic which have not been reported.

Williams and Schistad, writing in 1964, were optimistic about total cystectomy

---

*Flocks and Culp; Higgins; Kretschmer; Legier; Marshall; Meisel, Heath, and Miller; Parker, Smith, and Rathmell; Pettersson; Ramey and associates; Smith; Swinney; Thompson and Coppridge; Weaver, Card, and Rueb)

(and diversion) in children when the lesion is primary in the bladder. They reported that, in their series of 14 patients, 6 of 10 operated on more than 3 years previously were alive, well, and free of recurrence. In contrast, they stated that all forms of treatment had been a complete failure in cases of prostatic rhabdomyosarcoma.

In a more recent communication, Williams and Young reported survival of 8 of 15 children with rhabdomyosarcoma of the bladder but only 1 survival when the lesion was in the prostate. Apparently the lesion is radioresistant. The polypoid (botryoid) type of lesion appears to have much better prognosis than the solid type. In girls, because the vulva and vagina tend to be involved, complete vulvectomy with complete excision of bladder, urethra, uterus, and vagina is recommended. In boys the prostate and urethra to the level of the perineoscrotal junction are removed along with the bladder. Goodwin, Mims, and Young recently reported a 5-year survival in a 9-year-old boy with rhabdomyosarcoma of the prostate. Treatment consisted of radical surgery with diversion, irradiation, actinomycin D therapy, and intra-arterial administration of nitrogen mustard along with hypothermia.

Metastatic Tumors of the Bladder

Metastatic lesions from distant foci may involve the bladder the same as they do the renal pelvis and ureter (see pages 1184–1185). Goldstein collected 146 cases from the literature. The most common primary site in descending order of frequency were skin (malignant melanoma), stomach, breast, kidney, and lung. For an in depth consideration of **melanoma** of the genitourinary tract the reader is referred to the 1965 article of Das Gupta and Grabstald. Walsh and associates reviewed the literature in 1966 and stated that 23 cases had been reported. Of every 100 patients dying of malignant melanoma,

50% have metastasis to the adrenal, 45% to the kidney, and 18% to the bladder.

Benign Tumors of the Bladder

Benign tumors of the bladder are rare and relatively unimportant. **Pheochromocytoma** and nonfunctioning paraganglioma (**chemodectoma**) of the bladder wall have been discussed previously (page 1231). Invasion of the bladder by **neurofibromatosis** (von Recklinghausen's disease) has been reported in more than 30 cases. Torres and Bennett stated that 11 of 32 patients were children, and 22 of 32 also had cutaneous evidence of the disease. In three cases there was histologic evidence of malignancy but no evidence of metastasis. In the case of Deniz, Shimkus, and Weller, the disease originally involved the uterus and, following hysterectomy, recurred in the pelvis and invaded the bladder. Labardini, Kallet, and Cerny described a case of urogenital neurofibromatosis involving the bladder, urethra, and clitoris that simulated an intersex problem. The process tends to infiltrate the bladder wall so that on cystoscopy it appears as generalized edema and thickening. The process may be limited to one segment, or the entire bladder may be involved, with reduction in capacity of the bladder and ureteral obstruction. **Myxoma, fibroma, fibromyoma, myoma,** and **dermoid cyst** have all been reported.

Congenital vascular tumors such as **hemangioma** and **lymphangioma** of the bladder are encountered in both children and adults. In 1958 Liang was able to find 51 cases in the literature, approximately half being in the first two decades of life. Associated visceral and cutaneous hemangiomas are present in approximately 25% of cases. Gross hematuria is almost always the presenting symptom. *Cystoscopically* the lesion appears bluish, irregular in outline, sessile, and soft (Litin and associates). The lesions vary greatly in size, from those that are small and discrete to those so large that they extend through the bladder wall with the extravesical projection being larger than the intravesical. Microscopically the lesions are usually of the cavernous variety. If the lesion is large enough it may be demonstrated by a cystogram (Fig. 10–334). Treatment is usually surgical excision, although external irradiation has also been used successfully (Liang).

(Text continued on page 1291.)

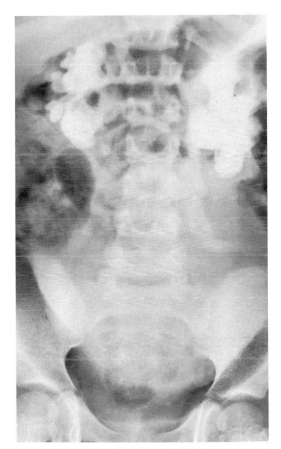

Figure 10–324. *Excretory urogram.* **Botryoid sarcoma of bladder** causing bilateral ureteral obstruction in boy, 5 years of age.

Fig. 10-325

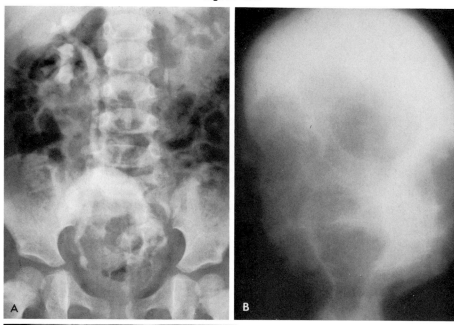

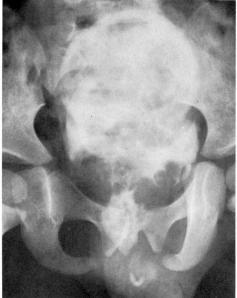

Fig. 10-326

Figure 10-325. Botryoid sarcoma of bladder in girl, 21 months of age. A, *Excretory urogram* showing filling defects from globular masses of tumor. B, *Cystogram* of excised bladder outlining grape-like masses of tumor as radiolucent circular shadows. Two years after operation patient was alive. (Courtesy of Dr. B. A. Smith.)

Figure 10-326. Botryoid sarcoma of bladder in boy, 2 years of age. *Excretory urogram*. Globular filling defects in lower half of bladder from extensive masses of tumor. Eight years after operation patient was alive. (Courtesy of Dr. B. A. Smith.)

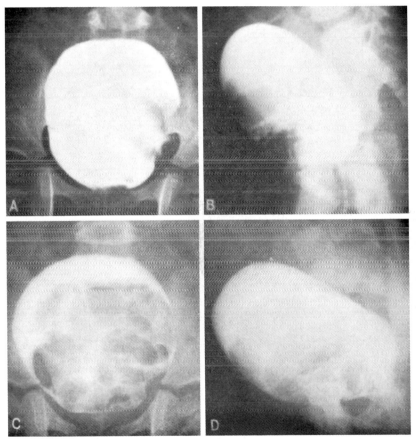

Figure 10–327. *Retrograde cystograms* of boy, 4 years of age, with rapidly growing **sarcoma of bladder.** **A** and **B,** *Anteroposterior* (**A**) *and lateral* (**B**) *views* showing filling defect from lesion. **C** and **D,** Same views 3 weeks later. Note great increase in size of tumor. (From Campbell, M.: Urology in Infancy and Childhood. In Urology, Philadelphia, W. B. Saunders Company, 1954, vol. II, pp. 1431–1665.)

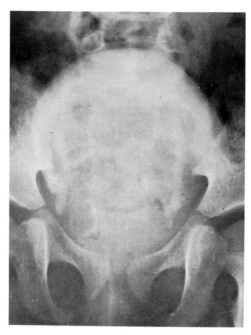

Figure 10–328. Large polypoid rhabdomyosarcoma (sarcoma botryoides) of bladder in girl, 2 years of age. *Cystogram.* Huge filling defect in bladder from tumor. Excretory urogram (not shown) revealed bilateral pyeloureterectasis from ureteral obstruction from tumor. (From Weaver, R. G., Card, R. Y., and Rueb, R. L.)

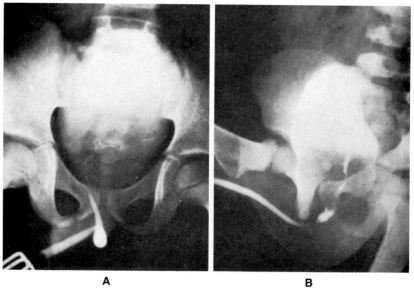

A   B

Figure 10–329. *Retrograde cystogram.* Sarcoma of prostate in boy, 2 years of age. **A,** *Anteroposterior view.* **B,** *Lateral view.* Note great elongation of prostatic urethra with upward displacement of bladder. (From Campbell, M.: Urology in Infancy and Childhood. In Urology, Philadelphia, W. B. Saunders Company, 1954, vol. II, pp. 1431–1665.)

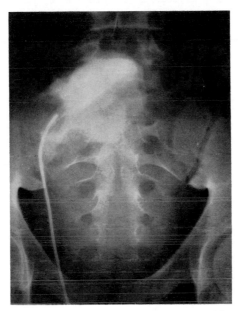

Figure 10–330. *Retrograde cystogram.* Extreme displacement of bladder out of bony pelvis due to large grade 4 malignant neoplasm, **probably sarcoma of prostate gland** in boy aged 15 years.

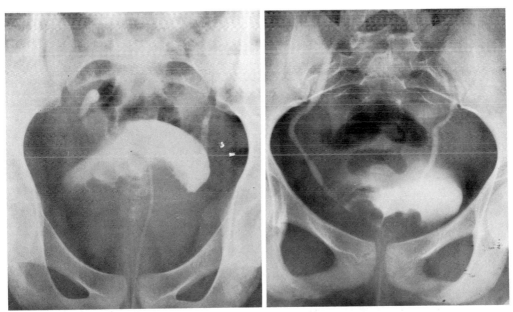

Fig. 10–331   Fig. 10–332

Figure 10–331. *Excretory urogram.* Botryoid (?) sarcoma of bladder neck and prostate in boy, 13 years of age. Marked filling defect in lower half of bladder with typical grape-like defects. No obstruction of ureters. Indwelling urethral catheter.

Figure 10–332. *Excretory urogram.* Botryoid sarcoma of vesical neck with no ureteral obstruction in girl, 15 years of age. Typical globular or grape-like filling defects in lower right half of bladder.

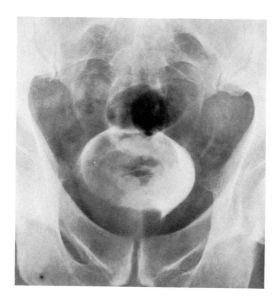

Figure 10–333. *Excretory urogram.* Sarcoma of prostate or bladder neck involving prostate in man, 54 years of age. Pedunculated type of lesion that cystoscopically appeared to be large right intravesical prostatic lobe attached in region of vesical neck at 8 o'clock position (see text for details).

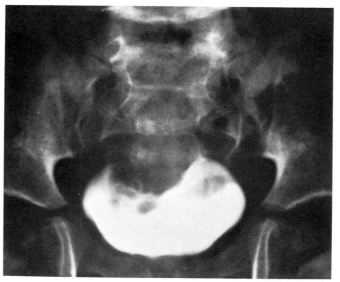

Figure 10–334. *Excretory urogram.* **Hemangioma-lymphangioma of bladder** in 23-month-old boy. Note large irregular filling defects in dome of bladder from tumor. (From Stanley, K. E., Jr.)

TUMORS OF THE URETHRA

Tumors of the Male Urethra
(Figs. 10–335 through 10–338)

Carcinoma

Carcinomas of the male urethra are relatively rare so that few urologists see enough cases to become proficient in their diagnosis and treatment. For this reason, many lesions are missed for varying lengths of time and not diagnosed until relatively late in the course of the disease.

As of 1966, more than 250 cases had been reported (Mandler and Pool). Kaplan, Bulkley, and Grayhack found 232 cases with enough data for evaluation. (They discarded 29 cases because of insufficient data.) At the Mayo Clinic during the 55-year period 1910 through 1964, 62 cases were recorded (Zaslow and Priestley reported 25 cases seen in the period 1910 through 1945; Mandler and Pool found 37 cases seen in the period 1946 through 1964).

In the 232 cases evaluated by Kaplan, Bulkley, and Grayhack the median age was 58 years (range 13 to 82). Between 50% and 60% of the carcinomas were located in the bulbomembranous urethra and approximately one third in the distal (pendulous) urethra. A few were found in the prostatic urethra, but in this location it is always difficult to distinguish a tumor of the bladder that has extended to the prostate from a primary transitional cell epithelioma of the prostate. The majority of urethral tumors are squamous cell epitheliomas (77%, Kaplan, Bulkley, and Grayhack; 67%, Mandler and Pool). The next most common is transitional cell epithelioma, while least common is adenocarcinoma. Almost all malignant lesions in the prostatic urethra are transitional cell epithelioma; almost all the adenocarcinomas are found in the bulb.

As is true of most malignant tumors, etiology is obscure. Kaplan, Bulkley, and Grayhack noted a history of venereal disease in 37% and a history of stricture in 35% of their 232 collected cases. For years it has been considered axiomatic that a stricture may predispose to tumor — that if a long-standing stricture suddenly requires more frequent dilations, the physician should investigate for carcinoma. As one looks at records of such cases, however, it begins to appear that often the primary cause of the "stricture" was a tumor which had been dilated periodically for years. Certainly any unusual characteristic developing in a "stricture," such as increased bleeding following dilation, inadequate relief from dilation, pain in the urethra, hematuria, or grossly bloody urethral discharge, swelling and palpable mass, periurethral "abscess" with spontaneous fistula, or increasing obstruction, should make the physician suspicious. As King stated, "the best means of a correct diagnosis is an investigator alert to the possibility of cancer of the urethra, aided by periodic examination of the Papanicolaou smear of the urinary sediment of patients with urethral stricture." Almost every urologist will be embarrassed at least once in his life from failure to think of the possibility of cancer in a patient that he has been treating for a long time for stricture or inflammatory disease of the urethra. A firm palpable mass may be present before any symptoms appear. The five most common **symptoms and findings** in 232 cases (Kaplan, Bulkley, and Grayhack) were as follows, in decreasing order of frequency: obstruction (47%), palpable mass (39%), periurethral abscess (31%), urethral discharge (22%), urethral fistula (20%). When looking over the histories of patients with urethral carcinoma, one is impressed with how often the diagnosis is "stumbled on" accidentally when the patient's complaints have not caused the physician to even consider the possibility of cancer.

Diagnosis is best made by careful **cystoscopic examination** with a panendoscope and by biopsy. A shaggy, eroded appearance of the area of "stricture" should alert the investigator; biopsy is usually required to be sure. When the biopsy is done cystoscopically it is easy to miss the area in question, thereby missing the diagnosis. Multiple attempts or open biopsy may be necessary. The **urethrogram** (Figs. 10–335 through 10–338) is only an additional help in diagnosis, which should be made by urethroscopy and biopsy.

Prognosis and Treatment. Generally speaking, tumors of the bulbomembranous (and perineal) urethra are more serious and have a much poorer prognosis than do tumors of the anterior (pendulous) urethra. Owing to paucity of experience by any one individual, treatment is far from standardized. At present, however, knowledgeable opinion favors the following:

1. For the pendulous urethra, the penis is removed, with just enough of the corpus spongiosum being saved for use as a perineal urethral stoma (Kaplan, Bulkley, and Grayhack; King; Marshall). Conservative treatment using radium for low-grade localized lesions of the terminal urethra (glans penis) has been advocated by some, but the ensuing radiation stricture makes it difficult to follow and determine whether tumor persists or recurs.

2. For tumors proximal to the penoscrotal junction (perineal urethra, bulbomembranous urethra) radical operation with removal of the penis, entire urethra, scrotum, prostate, and bladder with urinary diversion seems to be the procedure of choice (Kaplan, Bulkley, and Grayhack; King; Marshall). Some authors believe that irradiation may be as effective as radical surgery (Mandler and Pool).

Miscellaneous Tumors of the Urethra

Tumors of the urethra other than carcinoma are exceedingly rare and relatively unimportant. However, lesions such as rhabdomyosarcoma (Painter and associates) and hemangioma (Begley; Tilak), and secondary (metastatic) tumors from lesions of the prostate, bladder, and other organs, are occasionally encountered.

Tumors of the Female Urethra

Tumors of the female urethra do not lend themselves to urographic diagnosis. Careful examination of the urethral meatus, bimanual examination, and cystourethroscopic examination are usually sufficient for diagnosis. This subject has been discussed in detail by Grabstald and associates in a report of their experience with 79 cases at Memorial Hospital. The interested reader is referred to this excellent article. Their report points out that the prognosis is much better in the female than in the male, especially when the lesion is limited to the distal third of the urethra. Irradiation alone or irradiation plus local excision in such cases has proved satisfactory, as metastasis to pelvic and inguinal lymph nodes occurs late in the disease or not at all (Fricke and McMillan; Harrison; Uhle and Kohler).

Tumors other than carcinoma of the urethra are seen very rarely and are of little importance. For instance, Radman reported a pedunculated hemangioma protruding from the meatus which was attached to the urethra by a thin pedicle.

(Text continued on page 1296.)

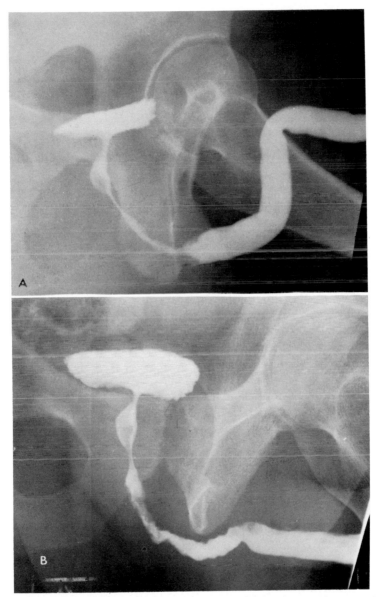

Figure 10–335. Adenocarcinoma of male perineal urethra. **A,** *Retrograde urethrogram.* Man aged 24 who was being treated for stricture of bulbous urethra. Perineal urethra looks like site of typical stricture, but juncture with normal urethra suggests filling defects which could be tumor. Cystoscopic biopsies of this area were reported negative. **B,** *Three months later.* There is now no question of diagnosis. Entire perineal urethra extending from apex of prostate to periscrotal junction is irregular with filling defects from tumor. Cystoscopic biopsy showed adenocarcinoma, grade 2. Patient died of pulmonary metastasis.

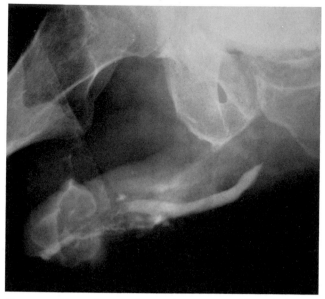

Figure 10–336. *Urethrogram.* **Recurring carcinoma** (squamous cell epithelioma, grade 2) **of pendulous urethra** in man aged 77.

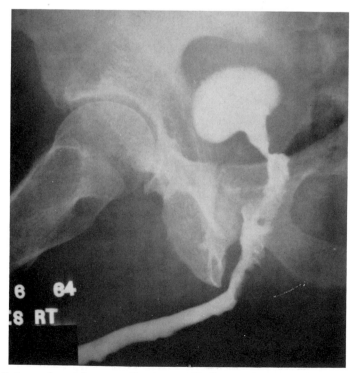

Figure 10–337. *Retrograde urethrogram.* **Carcinoma of bulbomembranous urethra** in man aged 55. Extensive tumor involving most of perineal urethra and extending just into apex of prostate. *Operation.* Radical removal. Infiltrative grade 1 squamous cell epithelioma. Growth penetrates through wall of urethra but does not penetrate perirectal tissue or rectum.

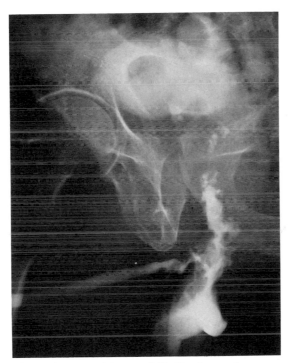

Figure 10–338.   *Retrograde urethrogram.* Man aged 71. Carcinoma (squamous cell epithelioma, grade 4) of bulbomembranous urethra invading prostate and associated with multiple perineal fistula. Contrast medium does not enter bladder. Multiple small prostatic calculi (contrast medium in bladder was from excretory urography done earlier).

TUMORS OF THE SEMINAL VESICLES

(Figs. 10–339 and 10–340)

Tumors of the seminal vesicles appear to be extremely rare. Dalgaard and Giertsen found a total of 34 cases reported up to 1956, but they accepted only 23 as bona fide primary lesions. Smith, Webb, and Price reported 2 cases in 1967 which they stated brought the total number of reported cases to 44, but they also questioned how many of these were primary in the seminal vesicles. Since then, two more cases have been reported (Awadalla, Hunt, and Miller; Hajdu and Faruque). Most authors suspect that the condition may be more common than is appreciated because proof of diagnosis is usually difficult.

Most tumors of the seminal vesicles have proved to be adenocarcinoma of the papillary type; several have been mucus-secreting. Often the lesion is encountered accidentally during transurethral resection (Smith, Webb, and Price), open prostatectomy (Awadalla, Hunt, and Miller), or necropsy (Hajdu and Faruque). Patients in whom the diagnosis has been made or suspected before operation have complained of a wide variety of symptoms such as the passage of grayish-brown chunks of thick gelatin-like material during micturition (Smith, Webb, and Price). Oddly enough, hematospermia has not been a common symptom but intermittent episodes of gross hematuria are usually present. The patient may complain only of irritative and obstructive symptoms that suggest simple prostatic obstruction.

The lesion may be first suspected by digital rectal examination, which may reveal a firm, tense, sausage-shaped mass on one side adjacent to and immediately above the prostate. Often, however, palpation discloses only an irregular, hard, fixed mass that could conceivably be primary cancer of either the prostate or the rectum.

An *excretory urogram* may reveal obstruction to one or both ureters and some asymmetrical and irregular elevation of the base of the bladder.

Cystoscopy may be helpful by revealing unilateral elevation of the trigone, base of the bladder, or vesical neck with evidence of tumor tissue near the verumontanum. In one case (Smith, Webb, and Price) this was described as "tenacious gray material and proliferative epithelium," which was scraped off, revealing a dilated ejaculatory duct. Marshall on two occasions noted blood issuing from the ejaculatory duct.

Seminal vesiculography made by injecting the vas deferens on the suspected side has been helpful in a few cases by demonstrating obliteration, deformity, or a filling defect of one or both vesicles (Figs. 10–339 and 10–340). Apparently extension of the carcinoma to involve the opposite vesicle is relatively common; the ejaculatory duct seems to be involved relatively early in the disease.

The histologic grade of malignancy seems to vary considerably, as some patients with low-grade lesions may go along for years with little evidence of activity or progression while others manifest rapid progression. Metastasis is local, by direct extension to adjacent organs (such as the prostate) or to the pelvic lymph nodes and lungs. Metastasis to bone is uncommon but when it occurs is of the *lytic* type, which is a differential point in distinguishing primary cancer of the prostate wherein bony metastasis is common and of the *blastic* type.

Differential diagnosis must include, in addition to carcinoma of the prostate, inflammatory lesions of the seminal vesicle and sigmoid colon, müllerian duct cyst, cyst of the seminal vesicle, and tumors of the rectovesical septum.

Surgical excision, including removal of the prostate, appears to be the treatment of choice. Operation is usually done suprapubically or retropubically. Several apparent "cures" have been reported

(Ewell; Smith). Rodriguez Kees reported dramatic response to estrogen (10 mg of stilbestrol daily) by a patient whose tumor had recurred after partial surgical removal; irradiation was of no help and lung metastasis developed which disappeared after estrogen therapy was instituted.

TUMORS OF THE PROSTATE

Benign Adenofibromatous Hyperplasia and Carcinoma

This subject has been considered in Chapter 5 (pages 562 and 563). Although cystourethrography is used rather extensively in some urologic clinics in the diagnosis of this condition, at the Mayo Clinic we have never considered it a practical or economical method when simpler methods are available for diagnosis.

In **carcinoma of the prostate**, the plain film is of great importance in detecting osteoplastic metastasis, which is almost pathognomonic of this lesion (see discussion, Chapter 3, Figs. 3-202 through 3-218). The response of pulmonary metastasis to treatment of carcinoma is occasionally quite dramatic.

Sarcoma

This subject is considered above in this chapter under the heading "Nonepithelial Tumors (Sarcoma of the Bladder and Prostate; Botryoid Sarcoma, etc.)."

TUMORS OF THE TESTES
(Figs. 10–341 to 10–344)

Malignant neoplasms of the testes are of urographic interest only when they metastasize. Metastatic involvement of lymph nodes, when present, usually is found (1) along the iliac vessels (proximal to the junction of the upper and middle thirds) and (2) along the aorta and vena cava to a point approximately 2 cm above the renal pedicles. A large region on each side of the great vessels also may be involved (see "Lymphography" Chapter 19, pages 2027–2028, Figs. 19–12, 19–13, 19–15, 19–19, and 19–20). Obviously, enlarged lymph nodes in these regions can encroach on, displace, or obstruct either ureter, and by so doing produce ureteropyelectasis of varying degree or absence of ureteral visualization in the urogram. This situation does occur not infrequently (Figs. 10–341 through 10–344).

(References begin on page 1301.)

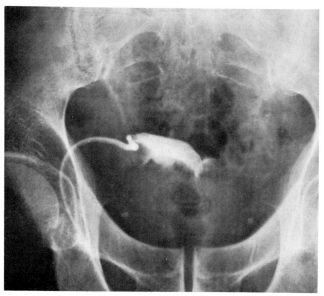

Figure 10–339. *Right seminal vesiculogram.* **Adenocarcinoma of seminal vesicle.** Note bizarre collection of contrast medium with no normal vesicular pattern. (From Smith, B. A., Jr., Webb, E. A., and Price, W. E.)

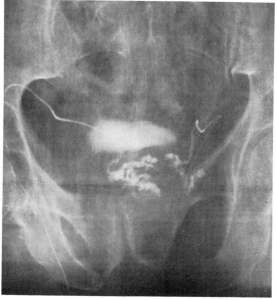

Figure 10–340. **Carcinoma of left seminal vesicle** in man aged 74. Right vas only was injected with contrast medium yet both vasa are outlined. Note large filling defect in left vesicle and displacement and deformity of right. At operation, right vas and vesicle were fused together and were involved from extension of tumor from left vesicle. Metastatically involved nodes are present at bifurcation of each common iliac artery. (From Smith, B. A., Jr., Webb, E. A., and Price, W. E.)

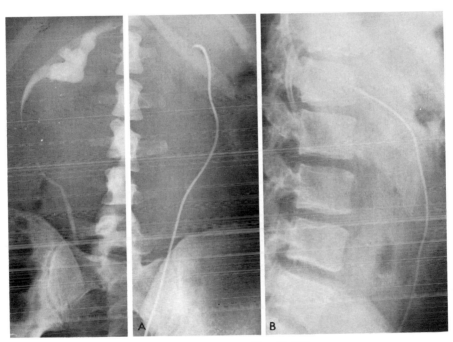

Fig. 10–341   Fig. 10–342

Figure 10–341. Testicular tumor with abdominal metastasis. *Excretory urogram.* Marked lateral displacement of right ureter and lateral and upward displacement of right kidney from enlargement of retroperitoneal nodes due to metastasis from grade 3 adenocarcinoma of right testis.

Figure 10–342. Testicular tumor with obstruction and displacement of left ureter and kidney from enlarged metastatic periaortic lymph nodes. An excretory urogram showed marked delay in visualization of left kidney, with hydronephrosis. **A,** *Plain film, anteroposterior view.* Opaque catheter shows lateral displacement of left ureter. **B,** *Lateral view* shows that ureter has been displaced anteriorly from enlarged retroperitoneal nodes.

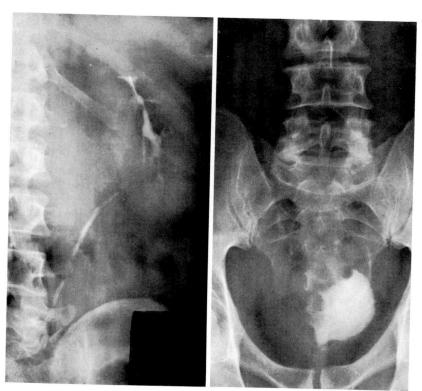

Fig. 10–343   Fig. 10–344

Figure 10–343.   Testicular tumor with metastasis. *Excretory urogram.* Lateral displacement of left kidney and ureter from enlargement of retroperitoneal nodes, due to metastasis from tumor of left testis.

Figure 10–344.   Testicular tumor with metastasis. *Excretory urogram.* Extensive and unusual type of metastasis to pelvis from testicular tumor. Metastatic mass displaces bladder to left of midline. Testicular tumor had been removed 3 years previously elsewhere. (Results of microscopic examination not available.) Excretory urogram did not show any obstruction to upper part of urinary tract on either side.

REFERENCES

Tumors of the Renal Cortex

Abrams, H. L., Boijsen, E., and Borgström, K.-E.: Effect of Epinephrine on the Renal Circulation: Angiographic Observations. Radiology 79:911-922 (Dec.) 1962.

Addison, N. V., and Peach, B.: Smooth Muscle Tumours of the Kidney: (Report on Two Cases). Brit. J. Urol. 38:382-387 (Aug.) 1966.

Anderson, W. A. D.: Pathology. Ed. 3, St. Louis, C. V. Mosby Company, 1957, 1402 pp.

Apitz, K.: Die Geschwülste und Gewebsmissbildungen der Nierenrinde: Die intrarenalen Nebenniereninseln. Arch. path. Anat. 311:285-305, 1943.

Appel, S. D., and Schoenberg, H. W.: Myxoma of the Renal Sinus. J. Urol. 100:254-256 (Sept.) 1968.

Bailey, O. T., and Harrison, J. H.: Large Benign Renal Neoplasms: Their Pathology and Clinical Behavior, With Report of Five Cases. J. Urol. 38:509-529 (Dec.) 1937.

Bauer, F. C., Jr., Murray, D. E., and Hirsch, E. F.: Solitary Adenoma of the Kidney. J. Urol. 79:377-382 (Mar.) 1958.

Bazaz-Malik, G., and Gupta, D. N.: Leiomyosarcoma of Kidney: Report of a Case and Review of the Literature. J. Urol. 95:754-758 (June) 1966.

Becker, J. A., Fleming, R., Kanter, I., and Melicow, M.: Misleading Appearances in Renal Angiography. Radiology 88:691-700 (Apr.) 1967.

Boijsen, E., and Folin, J.: Angiography in the Diagnosis of Renal Carcinoma. Radiologe 1:173-191, 1961.

Bosniak, M. A., and Faegenburg, D.: The Thick-Wall Sign: An Important Finding in Nephrotomography. Radiology 84:692-698 (Apr.) 1965.

Chynn, K. Y., and Evans, J. A.: Nephrotomography in the Differentiation of Renal Cyst From Neoplasm: A Review of 500 Cases. J. Urol. 83:21-24 (Jan.) 1960.

Colvin, S. H., Jr.: Certain Capsular and Subcapsular Mixed Tumors of the Kidney Herein Called "Capsuloma." J. Urol. 48:585-600 (Dec.) 1942.

Creevy, C. D.: Adenoma of the Kidney: Report of a Case With a Discussion of Its Relationship to Carcinoma (Hypernephroma). Am. J. Cancer 15:2309-2318, 1931.

Cristol, D. S., McDonald, J. R., and Emmett, J. L.: Renal Adenomas in Hypernephromatous Kidneys: A Study of Their Incidence, Nature and Relationship. J. Urol. 55:18-27 (Jan.) 1946.

Demel, R.: Nierentumoren. Beitr. klin. Chir. 158:527-557, 1933.

deVeer, J. A., and Hamm, F. C.: Tumors of the Kidney. I. Adenomas and Carcinomas Derived From Renal Parenchyma. II. Tumors Derived From Epithelium of the Renal Pelvis and Compounded Tumors Derived From Epithelium of Renal Pelvis and Parenchyma. Brooklyn Hosp. J. 8:53-84; 187-222, 1950.

Dubilier, W., Jr., and Evans, J. A.: Peripelvic Cysts of the Kidney. Radiology 71:404-408 (Sept.) 1958.

Emmett, J. L., Levine, S. R., and Woolner, L. B.: Coexistence of Renal Cyst and Tumour: Incidence in 1,007 Cases. Brit. J. Urol. 35:403-410 (Dec.) 1963.

Evans, J. A.: Nephrotomography in the Investigation of Renal Masses. Radiology 69:684-689 (Nov.) 1957.

Evans, J. A., Dubilier, W., Jr., and Monteith, J. C.: Nephrotomography: A Preliminary Report. Am. J. Roentgenol. 71:213-223 (Feb.) 1954.

Evans, J. A., Monteith, J. C., and Dubilier, W., Jr.: Nephrotomography. Radiology 64:655-663 (May) 1955.

Evans, J. A., and Poker, N.: Newer Roentgenographic Techniques in the Diagnosis of Retroperitoneal Tumors. J.A.M.A. 161:1128-1132 (July 21) 1956.

Ferris, E. J., Bosniak, M. A., and O'Connor, J. F.: An Angiographic Sign Demonstrating Extension of Renal Carcinoma Into the Renal Vein and Vena Cava. Am. J. Roentgenol. 102:384-391 (Feb.) 1968.

Folin, J.: Angiography in Renal Tumours: Its Value in Diagnosis and Differential Diagnosis as a Complement to Conventional Methods. Acta radiol., Suppl. 267, 1967, pp. 1-96.

Foster, D. G.: Large Benign Renal Tumors: A Review of the Literature and Report of a Case in Childhood. J. Urol. 76:231-243 (Sept.) 1956.

Freund, M. E., Crocker, Diane W., and Harrison, J. H.: Neurofibroma Arising in a Solitary Kidney. J. Urol. 98:318-321 (Sept.) 1967.

Fuchsman, J. J., and Angrist, A.: Benign Renal Tumors. J. Urol. 59:167-173 (Feb.) 1948.

Gall, E. A., and Mallory, T. B.: Malignant Lymphoma: Clinico-pathologic Survey of 618 Cases. Am. J. Path. 18:381-415 (May) 1942.

Gibson, T. E.: Lymphosarcoma of the Kidney. J. Urol. 60:838-854 (Dec.) 1948.

Gillies, C. L.: Malignant Tumors of the Kidney in Adults. Am. J. Roentgenol. 43:629-635 (May) 1940.

Gordon-Taylor, G.: Gigantic Benign Tumor of the Kidney Weighing 22 Pounds. Nephrectomy: Cure. Brit. J. Surg. 17:551-554 (Jan.) 1930.

Gowdey, J. F., and Neuhauser, E. B. D.: The Roentgen Diagnosis of Diffuse Leukemic Infiltration of the Kidneys in Children. Am. J. Roentgenol. 60:13-21 (July) 1948.

Grawitz, P.: Die sogenannten Lipome der Niere. Arch. path. Anat. 93:39-63, 1883.

Greene, L. F., and Rosenthal, M. H.: Multiple Hypernephromas of the Kidney in Association With Lindau's Disease. New England J. Med. 244:633-634, 1951.

Gruenwald, P.: The Interpretation of Certain Pathological Conditions of the Urogenital Tract on the Basis of Recent Advances in Embryology. Urol. & Cutan. Rev. 47:307-320 (Apr.) 1943.

Herbut, P. A.: Urologic Pathology. Philadelphia, Lea & Febiger, 1952, vol. 1, pp. 591-605.

Judd, E. S., and Simon, H. E.: Angioma of the Kidney. Surg., Gynec. & Obst. 46:711-713 (May) 1928.

Kahn, P. C., and Wise, H. M., Jr.: The Use of Epinephrine in Selective Angiography of Renal Masses. J. Urol. 99:133-138 (Feb.) 1968.

Kaplan, C., Sayre, G. P., and Greene, L. F.: Bilateral Nephrogenic Carcinomas in Lindau-von Hippel Disease. J. Urol. 86:36-42 (July) 1961.

Kernohan, J. W., Woltman, H. W., and Adson, A. W.: Intramedullary Tumors of the Spinal Cord: A Review of Fifty-one Cases, With Attempt at Histologic Classification. Arch. Neurol. & Psychiat. 25:679-699, 1931.

Khorsand, D.: Carcinoma Within Solitary Renal Cysts. J. Urol. 93:440-444 (Apr.) 1965.

Kincaid, O. W.: Renal Angiography. Chicago, Year Book Medical Publishers, Inc., 1966, 275 pp.

Klinger, M. E.: Secondary Tumors of the Genitourinary Tract. J. Urol. 65:144-153 (Jan.) 1951.

Klotz, P. G.: Hypernephroma in a Solitary Kidney Treated by Partial Nephrectomy: A Case Report. J. Urol. 84:456-459 (Sept.) 1960.

Kozoll, D. D., and Kirshbaum, J. D.: Relationship of Benign and Malignant Hypernephroid Tumors of Kidney: Clinical and Pathological Study of 77 Cases in 12,885 Necropsies. J. Urol. 44:435-449 (Oct.) 1940.

Levine, S. R., Witten, D. M., and Greene, L. F.: Nephrotomography in Lindau–Von Hippel's Disease. J. Urol. 93:660-662 (June) 1965.

Lindau, A.: Studien über Kleinhirncysten: Bau, Pathogenese und Beziehungen zur Angiomatosis Retinae. Acta path. et microbiol. scandinav. Suppl. 1, 1926, pp. 1-128.

Lucké, B., and Schlumberger, H. G.: Tumors of the Kidney, Renal Pelvis and Ureter. Atlas of Tumor Pathology, Armed Forces Institute of Pathology, Washington, D.C., 1957, Section 8, Fascicle 30, 208 pp.

Martínez-Maldonado, M., and Ramírez de Arellano, G. A.: Renal Involvement in Malignant Lymphomas: A Survey of 49 Cases. J. Urol. 95:485-488 (Apr.) 1966.

McDonald, J. R., and Priestley, J. T.: Malignant Tumors of the Kidney: Surgical and Prognostic Significance of Tumor Thrombosis of the Renal Vein. Surg., Gynec. & Obst. 77:295-306 (Sept.) 1943.

Newcomb, W. D.: The Search for Truth, With Special Reference to the Frequency of Gastric Ulcer — Cancer and the Origin of Grawitz Tumours of the Kidney. Proc. Roy. Soc. Med. 30:113-136 (Oct. 13) 1937.

Newsam, J. E., and Tulloch, W. S.: Metastatic Tumours in the Kidney. Brit. J. Urol. 38:1-6, 1966.

Olsson, O.: Angiography in Kidney Masses. In Viamonte, M., Jr., and Parks, R. E.: Progress in Angiography. Springfield, Illinois, Charles C Thomas, Publisher, 1964, pp. 314-345.

Park, W. W., and Lees, J. C.: Choriocarcinoma: A General Review, With an Analysis of Five Hundred Sixteen Cases. Arch. Path. 49:73-104 (Jan.) 1950.

Patrick, C. E., Norton, J. H., and Dacso, M. R.: Choriocarcinoma in Kidney: Case Report. J. Urol. 97:444-448 (Mar.) 1967.

Pease, G. L., and McDonald, J. R.: Lymphoblastomatous Involvement of Nonlymphoid Organs. Am. J. Clin. Path. 17:181-196 (Mar.) 1947.

Rabinowitz, J. G., Wolf, B. S., and Goldman, R. H.: Roentgen Features of Renal Adenomas. Radiology 84:263-269 (Feb.) 1965.

Rappoport, A. E.: Hematuria due to Papillary Hemangioma of the Renal Pelvis. Arch. Path. 40:84-87 (Aug.) 1945.

Riches, E. W., Griffiths, I. H., and Thackray, A. C.: New Growths of the Kidney and Ureter. Brit. J. Urol. 23:297-356 (Dec.) 1951.

Richmond, J., Sherman, R. S., Diamond, H. D., and Craver, L. F.: Renal Lesions Associated With Malignant Lymphomas. Am. J. Med. 32:184-207 (Feb.) 1962.

Ridlon, H. C., and McAdams, G. B.: Breast Carcinoma Metastatic to Kidney. J. Urol. 98:328-330 (Sept.) 1967.

Riley, A., and Swann, W. J., Jr.: Angioma of the Kidney. Urol. & Cutan. Rev. 45:377-382 (June) 1941.

Rives, H. F., and Pool, T. L.: Hemangioma of the Kidney. J.A.M.A. 125:1187-1188 (Aug. 26) 1944.

Robertson, T. D., and Hand, J. R.: Primary Intrarenal Lipoma of Surgical Significance. J. Urol. 46:458-474 (Sept.) 1941.

Seltzer, R. A., and Wenlund, D. E.: Renal Lymphoma: Arteriographic Studies. Am. J. Roentgenol. 101:692-695 (Nov.) 1967.

Shapiro, J. H., Ramsay, C. G., Jacobson, H. G., Botstein, C. C., and Allen, L. B.: Renal Involvement in Lymphomas and Leukemias in Adults. Am. J. Roentgenol. 88:928-941 (Nov.) 1962.

Simon, H. E.: Benign Tumors of the Kidney. South. Surgeon 2:67-73 (Mar.) 1933.

Simpson, W.: Curvilinear Calcification in Renal Carcinomata. Brit. J. Urol. 38:129-132 (Apr.) 1966.

Southwood, W. F. W., and Marshall, V. G.: A Clinical Evaluation of Nephrotomography. Brit. J. Urol. 30:127-141, 1958.

Spillane, R. J., Singiser, J. A., and Prather, G. C.: Fibromyxolipoma of the Kidney. J. Urol. 68:811-814 (Nov.) 1952.

Stout, A. P.: Hemangiopericytoma, a Study of Twenty-five New Cases. Cancer 2:1027-1054 (Nov.) 1949.

Stout, A. P., and Murray, M. R.: Hemangiopericytoma: Vascular Tumor Featuring Zimmerman's Pericytes. Ann. Surg. 116:26-33 (July) 1942.

Symmers, D.: Lymphoid Diseases: Hodgkin's Granuloma, Giant Follicular Lymphadenopathy, Lymphoid Leukemia, Lymphosarcoma and Gastrointestinal Pseudoleukemia. Arch. Path. 45:73-131 (Jan.) 1948.

Tahara, C., and Hess, E.: Massive Renal Fibrolipoma: Report of 2 Cases. J. Urol. 54:107-115 (Aug.) 1945.

Thompson, G. J., and Culp, O. S.: Perplexing Cystic Masses Near the Kidney. J. Urol. 89:370-376 (Mar.) 1963.

Villegas, A. C.: Bilateral Primary Malignant Renal Tumors of Dissimilar Histogenesis: Report of 2 Cases and Review of the Literature. J. Urol. 98:450-455 (Oct.) 1967.

von Hippel, E.: Die anatomische Grundlage der von mir Beschriebenen "sehr seltenen Erkrankung der Netzhaut." von Graefes Arch. Ophth. 79:350-377, 1911.

Walker, G.: Sarcoma of the Kidney in Children: A Critical Review of the Pathology, Symptomatology, Prognosis and Operative Treatment as Seen in One Hundred and Forty-five Cases. Ann. Surg. 26:529-602, 1897.

Watson, E. M., Sauer, H. R., and Sadugor, M. G.: Manifestations of the Lymphoblastomas in the Genito-urinary Tract. J. Urol. 61:626-642 (Mar.) 1949.

Watson, R. C., Fleming, R. J., and Evans, J. A.: Arteriography in the Diagnosis of Renal Carcinoma: Review of 100 Cases. Radiology 91:888-897 (Nov.) 1968.

Weisel, W., Dockerty, M. B., and Priestley, J. T.: Sarcoma of the Kidney. J. Urol. 50:564-573 (Nov.) 1943.

Witten, D. M., Greene, L. F., and Emmett, J. L.: An Evaluation of Nephrotomography in Urologic Patients. Am. J. Roentgenol. 90:115-123 (July) 1963.

Hamartoma and Tuberous Sclerosis

Adelman, B. P.: Angiomyolipoma of the Kidney. Am. J. Roentgenol. 95:403-405 (Oct.) 1965.

Albrecht-München: Ueber Hamartome. Verhandl. deutsch. Gesellsch. inn. Med. 7:153-157, 1904.

Allen, T. D., and Risk, W.: Renal Angiomyolipoma. J. Urol. 94:203-207 (Sept.) 1965.

Beck, R. E., and Hammond, R. C.: Renal and Osseous Manifestations of Tuberous Sclerosis: Case Report. J. Urol. 77:578-582 (Apr.) 1957.

Bell, E. T.: Renal Diseases Philadelphia, Lea & Febiger, 1946, 434 pp.

Bernstein, L., and Pitegoff, G. I.: Tuberous Sclerosis: Two Cases of Subtentorial Calcification. Connecticut M. J. 15:1051-1057 (Nov.) 1951.

Boggs, L. K., and Kimmelstiel, P.: Benign Multilocular Cystic Nephroma: Report of Two Cases of So-called Multilocular Cyst of the Kidney. J. Urol. 76:530-541 (Nov.) 1956.

Bourneville, D. M.: Contributions à l'étude de l'idiotie: Sclérose tubéreuse des circonvolutions cérébrales, idiotie et épilepsie hémiplegique. Arch. de neurol. 1:81-91, 1880.

Dickerson, W. W.: Familial Occurrence of Tuberous Sclerosis. A.M.A. Arch. Neurol. & Psychiat. 65:683-702 (June) 1951.

Golji, H.: Tuberous Sclerosis and Renal Neoplasms. J. Urol. 85:919-923 (June) 1961.

Heckel, N. J., and Penick, G. D.: A Mixed Tumor of the Kidney: Lipomyo-hemangioma. J. Urol. 59:572-576 (Apr.) 1948.

Holt, J. F., and Dickerson, W. W.: The Osseous Lesions of Tuberous Sclerosis. Radiology 58:1-7 (Jan.) 1952.

Inglis, K.: Relation of Renal Lesions to Cerebral Lesions in Tuberous Sclerosis Complex. Am. J. Path. 30:739-755 (July-Aug.) 1954.

Keshin, J. G.: Three Cases of Renal Hamartoma: Two Cases Presenting With Spontaneous Rupture and Massive Retroperitoneal Hemorrhage. J. Urol. 94:336-341 (Oct.) 1965.

Khilnani, M. T., and Wolf, B. S.: Hamartolipoma of the Kidney: Clinical and Roentgen Features. Am. J. Roentgenol. 86:830-841 (Nov.) 1961.

Klapproth, H. J., Poutasse, E. F., and Hazard, J. B.: Renal Angiomyolipomas: Report of Four Cases. A.M.A. Arch. Path. 67:400-411 (Apr.) 1959.

Love, L., and Frank, Stasia J.: Angiographic Features of Angiomyolipoma of the Kidney. Am. J. Roentgenol. 95:406-408 (Oct.) 1965.

Moolten, S. E.: Hamartial Nature of the Tuberous Sclerosis Complex and Its Bearing on the Tumor Problem: Report of a Case With Tumor Anomaly of the Kidney and Adenoma Sebaceum. Arch. Int. Med. 69:589-623 (Apr.) 1942.

Morgan, G. S., Straumfjord, J. V., and Hall, E. J.: Angiomyolipoma of the Kidney. J. Urol. 65:525-527 (Apr.) 1951.

Price, E. B., Jr., and Mostofi, F. K.: Symptomatic Angiomyolipoma of the Kidney. Cancer 18:761-774 (June) 1965.

Rusche, C.: Renal Hamartoma (Angiomyolipoma): Report of 3 Cases. J. Urol. 67:823-831 (June) 1952.

Seabury, J. C., Jr., Ensor, R. D., and Wolfe, W. G.: Angiomyolipoma of the Kidney: A Benign Tumor Demonstrating Neo-vascularization by Arteriography; Report of 2 Cases. J. Urol. 98:562-565 (Nov.) 1967.

Taylor, J. N., and Genters, K.: Renal Angiomyolipoma and Tuberous Sclerosis. J. Urol. 79:685-696 (Apr.) 1958.

Wechsler, I. S.: A Textbook of Clinical Neurology: With an Introduction to the History of Neurology. Ed. 6, Philadelphia, W. B. Saunders Company, 1947, pp. 571-572.

Tumors of the Renal Pelvis and Ureter

Abeshouse, B. S.: Primary Benign and Malignant Tumors of the Ureter. Am. J. Surg. 91:237-271 (Feb.) 1956.

Ackerman, L. V.: Mucinous Adenocarcinoma of the Pelvis of the Kidney. J. Urol. 55:36-45 (Jan.) 1946.

Alznauer, R. L.: Leiomyosarcoma of Right Ureter: Report of Case. Arch. Path. 59:94-99 (Jan.) 1955.

Anderson, J. B., Lee, J. J., Hancock, R. A., and Black, S. R.: Hemangioma of the Kidney Pelvis. J. Urol. 70:869-873 (Dec.) 1953.

Auerbach, S., Lewis, H. Y., and McDonald, J. R.: Recurrent Polypoid Hamartoma and Epithelial Cell Nests in the Ureter and Renal Pelvis of an Adolescent. J. Urol. 95:691-696 (May) 1966.

Barroso, C. H., Jr., Florence, T. J., and Scott, C., Jr.: Bilateral Papillary Carcinomas of the Ureters: Presentation of a Case and 2-Year Followup Report. J. Urol. 96:451-454 (Oct.) 1966.

Bergman, H., Friedenberg, R. M., and Sayegh, V.: New Roentgenologic Signs of Carcinoma of the Ureter. Am. J. Roentgenol. 86:707-717 (Oct.) 1961.

Brock, D. R.: Benign Polyp of Ureter. J. Urol. 83:572-574 (May) 1960.

Brodny, M. L., and Hershman, H.: Pedunculated Hemangioma of the Ureter. J. Urol. 71:539-543 (May) 1954.

Bustos, F., Lichtwardt, J. R., and Lichtwardt, H. E.: Benign Non-epithelial Tumors of the Ureter. J. Urol. (In press.)

Charlton, C. A. C., and Richardson, W. W.: Squamous Cell Carcinoma of an Ectopic Kidney With Staghorn Calculus: Case Report. Brit. J. Urol. 38:428-431, 1966.

Colston, J. A., Sr.: Followup Report on a Case of Bilateral Papillary Carcinoma of Renal Pelvis. J. Urol. 83:355-359 (Apr.) 1960.

Colston, J. A. C., and Arcadi, J. A.: Bilateral Renal Papillomas: Transpelvic Electro-resection With Preservation of Kidney. Contralateral Nephrectomy: 4-Year Survival. Tr. Am. A. Genito.-Urin. Surg. 46:134-141, 1954.

Compere, D. E., Begley, G. F., Isaacks, H. E., Frazier, T. H., and Dryden, C. B.: Ureteral Polyps. J. Urol. 79:209-214 (Feb.) 1958.

Cooney, C. J.: Fibroma of the Ureter. J. Urol. 47:651-657 (May) 1942.

Crassweller, P. O.: Bilateral Primary Carcinoma of the Ureter With Use of Ileal Graft for Ureteral Replacement: Case Report. Brit. J. Urol. 3:152-160, 1958.

Culp, O. S.: Treatment of Tumors of the Renal Pelvis and Ureter. Tr. Am. A. Genito.-Urin. Surg. 47:101-112, 1955.

Das Gupta, T., and Grabstald, H.: Melanoma of the Genitourinary Tract. J. Urol. 93:607-614 (May) 1965.

D'Aunoy, R., and Zoeller, A.: Primary Carcinoma of the Ureter: Report of a Case and Review of the Literature. Arch. Path. 9:17-30 (Jan.) 1930.

Evans, A. T., and Stevens, R. K.: Fibroepithelial Polyps of Ureter and Renal Pelvis: A Case Report. J. Urol. 86:313-315 (Sept.) 1961.

Fein, R. L., and Hamm, F. C.: Hemangiosarcoma of the Ureter: A Case Report. J. Urol. 93:684-686 (June) 1965a.

Fein, R. L., and Hamm, F. C.: Malignant Schwannoma of the Renal Pelvis: A Review of the Literature and a Case Report. J. Urol. 94:356-361 (Oct.) 1965b.

Felber, E.: Asynchronous Bilateral Benign Papilloma of the Ureter With Subsequent Cancer of Ureteral Stump, Bladder and Vagina. J.M.A. Georgia 42:198-200 (Apr.) 1953.

Forssman, W.: Fibromatöser Ureterpolyp. Ztschr. Urol. 44:708-710, 1951.

Gaca, A.: Das doppelseitige papilläre Harnleiterkarzinom. Ztschr. Urol. 53:261-265 (May) 1960.

Gahagan, H. Q., and Reed, W. K.: Squamous Cell Carcinoma of the Renal Pelvis: Three Case Reports and Review of the Literature. J. Urol. 62:139-151 (Aug.) 1949.

Galbraith, W. W.: Pedunculated Vascular Tumour of the Ureter. Brit. J. Urol. 22:195-200 (Sept.) 1950.

Gilbert, J. B., and MacMillan, S. F.: Cancer of Kidney: Squamous-Cell Carcinoma of the Renal Pelvis With Special Reference to Etiology. Ann. Surg. 100:429-444 (Sept.) 1934.

Grace, D. A., Taylor, W. N., Taylor, J. N., and Winter, C. C.: Carcinoma of the Renal Pelvis: A 15-Year Review. J. Urol. 98:566-569 (Nov.) 1967.

Gracia, V., and Bradfield, E. O.: Simultaneous Bilateral Transitional Cell Carcinoma of the Ureter: A Case Report. J. Urol. 79:925-928 (June) 1958.

Harbaugh, J. T.: Botryoid Sarcoma of the Renal Pelvis: A Case Report. J. Urol. 100:424-426 (Oct.) 1968.

Heslin, J. E., Milner, W. A., and Garlick, W. B.: Lower Urinary Tract Implants or Metastases From Clear Cell Carcinoma of the Kidney. J. Urol. 73:39-46 (Jan.) 1955.

Hovenanian, M. S.: Implantation of Renal Parenchymal Carcinoma. J. Urol. 64:188-192 (Aug.) 1950.

Howard, T. L.: Giant Polyp of Ureter. J. Urol. 79:397-402 (Mar.) 1958.

Howell, R. D.: Ureteral Implantation of Renal Adenocarcinoma. J. Urol. 66:561-564 (Oct.) 1951.

Immergut, S., and Cottler, Z. R.: Intrapelvic Fibroma. J. Urol. 66:673-676 (Nov.) 1951.

Kaplan, J. H., McDonald, J. R., and Thompson, G. J.: Multicentric Origin of Papillary Tumors of the Urinary Tract. J. Urol. 66:792-804 (Dec.) 1951.

Klinger, M. E.: Secondary Tumors of the Genitourinary Tract. J. Urol. 65:144-153 (Jan.) 1951.

Kraus, J. E.: Primary Sarcoma of the Ureter. Urol. & Cutan. Rev. 48:522-525 (Nov.) 1944.

MacAlpine, J. B.: Implantation of Secondaries From a Renal Carcinoma (Hypernephroma) Within the Ureteric Lumen. Brit. J. Surg. 36:164-168 (Oct.) 1948.

McCrea, L. E., and Peale, A. R.: Metastatic Carcinoma to the Ureter. Urol. & Cutan. Rev. 55:11-22 (Jan.) 1951.

McDonald, J. R., and Priestley, J. T.: Carcinoma of the Renal Pelvis: Histopathologic Study of Seventy-five Cases With Special Reference to Prognosis. J. Urol. 51:245-258 (Mar.) 1944.

Mirabile, C. S., and Spillane, R. J.: Metastatic Adenocarcinoma of the Ureter With Obstruction: Case Report. J. Urol. 70:187-190 (Aug.) 1953.

Newman, D. M., Allen, L. E., Wishard, W. N., Jr., Nourse, M. H., and Mertz, J. H. O.: Transitional Cell Carcinoma of the Upper Urinary Tract. J. Urol. 98:322-327 (Sept.) 1967.

Palmer, J. K., and Greene, L. F.: Benign Fibromucous Polyp of the Ureter: Report of a Case. Surgery 22:562-565 (Sept.) 1947.

Perlmutter, A. D., Retik, A. B., and Harrison, J. H.: Simultaneous Bilateral Carcinoma of the Ureter Present for Five Years Before Surgery. J. Urol. 93:582-587 (May) 1965.

Plaut, A.: Diffuses dickdarmähnliches Adenom des Nierenbeckens mit geschwulstartiger Wucherung von Gefässmuskulatur. Ztschr. f. Urol. Chir. 26:562-578, 1929.

Porras, E.: Metastatic Carcinoma of the Ureter: Case Report. Urol. & Cutan. Rev. 55:141-144 (Mar.) 1951.

Potampa, P. B., and Schneider, I. J.: Bilateral True Primary Papillary Carcinoma of Kidneys. J. Urol. 86:522-524 (Nov.) 1961.

Presman, D. A., and Ehrlich, L.: Metastatic Tumors of the Ureter. J. Urol. 59:312-325 (Mar.) 1948.

Putschar, W. G. J., and Irwin, G. G.: Pancreatic Carcinoma Involving Urinary Tract: Report of Two Autopsy Cases. Urol. & Cutan. Rev. 48:544-548 (Nov.) 1944.

Rademaker, L.: Primary Sarcoma of the Ureter: Case Report and Review of the Literature. Am. J. Surg. n.s. 62:402-406 (Dec.) 1943.

Ragins, A. B., and Rolnick, H. C.: Mucus Producing Adenocarcinoma of the Renal Pelvis. J. Urol. 63:66-73 (Jan.) 1950.

Ratliff, R. K., Banum, W. C., and Butler, W. J.: Bilateral Primary Carcinoma of the Ureter: A Case Report. Cancer 2:815-818 (Sept.) 1949.

Ravich, A.: Neurofibroma of the Ureter: Report of a Case With Operation and Recovery. Arch. Surg. 30:442-448 (Mar.) 1935.

Renner, M. J.: Primary Malignant Tumors of the Ureter. Surg., Gynec. & Obst. 52:793-803 (Apr.) 1931.

Robbins, J. J., and Lich, R., Jr.: Metastatic Carcinoma of the Ureter. J. Urol. 75:242-243 (Feb.) 1956.

Roen, P. R., and Kandalaft, S.: Primary Benign Mesodermal Ureteral Tumor. J. Urol. 96:890-891 (Dec.) 1966.

Rossien, A. X., and Russell, T. H.: Leiomyosarcoma

Involving the Right Ureter. Arch. Path. *41*:655-660 (June) 1946.

Samellas, W., and Marks, A. R.: Metastatic Melanoma of the Urinary Tract. J. Urol. 85:21-23 (Jan.) 1961.

Schneiderman, C., Simon, M., and Sedlezky, I.: Benign Polyp of the Ureter. Brit. J. Urol. *31*:168-175 (June) 1959.

Senger, F. L., and Furey, C. A., Jr.: Primary Ureteral Tumors With a Review of the Literature Since 1943. J. Urol. 69:243-258 (Feb.) 1953.

Stearns, D. B., Farmer, D. A., and Gordon, S. K.: Ureteral Metastasis Secondary to Gastric Carcinoma: Case Report. J. Urol. *80*:214-217 (Oct.) 1958.

Stone, F. D., and Baer, R. A.: Personal communication to Lucké and Schlumberger.

Suzuki, H., and Siminovitch, M.: Primary Mucus-Producing Adenocarcinoma of the Renal Pelvis. Report of a Case. J. Urol. 93:562-566 (May) 1965.

Thompson, I. M., Schneider, J., and Kavan, L. C.: Bilateral Squamous Cell Carcinoma of Kidneys. J. Urol. 79:807-810 (May) 1958.

Utz, D. C., and McDonald, J. R.: Squamous Cell Carcinoma of the Kidney. J. Urol. 78:540-552 (Nov.) 1957.

Utz, D. C., Brunsting, C. D., and Harrison, E. G., Jr.: Bilateral Ureteral and Vesical Carcinomas Occurring Asynchronously: Report of a Case. J. Urol. 88:488-493 (Oct.) 1962.

Walsh, E. J., Ockuly, E. A., Ockuly, E. F., and Ockuly, J. J.: Treatment of Metastatic Melanoma of the Bladder. J. Urol. 96:472-478 (Oct.) 1966.

Whitlock, G. F., McDonald, J. R., and Cook, E. N.: Primary Carcinoma of the Ureter: A Pathologic and Prognostic Study. J. Urol. 73:245-253 (Feb.) 1955.

Wöller, A.: Hämangiom des Ureters. Ztschr. Urol. *46*:668-670, 1953.

Wood, L. G., and Howe, G. E.: Primary Tumors of the Ureter: Case Reports. J. Urol. 79:418-430 (Mar.) 1958.

Young, I. S.: Ureteral Implant From Renal Adenocarcinoma: Report of a Case and Review of the Literature. J. Urol. 98:661-663 (Dec.) 1967.

Wilms' Tumor; Adrenal Tumors and Neuroblastoma

Altman, D. H.: Actinomycin D and Roentgen-Ray Therapy in the Treatment of Metastatic Wilms' Tumor. Am. J. Roentgenol. 86:673-681 (Oct.) 1961.

Anderson, E. E., Harper, J. M., Small, M. P., and Atwill, W. H.: Bilateral Diffuse Wilms Tumor: A 5-Year Survival. J. Urol. 99:707-709 (June) 1968.

Armstrong, M. D., McMillan, A., and Shaw, K. W. F.: 3-Methoxy-4-hydroxy-D-mandelic Acid: A Urinary Metabolite of Nor-epinephrine. Biochim. et biophys. acta 25:422-423 (Aug.) 1957.

Baert, L., Verduyn, H., and Vereecken, R.: Wilms Tumors (Nephroblastomas): Report of 57 Histologically Proved Cases. J. Urol. 96:871-874 (Dec.) 1966.

Bell, M.: The Clinical Chemistry of Neuroblastomas. In Varley, H., and Gowenlock, A. H.: The Clinical Chemistry of Monamines. Amsterdam, Elsevier Publishing Company, 1963, pp. 82-91.

Bell, M.: Observations on the Biochemical Diagnosis of Neuroblastoma. In Bohuon, C.: Recent Results in Cancer Research. 2. Neuroblastoma-Biochemical Studies. Berlin, Springer-Verlag, 1966, pp. 42-51.

Berry, K. W., Jr., and Scott, E. V. Z.: Pheochromocytoma of the Bladder. J. Urol. 85:156-158 (Feb.) 1961.

Bielschowsky, M.: Neuroblastic Tumors of the Sympathetic Nervous System. In Penfield, W.: Cytology and Cellular Pathology of the Nervous System. New York, Paul B. Hoeber, Inc., 1932, vol. 3, pp. 1085-1094.

Bishop, H. C., and Hope, J. W.: Bilateral Wilms' Tumors. J. Pediat. Surg. *1*:476-487 (Oct.) 1966.

Bodian, M.: Neuroblastoma. Arch. Dis. Childhood 38:606-619 (Dec.) 1963.

Bodian, M., and White, L. L. R.: Neuroblastoma: A General Review. Brit. Emp. Cancer Campaign 32:195-202, 1954.

Bodian, M., and White, L. L. R.: The Treatment of Neuroblastoma With Vitamin B$_{12}$. Brit. Emp. Cancer Campaign 31:213-216, 1956.

Duijsen, E., Williams, C. M., and Judkins, M. P.: Angiography of Pheochromocytoma. Am. J. Roentgenol. 98:225-232 (Sept.) 1966.

Bourne, R. B., and Beltaos, E.: Pheochromocytoma of the Bladder: Case Report and Summary of Literature. J. Urol. 98:361-364 (Sept.) 1967.

Caffey, J. P.: Pediatric X-ray Diagnosis. Ed. 4, Chicago, Year Book Medical Publishers, Inc., 1961, pp. 730-733.

Cohen, S. M., and Persky, L.: Malignant Non-chromaffin Paraganglioma With Metastasis to the Kidney. J. Urol. 96:122-126 (Aug.) 1966.

Collins, V. P.: Wilms' Tumor: Its Behavior and Prognosis. J. Louisiana M. Soc. 107:474-480 (Dec.) 1955.

Collins, V. P.: The Treatment of Wilms' Tumor. Cancer 11:89-94 (Jan.-Feb.) 1958.

Collins, V. P., Leffler, R. K., and Tivey, H.: Observations on the Growth Rates of Human Tumors. Am. J. Roentgenol. 76:988-1000 (Nov.) 1956.

Cope, O., and Raker, J. W.: Cushing's Disease. New England J. Med. 253:119-127; 165-173, 1955.

Crout, J. R., Pisano, J. J., and Sjoerdsma, A.: Urinary Excretion of Catecholamines and Their Metabolites in Pheochromocytoma. Am. Heart J. 61:375-381 (Mar.) 1961.

Culp, O. S., and Hartman, F. W.: Mesoblastic Nephroma in Adults: A Clinico-pathologic Study of Wilms' Tumors and Related Renal Neoplasms. J. Urol. 60:552-576 (Oct.) 1948.

Cushing, H., and Wolbach, S. B.: The Transformation of Malignant Paravertebral Sympathicoblastoma Into a Benign Ganglioneuroma. Am. J. Path. 3:203-216 (May) 1927.

Dockerty, M. B.: Pathology of Adrenal Tumors. Clin. Soc. Genito-Urin. Surgeons 27:40-41 (Feb. 27-28) 1948.

Edsman, G.: Angionephrography and Suprarenal Angiography: A Roentgenographic Study of the Normal Kidney: Expansive Renal and Suprarenal Lesions and Renal Aneurysms. Acta radiol. Suppl. 155, 1957, pp. 1-141.

Farber, S.: Carcinolytic Action of Antibiotics: Puromycin and Actinomycin D. (Abstr.) Am. J. Path. 31:582, 1955.

Farber, S.: Chemotherapy in the Treatment of Leukemia and Wilms' Tumor. J.A.M.A. *198*:826-836 (Nov. 21) 1966.

Farber, S., D'Angio, G., Evans, Audrey, and Mitus, Anna: Clinical Studies of Actinomycin D With Special Reference to Wilms' Tumor in Children. Ann. New York Acad. Sc. 89:421-424 (Oct.) 1960.

Farber, S., Toch, R., Sears, E. M., and Pinkel, D.: Advances of Chemotherapy of Cancer in Man. Advances in Cancer Research. New York, Academic Press, Inc., 1956, vol. 4, p. 49.

Farley, S. E., and Smith, C. L.: Unusual Location of Pheochromocytoma in the Urinary Bladder. J. Urol. *81*:130-132 (Jan.) 1959.

Ferris, D. O., and Beare, J. B.: Wilms' Tumor: Report of a Case With Unusual Postoperative Metastasis. Proc. Staff Meet., Mayo Clin. 22:94-98 (Mar. 5) 1947.

Garcia, M., Douglass, C., and Schlosser, J. V.: Classification and Prognosis in Wilms's Tumor. Radiology *80*:574-580 (Apr.) 1963.

Garrett, R. A., Donohue, J. P., and Arnold, T. L.: Metastatic Renal Embryoma: Survival Following Therapy. J. Urol. 98:444-449 (Oct.) 1967.

Gifford, R. W., Jr., Kvale, W. F., Maher, F. T., Roth, Grace M., and Priestley, J. T.: Clinical Experiences With Pheochromocytoma: A Review of 71 Cases. In Brest, A. N., and Moyer, J. H.: Hypertension: Recent Advances. The Second Hahnemann Symposium on Hypertensive Disease. Philadelphia, Lea & Febiger, 1961, pp. 586-599.

Gifford, R. W., Jr., Kvale, W. F., Maher, F. T., Roth, Grace M., and Priestley, J. T.: Clinical Features, Diagnosis and Treatment of Pheochromocytoma: A Review of 76 Cases. Mayo Clin. Proc. 39:281-302 (Apr.) 1964.

Glenn, J. J., and Rhame, R. C.: Wilms' Tumor: Epidemiological Experience. J. Urol. 85:911-918 (June) 1961.

Goldberg, L. G., and Diaz, A.: Bilateral Wilms' Tumor. J. Urol. 86:211-214 (Aug.) 1961.

Gross, R. E., and Neuhauser, E. B. D.: Treatment of Mixed Tumors of Kidney in Childhood. Pediatrics 6:843-852 (Dec.) 1950.

Gyepes, M. T., and Burko, H.: Diffuse Bilateral Wilms's Tumor Simulating Multicystic Renal Disease. Radiology 82:1029-1031 (June) 1964.

Hardwick, D. F., and Stowens, D.: Wilms' Tumors. J. Urol. 85:903-910 (June) 1961.

Harrison, J. H., and Jenkins, D.: The Adrenals. In Campbell, M.: Urology. Philadelphia, W. B. Saunders Company, 1954, vol. 3, pp. 2283-2356.

Hartman, G. W., Witten, D. M., and Weeks, R. E.: The Role of Nephrotomography in the Diagnosis of Adrenal Tumors. Radiology 86:1030-1034 (June) 1966.

Hinman, F., Jr., Steinbach, H. L., and Forsham, P. H.: Preoperative Differentiation Between Hyperplasia and Tumor in Cushing's Syndrome. J. Urol. 77:329-338 (Mar.) 1957.

Hope, J. W., and Borns, Patricia F.: Radiologic Diagnosis of Primary and Metastatic Cancer in Infants and Children. R. Clin. North America 3:353-374 (Dec.) 1965.

Hope, J. W., and Koop, C. E.: Abdominal Tumors in Infants and Children. In Cornwall, W.: Medical Radiography and Photography. Rochester, New York, Eastman Kodak Company, 1962, vol. 38, pp. 6-57.

Iannaccone, A., Gabrilove, J. L., Brahms, S. A., and Soffer, L. J.: The Roentgen Diagnosis of Adrenal Tumor in Cushing's Syndrome. A.M.A. Arch. Int. Med. *105*:257-263 (Feb.) 1960.

James, D. H., Jr., Hustu, O., Wrenn, E. L., Jr., and Pinkel, D.: Combination Chemotherapy of Childhood Neuroblastoma. J.A.M.A. *194*:123-126 (Oct. 11) 1965.

Joelson, F. J., Persky, L., and Rose, F. A.: Radiographic Diagnosis of Tumors of the Adrenal Gland. Radiology 62:488-495, 1954.

Kahn, P. C., and Nickrosz, L. V.: Selective Angiography of the Adrenal Glands. Am. J. Roentgenol. *101*:739-749 (Nov.) 1967.

Kaplan, J. H., and Greene, L. F.: The Urographic Findings in Cases of Tumor of the Suprarenal Gland. S. Clin. North America 28:1071-1078 (Aug.) 1948.

Karsner, H. T.: Tumors of the Adrenal: Atlas of Tumor Pathology. Armed Forces Institute of Pathology, Washington, D.C., 1950, Section VIII, Fascicle 29, 60 pp.

Kelleher, J., Walters, G., Robinson, R., and Smith, P.: Chemical Tests for Phaeochromocytoma. J. Clin. Path. 17:399-404 (July) 1964.

Kinzel, R. C., Mills, S. D., Childs, D. S., Jr., and DeWeerd, J. H.: Wilms's Tumor: A Review of 47 Cases. J.A.M.A. *174*:1925-1929 (Dec. 10) 1960.

Klapproth, H. J.: Wilms' Tumor: A Report of 45 Cases and an Analysis of 1,351 Cases Reported in the World Literature From 1940 to 1958. J. Urol. *81*:633-648 (May) 1959.

Köhler, R., and Holsti, L. R.: Angiographic Localization of Suprarenal Tumours. Acta radiol. [Diag.] 4:21-32, 1966.

Koop, C. E.: Nephroblastoma and Neuroblastoma in Children. Am. J. Surg. *101*:566-570 (May) 1961.

Koop, C. E., Hope, J. W., and Abir, E.: Management of Nephroblastoma (Wilms' Tumor) and Abdominal Neuroblastoma. CA *14*:178-186 (Sept.-Oct.) 1964.

Koop, C. E., Kiesewetter, W. B., and Horn, R. C.: Neuroblastoma in Childhood: An Evaluation of Surgical Management. Pediatrics *16*:652-657 (Nov.) 1955.

Kvale, W. F., and Roth, G. M.: Paroxysmal and Persistent Hypertension as the Result of Pheochromocytoma. M. Clin. North America 45:467-478 (Mar.) 1961.

Ladd, W. E., and Gross, R. E.: Abdominal Surgery of Infancy and Childhood. Philadelphia, W. B. Saunders Company, 1941, pp. 411-426.

Ladd, W. E., and White, R. R.: Embryoma of the Kidney (Wilms' Tumor). J.A.M.A. *117*:1858-1863 (Nov. 29) 1941.

Lagergren, C.: Angiographic Changes in the Adrenal Glands. Am. J. Roentgenol. *101*:732-738 (Nov.) 1967.

Lalli, A. F., Åhström, L., Ericsson, N. O., and Rudhe, U.: Nephroblastoma (Wilms's Tumor): Urographic Diagnosis and Prognosis. Radiology 87:495-500 (Sept.) 1966.

Lang, E. K., Nourse, M., Mertz, J., McCallum, D., and Wishard, W. N.: The Diagnosis of Suprarenal Mass Lesions by Retroperitoneal Gas Studies and

Arteriography. Am. J. Roentgenol. *98*:215-221 (Sept.) 1966.

Lathem, J. E., and Hunt, L. D.: Pheochromocytoma of the Urinary Bladder. J.A.M.A. *197*:588-590 (Aug. 15) 1966.

Lattimer, J. K., Melicow, M. M., and Uson, A. C.: Wilms' Tumor: Report of 71 Cases. J. Urol. *80*:401-416 (Dec.) 1958.

Liddle, G. W.: Tests of Pituitary-Adrenal Suppressibility in the Diagnosis of Cushing's Syndrome. J. Clin. Endocrinol. *20*:1539-1560 (Dec.) 1960.

Liddle, G. W., Estep, H. L., Kendall, J. W., Jr., Williams, W. C., Jr., and Townes, A. W.: Clinical Application of a New Test of Pituitary Reserve. J. Clin. Endocrinol. *19*:875-894 (Aug.) 1959.

Liebner, E. J., Kirkpatrick, G. P., and Rosenthal, I. M.: Various Childhood Tumors: Treatment With Actinomycin D and X-ray Therapy. Illinois M. J. *121*:531-537 (May) 1962.

Lumb, B. R. B., and Gresham, G. A.: Pheochromocytoma of the Urinary Bladder. Lancet *1*.81-82 (Jan.) 1958.

Mason, G. A., Hart-Mercer, J., Millar, E. Joan, Strang, L. B., and Wynne, N. A.: Adrenaline-Secreting Neuroblastoma in an Infant. Lancet *2*:322-325 (Aug. 17) 1957.

Moloney, G. E., Cowdell, R. H., and Lewis, C. L.: Malignant Phaeochromocytoma of the Bladder. Brit. J. Urol. *38*:461-470 (Aug.) 1966.

Moore, G. E., DiPaolo, J. A., and Kondo, Tatsuhei: The Chemotherapeutic Effects and Complications of Actinomycin D in Patients With Advanced Cancer. Cancer *11*:1204-1214 (Nov.-Dec.) 1958.

Pavlatos, F. Ch., Smilo, R. P., and Forsham, P. H.: A Rapid Screening Test for Cushing's Syndrome. J.A.M.A. *193*:720-723 (Aug. 30) 1965.

Pinkel, D.: Cyclophosphamide in Childhood Cancer. (Abstr.) Proc. Am. A. Cancer Res. *3*:142 (Mar.) 1960.

Platz, C. M., Knowlton, A. T., and Ragan, C.: Natural History of Cushing's Syndrome. Am. J. Med. *12*:597, 1952.

Poutasse, E. F.: Value and Limitation of Roentgenographic Diagnosis of Adrenal Disease. J. Urol. *73*:891, 1955.

Priestley, J. T., and Salassa, R. M.: Lesions of the Adrenal Glands of Surgical Significance. Postgrad. Med. *13*:500-506 (June) 1953.

Pugh, R. C. B.: Pheochromocytoma of the Bladder. Brit. J. Urol. *30*:432-435, 1958.

Pugh, R. C. B., Gresham, G. A., and Mullaney, J.: Phaeochromocytoma of the Urinary Bladder. J. Path. & Bact. *79*:89-107 (Jan.) 1960.

Rabin, C. B.: Chromaffin Cell Tumor of the Suprarenal Medulla (Pheochromocytoma). Arch. Path. *7*:228-243 (Feb.) 1929.

Reiser, M. P., and Creevy, C. D.: Wilms' Tumors. Urol. Survey *2*:413-431, 1952.

Reuter, S. R., Blair, J. A., Schteingart, D. E., and Bookstein, J. J.: Adrenal Venography. Radiology *89*:805-814 (Nov.) 1967.

Robbins, S. L.: Pathology. Ed. 3, Philadelphia, W. B. Saunders Company, 1967, vol. 2, pp. 1235-1239.

Rosenberg, L. M.: Pheochromocytoma of the Urinary Bladder: Report of a Case. New England J. Med. *257*:1212-1215 (Dec. 19) 1957.

Ross, P.: Calcification in Liver Metastases From Neuroblastoma. Radiology *85*:1074-1079 (Dec.) 1965.

Rubin, P., Bell, M., Koop, C. E., Tefft, M., Wittenborg, M. H., Sinks, L. F., and Woodruff, M. W.: Cancer of the Urogenital Tract: Wilms' Tumor and Neuroblastoma. [1] Neuroblastoma. J.A.M.A. *205*:153-166 (July 15) 1968a.

Rubin, P., Hope, J. W., Lattimer, J. K., Conway, G. F., and D'Angio, G. J.: Cancer of the Urogenital Tract: Wilms' Tumor and Neuroblastoma. [2] Wilms' Tumor. J.A.M.A. *204*:981-990 (June 10) 1968b.

Salassa, R. M., Mason, H. L., Mattox, V. R., Power, M. H., Orvis, A. L., and Sprague, R. G.: Effects of Aldosterone on Water, Electrolyte, and Nitrogen Balances in Addison's Disease. Proc. Central Soc. Clin. Research *28*:67-68, 1955.

Scott, L. S.: Bilateral Wilms' Tumour. Brit. J. Surg. *42*:513-516, 1954-1955.

Scott, W. W., and Eversole, S. L.: Pheochromocytoma of the Urinary Bladder. J. Urol. *83*:656-664 (May) 1960.

Sheps, S. G.: Pheochromocytoma. In Moyer, J. H., and Brest, A. N.: Cardiovascular Disorders. Philadelphia, F. A. Davis Company, 1968, pp. 979-989.

Sheps, S. G., Kottke, B. A., Tyce, Gertrude M., and Flock, Eunice V.: Effect of Methyldopa on the Metabolism of Catecholamines and Tryptophan in Metastatic Pheochromocytoma: Report of Two Cases. Am. J. Cardiol. *14*:641-649 (Nov.) 1964.

Sheps, S. G., and Maher, F. T.: Comparison of the Histamine and Tyramine Hydrochloride Tests in the Diagnosis of Pheochromocytoma. J.A.M.A. *195*:265-267 (Jan. 24) 1966.

Sheps, S. G., and Maher, F. T.: Histamine and Glucagon Tests in Diagnosis of Pheochromocytoma. J.A.M.A. *205*:895-899 (Sept. 23) 1968.

Sheps, S. G., Tyce, Gertrude M., and Flock, Eunice V.: Current Experience in the Diagnosis of Pheochromocytoma. (Abstr.) Circulation 32(Suppl. 2):195, 1965.

Sivak, G. C.: Pheochromocytoma of Bladder. J. Urol. *86*:568-571 (Nov.) 1961.

Sjoerdsma, A.: Sympatho-adrenal System. In Beeson, P. B., and McDermott, W.: Cecil-Loeb Textbook of Medicine. Ed. 12, Philadelphia, W. B. Saunders Company, 1967, vol. 2, pp. 1351-1352.

Sober, I., and Hirsch, M.: Embryoma of Kidney in Newborn Infant: Case Report. J. Urol. *93*:449-451 (Apr.) 1965.

Sprague, R. G.: Adrenalectomy, In Moon, H. D.: The Adrenal Cortex, by 19 Authors. New York, Paul B. Hoeber, Inc., 1961, pp. 268-277.

Sprague, R. G., Kvale, W. F., and Priestley, J. T.: Management of Certain Hyperfunctioning Lesions of the Adrenal Cortex and Medulla. J.A.M.A. *151*:629-639 (Feb. 21) 1953.

Sprague, R. G., and Priestley, J. T.: Cushing's Syndrome. In Conn, H. F.: Current Therapy. Philadelphia, W. B. Saunders Company, 1958, pp. 353-355.

Sprague, R. G., Weeks, R. E., Priestley, J. T., and Salassa, R. M.: Treatment of Cushing's Syndrome by Adrenalectomy. In Gardiner-Hill, H.: Modern Trends in Endocrinology. New York, Paul B. Hoeber, Inc., 1961, pp. 84-89.

Stein, J. J., and Goodwin, W. E.: Bilateral Wilms'

Tumor, Including Report of a Patient Surviving Ten Years After Treatment. Am. J. Roentgenol. 96:626-634 (Mar.) 1966.

Steinbach, H. L., and Smith, D. R.: Extraperitoneal Pneumography in Diagnosis of Retroperitoneal Tumors. A.M.A. Arch. Surg. 70:161-190, 1955.

Straube, K. R., and Hodges, C. V.: Pheochromocytoma Causing Renal Hypertension. Am. J. Roentgenol. 98:222-224 (Sept.) 1966.

Tan, C. T. C., Dargeon, H. W., and Burchenal, J. H.: The Effect of Actinomycin D on Cancer in Childhood. Pediatrics 24:544-561 (Oct.) 1959.

Tan, T., and Young, B. W.: Pheochromocytoma of the Bladder: Case Report. J. Urol. 87:63-67 (Jan.) 1962.

Thomas, J. E., Rooke, E. D., and Kvale, W. F.: The Neurologist's Experience With Pheochromocytoma: A Review of 100 Cases. J.A.M.A. 197:754-758 (Sept. 5) 1966.

Van Buskirk, K. E., O'Shaughnessy, E. J., Hano, Jessie, and Finder, R. J.: Pheochromocytoma of the Bladder. J.A.M.A. 196:293-294 (Apr. 18) 1966.

Voorhess, M. L., and Gardner, L. I.: Value of Serial Catecholamine Determinations in Children With Neuroblastoma: Report of a Case. Pediatrics 30:241-246 (Aug.) 1962.

Walters, W.: Diagnostic Clinic on Surgical Lesion of the Adrenal Gland. Postgrad. Med. 20:399-406 (Oct.) 1956.

Walters, W., and Sprague, R. G.: Hyperfunctioning Tumors of the Adrenal Cortex: Study of Nine Cases. J.A.M.A. 141:653-656 (Nov. 5) 1949.

Whitmore, W. F., Jr.: Nephroblastoma (Wilms's Tumor). In Pack, G. T., and Ariel, I. M.: Treatment of Cancer and Allied Diseases: Tumors of the Male Genitalia and the Urinary System. Ed. 2, New York, Paul B. Hoeber, Inc., 1962, vol. VII, pp. 281-294.

Williams, C. M., and Greer, M.: Homovanillic Acid and Vanilmandelic Acid in Diagnosis of Neuroblastoma. J.A.M.A. 183:836-840 (Mar. 9) 1963.

Willis, R. A.: The Spread of Tumours in the Human Body. London, Butterworth & Co., Ltd., 1952, 447 pp.

Wilms, M.: Die Mischgeschwülste. Heft 1: Die Mischgeschwülste der Niere. Leipzig, Arthur Georgi, 1899, p. 90.

Wurtman, R. J.: Catecholamines. New England J. Med. 273:637-646 (Sept. 16) 1965.

Wyatt, G. M., and Farber, S.: Neuroblastoma Sympatheticum: Roentgenological Appearances and Radiation Treatment. Am. J. Roentgenol. 46:485-495 (Oct.) 1941.

Young, R. B., Steiker, D. D., Bongiovanni, A. M., Koop, C. E., and Eberlein, W. R.: Urinary Vanilmandelic Acid (VMA) Excretion in Children: Use of a Simple Semiquantitative Test. J. Pediat. 62:844-854 (June) 1963.

Zimmerman, I. J., Biron, R. E., and MacMahon, H. E.: Pheochromocytoma of the Urinary Bladder. New England J. Med. 249:25-26 (July 2) 1953.

Retroperitoneal Tumors and Cysts; Presacral Tumors

Ackerman, L. V.: Tumors of the Retroperitoneum, Mesentery and Peritoneum. Atlas of Tumor Pathology. Armed Forces Institute of Pathology, Washington, D.C., 1954, Section VI, Fascicles 23 and 24, 136 pp.

Adson, A. W., Moersch, F. P., and Kernohan, J. W.: Neurogenic Tumors Arising From the Sacrum. Arch. Neurol. & Psychiat. 41:535-555 (Mar.) 1939.

Albers, D. D., Milla, A. B., and Vickers, P. M.: Presacral Tumor With a Large Dystrophic Calcification Confused With Urologic Disease: Case Report. J. Urol. 82:384-386 (Sept.) 1959.

Batsakis, J. G.: Urogenital Rhabdomyosarcoma: Histogenesis and Classification. J. Urol. 90:180-186 (Aug.) 1963.

Beeson, P. B., and McDermott, W.: Cecil-Loeb Textbook of Medicine. Ed. 12, Philadelphia, W. B. Saunders Company, 1967, 2 vol., 1738 pp.

Bodian, M.: Quoted by Hatteland and Knutrud.

Bremer, F. L.: Quoted by Gross, R. E., Clatsworthy, H. W., Jr., and Meeker, I. A., Jr.

Camp, J. D., and Good, C. A., Jr.: The Roentgenologic Diagnosis of Tumors Involving the Sacrum. Radiology 31:398-403 (Oct.) 1938.

Dahlin, D. C., and MacCarty, C. S.: Chordoma: A Study of Fifty-nine Cases. Cancer 5:1170-1178 (Nov.) 1952.

Deming, C. L.: Tumors of the Urogenital Tract. In Campbell, M.: Urology. Philadelphia, W. B. Saunders Company, 1954, vol. 2, pp. 969; 1004-1005.

Deniz, E., Shimkus, G. J., and Weller, C. G.: Pelvic Neurofibromatosis: Localized Von Recklinghausen's Disease of the Bladder. J. Urol. 96:906-909 (Dec.) 1966.

DeWeerd, J. H., and Dockerty, M. B.: Lipomatous Retroperitoneal Tumors. Am. J. Surg. 84:397-407 (Oct.) 1952.

Edson, M. J., Friedman, J., and Richardson, J. F.: Perivesical Liposarcoma: A Case Report. J. Urol. 85:767-770 (May) 1961.

Erb, K. H.: Ein Neurinom des Nervus obturatorius unter dem Bilde einer tiefgelegenen Cyste der Adduktorengegend. Deutsche Ztschr. f. Chir. 183:414-418, 1924.

Farrell, W. J.: Deformity of the Bladder Secondary to Pelvic Lymphoma. Radiology 85:898-903 (Nov.) 1965.

Frank, R. T.: Hemangioma of the Pelvic Connective Tissue. Am. J. Obst. & Gynec. 20:81-84 (July) 1930.

Greene, L. F.: Extreme Renal Displacement due to Retroperitoneal Tumors. J. Urol. 59:174-178 (Feb.) 1948.

Gross, R. E., Clatsworthy, H. W., Jr., and Meeker, I. A., Jr.: Sacrococcygeal Teratomas in Infants and Children: A Report of 40 Cases. Surg., Gynec. & Obst. 92:341-354 (Mar.) 1951.

Gwinn, J. L., Dockerty, M. B., and Kennedy, R. L. J.: Presacral Teratomas in Infancy and Childhood. Pediatrics 16:239-249 (Aug.) 1955.

Hanbery, J. W., Senz, E. H., and Jeffrey, R. A.: Sacrococcygeal Teratomas in Infancy and Childhood. Stanford M. Bull. 16:154-168 (Aug.) 1958.

Harvey, W. F., and Dawson, E. K.: Chordoma. Edinburgh M. J. 48:713-730 (Nov.) 1941.

Hatteland, K., and Knutrud, O.: Sacrococcygeal Teratomata in Children. Acta chir. scandinav. 119:444-452 (Sept.) 1960.

Jackman, R. J., Clark, P. L., and Smith, N. D.: Retrorectal Tumors. J.A.M.A. 145:956-962 (Mar. 31) 1951.

Krekeler, A.: Über ein Neurinom in der Wand des Mastdarms, Inaug.-Diss. Bonn., 1928.

Krumbien, C.: Über die "Band-oder Pallisadenstellung" der Kerne, eine Wuchsform des feinfibrillären mesenchymalen Gewebes: Zugleich eine Ableitung der Neurinome (Verocay) vom feinfibrillären Bindegewebe (Fibroma tenuifibrillare). Arch. path. Anat. 255:309-331, 1925.

Labardini, M. M., Kallet, H. A., and Cerny, J. C.: Urogenital Neurofibromatosis Simulating an Intersex Problem. J. Urol. 98:627-632 (Nov.) 1967.

MacCarty, C. S., Waugh, J. M., Mayo, C. W., and Coventry, M. B.: The Surgical Treatment of Presacral Tumors: A Combined Problem. Proc. Staff Meet., Mayo Clin. 27:73-84 (Feb. 13) 1952.

Mayo, C. W., Baker, G. S., and Smith, L. R.: Presacral Tumors: Differential Diagnosis and Report of Case. Proc. Staff Meet., Mayo Clin. 28:616-622 (Nov. 4) 1953.

Middeldorpf, K.: Zur Kenntniss der angeborenen Sacralgeschwülste. Arch. path. Anat. 101:37-44 (July) 1885.

Moreau, J., and Van Bogaert, L.: Les kystes des nerfs. Arch. franco-belges de chir. 26:864-894, 1923.

Pana, C.: Neurinoma del piccolo bacino con amiloidosi generalizzata. Osp. maggiore. 19:741-747, 1931.

Schulte, T. L., and Emmett, J. L.: Urography in the Differential Diagnosis of Retroperitoneal Tumors. J. Urol. 42:215-219 (Aug.) 1939.

Smith, G. G.: Neoplasms of the Kidney and Ureter: A Report of 40 Cases. Am. J. Surg. 30:130-140 (Oct.) 1935.

Stout, A. P.: Peripheral Manifestations of the Specific Nerve Sheath Tumor (Neurilemoma). Am. J. Cancer 24:751-796 (Aug.) 1935.

Stout, A. P.: Ganglioneuroma of the Sympathetic Nervous System. Surg., Gynec. & Obst. 84:101-110 (Jan.) 1947.

Stout, A. P.: Hemangiopericytoma: A Study of Twenty-five New Cases. Cancer 2:1027-1054 (Nov.) 1949.

Stout, A. P.: Quoted by Ackerman, L. V.

Stout, A. P., and Murray, M. R.: Hemangiopericytoma: Vascular Tumor Featuring Zimmermann's Pericytes. Ann. Surg. 116:26-33 (July) 1942.

Sweetser, T. H.: Retroperitoneal Tumors Influencing the Kidneys and Ureters. J. Urol. 47:619-631 (May) 1942.

Thompson, G. J., and Culp, O. S.: Perplexing Cystic Masses Near the Kidney. J. Urol. 89:370-376 (Mar.) 1963.

Whittaker, L. D., and Pemberton, J. deJ.: Tumors Ventral to the Sacrum. Ann. Surg. 107:96-106 (Jan.) 1938.

Windholz, F.: Roentgen Diagnosis of Retroperitoneal Lipoma. Am. J. Roentgenol. 56:594-600 (Nov.) 1946.

Wittenborg, M. H.: Roentgen Therapy in Neuroblastoma: A Review of 73 Cases. Radiology 54:679-687 (May) 1950.

Young, H. B.: Neurilemmoma of Pelvis Presenting With Acute Manifestations. Brit. J. Surg. 41:314-316 (Nov.) 1953.

Zimmerman, K. W.: Der feinere Bau der Blutcapillaren. Ztschr. f.d.ges. Anat. U. 68:29-109, 1923.

Epithelial Tumors of the Bladder

Bartley, O., and Eckerbom, H.: Perivesical Insufflation of Gas for Determination of Bladder Wall Thickness in Tumors of the Bladder. Acta radiol. 54:241-250 (Oct.) 1960.

Bartley, O., and Helander, C. G.: Double-Contrast Cystography in Tumors of the Urinary Bladder. Acta radiol. 54:161-169 (Sept.) 1960.

Boijsen, E., and Nilsson, J.: Angiography in the Diagnosis of Tumors of the Urinary Bladder. Acta radiol. 57:241-258 (July) 1962.

Braband, H.: The Incidence of Urographic Findings in Tumours of the Urinary Bladder. Brit. J. Radiol. 34:625-629 (Oct.) 1961.

Cobb, O. E., and Anderson, E. E.: Superimposition Cystography in the Diagnosis of Infiltrating Tumors of the Bladder. J. Urol. 94:569-572 (Nov.) 1965.

Connolly, J. G., Challis, T. W., Wallace, D. M., Bruce, A. W., and Fransman, S. L.: An Evaluation of the Fractionated Cystogram in the Assessment of Infiltrating Tumors of the Bladder. J. Urol. 98:356-360 (Sept.) 1967.

Cornell, S. H.: Angiography in the Staging of Bladder Carcinoma. J. Iowa M. Soc. 57:331-335 (Apr.) 1967.

Davidson, H. D., Witten, D. M., and Culp, O. S.: Roentgenologically Demonstrable Calcification in Tumors of the Bladder: Report of Three Cases. Am. J. Roentgenol. 95:450-454 (Oct.) 1965.

Franksson, C.: Tumours of the Urinary Bladder: A Pathological and Clinical Study of Four Hundred and Thirty-four Cases. Acta chir. scandinav. Suppl. 151, 1950, pp. 1-203.

Franksson, C., and Lindblom, K.: Roentgenographic Signs of Tumor Infiltration of the Wall of the Urinary Bladder. Acta radiol. 37:1-7 (Jan.) 1952.

Franksson, C., Lindblom, K., and Whitehouse, W.: The Reliability of Roentgen Signs of Varying Degrees of Malignancy of Bladder Tumors. Acta radiol. 45:266-272 (Apr.) 1956.

Goldstein, A. G.: Metastatic Carcinoma to the Bladder. J. Urol. 98:209-215 (Aug.) 1967.

Gosalbez, R., and Gil-Vernet, J. M.: Bladder Tomography: The Use of Air Intra- and Perivesically in the Radiologic Study of Bladder Tumors. J. Urol. 88:312-317 (Aug.) 1962.

Knappenberger, S. T., Uson, A. C., and Melicow, M. M.: Primary Neoplasms Occurring in Vesical Diverticula: A Report of 18 Cases. J. Urol. 83:153-159 (Feb.) 1960.

Lang, E. K., Wishard, W. N., Nourse, M., and Mertz, J. H. O.: Retrograde Arteriography in the Staging and Follow-up of Bladder Tumors. Radiology 80:267-269 (Feb.) 1963.

McDonald, J. R., and Thompson, G. J.: Carcinoma of the Urinary Bladder: A Pathologic Study With Special Reference to Invasiveness and Vascular Invasion. J. Urol. 60:435-445 (Sept.) 1948.

Nilson, A. E.: The Palpability of Infiltrative Bladder Tumours: A Diagnostic Comparison With Roentgenographic Findings. Acta chir. scandinav. 115:132-137, 1958.

Smith, W. H.: The Reliability of Excretion Urography in the Diagnosis of Bladder Tumors. J. Fac. Radiologists 6:48-54 (July) 1954.

Taylor, D. A., Macken, K. L., Veenema, R. J., and Bachman, A. L.: A Preliminary Report of a New Method for the Staging of Bladder Carcinoma Using a Triple Contrast Technique. Brit. J. Radiol. n.s. 38:667-672 (Sept.) 1965.

Wilchusky, B. L., and Lewin, J. R.: Cystoangiography for Determining the Extent of Bladder Tumors. Pennsylvania M. J. 69:51-53 (Feb.) 1966.

Wise, H. M., Jr., and Fainsinger, M. H.: Angiography in the Evaluation of Carcinoma of the Bladder. J.A.M.A. 192:1027-1031 (June 21) 1965.

Nonepithelial Tumors of Bladder and Prostate (Sarcoma; Sarcoma Botryoides)

Bhansali, S. K.: Sarcoma Botryoides of the Bladder in Infancy and Childhood. J. Urol. 87:871-875 (June) 1962.

Borski, A. A.: Lymphosarcoma of the Bladder. J. Urol. 84:551-554 (Oct.) 1960.

Brown, H. E.: Leiomyosarcoma of the Bladder: Followup Report of Two Cases With 4 and 10 Years' Survival. J. Urol. 94:247-251 (Sept.) 1965.

Danckers, U. F., Philipsborn, H. F., Baylor, J. E., and Burkhead, H. C.: Sarcomas of the Prostate, Periprostatic Tissue, and Bladder Neck in Children: Report of a New Case. Am. J. Roentgenol. 84:555-561 (Sept.) 1960.

Dockerty, M. B.: Personal communication to the author.

Evans, A. T., and Bell, T. E.: Rhabdomyosarcoma of the Bladder in Adult Patients: Report of Three Cases. J. Urol. 94:573-575 (Nov.) 1965.

Feggetter, G. Y.: Sarcoma of the Bladder. Brit. J. Surg. 25:382-387 (Oct.) 1937.

Flocks, R. H., and Culp, D. A.: Polypoid Fibromyxosarcoma of the Urinary Bladder in a Child. J. Urol. 73:299-306 (Feb.) 1955.

Goodwin, W. E., Mims, M. M., and Young, H. H., II: Rhabdomyosarcoma of the Prostate in a Child: First 5-Year Survival (Combined Treatment by Preoperative, Local Irradiation; Actinomycin D; Intra-arterial Nitrogen Mustard and Hypothermia; Radical Surgery and Ureterosigmoidostomy). J. Urol. 99:651-655 (May) 1968.

Graham, J. B., and Bulkley, G. J.: Angioma of the Bladder. J. Urol. 74:777-779 (Dec.) 1956.

Graves, R. S., and Coleman, M. W.: Sarcoma of the Prostate: An Unusual Survival. J. Urol. 72:731-734 (Oct.) 1954.

Hamlin, W. B., and Lund, P. K.: Carcinosarcoma of the Prostate: A Case Report. J. Urol. 97:518-522 (Mar.) 1967.

Hamsher, J. B., Farrar, T., and Moore, T. D.: Congenital Vascular Tumors and Malformations Involving Urinary Tract: Diagnosis and Surgical Management. J. Urol. 80:299-310 (Nov.) 1958.

Hellstrom, H. R., and Fisher, E. R.: Embryonal Rhabdomyosarcoma of the Bladder in the Aged. J. Urol. 86:336-339 (Sept.) 1961.

Higgins, T. T.: Rhabdo-myosarcoma of the Bladder. Brit. J. Urol. 24:158-159 (June) 1952.

Hunt, R. W.: Rhabdomyosarcoma in the Lower Urinary Tract. New York State J. Med. 43:513-517 (Mar. 15) 1943.

Joshi, D. P., Wessely, Zelma, Seerj, W. H., and Neier, C. R.: Rhabdomyosarcoma of the Bladder in an Adult: Case Report and Review of the Literature. J. Urol. 96:214-217 (Aug.) 1966.

Kafka, V., Krolupper, M., and Palecek, L.: Rhabdomyosarcoma of the Bladder in Childhood: Report of a Successfully Treated Case. J. Urol. 96:210-213 (Aug.) 1966.

Khoury, E. N., and Speer, F. D.: Rhabdomyosarcoma of the Urinary Bladder: A Clinicopathological Case Report With a Review of the Literature, Including a Tabulation of Rhabdomyosarcoma of Prostate. J. Urol. 51:505-516 (May) 1944.

Kretschmer, H. L.: Rhabdomyosarcoma of the Bladder: Report of a Case and Review of the Literature. Arch. Path. 44:350-355 (Oct.) 1947.

Legier, J. F.: Botryoid Sarcoma and Rhabdomyosarcoma of the Bladder: Review of the Literature and Report of 3 Cases. J. Urol. 86:583-590 (Nov.) 1961.

Liang, D. S.: Hemangioma of the Bladder. J. Urol. 79:956-960 (June) 1958.

Litin, R. B., Donahue, C. D., Overstreet, R. M., and Starr, G. F.: Hemangioma of the Bladder: Report of Two Cases. J. Urol. 85:556-558 (Apr.) 1961.

Longley, J.: Sarcoma of Prostate and Bladder. J. Urol. 73:417-423 (Feb.) 1955.

Marshall, V. F.: Pelvic Exenteration for Polypoid Myosarcoma (Sarcoma Botryoides) of the Urinary Bladder of an Infant. Cancer 9:620-621 (May-June) 1956.

McFarland, J.: Dysontogenetic and Mixed Tumors of the Urogenital Region: With a Report of a New Case of Sarcoma Botryoides Vaginal in a Child, and Comments Upon the Probable Nature of Sarcoma. Surg., Gynec. & Obst. 61:42-57 (July) 1935.

Meisel, H. J., Heath, W. H., and Miller, J. M.: Rhabdomyosarcoma of the Urinary Bladder: A Followup Note. J. Urol. 67:694 (May) 1952.

Melicow, M. M., Pelton, T. H., and Fish, G. W.: Sarcoma of the Prostate Gland: Review of Literature: Table of Classification; Report of Four Cases. J. Urol. 49:675-707 (May) 1943.

Mostofi, F. K., and Morse, W. H.: Polypoid Rhabdomyosarcoma (Sarcoma Botryoides) of Bladder in Children. J. Urol. 67:681-687 (May) 1952.

Murphy, G., and Bradley, J.: Primary Sarcoma of the Prostate. J. Urol. 85:973-976 (June) 1961.

Nicolai, C. H., and Spjut, H. J.: Primary Osteogenic Sarcoma of the Bladder. J. Urol. 82:497-499 (Oct.) 1959.

Ober, W. B., and Edgcomb, J. H.: Sarcoma Botryoides in Female Urogenital Tract. Cancer 7:75-91 (Jan.) 1954.

Ober, W. B., Smith, J. A., and Rouillard, F. C.: Congenital Sarcoma Botryoides of the Vagina: Report of 2 Cases. Cancer 11:620-623 (May-June) 1958.

Parker, P., Smith, P. L., and Rathmell, T. K.: Sarcoma Botryoides of the Bladder: Successful Therapy by Cystectomy. J. Urol. 82:494-496 (Oct.) 1959.

Pettersson, G.: Two Cases of Primary Tumours of the Bladder in Infants. Acta chir. scandinav. 107:534-538, 1954.

Prince, C. L., and Vest, S. A.: Leiomyosarcoma of the Prostate: Report of a Case and Critical Review. J. Urol. 46:1129-1143 (Dec.) 1941.

Ramey, W. P., Ashburn, L. L., Grabstald, H., and

Haines, J. S.: Myosarcoma of the Urinary Bladder. J. Urol. 70:906-913 (Dec.) 1953.

Siegel, J.: Sarcoma of the Prostate: A Report of Four Cases and a Review of Current Therapy. J. Urol. 89:78-83 (Jan.) 1963.

Slotkin, E. A., and Davis, R. D.: Rhabdomyosarcoma of the Bladder. New York J. Med. 54:2837-2840 (Oct. 15) 1954.

Smith, B. A., Jr.: Sarcoma Botryoides—Rhabdomyosarcoma of the Bladder. J. Urol. 82:101-104 (July) 1959.

Stanley, K. E., Jr.: Hemangioma-Lymphangioma of the Bladder in a Child: Report of a Case With Associated Hemangiomas of the External Genitalia. J. Urol. 96:51-54 (July) 1966.

Staple, T. W., and McAlister, W. H.: Hemangioma of the Bladder. Am. J. Roentgenol. 92:375-377 (Aug.) 1964.

Swinney, J.: Rhabdomyosarcoma of the Urinary Bladder in Children. Urol. & Cutan. Rev. 55:530-532 (Sept.) 1951.

Thompson, I. M., and Coppridge, A. J.: Bladder Sarcoma. J. Urol. 82:329-332 (Sept.) 1959.

Torres, H., and Bennett, M. J.: Neurofibromatosis of the Bladder: Case Report and Review of the Literature. J. Urol. 96:910-912 (Dec.) 1966.

Torres, L. F., Estrada, J. Y., and Esquivel, E. L., Jr.: Sarcoma of the Prostate Gland: Report of Four Cases. J. Urol. 96:380-384 (Sept.) 1966.

Weaver, R. C., Card, R. Y., and Rueb, R. L.: Polypoid Rhabdomyosarcoma of the Bladder. J. Urol. 85:297-300 (Mar.) 1961.

White, L. L. R.: Embryonic Sarcoma of the Urogenital Sinus. Thesis, University of Wales, 1955. Cited by Williams, D. I., and Schistad, G.

Williams, D. I., and Schistad, G.: Lower Urinary Tract Tumours in Children. Brit. J. Urol. 36:51-65, 1964.

Williams, D. I., and Young, D. G.: Malignant Tumours of the Genito-urinary Tract in Childhood. Practitioner 200:678-685 (May) 1968.

Tumors of the Urethra

Begley, B. J.: Hemangioma of the Male Urethra: Treatment by Johanson-Denis Browne Technique. J. Urol. 84:111-112 (July) 1960.

Fricke, R. E., and McMillan, J. T.: Radium Therapy in Carcinoma of the Female Urethra. Radiology 52:533-537 (Apr.) 1949.

Grabstald, H., Hilaris, B., Henschke, U., and Whitmore, W. F., Jr.: Cancer of the Female Urethra. J.A.M.A. 197:835-842 (Sept. 12) 1966.

Harrison, J. H.: Carcinoma of the Female Urethra. (Editorial.) J.A.M.A. 197:198 (Sept. 12) 1966.

Kaplan, G. W., Bulkley, G. J., and Grayhack, J. T.: Carcinoma of the Male Urethra. J. Urol. 98:365-371 (Sept.) 1967.

King, L. R.: Carcinoma of the Urethra in Male Patients. J. Urol. 91:555-559 (May) 1964.

Mandler, J. I., and Pool, T. L.: Primary Carcinoma of the Male Urethra. J. Urol. 96:67-73 (July) 1966.

Marshall, V. F.: Radical Excision of Locally Extensive Carcinoma of the Deep Male Urethra. J. Urol. 78:252-264 (Sept.) 1957.

Painter, M. R., O'Shaughnessy, E. J., Larson, P. H., and Ribbe, R. E.: Rhabdomyosarcoma of the Male Urethra. J. Urol. 99:455-457 (Apr.) 1968.

Radman, H. M.: Urethral Hemangioma. J. Urol. 94:580-581 (Nov.) 1965.

Tilak, G. H.: Multiple Hemangiomas of the Male Urethra—Treatment by Denis Browne-Swinney-Johanson Urethroplasty. J. Urol. 97:96-97 (Jan.) 1967.

Uhle, C. A. W., and Kohler, F. P.: Carcinoma of the Female Urethra: Report of 2 Cases of the Urethrovestibular Epidermoid Group. J. Urol. 95:378-383 (Mar.) 1966.

Zaslow, J., and Priestley, J. T.: Primary Carcinoma of the Male Urethra. J. Urol. 58:207-211 (Sept.) 1947.

Tumors of the Seminal Vesicle

Awadalla, O., Hunt, A. C., and Miller, A.: Primary Carcinoma of the Seminal Vesicle. Brit. J. Urol. 40:574-579 (Oct.) 1968.

Dalgaard, J. B., and Giertsen, J. C.: Primary Carcinoma of the Seminal Vesicle: Case and Survey. Acta path. et microbiol. scandinav. 39:255-267, 1956.

Dawson, E. K., and Mckie, D. E. C.: Primary Carcinoma of the Seminal Vesicles. J. Roy. Coll. Surgeons Edinburgh 10:235-238 (Apr.) 1965.

Ewell, C. H.: Seminal Vesicle Carcinoma. J. Urol. 89:908-912 (June) 1963.

Hajdu, S. I., and Faruque, A. A.: Adenocarcinoma of the Seminal Vesicle. J. Urol. 99:798-801 (June) 1968.

Lazarus, J. A.: Primary Malignant Tumors of the Retrovesical Region With Special Reference to Malignant Tumors of the Seminal Vesicles: Report of a Case of Retrovesical Sarcoma. J. Urol. 55:190-205 (Feb.) 1946.

Marshall, D. F., Leary, C. C., O'Donnell, E. E., and Geer, C. I.: Seminal Vesicle Carcinoma. J. Maine M. A. 52:145-147 (May) 1961.

Roberts, L. C., Coppridge, W. M., and Hughes, J.: Tumors and Cysts of the Male Pelvis Which Interfere With Urination. J. Urol. 79:159-164 (Jan.) 1958.

Rodriguez Kees, O. S.: Clinical Improvement Following Estrogenic Therapy in a Case of Primary Adenocarcinoma of the Seminal Vesicle. J. Urol. 91:665-670 (June) 1964.

Smith, B. A., Jr.: Carcinoma of the Seminal Vesicle: Report of Two Cases. J. Urol. 72:67-76 (July) 1954.

Smith, B. A., Jr., Webb, E. A., and Price, W. E.: Carcinoma of the Seminal Vesicle. J. Urol. 97:743-750 (Apr.) 1967.

CHAPTER 11

Embryology of the Genitourinary Tract*

EMBRYOLOGY OF THE KIDNEY AND URETER

The Kidney: Early Phases

The duct which drains the mesonephros (wolffian body) is called the *mesonephric* or *wolffian* duct. It originates as the pronephric duct which grows caudad, reaching and emptying into the cloaca at about the 4-mm stage. When mesonephric tubules become connected to the pronephric duct, its name is changed to mesonephric duct. The cloaca divides into a ventral segment, forming the bladder and the urogenital sinus, and a dorsal segment which becomes the rectum. Even before the cloaca divides, a bud appears on the dorsal surface of the wolffian duct a short distance from the cloacal wall. This is called the *ureteral bud* and is the anlage of the adult ureter. The cranial end of the ureteral bud grows cranially into a mass of undifferentiated mesoderm which soon becomes specialized to form the renal mesenchyme or anlage of the kidney proper. At approximately the 10-mm stage the cephalic end of the ureteral bud divides into two branches which are the forerunners of the two major calyces (Fig. 11–1). At this stage the renal mesenchyme,

which caps the branching ureter, has assumed a definite "bean" form. The two kidneys at this stage lie close together (almost in apposition and parallel to each other) and are at the level of the second sacral segment. Their upper poles reach to the brim of the true pelvis. The point of bifurcation of the ureteral bud becomes the future renal pelvis.

Further description of the subsequent branching to the ureter is best left to Arey, who said:

Of the first two [primary divisions of the ureter] one is cranial, the other is caudal in position and between these, two others usually appear [Fig. 11–2]. From an ampullary enlargement at the end of each primary tubule sprout off two, three or four secondary tubules. These in turn give rise to tertiary tubules and the process is repeated until the fifth month of fetal life, when it is estimated that twelve generations of tubules have been developed. The pelvis and the primary and secondary tubules enlarge greatly during development. The two primary expansions become the *major calyces* and the secondary tubules opening into them form the *minor calyces*. The tubules of the third and fourth orders are taken up into the walls of the enlarged secondary tubules so that the tubules of the fifth order, twenty to thirty in number, open into the minor calyces as *papillary ducts*. The remaining orders of tu-

---

*Only the embryology pertinent to the anomalies discussed in Chapter 12 is included here.

1313

bules constitute the *collecting tubules* which form the greater part of the medulla of the adult kidney.

The renal cortex is formed from the renal mesenchyme, which gives rise to the glomeruli and uriniferous tubules (proximal and distal convoluted tubules and loops of Henle).

Failure of the uriniferous tubules (originating from nephrogenic blastema) to connect with the collecting tubules (derived from the ureteric bud) is the most commonly accepted explanation of *polycystic disease of the kidneys*. However, McKenna and Kampmeier, in 1934, advanced a different explanation based on Kampmeier's original concept of three zones in the developing cortex of the kidney, namely a vestigial zone, a provisional zone, and a growth zone (Fig. 11–3). Kampmeier expressed the belief that the tubules of the vestigial zone are rudimentary and disappear without a trace, those of the provisional zone unite with the collecting ducts only to break away from them again, and those of the growth zone form the definitive renal cortex. McKenna and Kampmeier stated that the uriniferous tubules of the provisional zone usually collapse and disappear after they lose their connections to the collecting tubules, but that some of them may persist and expand to form cysts. They explained all types of renal cysts (solitary, multiple, and polycystic disease) on this basis.

The Ureter

Returning now to the lower end of the ureter it will be recalled that originally the ureter sprouted from the dorsal surface of the wolffian duct just proximal to its junction with the cloaca. The ureter next shifts its position to the lateral aspect of the wolffian duct. The lower end of the duct, from which the ureter arises, expands and through a rather complicated form of growth is absorbed as a part of the bladder in its vesicourethral portion so that the ureter and the mesonephric duct open separately (Fig. 11–4A through D). This change is taking place at about the same time that the kidneys are undergoing rotation and ascent. The portion of the bladder that receives the ureters and wolffian ducts grows in an uneven manner so that the ureters migrate laterally and cranially while the distal ends of the wolffian ducts remain close together in the midline and appear to migrate somewhat distally, their orifices eventually being situated in the verumontanum in the distal portion of the floor of the prostatic urethra. Embryologically, therefore, an area bounded by the ureteral orifices and the mesonephric (ejaculatory) ducts is thought to be of mesodermal origin, while the remainder of the bladder is of entodermal origin. There is still some difference of opinion concerning this last statement, however. This area of mesonephric tissue in the male includes the trigone and proximal part of the prostatic urethra. In the female it includes the trigone and almost all of the urethra.

Incomplete Ureteral Duplication (Bifid Ureter)

Abnormal bifurcation or splitting of the ureteral bud is thought to account for incomplete ureteral duplication, in which case the two ureters join to form a common ureter with only one ureteral orifice (Fig. 11–5). If the branching is high so that the point of juncture is at or just below the ureteropelvic juncture, the condition is called a *bifid pelvis. Trifid pelvis* and triplicated ureter are encountered occasionally.

Complete Ureteral Duplication

Complete duplication of the ureter (double ureter) each of which has its own separate ureteral orifice is the result of two separate ureteral buds sprouting from the wolffian duct (Fig. 11–6A through D). Logically, the ureteral bud sprouting from the highest level on the wolffian duct should serve the upper renal pelvis; the lower, the lower renal pelvis. Clinically, however, the *lower,* more medially situated ureteral orifice almost always serves the upper renal pelvis, whereas the upper (more cranially and laterally situated orifice) serves the lower pelvis. This situation comes about in the following manner: As mentioned previously, the portion of the bladder which contains the wolffian duct and ureter grows in an uneven manner so that the ureter migrates laterally and cranially. Referring again to Figure 11–6, the lower ureter is first absorbed into the bladder, while the upper ureter is carried caudally by the migrating mesonephric duct, and only as still more of the duct is absorbed into the bladder or urethra does this ureter attain its independent opening. Because of this, the orifice serving the lower renal pelvis is always situated cranial and lateral to the orifice serving the *upper* ureter and renal pelvis. This is known as the *Weigert-Meyers rule.* Only rare instances have been reported in which this rule did not hold. The two ureters course downward side by side to the pelvis, and just before the bladder is reached, the ureter from the lower pelvis crosses the other to enter the bladder, while the other ureter continues on to enter at a lower and more medial position. As will be mentioned subsequently, in the completely duplicated ureter, whenever one ureteral orifice is in an ectopic (extravesical) location the lower or ectopic orifice always serves the upper renal pelvis.

A rare type of ureteral duplication is the inverted **Y** in which two ureteral orifices are present but the duplicated ureters join to form a common ureter before reaching the single renal pelvis. This condition is thought to result from two ureteral buds sprouting from the wolffian duct. Just how they fuse to become one ureter is not clear.

(*Text continued on page 1319.*)

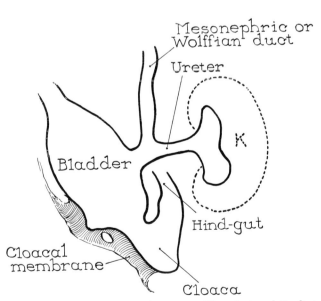

Figure 11–1. Sprouting of ureter from mesonephric or wolffian duct and its division into two branches which are forerunners of two major calyces. Renal mesenchyme, which caps branching ureter, has assumed definite "bean" form. (See text.) (Redrawn from Arey, L. B.)

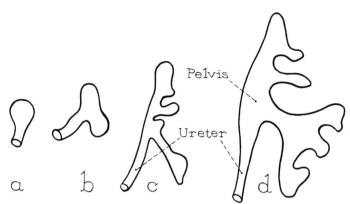

Figure 11–2. Branching of ureteral bud to form major and minor calyces. (See text.) (From Arey, L. B.)

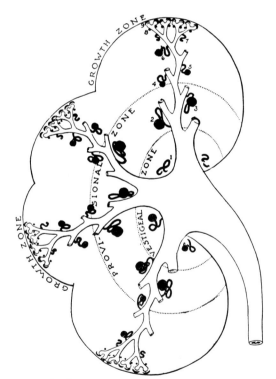

Figure 11–3. The three zones in development of uriniferous tubules. (From Kampmeier, O. F.)

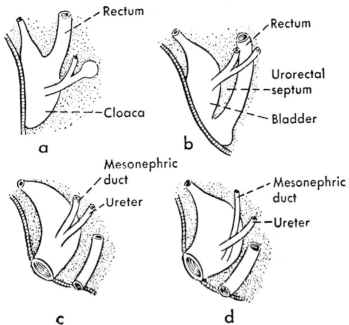

Figure 11–4.   Method of subdivision of cloaca and separation of openings of mesonephric duct (vas deferens in male) and ureter. A, Primitive condition. B, Urorectal septum has separated rectum from urinary bladder. C, Common stem of mesonephric duct and ureter has been largely absorbed into wall of bladder. D, Differential growth of wall of bladder is carrying mesonephric duct distally toward urethra. (From Hollinshead, W. H.)

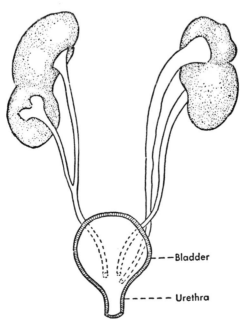

Figure 11–5.   Bifid, double or duplicated ureter. Incomplete duplication of right ureter, complete duplication of left ureter. (From Hollinshead, W. H.)

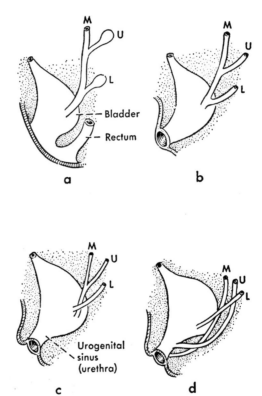

Figure 11–6. A to D, Development of complete ureteral duplication demonstrating reason why lower, most medial ureteral orifice connects with ureter which serves upper renal pelvis. M = mesonephric (wolffian duct); U = upper ureter (serving lower renal pelvis); L = lower ureter (serving upper renal pelvis). (From Hollinshead, W. H.)

Ectopic Ureteral Orifices

It is customary to limit the term *ectopic ureter* to a ureter that has an opening in some location other than the bladder. In the male, ectopic ureteral orifices may be found in the vesical neck, prostatic urethra, seminal vesicles, vas deferens, ejaculatory ducts, and, rarely, the rectum. In the female, they may be found in the vesical neck, urethra, vestibule, vagina, cervix, uterus, and rectum (Fig. 11–7A and B). In the male, ectopic ureters always open at some site cranial to the external urethral sphincter so that incontinence is rarely, if ever, a symptom. In the female, on the other hand, the ectopic orifice is frequently situated distal to or beyond the jurisdiction of the external sphincter so that incontinence of urine is a common complaint.

Approximately 30% of ectopic ureters are single ureters, whereas 70% are associated with ureteral duplication. As stated previously, if duplication is present, the ureter with the ectopic orifice is always the one that serves the upper renal pelvis.

After a survey of the literature, Kjellberg, Ericsson, and Rudhe found the relative incidence of the sites of ectopic ureteral orifices to be as follows:

Males:

Posterior urethra	54%
Seminal vesicles	28%
Vas deferens	10%
Ejaculatory ducts	8%

Females:

Vestibule	38%
Urethra	32%
Vagina	27%
Uterus	3%

When ectopic ureteral orifices are found in the vesical neck, prostatic urethra, seminal vesicles, vas deferens, or ejaculatory ducts of the male, or in the vesical neck, urethra, or vestibule of the female, the embryologic explanation is simple, because all of these structures have developed from the wolffian ducts or urogenital sinus.

When ectopic ureters are found in the fallopian tubes, uterus, cervix, or vagina, the explanation is more difficult, as those structures are formed from the paired müllerian ducts. In such a situation the most common explanation centers around Gartner's ducts, which are the remnants of the wolffian ducts in the female. It has been demonstrated that vestigial remnants of the wolffian ducts in the female may be found along a line running from the hymen (homologue of the verumontanum) through the anterior and lateral walls of the vagina, through the cervix, the wall of the uterus, and between the layers of the broad ligament to the epoophoron (Figs. 11–8 and 11–9). Inasmuch as the ureters arise from the wolffian duct, it seems reasonable to assume that their openings could be found anywhere along its course.

Another explanation, favored by Kjellberg, Ericsson, and Rudhe, calls attention to the intimate relationship of the wolffian and müllerian ducts during their embryologic development. They cited the work of Gruenwald who demonstrated that the müllerian duct actually grows *inside* the basal membrane of the wolffian duct and may be derived from the cells of the wolffian duct. Such a common origin and close association, therefore, could explain the presence of a wolffian duct structure (ureter) terminating in some organ formed by the müllerian ducts (vagina, cervix, uterus, or fallopian tubes).

As mentioned previously, in rare instances ectopic ureteral openings in the rectum have been reported. The best explanation advanced for this error of development is a faulty division of the cloaca by the urorectal septum.

(Text continued on page 1322.)

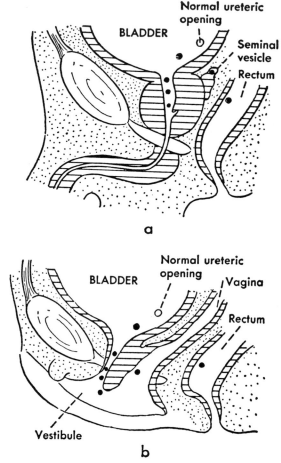

a

b

Figure 11–7.   Possible abnormal sites of ureteral orifices. A, Male. B, Female. (From Hollinshead, W. H.)

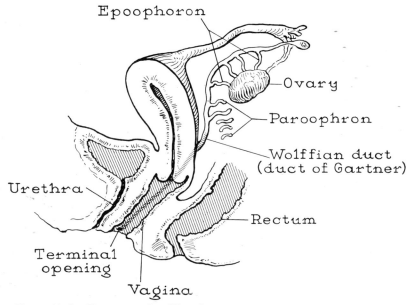

Figure 11–8.   Remnants of wolffian duct in female. (Redrawn from Keith, A.)

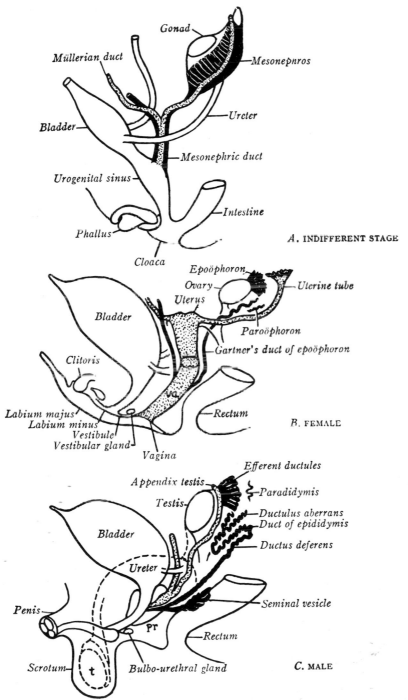

Figure 11–9.   Diagrams illustrating transformation of an indifferent, primitive genital system into definitive male and female types (Thompson). (From Arey, L. B.)

Ascent and Rotation of the Kidneys

NORMAL

Approximately between the 14- and the 30-mm stage of the embryo, ascent of the kidneys occurs. The definitive kidney formed by the union of the ureteric bud and nephrogenic blastema at first lies far caudally in the body (Fig. 11–10). To attain the normal position in the adult, the kidneys must migrate upward out of the pelvis and into the abdominal cavity. Whether the kidneys actually ascend or merely remain stationary while the body grows caudally is still a controversial point. During its so-called ascent the kidney is supplied in succession by arteries located higher and higher in the nephrogenic ridge.

In addition to ascent the kidney also undergoes rotation. The renal pelvis, which originally lay on the ventral surface of the kidney (forward), finally comes to face medially in the adult. At about the 25- to 30-mm stage the kidneys have reached their normal adult positions on each side of the second lumbar vertebra. When they have reached this position, permanent vascularization of the kidneys occurs.

ABNORMAL

Simple Renal Ectopia

Simple renal ectopia (kidney situated on its normal side but below its normal adult level) results from failure of normal ascent. A minimal degree of ectopia may be difficult to distinguish from secondary ptosis. The length of the ureter may help in differentiation. Also, the presence of some degree of malrotation tends to speak for ectopia rather than ptosis as does an anomalous type of blood supply, usually from multiple vessels. *It is of interest that in most cases of renal ectopia the adrenal gland is in normal position.*

Crossed Renal Ectopia

If, in addition to incomplete ascent, a kidney migrates to the opposite side of the vertebral column, the condition is spoken of as *crossed renal ectopia*. The crossed kidney usually lies below the other, although in rare instances it may lie medial or superior to it. In most cases malrotation is associated, the commonest condition being an anteriorly (forward) placed pelvis. In some cases the pelvis of the upper, normally situated kidney is projected anteromedially, and that of the lower kidney is projected anterolaterally. The descriptive term, *sigmoid kidney*, is applied to this condition. In the large majority of cases of crossed ectopia, kidneys are fused and the condition is called *crossed renal ectopia with fusion or unilateral fused kidney* (Fig. 11–11). The ureter serving the crossed kidney crosses the midline to enter the bladder on its normal side.

Malrotation (Abnormal Rotation; Incomplete Rotation)

Anomalous types of rotation are most frequently associated with ectopia but also may be present in normally placed kidneys. The most common type of malrotation is the persistent anterior position of the renal pelvis or some variation between the fetal anterior and the adult medial positions. Four major types of anomalous rotation have been described (Braasch; Weyrauch), namely, nonrotation, incomplete rotation, reverse rotation, and excessive rotation. As mentioned earlier, the most commonly encountered anomalies are the nonrotation (pelvis forward or ventral) and incomplete rotation, in which case the pelvis is between the forward (ventral) and medial positions. Reverse and excessive rotations (Fig. 11–12) are rare. It is obvious from Figure 11–12 that reverse rotations cannot be distinguished from excessive rotations from the pyelograms alone. Surgical exploration to determine the disposition of the renal vessels is necessary. In reverse rotation the renal vessels are twisted anteriorly around the kidney; in excessive rotation they are carried posteriorly to the kidney.

FUSION AND DUPLICATION OF THE KIDNEYS

Horseshoe Kidney, Unilateral Fused Kidney, and Cake Kidney

Fusion of the renal masses has already been mentioned in conjunction with crossed renal ectopia with fusion (unilateral fused kidney). The commonest type of fusion is *horseshoe kidney* (Fig. 11–13). In more than 90% of cases fusion is at the lower poles, and the area of fusion (isthmus) across the midline corresponds to the toe of a horseshoe. The isthmus may be composed of renal parenchyma or rather seldom simply of a band of fibrous tissue. Horseshoe kidneys usually lie rather low in the abdomen, the isthmus lying in the region of the aortic bifurcation. This isthmus almost always lies in front of the great vessels, but rare cases have been reported in which it lay either behind both the great vessels or behind the vena cava but in front of the aorta. In most cases the superior hypogastric sympathetic plexuses lie in front of the isthmus. The pelves are situated ventrally and usually lie anterior to the renal vessels. The renal vessels vary considerably in position, size, and number. In almost all cases the course of the ureters is downward, anterior to the renal substance and isthmus.

A less common type of fusion is the single disk known as a *cake, disk,* or *lump kidney* (Fig. 11–14A and B). It is usually situated lower than the horseshoe kidney and lies over the sacrum. This condition has also been called *fused pelvic kidneys.*

Renal Reduplication: Supernumerary Kidneys and Double Fused Kidneys

The problem of renal reduplication (double pelves or double fused kidneys) has been alluded to in the discussion of incomplete and complete ureteral duplication. In the case of incomplete duplication, abnormal formation or splitting of the ureteral bud occurred; in the case of complete duplication two ureteric buds arose from different positions on the wolffian duct. In either case, two renal pelves resulted, and each was capped with a nephrogenic blastemal mass. In nearly every case these masses fuse and become one kidney (Fig. 11–15). In rare cases they remain separate, resulting in a *supernumerary kidney* (Kretschmer) (Fig. 11–16), *which is the rarest of all renal anomalies.* In the illustration (Fig. 11–16) the ureter to the upper kidney joins the pelvis of the lower. More often, the two ureters join at some point above the bladder.

(Text continued on page 1327.)

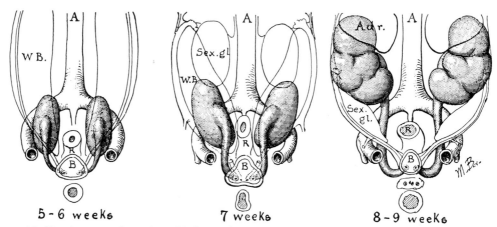

Figure 11–10. Ascent and rotation of kidneys. (See text.) (From Kelly, H. A., and Burnam, C. F.: Diseases of the Kidneys, Ureters, and Bladder, With Special Reference to the Diseases in Women. New York, D. Appleton and Company, 1914.)

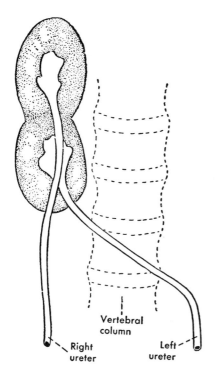

Figure 11–11. Crossed renal ectopia with fusion (unilateral fused kidney). (From Hollinshead, W. H.)

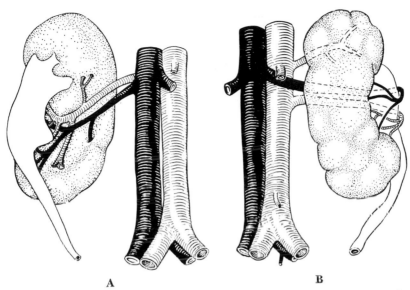

A   B

Figure 11–12. Abnormal renal rotation (malrotation). **A,** Reverse rotation. **B,** Hyperrotation. (After Weyrauch, H. M., by permission of Surg., Gynec. & Obst.)

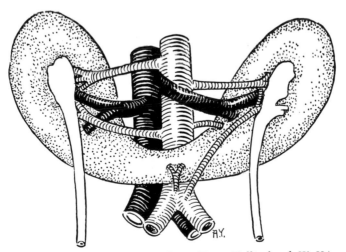

Figure 11–13. Horseshoe kidney. (From Hollinshead, W. H.)

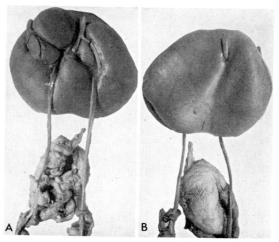

Figure 11–14. A and B, Cake, disk, or lump kidney. (From Campbell, M. F.)

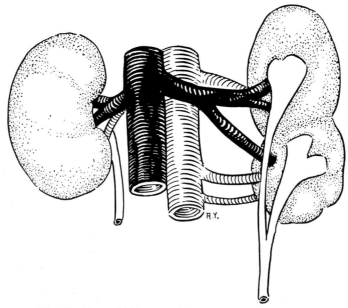

Figure 11–15. Duplicated kidney with fusion. (From Hollinshead, W. H.)

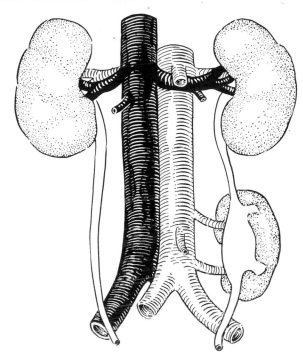

Figure 11–16. Supernumerary kidney. (Redrawn from Kretschmer, H. L. By permission of Surg., Gynec. & Obst.)

Miscellaneous Anomalies

Blind-Ending Ureter (Ureteral Diverticulum)

A blind ending is seen occasionally in a branch of a duplicated or bifid ureter. It is difficult to know whether the condition is acquired and represents a diverticulum or whether it is congenital and represents a ureteral reduplication in which no nephrogenic blastema formed to cap the ureter.

Renal Agenesis (Congenital Solitary Kidney)

In the vast majority of cases of renal agenesis the ureter is also absent, which suggests that the most likely explanation for the condition is primary failure of the ureteric bud to develop. Other suggested reasons are failure of the nephrogenic blastema to form or failure of the vascular sup-

ply. If the genital apparatus on the same side is absent also, the condition may be ascribed to failure of the wolffian duct to develop. *Hemiatrophy of the trigone* is found in some cases, but the suprarenal gland is always present and in its normal position.

Retrocaval Ureter (Postcaval Ureter; Circumcaval Ureter; Preureteric Vena Cava)

In this anomalous condition the ureter from a normal position in its upper third turns abruptly medial and passes behind the vena cava, then passes forward between the vena cava and aorta, then across the front of the vena cava to reach its normal position lateral to the vena cava. In its course it makes a "hook" around the vena cava (Fig. 11–17). The embryologic error here is probably one of the vena cava rather than of the ureter. In all reported cases except one the condition has been on the right side. Hollinshead described the origin of this anomaly as follows:

Without going into details, it can be stated that most of the infrarenal segment of the inferior vena cava is usually formed from a persistent venous channel (supracardinal vein) which lies dorsal to the ureter, but that during the development of the inferior vena cava there is also a subcardinal vein which lies ventral to the ureter [Fig. 11–18A, B, and C]; if the subcardinal vein persists as the infrarenal segment of the vena cava then the ureter passes behind the definitive vein, but in front of the dorsally formed iliac vein, and necessarily makes a hook around this anomalously formed vena cava as the vessel is shifted toward the midline. The majority of retrocaval ureters occur, then, because of the persistence of a ventral venous element and the disappearance of a dorsal element; occasionally, as in the case reported by Gruenwald and Surks, both dorsal and ventral elements persist simultaneously, so that the retrocaval ureter actually passes between two portions of the vena cava, an anterior and posterior. Again, however, it is the persistence of the ventral portion that causes the anomaly.

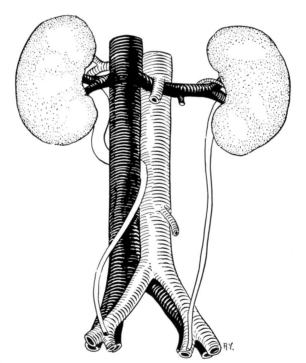

Figure 11–17.　Retrocaval ureter. (From Hollinshead, W. H.)

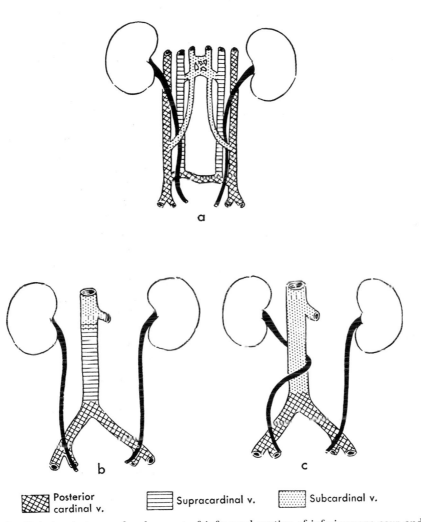

Posterior cardinal v.   Supracardinal v.   Subcardinal v.

Figure 11–18. Relation between development of infrarenal portion of inferior vena cava and retrocaval ureter. **A,** Primitive condition, with ureter winding between three cardinal veins. **B,** Usual method of formation of vena cava from right supracardinal vein (dorsal to ureter) has left ureter free. **C,** Subcardinal vein, ventral to ureter, has formed main portion of vena cava. (From Hollinshead, W. H.)

THE BLADDER, URETHRA, AND GENITALIA

CLOACA

The primitive cloaca (Fig. 11–19A through D) is formed by the distal part of the digestive tract, the hind gut. It receives the allantois (allantoic stalk) and the pared wolffian ducts (with their ureteral buds). It is separated from the outside by the *cloacal membrane.* The *urorectal septum* (urogenital septum, urogenital fold, or mesoderm) grows toward the cloacal membrane separating the cloaca into the *rectum* (posterior) and the *urogenital sinus** (Fig. 11–20A through D). The site of the fusion of the urorectal septum with the cloacal membrane becomes the *perineal body.* The part of the cloacal membrane anterior to the point of fusion is called the *urogenital membrane;* the part posterior, the *anal membrane.*† The connection between the rectum and urogenital sinus (just before they are completely divided from each other by the urorectal septum) is called the *cloacal duct.*

UROGENITAL SINUS

The urogenital sinus may be subdivided into two parts: 1. The proximal portion above the opening of the wolffian ducts (Müller's tubercle in the undifferentiated embryo, the seminal colliculus or verumontanum in the adult male, or the hymen in the female) develops into the bladder and prostatic urethra in the male and the bladder and entire urethra in the female. 2. The distal portion (the *urogenital sinus proper* or *definitive urogenital sinus*) becomes the remainder of the *urethra* (the cavernous urethra extending to the glans penis) in the male, and is represented by the introitus or vestibule in the female.

The narrowed apex of the bladder continuous with the allantoic stalk at the umbilicus is called the *urachus.* In an early developmental stage this structure undergoes regression normally resulting in complete obliteration. Failure to obliterate results in a *patent urachus (urachal fistula)* or *urachal cysts* (Fig. 11–21A through D).

There is some difference of opinion concerning the origin of the bladder. The most widely accepted view (Arey) is that in man the bladder is entirely cloacal in origin, that is, from the urogenital sinus. Another view (Krasa and Paschkis) is that part of the bladder is derived from the allantois. Kjellberg, Ericsson, and Rudhe have postulated that the part of the bladder lying above the trigone is of allantoic origin, whereas the part below is of cloacal origin. They have presented urographic and clinical evidence to support the thesis that the level of the trigone, which they stipulated as being at the first and second sacral vertebrae, is also the level of the juncture of the rectum (which is of cloacal origin) and the colon, which arises from the hind gut. In the adult, they stated that this junction is marked by the transverse folds (plica transversalis) of the upper part of the rectum. They emphasized the close relationship between the rectum (below the transverse folds) and the trigone and prostatic urethra and called attention to the fact that in cases of rectal atresia (imperforate anus) in which fistulous communications are common between the rectum and bladder or urethra, the literature contains no report in which the site of fistulous communication was at a higher level than the trigone. In most cases, of course, it involves the prostatic or membranous urethra in the region of the semi-

---

*Another explanation suggests that the urogenital septum is formed by urogenital folds growing from either side of the cloaca toward the midline and then fusing from above downward. Ladd and Gross stated that failure of fusion of these folds at various levels best explains the occurrence of multiple fistulae between the rectum and the urinary tract.

†This concept has been challenged by Tench, who concluded that the cloacal membrane ruptures before the urorectal septum reaches it so that there is really no separate anal membrane.

nal colliculus (verumontanum) or an area just distal to it.

Relation of Müllerian Ducts and Their Derivatives to the Urogenital Sinus

The paired müllerian ducts arise from the urogenital ridge near the cranial ends of the mesonephros lateral to the mesonephric (wolffian) ducts. The cranial ends of the ducts remain open and in the adult become the ostia of the fallopian tubes. The solid caudal tips grow caudally beside the wolffian ducts. At first they are lateral in position, but lower they turn medially to cross the wolffian ducts anteriorly, where they approach each other in the midline. At this point, lying between the wolffian ducts, they fuse and reach the posterior wall of the urogenital sinus where they terminate in Müller's tubercle, which is the point at which they communicate with the urogenital sinus. In the adult female, the cranial ends of the müllerian ducts become the fallopian tubes and the distal fused ducts become the *uterus* and *vagina* with Müller's tubercle marking the future position of the *hymen*. In the male, the terminal fused müllerian ducts persist as the *prostatic utricle* (*sinus pocularis* or *vagina masculina*), while the remainder of the ducts for the most part disintegrate. Remnants, however, may persist as the *appendix testis* (see Fig. 11-9, page 1321).

Persistent Urogenital Sinus: Embryologic Explanation of Clinical Findings

Originally the openings of both the wolffian and müllerian ducts lie close together at Müller's tubercle, where they communicate with the upper part of the urogenital sinus. The pared müllerian ducts become the vagina. The manner in which the opening of the vagina (at Müller's tubercle) ultimately "moves downward" until it finally has its own separate opening to the outside, instead of a common opening with the urethra (urogenital sinus), has been variously described. Keith visualized a rapid growth of mesodermal tissue around the terminal wolffian and müllerian ducts pushing downward that part of the cloaca (urogenital sinus) in which they end (Fig. 11-22). Arey said, "The intervening stretch of urogenital sinus (between Müller's tubercle and the outside) thereafter undergoes a great relative shortening to become the shallow vaginal vestibule into which both urethra and vagina open independently" (Fig. 11-23A and B). Wilkins described "... growth and elongation of the anterior wall of the vagina so as to carry the communication (of the vagina and the urogenital sinus) downward toward the perineum. At about the 162-mm stage the urethral and vaginal orifices become separated" (Fig. 11-24).

These classic descriptions subscribe to the common view that the vagina is formed entirely from the paired müllerian ducts and that the point of junction of the vagina and urogenital sinus is at Müller's tubercle (prostatic utricle in the male and region of hymen in the female). This concept also assumes that this point (Müller's tubercle) is the boundary line between the proximal portion of the urogenital sinus above (which forms the bladder and prostatic urethra in the male and the entire urethra in the female) and the distal portion (urogenital sinus proper or definitive urogenital sinus), which forms the bulbous and cavernous urethra in the male and the introitus in the female. This concept has been challenged by Kjellberg, Ericsson, and Rudhe who expressed the view that there is sufficient evidence to show (1) that the terminal portion of the vagina is formed from the urogenital sinus and only the upper part from the paired müllerian ducts, and (2) that the boundary line between the two divisions of the urogenital sinus is not Müller's tubercle but rather a point further distal which would correspond to the bulbous urethra in the male. They have supported the thesis of Politzer, who described an outpouching (rump or

Kaudalzapfen) from the floor of the distal ("definitive") urogenital sinus considerably below Müller's tubercle (which would correspond to the bulbous urethra in the adult male). This outpouching grows cranially and fuses with the paired müllerian ducts or vaginal plate to form the definitive vagina. They pointed out that with this hypothesis there would be no necessity to try to explain so great a shortening of the definitive urogenital sinus in the female. *Also, it would explain the high incidence of abortive vaginas which open into the bulbous urethra in males with hypospadias and the location of the junction of the vagina and urethra, which so often appears to be considerably distal to the expected site of Müller's tubercle in female pseudohermaphrodite with persistent urogenital sinus.* In fact the junction is often found fairly close to the perineal hypospadiac meatus. Kjellberg, Ericsson, and Rudhe quote Hart as stating that in the adult the appearance of the vaginal mucosa and rugae differs definitely in these two parts of the vagina.*

Koff expressed the view that the major portion of the vagina is formed from the lower fused ends of the müllerian ducts but that a small distal portion is contributed by the urogenital sinus. He described the solid lower end of the uterovaginal canal abutting against paired *sinovaginal bulbs* (Fig. 11–25A, B, and C). These sinovaginal bulbs are proliferations of the epithelium of the urogenital sinus. Canalization of the vagina occurs eventually and the part of the canal which tunnels through the *sinovaginal bulb* represents the portion of the vagina contributed by the urogenital sinus; its length depends on the thickness of the sinovaginal bulb. This

concept, however, supports the classic concept that Müller's tubercle is the boundary line between the proximal and distal definitive urogenital sinus.

Embryology of the Urethra

As mentioned previously, the *definitive urogenital sinus* below the openings of the wolffian ducts (seminal colliculus) becomes the *cavernous urethra* in the male, which extends from the membranous urethra to the glans penis.

At the 8-mm stage, the urogenital membrane (anterior half of the cloacal membrane) becomes surrounded by a mound of tissue known as the *genital tubercle*. This tissue assumes the form of folds (urogenital folds) on each side of a groove called the *urogenital groove* or *urogenital sulcus*. The floor of this sulcus is formed by the unruptured *urogenital membrane* (Fig. 11–26A through F). The genital tubercle gradually elongates into a more or less cylindrical phallus (penis in male, clitoris in female), during which time the urogenital sinus grows with it to form the lining of the future cavernous urethra (Fig. 11–27). At about the 15-mm stage the urogenital membrane in the floor of the sulcus breaks down, providing the urogenital sinus with an opening to the outside; its external orifice is now the urethral sulcus.

In the male, the edges of the urethral sulcus (the urogenital folds) progressively fold together and fuse in the midline from behind forward until the entire sulcus to the glans penis is completely enclosed to form the cavernous urethra. The fused edges of the urogenital folds constitute the median raphe. Failure of closure results in varying degrees of *hypospadias*.

In the female, the phallus remains rather small and becomes the clitoris. The urethral sulcus remains shorter and never extends on to the glans, as in the male, but remains open as the *vestibule*, the urethral folds becoming the *labia minora*.

(Text continued on page 1340.)

---

*An interesting sidelight concerning this concept is Arey's statement: "Its [the vagina's] permanent lining was formerly believed to be the original epithelium [of the müllerian ducts], but it is now known [Meyer; Vilas] . . . that the entodermal epithelium of the urogenital sinus invades this level of the genital cord and replaces the müllerian epithelium wholly or in part."

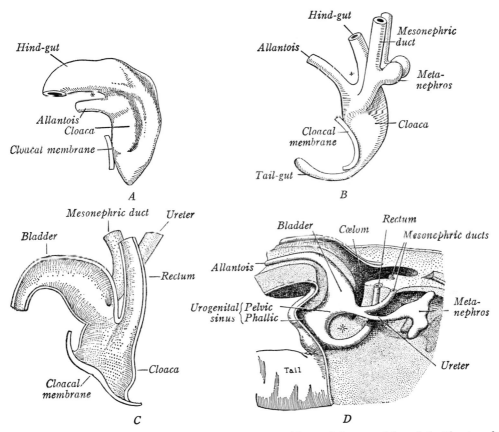

Figure 11–19. Partial division of human cloaca, illustrated by models viewed from left side. **A** and **B**, At 3.5 and 4 mm, respectively (after Pohlman; × 50). **C**, At 8 mm (× 50). **D**, At 11 mm (after Keibel; × 25). Asterisk indicates position of cloacal septum in **A** and **B**. (From Arey, L. B.)

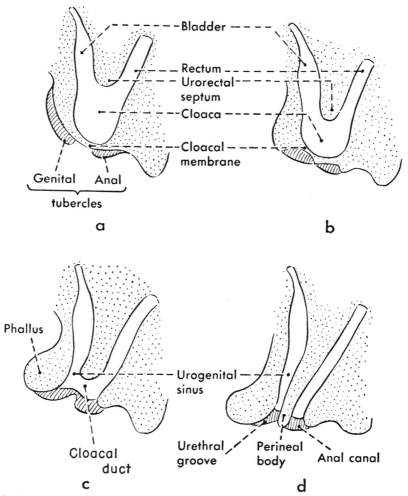

Figure 11–20. Division of cloaca into urogenital sinus, rectum, and anus. Note that paired genital tubercules (in **A**) have fused with each other (in **B** and **C**) to form phallus. (From Hollinshead, W. H.)

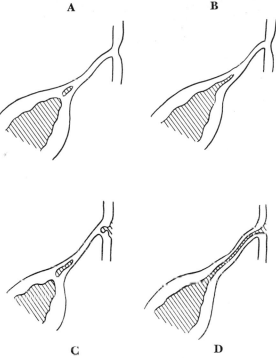

Figure 11 21. Variations in the urachus. **A**, Cavity of urachus not continuous with that of bladder (most common variety; 66% according to Begg). **B**, Lumen of urachus opens into bladder (approximately one third of cases). **C**, Persistent remains of urachus at umbilicus; it may or may not be cystically dilated and may or may not open at umbilicus. **D**, Patent urachus (rare). (From Hollinshead, W. H.)

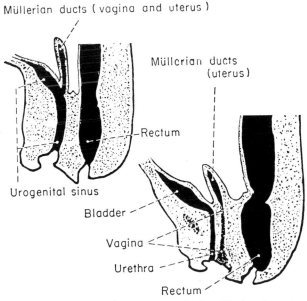

Figure 11–22. Diagrams illustrating normal manner in which müllerian ducts (uterus and vagina) become separated from and lose their communication with urogenital sinus (bladder and urethra). (Adapted from Keith, A.)

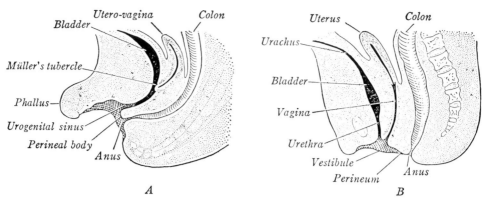

Figure 11–23. Sagittal sections of female fetuses, demonstrating relative shortening through which tubular urogenital sinus becomes shallow vestibule. A, At 10 weeks (× 4). B, At 5 months (× 1). (From Arey, L. B.)

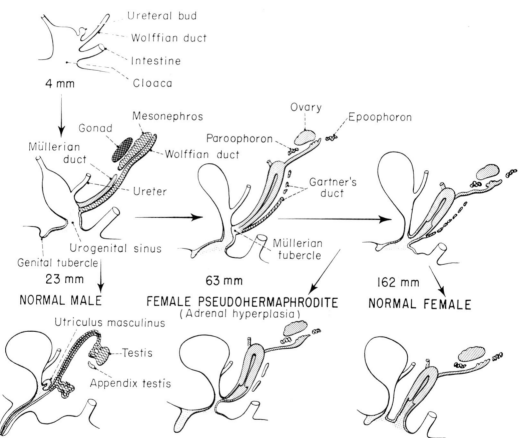

Figure 11–24. Sex differentiation of genital tract showing effects of congenital adrenal hyperplasia in females. At stage of 23-mm embryo, gonads do not yet show sex differentiation. Both wolffian and müllerian ducts are present after budding from urogenital sinus. By 63-mm stage, gonads and genital ducts have undergone male or female differentiation. In female, müllerian duct has developed into uterus and fallopian tubes, and wolffian duct has disintegrated, leaving only vestigial remains as Gartner's duct. After 63-mm stage, further female development consists of canalization of müllerian tubercle to establish communication between vagina and urogenital sinus. There is growth and elongation of anterior wall of vagina to carry communication downward toward perineum. At about 162-mm stage urethral and vaginal orifices become separated.

Since female patients with congenital adrenal hyperplasia show no persistence of male genital ducts but have persistent urogenital sinus, it is probable that masculinizing effects of lesion become manifest after 63-mm stage and before 162-mm stage. (Adapted from Wilkins, L.)

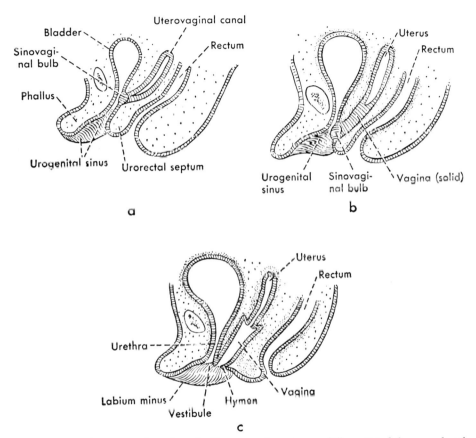

Figure 11–25. Development of vagina. **A,** Uterus and vagina undifferentiated from each other. Solid lower end of uterovaginal canal abuts paired sinovaginal bulbs, which are proliferations of epithelium of urogenital sinus. **B,** Vaginal epithelium has proliferated to occlude vaginal cavity completely, and relative decrease in depth of urogenital sinus below sinovaginal bulbs is bringing vagina closer to exterior. **C,** Vaginal cavity is reestablished; upper part of urogenital sinus has formed urethra, and lower part has become shallow vestibule into which both urethra and vagina open. (From Hollinshead, W. H.)

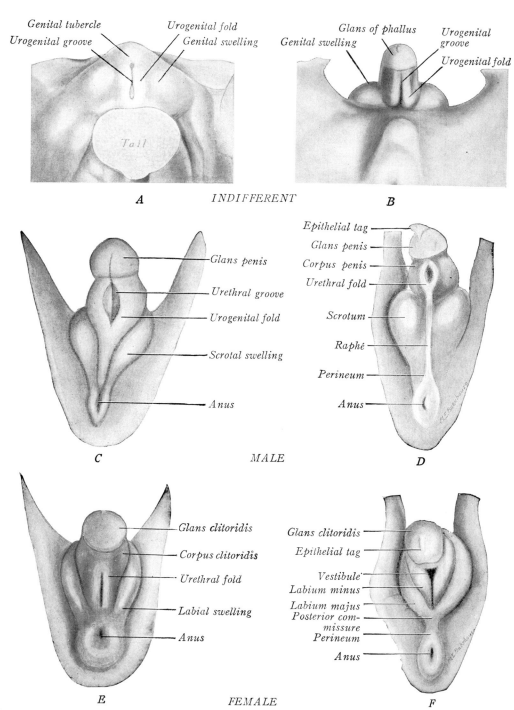

Figure 11–26. Differentiation of human external genitalia (after Spaulding). **A** and **B**, Indifferent period, at nearly 7 and nearly 8 weeks (× 15). **C** and **D**, Male, at 10 and 12 weeks (× 8). **E** and **F**, Female, at 10 and 12 weeks (× 8). (From Arey, L. B.)

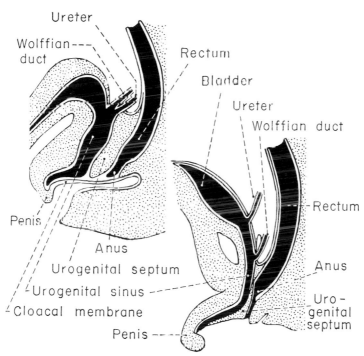

Figure 11–27. Late stages in division of cloaca into urogenital sinus and rectum and anus. Diagrams illustrate manner in which urogenital sinus grows into phallus (penis) to form lining of future cavernous urethra. (Adapted from Keith, A.)

ANOMALIES OF ANUS AND RECTUM ASSOCIATED WITH RECTOVES- ICAL, RECTO-URETHRAL, AND RECTOVAGINAL FISTULAE*

Fistulous communication between the rectum and bladder or urethra in the male with rectal atresia (imperforate anus) is common. In Gross's series of cases it amounted to 42%. In the female, however, it is almost nonexistent, apparently because of the interposition of the vagina and uterus. As a result, the incidence of rectovaginal fistulae in such cases is high. In Gross's series, it was 60%. A knowledge of the problem of congenital rectovesical or recto-urethral fistulae by the urologist is important because all too often the urologist may think that these fistulae are the result of a false passage of instruments during cystoscopy.

THE MALE

The normal division of the cloaca into a rectum (posterior) and bladder and urethra (anterior) is shown in Figure 11–28A through D (see also Fig. 11–20). Failure of closure of the cloacal duct because the urogenital septum did not grow all the way down to the cloacal membrane is given as the usual cause of rectovesical or recto-urethral fistula. As mentioned previously (footnote, page 1330), the concept of the division of the cloaca occurring as a result of infoldings from side-to-side meeting in the midline and fusing from above downward seems a better explanation of fistulae at various levels.

THE FEMALE

In the female the explanation is more difficult and involved. Rectovaginal fistulae

*This discussion follows the heretofore conventional teaching of this subject. For an entirely new concept of this complicated problem the reader is referred to the contribution of Dr. C. E. Shopfner (Chapter 12, page 1588) entitled "Urologic Aspects of Ectopic Anus (Imperforate Anus, Anal Atresia)."

apparently represent more than developmental arrest. As mentioned previously, according to the classic view, the müllerian ducts join the urogenital sinus at Müller's tubercle (level of the utricle in the adult male, hymen in the adult female). One would expect, therefore, that fistulae should most commonly be between the rectum and vestibule (distal to the hymen). Most fistulae, however, are rectovaginal. Ladd and Gross's explanation seems plausible. They stated that the downward extension of the müllerian ducts is "at the expense of the posterior wall of the urogenital sinus" (Fig. 11–29A through E), so that they take over any fistula existing between the rectum and the urogenital sinus. Kjellberg and associates' explanation that the vagina develops not only from the müllerian ducts but also from an outpouching of the urogenital sinus may somewhat simplify the explanation.

Ladd and Gross's classification of anorectal malformations is shown in Figure 11–30. Type 1 is incomplete rupture of the anal membrane or stenosis at any level from 1 to 4 cm above the anus. Type 2 is imperforate anus, the obstruction amounting only to a persistent membrane. Type 3, which is by far the most common type (117 of 162 cases), is an imperforate anus, but the rectal pouch ends blindly well above it and completely separated from it. In Type 4 the rectal pouch ends blindly above a normal anus. Kjellberg and associates reported finding only two types in their series of 38 cases: (1) The lumen was constricted or obliterated at the level of the second sacral vertebra and the vesical trigone, which they considered the junction of the primitive cloaca below and hind gut (colon) above, and (2) the occlusion was just proximal to the proctodeum.

The types of rectovesical, recto-urethral, and rectovaginal fistulae encountered in Ladd and Gross's series of cases are shown in Figures 11–31 and 11–32. As pointed out by Kjellberg's group the fistula is almost never above the trigone in the male. In Gross's series of 169 fistulae in males,

56 involved the trigone, 59 the prostatic or membranous urethra, and 54 were rectoperineal, most of which were located just behind the penoscrotal junction. Of 193 fistulae in females, 143 were rectovaginal and most involved the posterior wall of the lower third of the vagina. Forty-nine were rectoperineal, while only one was rectovesical and it was associated with a rectovaginal fistula also.

(Text continued on page 1344.)

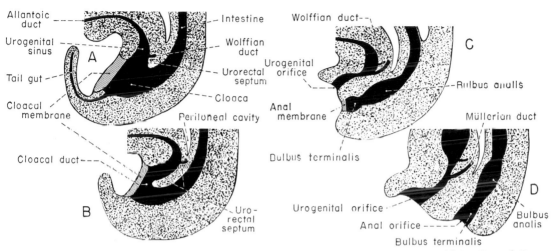

Figure 11–28. A to D, Normal development of rectum and anus. (Adapted from Ladd, W. E., and Gross, R. E.)

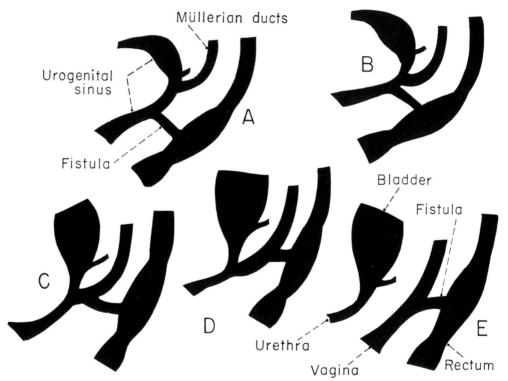

Figure 11–29. **Method of production of rectovaginal fistulae.** As müllerian ducts descend, they encounter and acquire any existing rectal fistula. **A,** 22-mm stage (7 weeks).**B, C, D,** and **E,** Successive stages in development of müllerian system and its separation from urinary apparatus. (Adapted from Ladd, W. E., and Gross, R. E.)

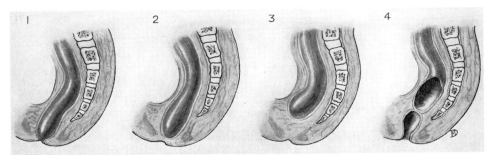

Figure 11-30. Types of anal and rectal abnormalities. Type 1, Stenosis at anus. Type 2, Imperforate anus. Obstruction only by persistent membrane. Type 3, imperforate anus. Rectal pouch ending blindly some distance above anus. Type 4, Anus and anal pouch normal. Rectal pouch ends blindly in hollow of sacrum. (From Gross, R. E.)

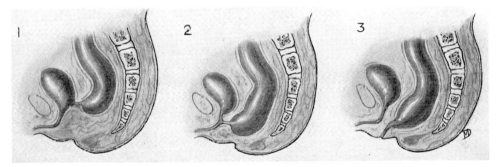

Figure 11-31. Types of fistulae encountered in male patients. Type 1, Rectovesical fistula. Type 2, Rectourethral communication. Type 3, Rectoperineal fistula (opening being in front of area where anus should normally open). (From Gross, R. E.)

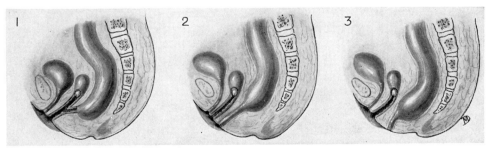

Figure 11-32. Types of fistulae encountered in female patients. Type 1, Rectovaginal fistula. Type 2, Rectofossa navicularis fistula. Type 3, Rectoperineal fistula. (From Gross, R. E.)

INTERSEXUALITY INCLUDING HYPOSPADIAS*

Abnormalities in sexual differentiation, commonly referred to as *intersex states,* present a most complex subject which cannot be considered in any detail in a book of this kind. The only reason for its consideration here is the high incidence in these cases of *persistent urogenital sinus* (common outlet for the urethra and vagina), which is often best demonstrated by urographic techniques.

Sexual differentiation of the genital ducts in the fetus is thought to be controlled by (1) male or female hormones formed in the embryonic gonad, (2) genetic factors at the time of fertilization of the ovum, or (3) a combination of both. The simplest classification of intersex based on gonadal tissue present divides the cases into two groups, namely (1) *pseudohermaphrodites,* either male (with testes) or female (with ovaries), and (2) *true hermaphrodites* with gonads of both sexes (an ovary and testis, ovotestes, or a combination of both).

Female Pseudohermaphroditism (Female Intersex With Ovaries; Masculinization of the Female)

The overwhelming majority of these abnormalities are the result of excessive androgen secretion by hyperfunctioning adrenal glands during intra-uterine development. This condition is called *adrenogenital syndrome.* It can be distinguished from the nonhormonal condition by determination of the 17-ketosteroids and pregnanetriol in the 24-hour excretion of urine. In the adrenogenital syndrome, excretion

---

*Gonadal classification of sex is now considered only one of many factors which enter into the problem of sexual differentiation. Modern concepts of sex assignment include chromosomal sex, external and internal genitalia anatomy, urinary hormonal excretion, sex of rearing, gender role, and so on. For a comprehensive discussion of this problem including newer methods of genitography the reader is referred to the contribution of Dr. C. E. Shopfner (Chapter 12, page 1573) entitled "Intersexuality: Genitography in the Intersexual State."

of these substances is always high. The characteristic deformity is an *enlarged clitoris* (which may have the appearance of a penis with perineal hypospadias) and a *persistent urogenital sinus* in which the vagina is still attached to the urethra so that they empty to the outside through a common opening. The vagina above is attached in a normal manner to the uterus and tubes, and the ovaries are in their normal position. A urogenital sinus may be demonstrated by urethroscopy but may be overlooked unless a urethrogram is made. A persistent urogenital sinus may vary somewhat in contour and arrangement. In all cases, of course, the urethra and vagina join and utilize a common tube or outlet to the outside. This common outlet is known as the *urogenital sinus.* As pointed out by Paquin and associates, in some cases the urogenital sinus appears to be simply a continuation of the urethra with the vagina opening on an angle into its posterior wall (Fig. 11–33). In other cases the urogenital sinus is large and appears to be the continuation of the vagina with the urethra coming in at an angle and joining the sinus on its anterior wall (Fig. 11–34). The juncture of the vagina with the urogenital sinus may be close to the surface of the perineum so that the urogenital sinus is short, or it may be more proximal so that the urogenital sinus may be relatively long. Treatment consists of reducing the excessive androgen excretion of the hyperfunctioning adrenal cortex with cortisone. This results in cessation of growth of the clitoris. The urogenital sinus can be corrected surgically at any time to provide a normal separate vaginal opening which will permit normal sexual intercourse.

The question is often asked why some remnants of the male genital duct system, such as seminal colliculus (verumontanum), ejaculatory ducts, and prostate, are never found in these cases. Wilkins pointed out that in the female embryo, atrophy of the male genital duct system is usually complete by the 63-mm stage (12th week), well before the separation of the vagina from the urogenital sinus, which is completed about the 162-mm stage (20th week; see Fig. 11–24). The androgenic stimulation from the hyperfunctioning adrenal cortex apparently always begins after the 12th week. Similar abnormalities may result from maternal ingestion of androgens or certain progestational steroids during pregnancy.

Male Pseudohermaphroditism; Hypospadias (Male Intersex With Testes; Feminization of the Male)

In this condition there is no evidence of hormonal reversal from excessive androgen or estrogen excretion. It is most likely the result of genetic aberration. This type of patient usually is a *cryptorchid, hypospadiac male*. The mildest anomalies in this category are, of course, the commonly seen cases of hypospadias. Money and associates put the cryptorchid hypospadiac male in a separate category, pointing out that "historically hypospadiacs have not been called hermaphrodites unless the hypospadias is extreme, the scrotum bifid, and the testes undescended." If a persistent urogenital sinus is present, however, with some form of vagina joining the urethra, there seems to be little doubt that the condition should be labeled intersex or pseudohermaphroditism. In an excellent discussion of this subject, Paquin and associates stated, "In practice, however, the radiographic determination of the müllerian derivative is essential for the diagnosis of male pseudohermaphroditism. However, it is our opinion that hypospadiacs represent, in fact, a form of male pseudohermaphroditism. In hypospadiacs, Howard pointed out that the more proximal the urethral meatus, the more bifid the scrotum, and the higher the testes, the greater will be the size of the internal genitalia derived from the müllerian ducts."

The müllerian duct derivatives usually consist of some form of a rudimentary vagina, vaginal pouch, or vagina-like recess of 1 to 10 cm in length, which comes off the posterior surface of the bulbous urethra (Fig. 11–35). In advanced conditions a uterus and tubes may be attached, but there are never any ovaries. Gross advised that all cases of hypospadias in which the hypospadiac meatus is at, or proximal to, the penoscrotal junction should be investigated. The presence of stigmata of sexual maldevelopment, such as bifid scrotum or cryptorchidism, should increase one's suspicions. Kjellberg, Ericsson, and Rudhe said that in most cases of perineal hypospadias a rudimentary vagina connected to the bulbous urethra can be demonstrated if the patient is subjected to either retrograde or micturition urethrography. They also mentioned that in their cases they have been unable to visualize a verumontanum.

True Hermaphroditism

True hermaphroditism implies that both male and female gonads are present in each case (ovary and testes, ovotestes, or a combination of both). Such cases are relatively rare when compared to the more common pseudohermaphrodites. The types of genital derangements possible in this situation are myriad and could not possibly be described here.* As in the case of pseudohermaphroditism, persistent urogenital sinus is a common finding in these cases and is best demonstrated by urethrography (Fig. 11–36).

THE COMPLEX PROBLEM OF MANAGEMENT OF INTERSEXUALITY

Although the subject of management and treatment of intersexuality is not with-

---

*An excellent description of the reported cases of true hermaphroditism may be found in Lawson Wilkin's book, "The Diagnosis and Treatment of Endocrine Disorders in Childhood and Adolescence." Ed. 2, Charles C Thomas, Springfield, Illinois, 1957, Chapter 13, and in the book by H. W. Jones, Jr., and W. W. Scott on "Hermaphroditism, Genital Anomalies and Related Endocrine Disorders," Williams & Wilkins Company, Baltimore, 1958.

in the province of this book, a few general statements may not be out of order. In recent years our basic ideas of what sex is and how it is determined have undergone radical change. The brilliant discovery of Barr and Bertram (1949; 1956) that sex may be determined by the chromosomal pattern of an individual's somatic cells (skin biopsy and oral or vaginal smears) has challenged gonadal biopsy as the most important factor in the determination of sex. Certainly it has emphasized the necessity for careful consideration of many factors before one attempts to assign the sex to these unfortunate individuals. Among the other factors to be considered are the hormonal sex, the type of internal genitalia (duct structures), and the external genitalia (copulatory organs). The psychic pattern of the individual, which involves the sex of assignment during rearing, must be given

serious consideration. These complex factors require the cooperative effort of the pediatrician, the internist, the endocrinologist, the urologist, and the psychiatrist in making the final decision as to what sex should be assigned to the individual and what surgical procedures and endocrine treatment should be instituted to support it. The complicacy of the problem is well stated by Kiefer who said:

The definition (of sex) is as follows: Sex is the over-all state of body and mind by which the individual conforms to the male or female standards of normality in the named sex-determining factors. It is the algebraic summation of these factors in which no one factor supersedes the others. In other words, there is no single conclusive determining factor. Every individual we know is a mixture of characteristics of the male and female, and it is the algebraic sum or preponderance of all these factors which determine sex, and not any one of them.

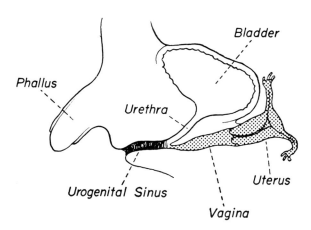

Figure 11-33. Persistent urogenital sinus. Here urogenital sinus and urethra appear to be continuous with vagina, opening into floor. This is commonest type encountered in male pseudohermaphrodites. (From Paquin, A. J., Baker, D. H., Finby, N., and Evans, J. A.)

Figure 11-34. Persistent urogenital sinus. Here urogenital sinus and vagina appear to be continuous and urethra opens at angle into roof of passage. This is commonest type encountered in female pseudohermaphrodites. (From Paquin, A. J., Baker, D. H., Finby, N., and Evans, J. A.)

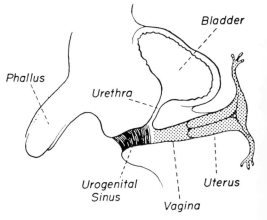

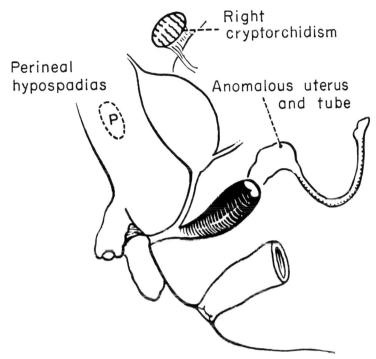

Figure 11-35. Male pseudohermaphrodite with persistence of müllerian duct structures. Hypospadias which represents orifice of urogenital sinus. Vagina (with anomalous uterus and tube) communicates with urethra (urogenital sinus). (From Gross, R. E., and Meeker, I. A., Jr.)

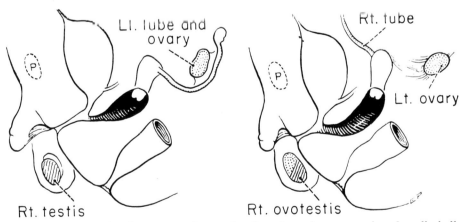

Figure 11-36. Example of findings in true hermaphrodites. In each are examples of small phallus, hypospadiac orifice of urogenital sinus, and normal vagina and uterus. In one, testis is present in scrotum and ovary in abdomen. In other, there is ovotestis in scrotum and ovary in abdomen. (From Gross, R. E., and Meeker, I. A., Jr.)

REFERENCES

Arey, L. B.: Developmental Anatomy, Ed. 6, Philadelphia, W. B. Saunders Company, 1954, pp. 325, 333, and 336.

Barr, M. L.: The Sex Chromatin and Its Bearing on Errors of Sex Development. Canad. M. A. J. 74:419–422 (Mar.) 1956.

Barr, M. L., and Bertram, E. G.: The Morphological Distinction Between Neurones of the Male and Female, and the Behaviour of the Nucleolar Satellite During Accelerated Nucleoprotein Synthesis. Nature 163:676–677 (Apr. 30) 1949.

Braasch, W. F.: Anomalous Renal Rotation and Associated Anomalies. J. Urol. 25:9–21 (Jan.) 1931.

Campbell, M. F.: Urology. Philadelphia, W. B. Saunders Company, vol. 1, 1954, p. 273.

Gross, R. E.: The Surgery of Infancy and Childhood. Philadelphia, W. B. Saunders Company, 1953, pp. 349–351.

Gross, R. E., and Meeker, I. A., Jr.: Abnormalities of Sexual Development: Observations From 75 Cases. Pediatrics 16:303–322 (Sept.) 1955.

Gruenwald, P.: The Relation of the Growing Müllerian Duct to the Wolffian Duct and Its Importance for the Genesis of Malformations. Anat. Rec. 81:1–16 (Sept.) 1941.

Gruenwald, P., and Surks, S. N.: Pre-ureteric Vena Cava and Its Embryological Explanation. J. Urol. 49:195–201 (Jan.) 1943.

Hart, D. B.: Adenoma Vaginae Diffusum (Adenomatosis Vaginae) With a Critical Discussion of Present Views of Vaginal and Hymeneal Development. Edinburgh M. J. 6:577–590, 1911.

Hollinshead, W. H.: Anatomy for Surgeons. New York, Hoeber-Harper, vol. 2, 1956, pp. 556, 564, 567–569, 733, 735, and 753.

Howard, F. S.: Hypospadias With Enlargement of Prostatic Utricle. Surg., Gynec. & Obst. 86:307–316 (Mar.) 1948.

Jones, H. W., Jr., and Scott, W. W.: Hermaphroditism, Genital Anomalies and Related Endocrine Disorders. Baltimore, Williams & Wilkins Company, 1958, 456 pp.

Kampmeier, O. F.: The Metanephros or So-called Permanent Kidney in Part Provisional and Vestigial. Anat. Rec. 33:115-120 (May) 1926.

Keith, A.: Human Embryology and Morphology. Ed. 5, Baltimore, William Wood & Company, 1933, 558 pp.

Kiefer, J. H.: Recent Advances in the Management of the Intersex Patient. J. Urol. 77:528–536 (Mar.) 1957.

Kjellberg, S. V., Ericsson, N. O., and Rudhe, U.: The Lower Urinary Tract in Childhood. Chicago, The Year Book Publishers, Inc., 1957, p. 104.

Koff, A. K.: Development of the Vagina in the Human Fetus. Contrib. Embryol. 24:59, 1933.

Krasa, F. C., and Paschkis, R.: Das Trigonum vesicae der Säugetiere: Eine vergleichendanatomische Studie. Ztschr. Urol. 6:1–53, 1921.

Kretschmer, H. L.: Supernumerary Kidney: Report of a Case With Review of the Literature. Surg., Gynec. & Obst. 49:818–831 (Dec.) 1929.

Ladd, W. E., and Gross, R. E.: Congenital Malformations of the Anus and Rectum: Report of 162 Cases. Am. J. Surg. 23:167–183 (Jan.) 1934.

McKenna, C. M., and Kampmeier, O. F.: A Consideration of the Development of Polycystic Kidney. J. Urol. 32:37–43 (July) 1934.

Meyer, R.: Zur Frage der Entwicklung der menschlichen Vagina: Altersklasse V und Übergangsfälle zu ihr. Rückbildung des Wolffschen Epithelgebietes. Reinfung des Epithels der Vagina, Bildung ihrer Lichtung, ihre Eröffnung in die Dorsalkammer des Sinus und deren Anstückung als retro-hymenaler Introitus vaginae unter Beteiligung der Wolffschen Epithelhöcker. Die Bildung des Hymens als selbständige Leistung des Vestibularepithels. Persistente Gefässstränge des Septum urorectale und Wolffsche Epithelhöcker als Kronzeugen für die Ortsgleichheit der Vaginalöffnung in den Sinus mit den ursprüglichen Enden der Müllerschen Gänge. Arch. f. Gynäk. 164:207–357, 1937.

Money, J., Hampson, J. G., and Hampson, J. L.: An Examination of Some Basic Sexual Concepts: The Evidence of Human Hermaphroditism. Bull. Johns Hopkins Hosp. 97:301–319, 1955.

Paquin, A. J., Jr., Baker, D. H., Finby, N., and Evans, J. A.: The Urogenital Sinus: Its Demonstration and Significance. J. Urol. 78:796–807 (Dec.) 1957.

Politzer, G.: Das Schicksal des Sinus urogenitalis beim Weibe. Ztschr. mikr. anat. Forsch. 59:6, 1952-1953.

Tench, E. M.: Development of the Anus in the Human Embryo. Am. J. Anat. 59:333–343 (July) 1936.

Vilas, E.: Über die Entwicklung der menschlichen Scheide. Ztschr. anat. 98:263–292, 1932.

Weyrauch, H. M.: Anomalies of Renal Rotation. Surg., Gynec. & Obst. 69:183–199 (Aug.) 1939.

Wilkins, L.: The Diagnosis and Treatment of Endocrine Disorders in Childhood and Adolescence. Ed. 2, Springfield, Illinois, Charles C Thomas, 1957, 526 pp.

INDEX

INDEX

Boldface numbers indicate pages on which illustrations appear.
Italic numbers indicate pages on which tables appear.

Amyloidosis, 1879–1887, **1888–1893**
  classification of, 1879–1881
  clinical aspects of, 1881–1882
  diagnosis of, 1882–1883
  etiology and pathogenesis of, 1879
  heredofamilial, 1881
  in children, 1882
  of genitourinary tract, 1883–1887, **1888–1893**
  primary vs. secondary, 1880
Anal plate, 1588, **1591**
Analgesic abuse, renal papillary necrosis and, 1895, 1896
Anastomosis
  pyelocutaneous, 1843, **1847**
  ureterocolic, 1800–1802, **1802–1818**
  uretero-ileal, 1819–1820, **1821–1842**
Anesthesia, for renal angiography, 100–101
Aneurysms
  gastroepiploic artery, **1940**
  iliac artery, 1678–1679
  intrarenal, renovascular hypertension and, 1627, **1629**
  of abdominal aorta, 1678–1679, **1681**
  renal artery, 1639–1642, **1643–1654**
    calcification of, confusing shadows from, 152, **157–160**
    classification of, 1639–1640
    clinical features of, 1640
    diagnosis of, 1640–1641
    dissectng, 1640, **1652, 1653**
      renal infarction from, 1628, **1630**
    etiologic factors in, 1640
    extraparenchymal, 1640, **1647–1654**
    intrarenal (intraparenchymal), 1639, **1643–1646**
    poststenotic, 1640, **1652**
    renal angiography in, 128, **131**
    treatment of, 1641–1642
    true vs. false, 1639
Angiogram, renal, normal, 123–125, **124–127**
Angiography
  aorticorenal, in renal artery occlusion, 1665
  aortorenal, in renovascular hypertension, 1617–1618
  renal, techniques and applications of, 97–137. See also *Renal angiography.*
Angiolipoleiomyoma, renal, **1060, 1065**
Angiolipomyoma, renal, **1060, 1061**
  tuberous sclerosis with, **1066, 1067**
Angioma, of renal cortex, 1050
Angiomyolipoma, renal, 1050, **1061, 1063, 1064**
Angiotomography, 100
Anomalies, 1349–1596. See also names of specific anomalous conditions.
  clinical classification of, 1350
  demonstration of, by excretory urography, 40, **41**
Antihistamines, reactions to contrast media and, 35
Anus
  anomalies of, fistula and, 1340–1341, **1342, 1343**
  ectopic, 1588–1596
    associated anomalies with, 1593, *1594*
    classification of, 1593, **1595**
    management of, 1594
    roentgenographic examination of, 1589–1590
  embryology of, 1330, **1334,** 1340, **1341**
  "imperforate," 1588, **1590**

Aorta, abdominal, aneurysms of, 1678–1679, **1681**
  aneurysm or calcification of, confusing shadows from, 152, **158–160**
Aortic arch arteritis, 1679, **1683**
Aorticorenal angiography, in renal artery occlusion, 1665
Aortography
  in retroperitoneal fibrosis, 1852
  in secondary renal calculi, 636, **645, 646**
  translumbar, 109–110, **115–118**
  vascular complications of, 122
Aortorenal angiography, in renovascular hypertension, 1617–1618
Aortorenal arteriography, 104, **111–113**
Appendix, malignant tumor of, calcified, 174, **176**
Arteriography
  aortorenal, 104, **111–113**
  in adrenal tumors, 1247, **1256**
  in evaluation of renal transplant, 1926, **1927–1929**
  in vesical tumors, 1273, **1277, 1278**
  renal, in renal cyst vs. renal tumor, 957, **967–969,** 1087, *1087,* **1100–1114**
    in renal injury, 1697, **1710–1719**
    in renal tuberculosis, 905
    in renal vein thrombosis, 1667
    selective, 108, **114, 115**
Arteriolar sclerosis, renovascular hypertension and, 1626, **1628**
Arteriovenous fistula
  intrarenal, renovascular hypertension and, 1627, **1629**
  of iliac and hypogastric vessels, 1678–1679, **1682**
  renal, 1655–1656, **1657–1664**
    excretory urography in, 1656
    renal angiography in, 129, **132**
  secondary to renal adenocarcinoma, 1655, **1662**
Arteritis, aortic arch, 1679, **1683**
  renal, syphilitic, 1679
Artery
  gastroepiploic, aneurysm of, **1940**
  iliac, aneurysms of, 1678–1679
    calcification of, confusing shadows from, 152, **155–157**
  impressions of, on renal pelvis, simulatng negative filling defects, 289, **293–295**
  renal. See *Renal artery(ies).*
Arthritis, sacro-iliac, in ankylosing spondylitis, 210, **212, 213**
Ascites, chylous, lymphography in, 2037
Atherosclerosis, causing renovascular hypertension, 1619–1620, **1622, 1623**
  renal angiography in, 127, **128, 129**
Atherosclerotic intrarenal artery aneurysms, 1639
Atonic bladder, 481, **483, 484**
Atresia, vaginal, hydrocolpos from, 1973, **1975**
Autonephrectomy, 889, **893, 894**

Backflow
  pyelointerstitial, 323, **331–333**
  pyelolymphatic, 324, **334, 335**
  pyelorenal, 323
  pyelosinous, 323
  pyelotubular, 323, **328**
  pyelovenous, 323, **330, 331**

Catheterization (*Continued*)
  ureteral, ureteral injury from, prevention of, 1726–1727
Cavernosaphenous shunt, for treatment of priapism, 1937
Cavernotomy, in tuberculous abscess, 913, **925, 926**
Cecal bladder, as substitute for urinary bladder, 1802, **1818**
Cervix, carcinoma of, urinary tract involvement from, 1973, **1976**
Chain cystourethrography, in stress incontinence, 1966, **1969–1971**
Children
  amyloidosis in, 1882
  chronic pyelonephritis in, 751
  congenital polycystic disease of, 982, **984–987**
    "adult type," 983
  cystourethrography in, 359, **363–365**
  delayed cystography in, for determination of urinary retention, 62
  excretory urography in, 39, 275, **278**
    dose for injection in, 27, 31
    filming techniques in, 20, **26**
  obstruction of ureteropelvic junction in, 408, **412–414**
  renal vein thrombosis in, 1666
  residual urine in, instillation of mineral or iodized oil in demonstration of, 63
  urethral polyps in, 543, **546**
  urethral strictures in, 544, **548–552**
Chlormerodrin scans, 2064, **2068**
Cholecystography, previous, confusing shadows from, 174, **177, 178**
Cholesteatoma, renal, 1864–1865, **1866, 1867**
Chondrosarcoma, 230, **233**
Chordoma, retroperitoneal, 1222
  roentgenographic appearance of, 230, **234, 235**
Choriocarcinoma, metastatic, of kidney, 1132, **1144**
Chromaffin paragangliomas, 1231
Chromaffinoma, 1230–1233, **1236, 1237, 1244, 1245**
Chromoscopy, in ectopic ureteral orifice, 1485
Chromosomal sex, 1574, **1574**
Chylous ascites, lymphography in, 2037
Chyluria, 1869–1872, **1873–1878**
  lymphography in, 1871, **1873–1878,** 2037
  pyelolymphatic backflow and, 324
Cinecystourethrography, voiding, 70–71. See also *Cystourethrography, voiding.*
Cinefluoroscopy, in ureteral reflux, 461
Circumcaval ureter, 1327, **1328, 1329,** 1472, **1478–1481**
Clitoris, in adrenogenital syndrome, 1344
Cloaca, embryology of, 1314, **1317, 1330, 1333, 1334**
Clothing, confusing shadows from, 152
Clubbing of renal calyces, 370, **375, 376**
Collecting tubules, embryology of, 1314
  urographic visualization of, 323, **326, 327**
Colon, carcinoma of, ureteral obstruction from, 440, **444, 445**
Colonic stoma, confusing shadows from, 152, **154**
Colostomy, sigmoid, cutaneous, ureterosigmoidostomy with, 1800–1801, **1813, 1814**
Conduit, ileal, 1819, **1821–1832**
  sigmoid, 1801, **1816, 1817**
Contrast media
  disparity in appearance of, in renovascular hypertension, 1611, **1613, 1614**

Contrast media (*Continued*)
  for excretory urography, 20, 27, **28**
    methods of administration of, 27, **29–32**
    reactions to, 30, 32
      allergic history and, 33, 34
      antihistamines for, 35
      cause of, 33
      sensitivity tests for, 34
      treatment of, 36
  for pneumography, 72
  for renal angiography, 101
    complications due to, 120–122
  for retrograde cystourethrography, 64–65
  for retrograde pyelography, 10–11, **11**
    injection methods in, 11–12
  incomplete filling with, arterial impressions simulating, 289, **293–295**
    distortion of pelvic outline from, 289, **290–293**
    in ureter, 338, 342–344, 432, **435–437**
  injection of, in lymphography, 2018–2019, **2023**
  simulation of, by opaque shadows, 152–190
Corpus cavernosography, in Peyronie's disease, 1933, **1934, 1935**
Corpus luteum cyst, ureteral obstruction from, 1974, **1977, 1979**
Cortex, renal. See *Renal cortex.*
Cortical hyperplasia, bilateral, 1233
Costal cartilage, confusing shadows from, 152, **153,** 609, **612**
Crescent sign of hydronephrosis, 372, **383**
Crohn's disease, 779, **786**
Cryptorchid male, 1345
Cushing's disease, adenoma of adrenal gland with, 1249, **1255**
  from carcinoma of adrenal cortex, **1241**
Cushing's syndrome, 1233, **1239, 1240**
Cutaneous amyloidosis, 1881
Cutaneous pyelostomy, 1843, **1847**
Cutaneous sigmoid colostomy, ureterosigmoidostomy with, 1800–1801, **1813, 1814**
Cutaneous ureterostomy, 1786–1787, **1791–1794**
  transureteroureterostomy and, 1787–1788, **1797–1799**
Cutaneous vesicostomy, 1786, **1788**
Cyst(s)
  adrenal, 1235, **1246, 1254**
  corpus luteum, ureteral obstruction from, 1974, **1977, 1979**
  dermoid, erosion of sacrum by, 231, **236**
    ovarian, confusing shadows from, 175, **188**
    retroperitoneal, 1222
  ectopic kidney with, 1378, **1391, 1392**
  hepatic, vs. retroperitoneal tumor, **1206, 1207**
  müllerian duct, 1557, **1560, 1561**
  of sacral nerve root, 231, **237**
  of seminal vesicles, 1558–1559, **1565, 1566**
  pancreatic, **1203**
  pelvic, deep, 1557–1559, **1560–1568**
  perinephric, traumatic, 1033–1034, **1035–1042**
  peripelvic, 976, **977–980**
    calyceal obstruction from, 394, **397**
    renal sinus lipomatosis simulating, 305, **312, 313**
  perirenal, traumatic, 1033–1034, **1035–1042**
  prostatic, 1559, **1567, 1568**
  pyelogenic, 394, **398–400, 402–404**
    stones in, 648

Cyst(s) (*Continued*)

   renal, 931–1042. See also *Cystic disease* and *Polycystic disease.*

     calcification in, **204**

     classification of, 931

     congenital, 981–1021. See also *Cystic disease, renal, congenital.*

     echinococcus, 1022–1024, **1024–1032**

     in duplex kidney, **1441**

     in renal duplication, 1453, **1467, 1468**

     management of, 970

     multilocular, 1007, **1009**

     multiple, 934, **949–953**

     nephrogenic polycythemia and, 933

     pyelogenic, stones in, 648

     renal angiography in, 133, **134**

     renal tuberculosis and, 896, **900**

     renovascular hypertension and, 1632–1633

     simple, 931–976

       histopathogenesis of, 932

       tumor incidence with, 932, **935**

       urographic diagnosis of, 933–935, **936–956**

     vs. renal tumor, 934, **954–956**, 1087, **1090–1114**

       arteriography in, 957, **967–969**

       nephrotomography in, 957, **958–966**

       percutaneous renal cystography in, 970, **971–976**

   retroperitoneal, 1190, **1200–1203**

   sebaceous, of scrotum, **1938**

   splenic, vs. retroperitoneal tumor, 1209

   urachal, 1330, **1335**, 1532, **1537**

Cystadenocarcinoma, papillary mucous, confusing shadows from, 189, **193, 194**

Cystadenoma

   of renal cortex, 1049–1050, **1053, 1056**

   ovarian, ureteral obstruction from, 1974, **1978**

   pancreatic, **1204**

   retroperitoneal, **1200**

Cystic adenoma, 820–821, **823, 824**

Cystic disease. See also *Polycystic disease.*

   of renal pyramids, 1013–1014, **1015–1021**

   renal, congenital, 981–1021

     classification and pathogenesis of, 981–982

     with lower urinary tract obstruction, 989

Cystic dysplasia, familial bilateral, 983, **986, 987**

Cystic lymphangioma, **1203**

Cystic necrotic adenoma of adrenal gland, 1235, **1246**

Cystine calculi, 608, **611**

Cystitis, 818–821, **822–824**

   amicrobic, 818, **822**

   eosinophilic, 819, **823**

   interstitial, 818–819

   panmural, 818–819

   tuberculous, 818

Cystitis cystica, 819–820

Cystitis emphysematosa, 787, 788, **795–797**

Cystitis glandularis, 820–821, **823, 824**

Cystitis granuloma, 820–821, **823, 824**

Cystocele, 1962, **1962–1964**

   stress incontinence with, **1970**

Cystogram, 58–63

   definition of, 7

   distortion of, by uterus, 350, **352, 353**

   errors in interpretation of, 351, **356, 357**

Cystography, 58–63

   air, 60

   delayed, 61

     for demonstration of urinary retention in children, 62

   excretory, 350–357

     definition of, 58

   in papillary vesical tumors, 1258, **1260–1262**

   in ureteral reflux, 461, **468–470**

   percutaneous renal, in renal cyst vs. renal tumor, 970, **971–976**

   retrograde, 350–357

     definition of, 58

     in vesical and ureteral hernias, 1860, **1861–1863**

     technique of, 59–60

   superimposition, 60

   triple-voiding, 62

Cystorectostomy, 1786, **1790**

Cystoscopy

   excretory urography prior to, 40

   in diagnosis of congenital vesical neck obstruction, 510

   in ectopic ureteral orifice, 1485

   urethroscopy and, in urethral diverticulum in female, 1955

Cystostomy, suprapubic, 1785–1786, **1788**

Cystourethrography, 63–71, 358–366

   chain, in stress incontinence, 1966, **1969–1971**

   evacuation, 63

     contrast media for, 65

     techniques of, 68–70

   expression, 63

     technique of Williams, 69, **70**

   in adult male, 358, **360–363**

   in female, 360, **366**

   in male infants and children, 359, **363–365**

   in urethral stricture, 585

   micturition, 63

     definition of, 59

   retrograde, contrast media for, 64–65

     definition of, 59

     technique of, 65–68

       Flock's, 63, 67

       in female, 66, **67**

       in male, 65, **69**

   voiding, 63, **70–71**

     in congenital anterior urethral valves, 528, **537–539**

     in congenital posterior urethral valves, 527, **529–537**

     in congenital urethral valves in females, 528, **540–542**

     in congenital vesical neck obstruction, 511, **518–523**

     in urethral diverticulum in female, 1955, **1960, 1961**

     technique of, 68, **69**

Davis, intubated ureterotomy technique of, Y-plasty and, for long constriction of ureter, 429

Delayed cystography, 61

   for demonstration of urinary retention in children, 62

Dermoid cyst(s)
  erosion of sacrum by, 231, **236**
  ovarian, confusing shadows from, 175, **188**
  retroperitoneal, 1222
Diabetes mellitus, renal papillary necrosis and, 1894
Diatrizoate, in GFR estimation, 2042, **2045–2048**
Disk kidney, 1323, **1326**, 1393, **1396**, **1401**
Diverticulitis, complicated by vesicocolic fistula, **1772**
  vesicosigmoidal fistula secondary to, **1769**
Diverticulum(a)
  calyceal, 394, **398–404**
    stones in, 648, **657**, **658**
  Hutch, 460–461, **466**
  ureteral, 1327, 1472, **1475–1477**
  urethral, ectopic ureteral orifice simulating, 1486, **1503**
    in female, 1954–1957, **1958–1961**
    in male, 581, **582–584**, 1548–1549, **1553–1556**
    urethral calculi due to, 736, **743**
  vesical, 553, **554–561**
    calculus in, 726, **733**, **734**
    tumors in, 1273, **1274–1276**
    ureteral obstruction from, 441, **447**
    with vesicocolic fistula, **1772**
  vesicourachal, 1531, **1535**, **1536**
Dopamine, 1231
Drip-infusion urography, 42–43, **44–49**
DTZ, in GFR estimation, 2042, **2045–2048**
Duplication. See names of duplicated organs.
Dysgenesis, renal, 1351–1354
Dysmorphism, lobar, in duplex kidney, 1436, **1448–1450**
Dysplasia
  cystic, familial bilateral, 983, **986**, **987**
  fibromuscular, hypertension and, **1613–1614**, 1620–1621, **1624**, **1625**
    renal angiography in, 128, **129–131**
  renal, congenital, simulating renal papillary necrosis, **1907**

Echinococcus cysts, 1022–1024, **1024–1032**
Ectasia, tubular, 323, **326**, **327**
Ectopia, renal, 1366, **1367**, **1368**
  crossed, 1322, **1324**
    with fusion, 1393, **1395–1405**
      vs. crossed ectopia without fusion, 1394
      with solitary kidney, 1378, **1380**, **1381**
      without fusion, 1378, **1379**, **1380**
    malrotation and, 1322, **1325**
    pathologic conditions associated with, 1378, **1385–1392**
    simple, 1322
    vs. nephroptosis, 340, **348**
    vs. ptosis, 1366, **1368–1371**
Ectopic anus, 1588–1596
  associated anomalies with, 1593, *1594*
  classification of, 1593, **1595**
  management of, **1594**
  roentgenographic examination of, 1589–1590
Ectopic bone formation in hilus of kidney, **1938**
Ectopic endometriosis, 1949–1953

Ectopic ureter, 1319
Ectopic ureteral orifice, 1319, **1320**, **1321**, 1435, 1483–1487, **1488–1505**
  as cause of vesicoureteral reflux, 453
  embryologic explanation for, 1483
  in female, 1484–1487, **1494–1505**
    atypical cases of, 1485, **1500–1502**
    diagnostic methods in, 1484–1485
    familial tendency in, 1486, **1492**, **1493**
    simulating urethral diverticulum, 1486, **1503**
  in male, 1506–1507, **1508–1512**
  sites of, 1483
  treatment of, 1522–1523, **1530**
  unilateral vs. bilateral, 1483, **1490–1493**
Ectopic ureterocele, 1520–1522, **1523–1529**
Edema of obscure origin, lymphography in, 2027, 2030
Effective renal plasma flow, measurement of, 2041
Ejaculatory ducts, demonstration of patency of, after suprapubic prostatectomy, **1936**, 1937
  obstruction of, 82, **88**
Embolic occlusion of renal artery, 1665, **1668**, **1671**, 1675
Embryologic anatomy of genital system, 1576, **1578**
Embryology of urinary tract, 1313–1347
Embryoma, malignant mixed, 1119–1122, **1123–1130**
Embryonal adenosarcoma, 1119–1122, **1123–1130**
Emphysema, renal and perirenal, 787, **793**
Enchondroma of bony pelvis, 230
Endolymphatic therapy, 2038
Endometrioma, 1949–1953
Endometriosis of urinary tract, 1949–1953
  renal, 1950, **1952**, **1953**
  ureteral, 1950, **1951**, **1952**
  vesical, 1949, **1951**
Eosinophilic cystitis, 819, **823**
Ependymoma, retroperitoneal, 1223
  roentgenographic appearance of, 230, **235**
Epididymography, 88–89, 89, **90**
Epinephrine, 1231
Epispadias, 1532–1533, **1538**
Epithelioma, squamous cell, of bladder, 1257–1259
  of renal pelvis, 1152, 1154, **1167**, **1168**
  of ureter, 1152
  transitional cell, of bladder, 1257–1259, **1260–1272**
    of renal pelvis, 1152, 1154, **1156–1166**
    of ureter, 1152
ERPF, measurement of, 2041
Evacuation cystourethrography, 63
  contrast media for, 65
  techniques of, 68–70
Ewing's giant cell tumors, retroperitoneal, 1223
Excretory cystography, 350–357
  definition of, 58
Excretory urography, 14–39
  as preliminary examination before cystoscopy, 40
  as test of renal function, 43, 50–53, **51**, **52**
  contrast media for, 20, 27, 28. See also under *Contrast media.*
  definition of, 7
  disadvantages of, 41
  fever and, 40
  filming technique in, 19–20, **21–26**
  history of, 1–4
  in adults, 275, **279**

Kidney(s) (*Continued*)
  size disparity in, in renovascular hypertension, 1611, **1612**
  solitary, compensatory hyperplasia of, 1352
    congenital, 1327
    crossed renal ectopy with, 1378, **1380, 1381**
    sponge, 1013–1014, **1015–1021**
  supernumerary, 1323, **1327**
    "free," 1351, **1356–1358**
  transplantation of, 1926–1932
    arteriographic evaluation of, 1926, **1927–1929**
    renal angiography and, 134
    urographic evaluation of, 1926–1927, **1929–1932**
  trauma to, 1695–1698, **1699–1725.** See also *Kidney(s), injury to.*
  traumatic infarction of, 1665
  tuberculosis of. See *Tuberculosis, renal.*
  tuberculous, silent, 889
  tumors of, 1047–1144. See also *Tumors, renal* and names of specific tumors.
  urinary diversion at level of, 1843, **1844–1847**
Kirwin, semisolid contrast medium of, 64
KUB, 4–7. See also *Plain film.*

Labia minora, embryology of, 1332
Laminated calculi, 608, **611,** 647, **649**
Leiomyoma, renal, **1059**
Leiomyosarcoma
  renal, 1117, **1117**
  retroperitoneal, 1190, **1193, 1197**
  vesical, vs. presacral tumor, 1225, **1229**
Leukemic infiltration of kidney, 1131, **1133, 1134**
Leukoplakia, of bladder, 1864, 1865, **1868**
  of renal pelvis, 1864–1865, **1866, 1867**
Ligaments, vertebral, calcification of, 210, **216**
Lindau–von Hippel disease, 1089, **1115, 1116**
Lipogranuloma, sclerosing, 1849–1852, **1853–1859**
Lipoma, of renal cortex, 1050
  retroperitoneal, 1190, **1198, 1199**
Lipomatosis, pelvic, 1940–1942, **1941**
  renal sinus, 304, **311–314**
Lipomyxosarcoma, renal, **1118**
  retroperitoneal, **1193**
Liposarcoma, renal, 1117
  retroperitoneal, 1190, **1196**
Lithopedion, 174, **177**
Liver
  calcification in, confusing shadows from, 161, **162, 163**
  carcinoma of, vs. retroperitoneal tumor, **1205**
  cyst of, vs. retroperitoneal tumor, **1206, 1207**
  polycystic disease of, vs. retroperitoneal tumor, **1207**
Lobar dysmorphism, in duplex kidney, 1436, **1448–1450**
Lowsley, semisolid contrast medium of, 64
L-shaped kidney, 1393, **1396**
Lump kidney, 1323, **1326,** 1393, **1396**
Lymph channels, cannulation of, for injection of contrast media in lymphography, 2018, **2022**
  lymphograms of, in normal state, 2019–2020, **2021, 2024–2026**
Lymph nodes
  calcified, confusing shadows from, 161, **170–172**

Lymph nodes (*Continued*)
  involvement of, by metastatic neoplasm, lymphography in, 2027–2028, **2030–2036**
  lymphograms of, in normal state, 2020, **2021**
  mesenteric, calcified, renal calculi and, 609, **613**
  tumors of, involving renal cortex, 1131
Lymphadenography. See *Lymphography.*
Lymphangiography. See *Lymphography.*
Lymphangioma
  cystic, **1203**
  renal, **1058**
  vesical, 1284, **1290**
Lymphatic fistula, lymphography in, 2037
Lymphedema, lymphography in, 2027, **2030**
Lymphoblastoma, involving renal cortex, 1131, **1136**
Lymphocysts, lymphography in, 2037
Lymphography and lymphograms, 2017–2038
  complications of, 2037–2038
  history and development of, 2017–2018
  in normal state, 2019–2020, **2021, 2024–2026**
  in pathologic states, 2027–2028, **2029–2036,** 2037
  in retroperitoneal fibrosis, 1851, **1859**
  indications for, *2029*
  technique of, 2018–2019, **2021–2024**
  terminology in, 2017
Lymphoma, lymphography in, 2027, **2029**
  malignant, involving renal cortex, 1131, **1135, 1138, 1141, 1142**
Lymphosarcoma
  involving renal cortex, 1131, **1136, 1137**
  lymphography in, 2027
  retroperitoneal, **1191, 1192, 1198**

Magnesium ammonium phosphate hexahydrate calculi, 608, **610**
Malacoplakia of urinary tract, 787, **792–793**
Masculinization of female, 1344
Matrix calculi, 608, **612**
McCarthy ejaculatory duct instrument, 81, **81**
Meatus, ureteral, iatrogenic stricture of, 440, **442, 443**
  urethral, congenital stenosis of, 543, **547, 548**
Medulla, adrenal, hormones of, 1231
  tumors of, 1230–1233, **1236, 1237**
  renal, 268, **271**
Medullary sponge kidney, 1013–1014, **1015–1021**
"Megacystis," 461
Megaloureter, ureteral stone in, **715**
Megalourethra, 1548, **1556**
Melanoma, involving urinary tract, 1185, **1187, 1188**
Membranous urethra, 359
Meningocele, 494, **498**
Meningomyelocele, 494
Mesenchymoma, benign, renal, 1050
Mesenteric lymph nodes, calcified, renal calculi and, 609, **613**
Mesonephric duct, embryology of, 1313, **1315**
Metanephrine, 1231
Metastasis
  osteolytic vs. osteoplastic, 238, **240–242**
  osteoplastic, from carcinoma of prostate, 238–239, **243–254**
  pulmonary, from prostatic carcinoma, 239, **254–256**
  to bone, castration and, 239, **252–254**

Ovary(ies) (*Continued*)
  abscess of, ureteropyelectasis from, **1981**
  carcinoma of, confusing shadows from, 175, **187**
  corpus luteum cyst of, ureteral obstruction from, 1974, **1977, 1979**
  cystadenoma of, ureteral obstruction from, 1974, **1978**
  dermoid cysts of, confusing shadows from, 175, **188**

Paget's disease, 239–240, **257–263**
Pancreas
  calcification of, confusing shadows from, 161, **168, 169**
  carcinoma of, secondary ureteral tumor and, 1184, **1186, 1187**
    ureteral obstruction from, 440, **445**
  cyst of, **1203**
  cystadenoma of, **1204**
Panmural cystitis, 818–819
Papillae, renal, 268, **271**
  atrophy of, 370, **375**
    obstructive pelviocalyceal dilatation mimicking, 370, **377**
  necrosis of, 1894–1898, 1899–1907. See also *Renal papillary necrosis.*
Papillary ducts, embryology of, 1313
Papillitis, necrotizing, 1894–1898, **1899–1907**
Papilloma, vesical, **1262**
  prostatic hypertrophy and, **1261**
Paquin ureteroneocystostomy for vesicoureteral reflux, 472, **477**
Para-aminohippuric acid, in GFR and ERPF determinations, 2041, **2044–2046**
Paraganglioma, chromaffin, 1231
  nonchromaffin, 1231, **1237**
Pararenal pseudocyst, 1033–1034, **1035–1042**
Pararenal pseudohydronephrosis, 1033–1034, **1035–1042**
Pararenal teratoma, 1222, **1226**
Parenchyma, renal. See *Renal parenchyma.*
Pelvic cysts, deep, 1557–1559, **1560–1568**
Pelvic inflammatory disease, ureteropyelectasis from, 1974, **1980**
Pelvic kidney, 1366–1367, **1372–1377**
  fused, *1323*, **1326**
  in pregnancy, 1378, **1385**
Pelvic lipomatosis, 1940–1942, **1941**
Pelviocalyceal system, 269
Pelvioileoneocystostomy, 1819–1820, **1838**
Pelvioileostomy, 1819, **1833–1836**
Pelvis
  bony, lesions of, 210–263
    congenital and degenerative, 224, **225–229**
    inflammatory, 210–212, **212–223**
    neoplastic, 230–231, **232–237**
    secondary, 238–240, **240–263**
  renal. See *Renal pelvis(es).*
  soft-tissue shadows of, 190, **198**
Penis
  amyloidosis of, 1886–1887
  carcinoma of, lymphography in, 2028, **2036**
  duplication of, vesical duplication with, 1534, **1546**
Penoscrotal junction, iatrogenic trauma to, 544, **552**
Percutaneous transaxillary catheterization, 109

Percutaneous transfemoral catheterization, 101–109, **105**
Periarteritis nodosa
  renal artery aneurysms from, 1639, **1646**
  renovascular hypertension and, 1627
  urinary tract involvement in, 1678, **1680**
Perineal sigmoidostomy, ureterorectostomy with, 1801, **1815**
Perinephric abscess, 800–802, **812–817**
  tuberculous, 896, **903**
Perinephric cyst, traumatic, 1033–1034, **1035–1042**
Perinephritis, 800–802
Perinephritis plastica, 1849–1852, **1853–1859**
Perineum, watering-pot, 1764
Peripelvic cysts, 976, **977–980**
  calyceal obstruction from, 394, **397**
  renal sinus lipomatosis simulating, 305, **312, 313**
Perirenal cyst, traumatic, 1033–1034, **1035–1042**
Perirenal fascitis, 1849–1852, **1853–1859**
Perirenal hematoma, from renal injury, 1698, **1722**
Perirenal insufflation, 72–77. See also *Pneumography.*
Peristalsis
  in calyces, 316, **321**
  in renal pelvis, 315, **319, 320**
  in ureter, 315
Peritonitis, tuberculous, lymph node calcification from, 161
Periureteral fascitis, 1849–1852, **1853–1859**
Periureteric fibrosis, 1849–1852, **1853–1859**
Periureteritis fibrosa (obliterans, plastica), 1849–1852, **1853–1859**
Peyronie's disease, corpus cavernosography in, 1933, **1934, 1935**
Phenacetin, renal papillary necrosis and, 1895, 1896, **1904**
Pheochromocytoma, 1230–1233, **1236, 1237, 1244, 1245, 1252, 1255**
Phlebography, vena cava, in renal vein thrombosis, 1667, **1677**
Phleboliths, confusing shadows from, 152, **155**
  vs. ureteral calculi, 609, **614**, 684, **689, 690**
Placenta, calcification of, in placental localization, 1984, **1987**
  localization of, by radioisotope techniques, 2071, **2072–2074**
    ultrasonic, 1991
Placenta previa, central and marginal, 1984, **1988, 1989**
Placentography, 1982–1984, **1985–1989**, 1990–1992, **1993–1996**
  anatomic considerations in, 1982–1983
  arterial and intravenous, 1990, **1994**
  contrast, 1984, **1988, 1989**
  direct, 1983, **1985, 1986**
  indirect, 1983–1984
  radioisotope method, 2071
  terminology of, 1982
  thermographic, 1991, **1995, 1996**
Plain film (KUB), 4–7
  definition of, 141
  examination of, 141–142, **144–146**
  good quality in, importance of, 143, **150, 151**
  in adrenal tumors, 1234
  in adult polycystic disease, 988
  in calculous disease, 607–609, **610–614**

Plain film (KUB) (*Continued*)
  in echinococcus cysts, 1023, **1025, 1026**
  in genitourinary bilharziasis, 839–840, **842–846**
  in genitourinary tuberculosis, 859–861, **862–870**
  in lesions of lumbar vertebrae and bony pelvis, 210–263
  in presacral tumors, 1224
  in renal artery occlusion, 1665
  in renal vein thrombosis, 1667
  in retroperitoneal fibrosis, 1851
  in simple renal cysts, 933, **936–939**
  in ureteral calculi, 684, **685–693**
  in urographic diagnosis, importance as preliminary procedure, 142–143, **147–149**
  necessity for, 4, **5,** 6
  shadows in. See *Shadows* and various sites.
  technique of, 6
    errors in, 143, **150**
Pneumography, 72–77, **76–79**
  complications of, 74
  contrast media for, 72
  gas embolism in, 74
  in adrenal tumors, 1234
  indications for and contraindications of, 75
  of adrenal gland, 75, **79**
  presacral, 73
  translumbar, 72
Politano-Leadbetter ureteroneocystostomy, for vesicoureteral reflux, 471, **475, 476**
Polyarteritis type of renal artery aneurysm, 1639, 1646
Polycystic disease. See also *Cystic disease.*
  congenital, 982–989
    of infants and children, 982, **984–987**
    hamartoma simulating, 1053, **1066, 1067**
    in adults, 987–989, **990–1006**
  in renal duplication, 1453, **1468**
  renal embryology and, 1314
Polycystography, 60, **61**
Polycythemia, nephrogenic, 933
Polyneuropathic amyloidosis, 1881
Polypoid fibromyxosarcoma, vesical, 1279
Polyps, ureteral, 1145, **1148, 1151**
  urethral, in boys, 543, **546**
Postcaval ureter, 1327, **1328, 1329,** 1472, **1478–1481**
Postnephrectomy renal arteriovenous fistula, 1655, **1657, 1658**
Pott's disease, tuberculous psoas abscess with, 896, 902
Pregnancy
  effects of, on ovarian vein, 1997
  pelvic kidneys in, 1378, **1385**
  pyeloureterectasis and pyelonephritis of, 775–776, **776–778.** See also *Right ovarian vein syndrome.*
  ureteral obstruction from, 441
Presacral insufflation, 72–77. See also *Pneumography.*
Presacral tumors, 230–231, **234–237,** 1223
Preureteric vena cava, 1327, **1329**
Priapism, cavernosaphenous shunt for, **1937**
Prostate
  abscess of, acute, 832, **834**
    chronic, 832, **834, 835**
  allergic granulomas of, 833, **836**
  amyloidosis of, 1885
  calcification of, 189
    in tuberculosis, 860, **868–870,** 907, **908**

Prostate (*Continued*)
  calculi of, **146,** 736, **737–742**
  carcinoma of, 1297
    causing bladder neck obstruction, 562, **575**
    lymphography in, 2028, **2036**
    metastasis to bone from, 238–240, **240–263**
    pulmonary metastasis from, 239, **254–256**
    ureteral obstruction from, 441, **446**
    vs. osteitis deformans, 239–240, **257–263**
  cysts of, 1559, **1567, 1568**
  hyperplasia of, adenofibromatous, 1297
    causing bladder neck obstruction, 562, **563–574**
    vesical papilloma and, **1261**
  hypertrophy of, vesical calculi and, 726, 730, 731
  sarcoma of, 1279–1282, **1288–1290**
Prostatectomy, suprapubic, demonstration of patency of ejaculatory ducts after, **1936,** 1937
Prostatic urethra, 359
  diverticulum of, 1549, **1556**
  ectopic ureteral orifice in, 1506, **1508**
  micturition and, 358, **362, 363**
  polyps of, in boys, 543, **546**
Prostatic utricle, dilatation of, 1557, **1563, 1564**
Prostatitis, 832
  granulomatous, 832–833, **835**
    allergic, 833, **836**
  tuberculous, 907, **909–911**
Protein-losing gastroenteropathy, lymphography in, 2037
Prune belly syndrome, 1569, **1570–1572**
Pseudocyst, pararenal, 1033–1034, **1035–1042**
Pseudoexstrophy of bladder, 1533, **1539**
Pseudohermaphroditism, female, 1336, 1344, 1346, 1580
    genitography in, **1579, 1587**
  male, 1345, 1346, 1347, 1580
Pseudohydronephrosis, pararenal, 1033–1034, **1035–1042**
Pseudomyxoma peritonaei, confusing shadows from, 189, **193, 194**
"Pseudotumor," in duplex kidney, 1436, **1448–1450**
  vs. renal tumor, 751, **768, 769**
Psoas abscess
  complicating parenchymal infections, 801
  tuberculous, 896, **902, 903**
  ureteral displacement and, **1776**
Ptosis, renal, 339–341, **346–349.** See also *Nephroptosis.*
Pulmonary metastasis, from prostatic carcinoma, 239, **254–256**
Pulseless disease, 1679, **1683**
Pyelectasis, 370–393. See also *Ureterectasis* and *Ureteropyelectasis.*
  advanced, **382**
  after ureterosigmoidostomy, 1809, **1811**
  clubbing of calyces with, **376**
  excretory urography in, 388, **389, 390**
  exstrophy of bladder with, **1544**
  horseshoe kidney with, 1419, **1421**
  in duplication of renal pelvis and ureter, 1453, **1460**
  in ectopic kidney, 1386, **1388**
  in ectopic ureterocele, **1527**
  minimal, 277, **373, 375**
  nonobstructive infective, 409
  obstruction at ureteropelvic junction and, 373